Integrating
Therapeutic
and
Complementary
Nutrition

Integrating Therapeutic and Complementary Nutrition

Edited by

Mary J. Marian
Pamela Williams-Mullen
Jennifer Muir Bowers

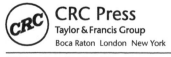

CRC Press
Taylor & Francis Group
Boca Raton London New York

CRC Press is an imprint of the
Taylor & Francis Group, an **informa** business

A TAYLOR & FRANCIS BOOK

CRC Press
Taylor & Francis Group
6000 Broken Sound Parkway NW, Suite 300
Boca Raton, FL 33487-2742

First issued in paperback 2019

ISBN-13: 978-0-8493-1612-8 (hbk)
ISBN-13: 978-0-367-39054-9 (pbk)

Library of Congress Card Number 2006004732

Library of Congress Cataloging-in-Publication Data

Integrating therapeutic and complementary nutrition / editors, Mary J. Marian, Pamela Avonne Williams, and Jennifer Muir Bowers.
    p. ; cm.
Includes bibliographical references and index.
ISBN-13: 978-0-8493-1612-8 (Hardcover : alk. paper)
ISBN-10: 0-8493-1612-X (Hardcover : alk. paper)
1. Diet therapy. 2. Alternative medicine. I. Marian, Mary, 1956-. II. Williams, Pamela Avonne. III. Bowers, Jennifer Muir.
[DNLM: 1. Diet Therapy--methods. 2. Complementary Therapies--methods. 3. Diet. 4. Nutrition Disorders--diet therapy. WB 400 I608 2006]

RM217.I65 2006
615.8'54--dc22   2006004732

Visit the Taylor & Francis Web site at
http://www.taylorandfrancis.com

and the CRC Press Web site at
http://www.crcpress.com

Foreword

Interest in complementary and alternative options to conventional healthcare has been steadily growing in the United States over the past two decades. In 1994 a strong grassroots movement culminated in a landmark federal legislation, the Dietary Supplement Health and Education Act (DSHEA), which made dietary supplements readily available to consumers for health applications of their choosing. At the same time, U.S. consumers became increasingly aware of centuries-old health systems in use elsewhere in the world. Many of these systems, such as traditional Chinese medicine and the Ayurvedic medical traditions of India, were considered alternative in the United States but were quite conventional and widely accepted as effective approaches to healthcare in their countries of origin.

The speed and tenacity with which complementary and alternative medicine (CAM) was embraced by American consumers took many within the U.S. healthcare system by surprise. For decades the United States had enjoyed a reputation of being on the cutting edge of medical technology and therapy, providing its citizens with an unprecedented level of sophisticated healthcare. Why were American consumers suddenly turning to remedies used by their ancestors? And why were they reluctant to disclose to their healthcare providers that they were exploring nonconventional therapies?

For many, it was about the growing sense of a lack of congruency between their personal values and those of America's healthcare system. It was about having options and the freedom to make one's own informed choices. It was also about establishing working partnerships with one's healthcare providers, about being heard. And, for those with chronic disorders for which modern medicine offered few effective solutions, it was about wanting to explore other options, about having choices and the ability to make those choices oneself. Fueled by the sheer number of well-educated, assertive, reluctantly aging "baby boomers" with significant discretionary income, what might have been a passing fad for another generation became a strong trend that has posed many challenges for consumers and healthcare professionals alike over the past two decades.

With these expanded options has come the responsibility for both the users of these options and their healthcare providers to become knowledgeable about the various types of complementary and alternative therapies available. In order to make informed decisions, credible information must be readily available as to which therapies are helpful for which conditions, which dietary supplements are appropriate and their effective dosages, and which manufacturers have established high-quality standards for their production processes. Reliable information is particularly critical for the safe, effective use of dietary supplements. Whereas many CAM approaches are complementary to conventional therapy or, at a minimum, unlikely to cause harm, dietary supplements and other nutritional therapies represent important exceptions. An uninformed choice with respect to nutrition-related options can potentially have far-reaching harmful consequences.

Until recently, there have been few credible resources available to guide either consumers or healthcare professionals in the use of CAM therapies, particularly concerning dietary supplements and other nutrition-related practices. *Integrating Therapeutic and Complementary Nutrition* by Marian, Williams, and Bowers fills a gap in the need for credible educational resources for healthcare professionals, particularly nutrition professionals. The editors have assembled a wide array of healthcare professionals knowledgeable about conventional nutrition therapy and the use of complementary and alternative approaches. Many are clinicians from the nutrition and medical specialties, others are university professors who conduct research and teach healthcare professionals, and still others have provided insight from the perspective of the industry–corporate representative. In each chapter the authors carefully detail the underlying processes involved in healthy function and the pathology characteristic of dysfunction (disease) with current medical nutrition therapy. They then move beyond the conventional approaches to include the popular complementary and alternative options used for each type of disease state, explaining what these CAM approaches are and the state of the science to date. (I do not think all the chapters cover efficacy and safety data.)

This book is a collection of scientific data, considered opinions, case studies, and answers to many of the more pressing questions about complementary and alternative therapy. It does not pretend to answer all the questions, but what it does do is tell us what is known and what is not known, what is proven and what is not. It is forthright in identifying therapies that are beneficial, those that are useless or harmful, and therapies for which we simply do not have enough information to make informed decisions. It separates effective uses of complementary and alternative therapies from misinformation. From the foundation provided here, clinicians, educators, and corporate executives alike will find reliable information upon which to base decisions. The purpose of this text is to bridge the gap between conventional and complementary nutrition approaches, with the ultimate goal of integrating the best of each into conventional care in order to provide optimal healthcare, a most worthy goal.

Ruth M. DeBusk, PhD, RD
Tallahassee, FL

Preface

The use of complementary and alternative medicine, also known as CAM, continues to increase worldwide as consumers are actively exploring and incorporating complementary and alternative practices into their lifestyles. The growing popularity of these practices is changing mainstream healthcare. In the United States, the Office of Alternative Medicine (OAM) within the National Institutes of Health (NIH) was established to investigate and evaluate promising unconventional medical practices as a result of the increasing interest and usage of CAM therapies by Americans. By October of 1998, the OAM was officially changed to the National Center for Complementary and Alternative Medicine (NCCAM). Today, many are calling for a convergence of traditional and complementary healthcare, in other words, integrating care to achieve the best positive clinical outcomes. The use of CAM therapies by individuals and patients reportedly does not reflect negative attitudes toward conventional medical care, but rather an orientation to self-care in the optimization of their health and well-being. However, fraudulent and dangerous CAM practices and therapies must be avoided as individuals apparently turn to CAM therapies as their health begins to decline. In order for healthcare providers to assist individuals in making safe, appropriate, and informed choices, practitioners in all settings must be aware of the indications and potential adverse interactions associated with CAM modalities.

Many CAM therapies such as acupuncture, aromatherapy, homeopathy, mind–body, botanical, and dietary supplements are commonly used to prevent certain diseases, enhance quality of life, and for healing purposes. Evidence is accumulating that many integrative therapies including nutrition can enhance conventional medical practice. Numerous research studies now support the critical role of nutrition in disease prevention and management.

Our goal was to create a text that integrates therapeutic and complementary nutrition and also serves as a preeminent resource for healthcare practitioners in all settings. This text will also provide a framework for integrating conventional nutrition together with complementary and alternative practices. Utilizing an evidence-based approach, an understanding of the pathophysiology and the integrated therapies recommended for disease prevention and management is provided. The chapters focus on the various stages of the life cycle, and the key functional processes that support wellness and the prevention or ameliorating dysfunction are also discussed. Through practice perspectives and case studies, the reader is presented with options for integrating conventional and alternative practices.

Editors

Mary Marian is currently a clinical nutrition research specialist and clinical lecturer with the College of Medicine and Arizona Cancer Center at the University of Arizona in Tucson. She is also a faculty member for the Program in Integrative Medicine at the University of Arizona. Her interests include nutrition for disease prevention, nutrition support, and integrative medicine. She has been a clinical dietitian for over 20 years. After completing her dietetic internship, she was a clinical dietitian and clinical nutrition manager at the University Medical Center (UMC) in Tucson, Arizona. Her clinical responsibilities included providing nutritional care to medical, surgical, trauma, and pediatric intensive care patients in addition to general surgery patients, liver and kidney transplants, and patients with cystic fibrosis. Since leaving UMC, Marian has been involved with teaching medical and dietetics students, residents, and fellows about the role of nutrition in disease prevention and treatment at the College of Medicine and with the Program in Integrative Medicine. She has been an advocate for educating medical students and physicians on the importance of nutrition in disease prevention as well as medical care.

Marian is involved with many nutrition organizations, including the American Dietetic Association, Dietitians in Nutrition Support (DNS), and the American Society for Parenteral and Enteral Nutrition (A.S.P.E.N.). Marian is the past-Chair of the DNS and currently is the secretary-cum-treasurer for A.S.P.E.N. She has also been active in the Southern Arizona Dietetic Association and the Arizona Dietetic Association.

Marian has served as an editor or coeditor for several textbooks and publications and has published many chapters and articles in peer-reviewed publications. She has also been a speaker on various nutrition topics at many local, state, national, and international conferences.

Marian's primary focus has been her family — husband Jim, son Scott, and daughter Brittney. In addition to her family, Marian enjoys traveling, skiing, working out, and friends.

Pamela Williams-Mullen is the nutrition specialist for the Huntington Beach Union High School District and the Westminster School District in Southern California. She is responsible for promoting nutrition and integrating nutrition education into the high school, middle school, and elementary school classes. For ten years, she has worked as a research scientist and a technical nutrition writer for Access Business Group, where she reviews research articles and creates technical documents on ingredients found in supplements. She also has over eight years of experience at the Charles R. Drew University of Medicine and Science as a clinical nutritionist and program director of the Bachelor's of Science Coordinated Program in Community Nutrition. Over the past 15 years, Williams-Mullen has made numerous presentations and written articles for professional publications and the general public covering nutrition and health topics for magazines and the Internet.

Williams-Mullen received her bachelor of science degree in home economics from Oakwood College and her master degree in public health nutrition and health education from Loma Linda University. She has also taken graduate courses in business and writing. She maintains her registration with the American Dietetic Association. Her interests include the prevention of obesity, diabetes and cancer; the impact of marketing on nutrition choices, phytochemicals, herbs and nutraceuticals; child and adolescent health; and nutrition education. Williams-Mullen is the wife of Stan and the mother of a teenage daughter, Erica.

Jennifer Muir Bowers, a registered dietitian, earned her Ph.D. in nutritional sciences, with a minor in microbiology and immunology, from the University of Arizona in Tucson. She finished her M.S. in nutrition at Texas Woman's University in Houston while completing a dietetic internship at the Houston Veterans Affairs Medical Center. She received a B.S. in dietetics from the University of Arizona. Dr. Bowers has more than 15 years of clinical nutrition experience, specializing in nutrition support and HIV/AIDS nutrition. Her clinical experience includes work at the Tucson Veterans Affairs Medical Center, Tucson General Hospital, Caremark, Inc., Pima County Health Department, and Special Immunology Associates Clinic.

Her works have appeared in peer-reviewed journals, books, and the lay literature. She has presented research at local, state, national and international conferences, including Canada, Switzerland, and France. She has received numerous awards and fellowships, including the Arizona Dietetic Association's Recognized Young Dietitian of the Year and the Emerging Leader Award, the E. Neige Todhunter Memorial Doctoral Fellowship, the Dietetic Educators of Practitioners Graduate Scholarship, the University of Arizona Food Science Fellowship, A+ Advisor Award for the College of Agriculture and Life Sciences, and Outstanding Student Organization Advisor Award from the University of Arizona. She has served in various positions for the HIV/AIDS Dietetic Practice Group and the Dietitians in Nutrition Support Dietetic Practice Group of the American Dietetic Association.

Dr. Bowers was a faculty member in the Department of Nutritional Sciences at the University of Arizona for over five years, where she advised students and taught undergraduate courses in clinical nutrition. Currently, Dr. Bowers teaches part-time for the University of Phoenix, Grand Caryon University, and Central Arizona College; works as a consultant on various writing and educational projects; and is a full-time mother to her daughter.

Contributors

Susan Allen-Evenson, RD, CCN
River Forest, Illinois, U.S.

Mary Atkinson, RD
Tucson Medical Center
Tucson, Arizona, U.S.

Ellen Augur, MBA, RD
Tucson Medical Center
Tucson, Arizona, U.S.

Andrea Avery, MD
University of California, Irvine
Orange, California, U.S.

Lisbeth Benoit, MS, CNS
San Clemente, California, U.S.

**Richard G. Berry, MD, FACP,
  FACGS, FAAETS**
UNC Chapel Hill and Signet Healthcare Inc,
Whiteville, North Carolina, U.S.

Jennifer Muir Bowers, PhD, RD
University of Phoenix
Oro Valley, Arizona, U.S.

Michael Buchwald, DC
Canyon Ranch Spa and Health Resort
Tucson, Arizona, U.S.

Paul J. Cimoch, MD, FACP
Center for Special Immunology
Fountain Valley, California, U.S.

Mari Clements, MS, RD, CDE, DAy
Swarthmore College
Swarthmore, Pennsylvania, U.S.

Aaron W. Crawford, PhD
Nutrilite Health Institute
Buena Park, California, U.S

Carlos DaSilva, MD, MPH
Staff Nephrologist-Commonwealth
  Nephrology Association
Boston, Massachusetts, U.S.

Jennifer Doley, RD, CNSD
Carondelet St. Mary's Hospital
Tucson, Arizona, U.S.

Amy A. Drescher, PhD, RD
General Clinical Research Center
University of Arizona
Tuscon, Arizona, U.S.

Pamela Echeverria, MS, RD, CNSD
Department of Pharmacy
Northwest Medical Center and Canyon
  Ranch Spa and Health Resort
Tucson, Arizona, U.S.

Kelly Eiden, MS, RD, LD, CNSD
Jewish Hospital College of Nursing and
  Allied Health
St. Louis, Missouri, U.S.

**M. Patricia Fuhrman, MS, RD, LD,
  FADA, CNSD**
Coram Healthcare,
St. Louis, Missouri, U.S.

Margaret Furtado, MS, RD, LD/N
Obesity Consult Center,
  Tufts–New England Medical Center
Boston, Massachusetts, U.S.

Joseph Genebriera, MD
Department of Dermatology
University of Alabama
Tuscaloosa, Alabama, U.S.

Ame Golaszewski, MS, RD, CNSD, DN
Clinical Nutrition Support Services
Hospital of the University of Pennsylvania
Philadelphia, Pennsylvania, U.S.

Nick Gonzalez, MD
New York, NY, U.S.

Philip J. Gregory, PharmD
Natural Medicines Comprehensive
  Database
Stockton, California, U.S.

David W. Grotto, RD, LD
Block Center for Integrative Cancer Care
Evanston, Illinois, U.S.

Roschelle Heuberger, PhD, RD
Department of Human Environmental
  Studies
Central Michigan University
Mt. Pleasant, Michigan, U.S.

Lisa High, MS, RD
Boulder, Colorado, U.S.

Melanie Hingle, MPH, RD
Department of Physiology
University of Arizona
Tucson, Arizona, U.S.

Duke Johnson, MD
Nutrilite Center for Optimal Health
Buena Park, California, U.S.

Renee M. Kishbaugh, DC
Tucson, Arizona, U.S.

Robert Lutz, MD, MPH
Nutritional Program in Health Sciences
  Department
Spokane, Washington, U.S.

Mary Marian, MS, RD
College of Medicine
University of Arizona
Tucson, Arizona, U.S.

John D. Mark, MD
Pediatric Pulmonary and
  Integrative Medicine
University of Arizona
Tucson, Arizona, U.S.

Leo McCluskey, MD
Hospital of the University of Pennsylvania
Philadelphia, Pennsylvania, U.S.

Cynthia Payne, MS, RD, CDE, FADA
University of Maryland School of Medicine
Baltimore, Maryland, U.S.

Deborah Pesicka, RD, CDE
University Medical Center
Tucson, Arizona, U.S.

Jill Place, MA, RD
Los Angeles, California, U.S.

Susan Roberts, MS, RD, CNSD
Baylor University Medical Center
Arlington, Texas, U.S.

Mary Krystofiak Russell, MS, RD, CNSD
University of Chicago Hospitals
Chicago, Illinois, U.S.

Jyotsna Sahni, MD
Preventive Medicine Women's Health
Canyon Ranch Spa and Health Resort
Tucson, Arizona, U.S.

Judith Shabert, MD, MPH
Kauai, Hawaii, U.S.

Ellyn Silverman, MPH, RD, PA
Center for Special Immunology
Fountain Valley, California, U.S.

Nanette Steinle, MD, RD
Division of Endocrinology, Diabetes,
  Nutrition and Obesity
University of Maryland School of Medicine
Baltimore, Maryland, U.S.

John Stroster
Department of Nutritional Sciences
University of Arizona
Tucson, Arizona, U.S.

Cynthia A. Thomson, PhD, RD, FADA
Department of Nutritional Sciences and
  Arizona Cancer Center
University of Arizona
Tucson, Arizona, U.S.

Riva Touger-Decker, PhD, RD, FADA
School of Health Related Professions
  and Associate Professor
New Jersey Dental School
University of Medicine and Dentistry
  of New Jersey
Newark, New Jersey, U.S.

Richard Wahl, MD
University of Arizona
Tucson, Arizona, U.S.

Pamela Williams, MPH, RD
Huntington Beach Union High School
  District
Westminster, California, U.S.

Douglas W. Wilmore, MD
Laboratories for Surgical
  Nutrition and Metabolism
Department of Surgery
Brigham and Women's Hospital
Harvard Medical School
Boston, Massachusetts, U.S.

Contents

1 Fundamentals of Integrative Nutrition

Cynthia A. Thomson and Robert Lutz

CONTENTS

INTRODUCTION

The phrase "integrative nutrition" is one that is not part of the common vernacular. Rather, it is a concept that, in keeping with the changing paradigm evident in current healthcare, suggests that nutritional science is likewise undergoing a parallel evolution that reflects a more holistic approach than what has historically been practiced. To best understand this, it is necessary to first look at the development of healthcare practice in this country.

MEDICAL PLURALISM IN AMERICA

From its earliest days, the practice of medicine in the United States has been pluralistic. Whereas what is currently referred to as conventional, regular, or biomedicine has become the dominant practice, numerous alternative or irregular practices have existed or evolved in America in the past. Some alternative forms of medicine, such as hydrotherapy and homeopathy, were imported by Europeans in the latter part of the 18th and early 19th centuries. Others, such as Thomsonianism or chiropractic, were developed in this country. A look at the history of medicine in the United States during the 19th and early part of the 20th centuries reveall a great diversity of medical practices available for individuals to choose from.

Two seminal events served to establish the dominance of biomedicine. The first was the establishment of the American Medical Association (AMA) in 1847 and its adoption of a Code of Ethics. This document encouraged consultation among regular physicians when challenging cases existed but strictly viewed consultation with physicians not aligned with the AMA as unethical. It was used to successfully argue against the licensing and certification of alternative practitioners, the exclusion of alternative practitioners from local and state medical societies, and to prevent them from receiving privileges and teaching responsibilities at hospitals and medical schools. The AMA provided cultural and political authority for "regulars."

The second major event was the release of the Flexner Report in 1910, which that served as the signature for reformation of medical education in the late 1800s. The Flexner Report, commissioned by the Carnegie Institute and the AMA, identified criteria that defined appropriate medical education. It critically evaluated the lack of uniform training for physicians and served to eliminate a significant number of "medical schools." It also reviewed alternative medical training facilities and often found them inadequate as well, allowing for further marginalization of alternative practitioners. It identified a four-year curriculum as appropriate for medical training, with the recently opened Johns Hopkins Medical School serving as the example. This document had significant political importance as it was effectively used to gain support from politicians and state and federal governments. Thus, by the early part of the 20th century, conventional medical practitioners had been effectively established as the dominant force in medicine in the United States.

RESURGENCE OF COMPLEMENTARY AND ALTERNATIVE MEDICINE

Medicine is a dynamic field and has seen significant changes over the decades. Technological advances and an increased understanding of the mechanisms of disease have served to positively affect the health of Americans, although it should be noted that the increase in life expectancy of the population as measured over the past century is more a reflection of advancements in public health, such as childhood immunizations and sanitation, than of improved medical technology.[1] The epidemiological transition that is a result of these advances has the downside of increasing the rates and duration of chronic disease currently experienced. With this have come escalating costs of healthcare. Efforts directed at decreasing the costs of healthcare have often proved frustrating to consumers at many levels. Alternatives have been sought, and thus a renewed interest has developed and increased steadily since the 1950s.[2]

In 1993, results of a national survey indicated that a significant percentage of Americans were currently using methods that were "not taught widely at US medical schools or generally available at US hospitals." This came to be described as complementary and alternative medicine (CAM). Often, individuals were making use of CAM at their own expense (as insurance companies rarely covered these practices). Many individuals reported using alternatives without discussing these practices with their physicians.[3] Of concern was potentially adverse interactions between conventionally prescribed medications and complementary and alternative practices (e.g., botanicals and nutritional supplements) that could go unrecognized by patients and their physicians.

What has proved vexing to conventional medicine is why these choices were made in spite of identified advances in conventional medical therapeutics. Theories forwarded to explain this phenomenon included (1) dissatisfaction with conventional treatment (perceived ineffectiveness, adverse side effects, impersonal, and costly); (2) need for personal control; and (3) philosophical congruence (CAM was more compatible with patients' values, worldview, philosophy, and beliefs concerning the nature and meaning of health and illness).

Interestingly, and contrary to the predominant view, it was the latter theory that was identified as most relevant to CAM use.[4] Increased usage of CAM was associated with poorer health status, reflecting a possible failure of conventional treatments and serving as a springboard for CAM use. Likewise, individuals who subscribed to a more holistic approach to life and their health may have been attracted to these therapies due to their greater acknowledgment of the role of mind and spirit than viewed by Western medicine. Additionally, a desire to find simpler and more natural approaches that often demonstrated fewer side effects was worth the out-of-pocket expense.

Although these findings were not necessarily new to healthcare providers, their magnitude was of significance to the healthcare industry. It represented a sizable proportion of expense, often out-of-pocket, that was equivalent to or in excess of that spent on conventional therapies. In spite of concerns raised about possible safety issues and lack of research for many of these CAM methods, interest and growth continued to increase, as demonstrated by follow-up data from Eisenberg's national survey of consumers 1998.[5] Recent data have confirmed the continued interest with 36% of adults using some form of CAM (this number rises to 62% if megavitamin therapy and prayer for health reasons are included).[6] This usage may, however, reflect a need to address rising costs of healthcare as much as personal beliefs and empowerment as previously identified.[7]

This phenomenon reflects a societal change whereby individuals, who have become healthcare consumers, feel the need to take an increased role in determining their healthcare choices. This new "reality" may be difficult for the conventional medical community to understand and accept. Current resistance to CAM is similar to that seen in earlier times as "regular" medical practitioners attempted to discredit "irregular" practices by claiming that only they practiced scientific medicine. Changes in medicine have historically come from within as new knowledge or research shapes clinical practice. In this current situation, interest in CAM has brought about a change in medical practice from *without*, as patient-consumers are determining what specific interventions will be incorporated into their individual treatment considerations.

This growth in self-care has paralleled the information explosion that has been facilitated by rapid access to in-depth information through the Internet. Individuals often present to their physician offices with information gleaned from searching the Web that may or may not be known to their providers. This has proved to be a double-edged sword, however, as quality of information is often suspect.[8] Thus, the need for healthcare providers to become educated in these CAM modalities has become real as the need for appropriate guidance in choosing among options has increased. Partnering, guidance, and exploration have increasing relevance, as decision making has become a shared effort.

ACCEPTANCE OF CAM

The scope of CAM practices is significant, with over 350 modalities listed under this heading.[9] To codify these practices, the National Center for Complementary and Alternative Medicine (NCCAM), established in 1992 as a branch of the National Institutes of Health (NIH), has identified five major categories of CAM therapy (Table 1.1).[10] Many of these practices are currently used within conventional practice or have become mainstream (e.g., physical therapy, support groups, cognitive–behavioral therapy). A listing of CAM healing systems and selective CAM modalities are also provided in Table 1.2 and Table 1.3.

The NIH also established the Office of Dietary Supplements (ODS) to evaluate the role of dietary supplements in disease prevention and physical and mental health. It serves as a clearinghouse for information and education about the risks and benefits of these substances, as well as providing extramural research funding.[11]

TABLE 1.1
NIH Classification of Complementary and Alternative Medicine

Mind–body practices (e.g., meditation, imagery, hypnosis, prayer, yoga, art therapies)
Alternative systems of medical practice (e.g., traditional Chinese medicine, Ayurveda, homeopathy, naturopathy, native American medicine, curanderismo)
Biologically based therapies (e.g., nutritional supplements, orthomolecular medicine [megavitamins], herbal medicine, shark cartilage, therapeutic diets)
Manipulative- and body-based methods (e.g., osteopathic manipulation, physical therapy, chiropractic, massage, rolfing, Feldenkrais)
Energy therapies
    Biofield therapies (e.g., Reiki, Qigong, therapeutic touch)
    Bioelectromagnetic-based therapies (e.g., magnet therapy, pulsed fields)

TABLE 1.2
Integrative Medicine Healing Systems

Conventional medicine
Traditional Chinese medicine
Ayurvedic medicine
Osteopathy
Chiropractic
Native American medicine
Herbal medicine
Naturopathy
Homeopathy

TABLE 1.3
Integrative Nutrition Therapies: Modalities

Nutrition biotherapy	Energy medicine
Behavioral interventions	Acupuncture
Massage	Herbal medicine
American Medical Association	Spiritual healing
Mind–body — biofeedback, meditation, imaging, hypnotherapy	Pet therapy
Detoxification	Qigong
	Feldenkrais
	Zen therapy

In March 2000, the White House Commission on Complementary and Alternative Medicine Policy was created. Its objective was to provide legislative and administrative recommendations to the President that would maximize the potential benefits of CAM. Its final report, issued in March 2002, identified ten recommendations[12]:

1. A wholeness orientation in healthcare delivery
2. Evidence of safety and efficacy
3. The healing capacity of the person
4. Respect for individuality
5. The right to choose treatment
6. An emphasis on health promotion and self-care
7. Partnerships as essential to integrated healthcare
8. Education as a fundamental healthcare service
9. Dissemination of comprehensive and timely information
10. Integral public involvement

Most recently, the Institute of Medicine convened a panel of experts to evaluate CAM within the United States.[13] It recommended that healthcare should be both comprehensive and evidence-based and CAM should be held to the same standards as conventional medicine. It acknowledged that new research methodologies might need to be identified. Importantly, it called upon the Federal Government to better regulate the dietary supplement industry and to adequately fund research in evaluating natural substances.

Whereas the emphasis has been on CAM, a shift towards integration of these practices with conventional therapies has been identified as the necessary evolution of this movement. As defined by NCCAM, integrative medicine (IM) "combines mainstream medical therapies and CAM therapies for which there is some high-quality scientific evidence of safety and effectiveness." This functional definition is lacking, however. It focuses on the elements of IM (i.e., conventional therapies, CAM therapies, high-quality evidence) without addressing the art and practice of integration. Medicine, as historically practiced, is an art rather than simply a vocation of rote practice. Individuals experience illnesses, while medicine diagnoses diseases. These illness experiences need to be understood within the context of the person's life. Acknowledgment of this context provides a greater understanding of how defined disease affects the person and it is in this way that a more holistic definition of IM provides an increased opportunity of healing.

INTEGRATIVE MEDICINE

Within this challenging environment the concept of IM has come to the forefront. Philosophically, it seeks to shift the orientation of medicine from disease-focused to one of healing by engaging the mind and spirit as well as the body. It emphasizes the supremacy of the patient–practitioner relationship as fundamental to facilitate healing, and espouses the Hippocratic dictum of *primum non nocere* in seeking the best and most safe treatment options. Recognizing that there are strengths and weaknesses inherent to each healing system incorporated, it seeks to identify what treatment options will best serve the individual in the specific situational context. Thus, IM practitioners serve as guides and partners with patients to navigate the everchanging seas of healthcare.[14]

WHAT IS HEALTH?

Fundamental to this changing paradigm of medicine is a reevaluation of what constitutes "health." Within the all too recent history of Western medicine, this term has been defined by what it is not — namely the absence of disease. Health-related research has primarily focused upon the physical/physiological component of health, consistent with a traditional definition of health as physical and mental well-being; freedom from disease, pain, or defect.[15] The World Health Organization (WHO),[16] in their classic definition provided in 1948, states that health is "a state of complete physical, social and mental well-being, and not merely the absence of disease or infirmity." This definition was further expanded upon in the WHO Ottawa Charter on Health Promotion. A more functional approach was provided to this working definition: "Health is a resource for everyday life, not the object of living. It is a positive concept emphasizing social and personal resources as well as physical capabilities."[17] Consistent with these concepts of health is that of IM that "engages the mind, spirit, and community as well as the body ... to stimulate the body's innate healing."[18]

INTEGRATIVE NUTRITION WITHIN THE CONTEXT OF INTEGRATIVE MEDICINE

Given the NCCAM definition of IM and the philosophical basis for its practice, the discipline of integrative nutrition begins to take shape. From the standpoint of the former, it should combine conventional nutritional practices with those of CAM for which there is "some high-quality scientific evidence of safety and effectiveness." This must be contextualized within the framework of acknowledging an individual's personal beliefs, the social and cultural environments in which nutritional practices will be performed, and should seek to address more than just the physical aspects of health and disease. Practitioners of integrative nutrition will seek to avoid dogmatic recommendations that are "cookbook." Rather, they will seek to understand the "hows" and the "whys" of the individual's current nutritional practices rather than just the "whats," and through partnering with the individual, serve as a guide to choosing health-promoting nutritional options that are congruent with the person's understanding of the importance of these choices. Making use of evidence, where it exists, and a willingness to explore areas where evidence may be lacking, practitioners can provide nutritional opportunities that can positively affect all aspects of an individual's health.

NUTRITION AND ALTERNATIVE HEALTH SYSTEMS

In contrast to Western medicine where nutrition is commonly viewed as an ancillary component of health recommendations, alternative systems of medicine (e.g., Ayurvedic, Chinese medicine) view dietary practices as integral to maintaining health and treating disease. This again serves to demonstrate the fundamental difference between conventional and alternative systems, namely the holistic approach of the latter and the dualistic (mind versus body) approach of the former. Ironically, Hippocrates, cited as the father of medicine, is quoted as saying, "Let food be your medicine." This phrase takes on increasing importance as evidence continues to grow to supporting the role of diet in disease. Estimates suggest that many of the leading causes of death in the United States can be attributed to poor nutritional practices. Over 30% of all cancers and over 50% of all cardiovascular diseases could be prevented through the acknowledgment and practice of optimal diet. Thus, the need to integrate nutrition into all health recommendations is apparent.

As an example of how diet is fundamental to alternative health systems, Ayurvedic medicine can be examined. Four diet-related principles serve as guidelines for wellness.[19]

1. An individual's best food choices are determined by their primary *dosha* (constitution)
2. Nutrition may be used as a therapeutic intervention
3. The taste of food defines its nutritional value
4. The act of eating is as important as what is eaten

In Ayurveda, individuals are described as constitutionally defined by the interrelationship of three organizing principles termed *doshas*. They reflect elements of body and mind, and homeostasis occurs when *doshas* are in balance; conversely an imbalance (either excess or deficiency, or a change in the underlying interrelationship) will result in symptoms or disease. *Doshas* reflect natural phenomena (e.g., *pitta* is seen in fire while *vata* is expressed through the wind and *kapha*, the earth), thus tying humans into their natural environment. They are also physiologically defined by their control over body systems — *vata* for motion (to include musculoskeletal movement, blood circulation, gastrointestinal peristalsis, and breathing); *pitta* for metabolism; and *kapha* for structure of organs and tissues. Individuals have a dominant *dosha* but will demonstrate elements of the others. The qualities associated with the *doshas* are fundamental to reestablishing balance — *vata* is described as cold, dry, and astringent; *pitta* is defined by heat and acidity; and *kapha* with cold, heaviness, and oiliness. *Vata* is the "lead" *dosha* and is the more common cause of imbalance than either *pitta* or *kapha*. Ayurvedic treatment involves diagnosing where the imbalance exists and addressing the underlying cause, rather than simply focusing upon symptoms.

Using the above information, Ayurvedic nutritional recommendations seek to restore homeostasis when imbalance exists. When excess in a *dosha* exists, the Ayurvedic physician will recommend the "opposite" to balance. For example, a *vata* person, characterized by cold, dryness, and astringency, will be best treated by warm sweet foods. *Vata* individuals may become imbalanced when they consume excess cold, dry, or astringent foods as well. Thus, food cannot only cause imbalance but may be used for treatment (restoring balance) as well. Finally, the Ayurvedic physicians emphasize *what* to eat as much as they emphasize *how* to eat. Eating should be a practice that is given full attention and mindfulness (i.e., eat slowly, peacefully, sitting) and the preparation of foods should likewise be given the same attention.

In a similar fashion to its progenitor discipline, Chinese medicine sees the role of nutrition and health or illness in a very broad context. Chinese medicine physicians, upon evaluating individuals, take a detailed history that will include significant dietary intakes, likes and dislikes, and seasonal and climatic variations in food choices. Nutritional practices are seen as more than just providing sustenance, but rather constitute a person's connection to his/her environment. Foods may be recommended for consumption, both therapeutically as well as constitutionally (e.g., garlic may be acutely prescribed for treatment of indigestion, but may be recommended to prevent infections as well). Disease is described in terms of imbalances and causative factors — external causes (e.g., climatic change), internal causes (e.g., emotions), or neither (e.g., behaviors). Dietary excess, cravings and addictions, and unhealthy and toxic foods may all be causative of symptoms or disease. The Chinese medicine physician will combine all elements of an individual's history with a few physical examination practices (e.g., pulse diagnosis at the wrist, evaluation of the tongue), and determine how best to treat the presenting symptoms.

Foods are described in Chinese medicine as yin or cold or cool (e.g., cucumber, melon); yang or hot or warm (e.g., peppers, ginger); or neutral (e.g., pineapple, Chinese yam). As in Ayurveda, opposites are used to treat excesses, and similars are used to treat deficiencies. Neutral foods are used when delineation between yin and yang is not possible.

Another food quality that is used in Chinese medicine is the determination of the flavor — sour, bitter, spicy, salty, and sweet. Each of these flavors specifically affects one or more of the "12 organs" of the human body. Sour foods work on the liver; bitter foods work at the level of the heart and affect Qi (energy); spicy foods affect the lungs and promote circulation of Qi; salty foods act upon the kidney; and sweet foods affect the spleen, serving to regulate Qi. Finally, bland foods may affect both the spleen and the stomach.

Also important to the Chinese medicine physician is the season in which foods are consumed. Historically, foods were only available at specific times of the year. Modernity has significantly affected this availability, and consumption of foods "out-of-season" may adversely affect health. In keeping with finding balance, the seasonal characteristic is treated with the opposite foodstuff. For example, summer heat should be treated with cool foods that are light and easily digested (e.g., cucumber). Conversely, winter cold should be balanced by consuming warm/hot foods such as soups, peppers, and ginger.[20]

INTEGRATIVE NUTRITION PRACTICE

Utilizing the above principles, integrative nutrition practitioners will necessarily look at dietary practices in a greatly expanded light than what is currently offered. Whereas current conventional nutritional practices seek to make recommendations based upon scientific research that has identified specific biochemical properties of foodstuffs, integrative nutrition will combine these data into therapeutic recommendations that will include personal choice (based upon social and cultural beliefs and practices), personal preferences, personal constitution, seasonal variation, and the nature and quality of foods. Suffice it to say that the challenges that confront such practitioners may be significant in light of the fact that food knowledge, as it currently exists, may need to be amended to incorporate different perspectives. Given that nutrition facts — including food nutrient composition — are now readily available to consumers, nutrition professionals will no longer serve as the reservoir of nutrition facts but rather will be challenged to serve as a resource for accurate, timely, and reliable nutrition information and, even more importantly, to practice the *art* of diet by facilitating healthy nutrition practices among consumers through the integration of the best of conventional and alternative nutritional medicine.

As important to making recommendations to individuals on food choices is that of encouraging an appreciation of food and what it represents. Food preparation and eating have become a mindless practice as Americans find themselves rushed for time and food is more and more readily available. Eating on the run, encouraged by the proliferation of take-out choices and fast food restaurants, has made eating something to be added to our daily "to do" list. The Slow Food movement,[21] growing out of Europeans' distaste for the Western diet exported from the United States throughout the world predominantly in the form of fast food chains, added to an appreciation for the bounty of locally grown and produced foods, has gained international support and is even making inroads in this country. Food preparation and consumption has a strong historical presence throughout the world, as seen in rituals and ceremonies. Feasts giving thanks for the harvest and meals used to celebrate holiday and festive events are but two examples of how food has been used as more than mere nourishment for the body. Such events demonstrate the importance of food to nurture the mind and the spirit as well. It, with the underlying conflict between this philosophy and current dietary practice, has fostered an integrative approach to nutrition that seeks to redefine how food and dietary practices are viewed.

CHALLENGES CONFRONT

Change is not always easily performed, and there are many challenges that confront individuals who desire to practice nutrition in a different way. The relationship that currently exists between nutritional sciences and medicine serves as one of the foremost challenges that will be confronted. IM has found itself criticized by conventional medicine for its lack of "evidence" and science. Nutrition science, and in particular dietetics, has also been the recipient of such disinterest by the medical profession. Fundamentally, however, the practice of integrative nutrition is nothing short of synonymous with good nutrition practiced in the context of good medicine, as it seeks to provide optimal treatment opportunities for individuals to maintain their health and to treat illness and disease. The realization that there are other equally effective systems of healing holds promise for the management of different conditions through providing an individual confronted with a medical problem a more extensive menu from which to choose. The role of the IM practitioner, similar to that of the integrative nutritionist, is to serve as a guide, and at times an interpreter, to the vast array of potential options that exist. Some options are indeed better than others, both in efficacy and in safety, and it is through a willingness to explore different methods of treatment that the integrative practitioner can best affect health.

To address the challenges that exist, integrative nutritionists must be willing to question the "evidence," from both conventional as well as alternative systems. Clinical experience and a long tradition of practice may serve as validation that some CAM therapies are safe and beneficial. Research that explores new ways of understanding alternative healing systems (e.g., acupuncture affects the flow of Qi versus the release of endorphins) may provide the evidence necessary for support of their use.

As previously alluded to, it will be necessary to reframe our current knowledge of foods and their beneficial qualities. It is not sufficient to know that allium vegetables may be beneficial for heart disease due to the presence of allicin; rather it will be necessary to frame this knowledge into the context that these foodstuffs have certain qualities that may optimize health through consideration of not only biological mechanisms but also an appreciation of the optimal time of year for consumption and the importance of preparation methods. Therefore, integrative nutrition professionals must be willing to expand their knowledge repertoire to include other elements of nutrition beyond biochemistry.

It is into the relative unknown that professionals who desire to practice in this new way must be willing to proceed. There is a basic ethical consideration that must be considered when practitioners decide to practice outside of the conventional norms. The Hippocratic dictum *primum non nocere* should always be at the forefront. Recommendations that are hierarchically determined based upon the determination of their role in prevention, support, or treatment may suggest the degree of reliance upon research-produced evidence. For example, whereas ecological data support a role for increased consumption of soy foods to *prevent* many diseases, the data are not as determinant. As these foodstuffs have many beneficial biochemical nutrients, recommendations for increasing consumption may be appropriate. To recommend their consumption to *treat* some forms of disease (e.g., prostate and breast cancer), however, warrants a greater corpus of research data before safety and efficacy can be appropriately understood.

WHY INTEGRATIVE NUTRITION?

As stated earlier, IM is a new reality. Thus, it appears logical that conventional dietetic professionals would want to get on board. However, the impetus goes much deeper. First, dietetic professionals are increasingly approached by their patients and clients with questions regarding dietary supplement use, alternative diets, and even potential benefits of integrating diet with other more traditional therapies such as Chinese medicine, homeopathy, and movement therapy. Second, there is increasing awareness that the ability to make and sustain changes in diet is central to improved health. Yet, dietetic counseling alone is unlikely to achieve optimal outcomes. Rather, it is through partnerships with medical professionals such as pharmacists, nurses, and physicians that we best serve our patients. Is this enough? Many now realize that expanding the care team even further, to include practitioners such as spiritual healers, acupuncturists, or visual imagery psychologists, is essential to optimize healthcare and individual wellness. For example, research has shown that dietetic professionals often fail at achieving and maintaining weight loss among their obese clients. Studies suggest that the addition of regular physical activity and behavior modification can significantly enhance the efficacy of diet-related therapy for weight loss. Integrative nutrition professionals would argue that the *status quo* is inadequate. Rather, they need to explore on an in-depth level the client's values, barriers, support mechanisms, as well as the biological markers of disease, in order to effectively integrate other potential therapies such as mind–body medicine, body-based manipulation, or spirituality which will produce optimal outcomes.

A third reason to consider an integrative approach of nutrition — if not you, then who? As IM is evolving, it is clear that nutritional care will have a central role. A variety of reasons exist to explain this. Nutrition has hung on the hems of conventional medicine for decades. Medical providers, at some level, understand the importance of diet in disease prevention and therapy, but without a mechanism to sufficiently charge for nutrition and diet therapy, most give it little focus in patients' care. In addition, as conventional practitioners enter a more integrative approach it is logical to initiate this process with something they have, some understanding of diet. Thus, dietetic professionals should be acutely aware that if they choose not to practice integratively there is a strong possibility that other healthcare providers will. Yet, the face of integrative practice is multifaceted, not territorial. Integrative practitioners generally do not aspire to be registered dietitians; most are seeking to establish a network of integrative practitioners — including integrative nutrition professionals — available to their patients.

GAINING COMPETENCY

Despite a desire to develop an integrative approach to nutritional care, many dietetic professionals remain confused as to the path to take. There is no definition of "integrative nutrition practitioner." Today, each practitioner is left to their own accord in defining the competencies and underpinnings of such a professional. In the fall of 2002, the American Dietetic Association (ADA) initiated a task force to develop competencies in CAM for dietetic professionals. Although their work remains under development, it is not without foundation. Over eight years ago, the ADA established a dietetic practice group focused on the practice or CAM. This practice group has been the leader in membership growth over the past several years, demonstrating the strong interest in integrative nutrition among dietetic professionals. In fact, in recent years the New Jersey Medical and Dental School became the first NIH CAM Center to be directed by a registered dietitian. Efforts have been made despite the fact that much work remains.

The White House Commission on Complementary and Alternative Medicine Policy, in Chapter 4 of the report, challenged education systems to move forward in this new realm of healthcare. Their recommendation was that, "the education and training of CAM and conventional practitioners should be designed to ensure public safety, improve health, and increase the availability of qualified and knowledgeable CAM and conventional practitioners and enhance collaboration among them." A 1997 survey of medical schools demonstrated that 67% of medical schools were offering elective courses or providing some CAM content in required courses.[22] This compares with slightly over 25% that offer nutrition. In November 2000, the Josiah Macy, Jr. Foundation convened an in-depth, multidisciplinary conference to further refine competency and training in CAM for healthcare professionals.[23] Importantly, the conference explicitly recommended that all healthcare professionals be adequately trained in CAM. But defining the curricula is another dimension. Many who have been involved in curriculum development understand the complexity not only of defining the desired change, but also in determining the "how to" of implementation. What is clear is that time is of the essence. At a minimum, dietetic professionals should be afforded the opportunity to learn what CAM is; what individual therapies are encompassed in CAM; the scientific and philosophical underpinnings of each therapy; the unique components of each therapy; current use and

TABLE 1.4
Four Levels of Competency Assessment

The *knows* level — refers to the recall of facts, principles, and theories
The *knows how* level — involves the ability to solve problems and describe procedures
The *shows how* level — usually involves human (standardized patient), mechanical, or computer simulations that
   involve demonstration of skills in a controlled setting
The *does* level — refers to observations of real practice

Source: From Epstein, R.M. and Hundert, E.M. *JAMA*, 287, 226–244, 2002.

rationale for use; as well as evidence-based efforts to evaluate the safety and efficacy of each therapy. Table 1.4 outlines the four levels of assessment that ideally should be included in the training of integrative nutrition professionals.

Dietetic professionals must also develop open approaches to counseling and assessment that foster patient sharing of information and interest in CAM therapies. However, for most dietetic professionals even this will be inadequate. Thorough, evidence-based education in the area of dietary supplements is essential for any dietetic professional entering clinical or research practice. Given the significant usage of dietary supplements by American consumers, the potential for harm as well as benefit, and the unique educational backgrounds of dietetic professionals, it seems imperative that all dietetic training programs provide students the knowledge and resources necessary to appropriately guide consumers through the myriad of supplements available on the market. In fact, dietetic professionals currently define the evaluation of dietary supplement use as the cornerstone of integrative nutritional practice — a skill that separates conventional dietetic practice from integrative practice. But to establish ourselves in this realm, we must first establish competence.

So what is competence? Professional competence is the habitual and judicious use of communication, knowledge, technical skills, clinical reasoning, emotions, values, and reflection in daily practice for the benefit of the individual and community served.[24] To build competence requires certain personal and professional characteristics that are outlined on the building blocks of Figure 1.1. In addition, there are core skills and behaviors that dietetic professionals will need to acquire (Table 1.5). Reviewing these core skills and behaviors it may seem that dietetic professionals already have such skills, however, careful assessment of the application of each of these skills and behaviors to *integrative* nutrition practice will provide unique challenges as well as opportunities. At a minimum, it will mean seeking out and competently completing professional development in the general study of CAM. This will include obtaining the knowledge and resources to identify and define CAM therapies. It will also entail collaboration with integrative and CAM practitioners, and acquisition of "hands-on" skills and competence in select areas of CAM practice, as dictated by one's customer, patient, or client.

Ethics

Ethics and quality should also guide integrative nutrition practice. Dietetic professionals should rely on their professional code of ethics to guide them as well as any applicable professional position statements or practice guidelines. For example, in the area of dietary supplements, the ADA in 2002 published specific guidelines for the recommendation or sale of dietary supplements that can serve to guide professionals as well as a practice paper in this area.[25,26] However, for many CAM therapies clear guidelines may not exist. In these cases,

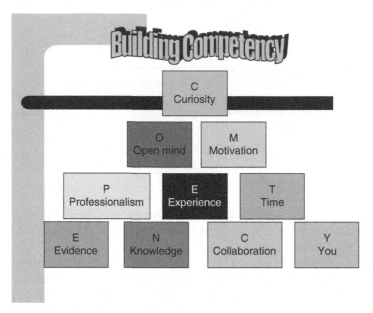

FIGURE 1.1 Professional and personal characteristics of competency building.

professionals should consider several factors when making recommendations or developing care plans. These should include: safety, efficacy, patient-centered application, timeliness and convenience, efficient in terms of reducing or minimizing waste of resources, and equitable (providing care to all regardless of gender, ethnicity, ability to pay, etc.) and should be inclusive of all conventional and CAM approaches that may be of benefit to the individual or community.

The decision to recommend or apply CAM therapies should not be taken lightly. Every effort to gain competence should be made and competence should be viewed as an evolving phenomenon. In addition, the integrative nutrition practitioner should be open to new ideas and philosophies that may even be in conflict with conventional wisdom. It is only through curiosity and challenge that new insights are born. Thus, to be close-minded implies incompetence. Table 1.6 lists several nutrition practices that either now or in the recent past have gained acceptance as potential therapies to promote improved health.

TABLE 1.5
Core Skills and Behaviors for Dietetic Practitioners to Acquire

CAM
    Ability to access high-quality, high-value information
    Ability to think critically
    Ability to advise patients intelligently
    Ability to communicate effectively with patients and peers
IM
    Ability to listen, understand, guide, and comfort patients
    Ability to facilitate change, when needed
    Respectful of humans' needs and experiences

TABLE 1.6
Conventional and Alternative Nutrition Practice

Conventional Nutrition Therapy	Integrative/Alternative Nutrition Therapy
Diabetic diet	Glycemic index
American Heart Association Step 1, Step 2	Atkins diet, Ornish diet, Pritichin
Low sodium diet for hypertension	DASH diet
American Cancer Society Dietary Guidelines	Macrobiotic diet
Food Guide Pyramid for rheumatoid arthritis	Anti-inflammatory diet with omega-3-fatty acids and select herbal supplements; intermittent fasting; vegetarianism
Food Guide Pyramid for epilepsy	Ketogenic diet
Energy restricted diet for weight loss	Individualized approach that includes dietary modification, mind–body, acupuncture, manipulation therapy, etc.

REFERENCES

1. Institute of Medicine. *The Future of the Public's Health in the 21st Century*. National Academy Press, Washington, D.C., 2003.
2. Kessler, R.C. et al. Long-term trends in the use of complementary and alternative medical therapies in the United States. *Ann. Intern. Med.*, 135, 262–268, 2001.
3. Eisenberg, D.M. et al. Unconventional medicine in the United States: prevalence, costs, and patterns of use. *New England J. Med.*, 328, 246–252, 1993.
4. Astin, J.A. Why patients use alternative medicine. *JAMA*, 279(19), 1548–1553, 1998.
5. Eisenberg, D.M., David, R.B., and Ettner, S.L. Trends in alternative medicine use in the United States, 1990–1997. *JAMA*, 280, 1569–1575, 1998.
6. Barnes, P. et al. Complementary and alternative medicine use among adults: United States, 2002. *CDC Advance Data Report #34*, 2004.
7. Pagan, J.A. and Pauly, M.V. Medical care and the use of complementary and alternative medicine. *Health Affairs*, 24(1), 255–262, 2005.
8. Walji, M. et al. Efficacy of quality criteria to identify potentially harmful information: a cross-sectional survey of complementary and alternative medicine web sites. *J. Med. Internet Res.*, 6(2), e21, 2004.
9. Jonas, W.B. and Levin, J.S., Eds. *Essentials of Complementary and Alternative Medicine*. Lippincott William & Wilkins, Philadelphia, 1999.
10. National Center for Complementary and Alternative Medicine (NCCAM). Available at http://nccam.nih.gov/health/whatiscam/#1. Accessed April 14, 2005.
11. Office of Dietary Supplements. Available at http://ods.od.nih.gov/. Accessed April 16, 2005.
12. White House Commission on Complementary and Alternative Medicine Policy. Available at http://whccamp.hhs.gov/finalreport.html. Accessed April 16, 2005.
13. IOM. *Complementary and Alternative Medicine in the United States*. National Academy Press, Washington, D.C., 2005.
14. Rees, L. and Weil, A. Integrated medicine. *Br. Med. J.*, 322, 119–120, 2002.
15. *Webster's New World Dictionary*. Prentice Hall/Macmillan Co., New York, 1994.
16. World Health Organization (WHO). Available at http://www.who.int/en/. Accessed April 16, 2005.
17. Ottawa Charter for Health Promotion. Ottawa, Ontario. Available at http://who.int/hpr/NPH/docs/ottawa_charter_hp.pdf. Accessed April 14, 2005.
18. Gaudet, T.W. Integrative medicine. *Integr. Med.*, 1(2), 67–73, 1998.
19. Sharma, H. and Clark, C. *Contemporary Ayurvedic*. Churchill Livingstone, New York, 1998.
20. Gao, D., Ed. *Chinese Medicine*. Thunder's Mouth Press, New York, 1997.
21. Slow Food. Available at http://www.slowfood.com/. Accessed April 16, 2005.
22. Wetzel, M.S., Eisenberg, D.M., and Kaptchuk, T.J. Courses involving complementary and alternative medicine at US medical schools. *JAMA*, 280, 784–787, 1998.

23. Education of Health professionals in Complementary/Alternative Medicine, Josiah Macy, Jr. Foundation 44 East 64th Street, New York, NY 10021, 2001.
24. Epstein, R.M. and Hundert, E.M. Defining and assessing professional competence. *JAMA*, 287, 226–244, 2002.
25. Thomson, C.A. et al. Proposed guidelines regarding the sale of dietary supplements. *J. Am. Diet. Assoc.*, 102(8), 1158–1164, 2002.
26. Thomson, C.A. et al. Practice Paper of the American Dietetic Association: dietary supplements. *J. Am. Diet. Assoc.*, 105(3), 460–470, 2005.

2 Ayurveda: The Mother of Traditional Medicine

Mari Clements

CONTENTS

AYURVEDA AS A COMPLEMENTARY MEDICINE SYSTEM

Ayurveda has been referred to as the mother of all traditional medicines because it has a documented history dating back 5000 years. Ayurveda, the "science or knowledge of life," is a comprehensive medical system that evolved within the Vedic, or spiritual, philosophy of India. Ayurveda encompasses internal medicine, surgery, pediatrics, rejuvenation, and psychology as well as other specialized branches of medicine. A separate but integral branch of Ayurveda is the science of yoga, which is also incorporated within Ayurveda as a whole.

Traditional Chinese medicine (TCM) was formally introduced into American culture during the early 1970s, which was an era of rich political and cultural exchange between China and the United States. TCM has remained a viable medical option in China despite the introduction of Western medicine into Chinese culture. Unfortunately, traditional Ayurveda was not so well preserved. In contrast, Ayurveda was suppressed for many years during the British colonial rule in India. The British did not allow Ayurveda to be taught in medical schools and closed many Ayurvedic teaching institutions. This forced Ayurvedic teachers and practitioners to teach and administer Ayurveda in secret. During the 20th century there has been a revival of Ayurveda, and new schools have been created.[1] The Ayurveda community in India has been working toward reestablishing itself in hospitals, clinics, and medical schools. Due to the dissolution of Ayurvedic medical schools in the past, the Ayurvedic community in India remains in a semidisjointed state. In the United States there are no set standards for Ayurvedic curriculum in schools and no established certification standards at this time. This has made it very challenging to find a reliable Ayurvedic practitioner or teacher. This may be one reason why it has taken a long time for Ayurveda to become recognized and accepted as a viable traditional medicine. Nonetheless, Ayurveda continues to embrace new scientific discoveries and to evolve as a medical system. The Ayurvedic system incorporates modern-day discoveries about the human body and nutrition into its ancient principles. In fact, much of what is known today by Ayurvedic practitioners was already understood thousands of years ago. The terminology was simply different.

Achieving balance within one's life is a primary focus of Ayurveda, for it is believed that the roots of disease lie within imbalances. This system offers principles in the art of daily living that help to maintain the quality and longevity of life. There is a "formula" within these principles that can be applied to daily life habits to help reestablish balance in a person's life. Ayurveda offers a wealth of healing modalities to assist with correcting imbalances, including diet, herbal therapy, massage therapy, yoga, and elimination therapies. Food is viewed as medicine and is considered one of the foremost approaches to health and longevity in Ayurveda. The diet and lifestyle recommendations of Ayurveda can be incorporated into virtually any aspect of a patient's medical plan.

Perhaps the most important component of Ayurveda is that each patient is treated as an individual, with individual needs. These needs require individually determined therapeutic recommendations. The foundation of Ayurveda aims to restore within a person the basic individual nature with which they were born. The premise is that people are healthiest and happiest when they live in harmony with their own true natures. The qualities of their natures are reflected in the universe that surrounds them. These qualities can be used to determine as well as to heal the imbalances and illnesses. To learn to apply the Ayurvedic principles, nutrition professionals need first to understand the qualities of a person's individual nature and the way these qualities manifest in the person's anatomy and physiology. These qualities provide practitioners with a basic language from which they can describe virtually any aspect of a person's life from the physical to the spiritual.

COSMIC PRINCIPLES OF AYURVEDA: AYURVEDA AS A REFLECTION OF MOTHER NATURE

There are five great elements within the natural world that represent the core qualities found in the human body. The five elements are: earth, water, fire, air, and ether. Each of these elements further represents the various forms of matter: solid, liquid, radiant, gaseous, and etheric forms, respectively.[2] The five elements are like metaphors that represent the state of density within matter, such as solid or liquid, or within fields of expression, such as stability versus flowing motion. Each element then encompasses both physical and descriptive expressions that can be applied in many different contexts.

> *Earth* manifests the quality of solidity, stability and giving resistance to action. *Water* manifests the quality of liquidity, a flowing motion and bringing forth life. *Fire* manifests the quality of light, perception, movement and transformation. *Air* manifests the quality of subtle movement, of direction, velocity and change. *Ether* manifests the quality of connection, communication and self-expression.

These five elements correspond with both the function and the form of the human body. Earth, with its properties of solidity and stability, is represented in the bones and promotes structure and stability in the body. Water, with its properties of liquidity, is represented in the plasma, blood, urine, sweat, saliva, and mucus. Fire, with its transformational abilities, manifests in the metabolic process and in the production of bodily heat. Air relates to any kind of movement in the body. Ether manifests as our emotions and thoughts.

Within the five elements there are 20 attributes, which consist of ten pairs of qualities and their opposite counterparts. These ten pairs are: cold/hot, wet/dry, heavy/light, gross/subtle, dense/flowing, static/mobile, dull/sharp, soft/hard, smooth/rough, and cloudy/clear. Ayurveda, similar to TCMs use of yin and yang to achieve balance, uses the concepts of opposite qualities to promote balance. The concept of opposites presupposes that like increases like and opposites cure or balance each other, particularly when there is a condition of excess. Disease ("dis-ease") of the mind or body generally manifests as an excessive amount of a certain quality or qualities that have accumulated in the body or mind. Where there is excessive accumulation, aggravation results and leads to the origin of disease. Similarly, foods, herbs, exercises, and lifestyle activities also consist of qualities and their counterparts, which make them valuable as tools for correcting imbalances within the body. By reestablishing balance, the excess that is promoting the imbalance and causing the illness is eliminated and health is restored.

DETERMINING BIOLOGICAL NATURE

Ayurveda categorizes the qualities from the five elements and the 20 attributes into a system or model, referred to as the science of the three biological humors, which are called "doshas." The three doshas are: *Vata*, *Pitta*, and *Kapha*. Learning the differences and essences of each dosha helps to simplify the application of Ayurveda.

- The Vata dosha is ruled by the elements of air and ether, which are represented by the attributes of dry, light, cold, rough, clear, subtle, and mobile.
- The Pitta dosha is ruled by the elements of fire and water represented by the attributes of somewhat oily, sharp, hot, light, mobile, and liquid.
- The Kapha dosha is ruled by earth and water, which is represented in the attributes of wet, cold, heavy, dull, sticky, cloudy, dense, soft, and firm.

Use the Ayurveda mind–body type questionnaire to determine personal dosha (see Table 2.1). Using the qualities of the three doshas, born of the five elements of nature and the 20 attributes, a balance can be established by increasing those qualities that a person has in short supply or by reducing those qualities that are in excess or by both. These qualities can be found within the food eaten, the activities in which a person participates, and the emotions expressed. Generally Ayurveda works toward reducing those qualities that are in excess. If someone is too Kapha in nature, they would participate in Kapha-reducing activities and eat Kapha-reducing foods. Whichever dosha is predominant becomes the dosha that needs to be balanced by applying the concept of opposite qualities. What someone craves and likes most should be avoided or at least limited in their diets and in their lives. See Table 2.2 for the symptoms of a dosha imbalance and Table 2.3 for a list of foods that can be used to increase or reduce a dosha.

DIGESTION: THE CORNERSTONE TO HEALTH

The key to health in Ayurveda is through the maintenance of *agni* ("aug-nee"), the biological fire that governs metabolism. Proper digestion, assimilation, and elimination of the food provide the foundation for all the other functions of the body. When the digestive fire (*agni*)

TABLE 2.1
Ayurveda Mind–Body Type Questionnaire

	V	P	K
Mental profile			
Mental activity	Restless, active mind	Sharp, assertive intellect	Calm, steady, slow
Concentration	Short term is best	Better than average	Long time focus
Comprehend new info	Quick to learn, quick to forget	Excellent comprehension	Slow to comprehend, good retention
Memory	Short term is best	Good general memory	Long term is best
Thoughts	Constantly changing	Fairly steady	Steady
Emotional temperament	Fearful, anxious, unpredictable	Aggressive, irritable, jealous	Calm, content, attached, greedy
Mood	Changes quickly	Slowly changing	Steady, unchanging
Mental subtotal	—	—	—
Behavioral profile			
Voice	Low, weak, hoarse	High pitch	Deep, pleasant, good tone
Speech	Fast, frequent, erratic	Moderate speed, sharp, clarity	Slow, definite, not talkative
Sleep	Interrupted, light	Sound, medium length	Sound, heavy, long
Impulsiveness	Very impulsive	Somewhat impulsive	Not impulsive
Sex drive	Variable — low	Moderate	Strong
Reaction to stress	Quickly excited	Moderate reaction	Slow to excite
Competition	Does not like competition	Is very competitive	Deals well with competition
Money	Does not save, spends quickly	Saves, also big spender	Saves and accumulates wealth
Friendships	Short-term friendship	Tends to be a loner	Long-term friendship
Weather	Aversion to cold	Aversion to hot	Aversion to damp and cool
Behavior subtotal	—	—	—
Digestion			
Eating	Quickly	Medium speed	Slowly
Hunger	Irregular	Sharp, needs food	Can easily miss meals
Food and drink	Prefers warm	Prefers cold	Prefers dry and warm
Bowel movements	Dry, hard, thin, constipation	Frequent, soft to normal	Heavy, slow, thick
Thirst	Very variable	Excessive	Scanty, little
Digestion subtotal	—	—	—
Physical profile			
Body type	Thin, very tall, or very short	Average size	Heavy set, stocky
Body weight	Thin, difficult to gain	Medium, gains and loses easily	Heavy, easy to gain
Skeletal structure	Small boned	Medium boned	Big bones
Veins and tendons	Very prominent	Fairly prominent	Well covered
Muscle tone	Lean	Medium with good definition	Bulkier muscles
Strength	Fair	Better than average	Excellent

TABLE 2.1 (Continued)
Ayurveda Mind–Body Type Questionnaire

	V	P	K
Amount of hair	Average	Thinning with age	Thick
Type of hair	Dry	Medium	Oily
Skin	Dry or rough	Soft, medium oily	Oily, moist, cool
Skin temperature	Cold hands and feet	Warm	Cool to touch
Complexion	Darker	Pinkish, ruddy complexion	Pale-white
Eyes	Small	Medium	Large
Size of teeth	Very large or very small	Small to medium	Medium to large
Physical subtotal	—	—	—
Add subtotals			
Mental	—	—	—
Behavioral	—	—	—
Digestion	—	—	—
Physical	—	—	—
Final total	—	—	—
Your body–mind type	VATA	PITTA	KAPHA
	Air and Ether	Fire and Water	Water and Earth

This questionnaire is most accurate if you allow someone who knows you well to review it after you have answered all the questions. Circle the answers under V, P, or K that best suit your long-term personality and body type. Try to select only one answer that best describes you, but if two answers apply equally, then circle both. Total the column at each line, carry the subtotals to the end of the questionnaire and add them to determine your dosha constitution.

Source: Adapted from Douillard J. *The 3-Season Diet* and *Body, Mind and Sport*. Three Rivers Press, New York, 2000

is impaired, the whole system is affected. There is a build up of toxins in the body, and this toxin accumulation is believed to be the root cause for all diseases. Food becomes the most important medicine because it has such a direct effect on *agni* and because more food than any other substance goes into our bodies. Digestion and elimination become good indicators of overall well-being. Problems in these areas signal the first stage of the disease process. Digestive problems such as heartburn, nausea, and bloating and elimination problems such as gas, constipation, and loose stools become useful indicators of overall health. Eating guidelines within Ayurveda are designed to optimize digestion and elimination, and each dosha has specific food and lifestyle recommendations associated with it (see Table 2.3 and Table 2.4).

AYURVEDA EATING GUIDELINES FOR THE PROMOTION OF HEALTHY DIGESTION AND ELIMINATION

Eat in a quiet environment: no television, loud music, or other distractions. Do not eat when emotionally disturbed or upset. Eat sitting down and with good posture. Eat when hungry: allow for 4–6 h before the next meal. Avoid drinking milk or icy cold beverages with meals. Drink warm beverages, sipped slowly and in limited amounts with meals. Eat slowly and chew food well. Eat lightly cooked, fresh, and warm foods. Eat until two thirds to three fourths full. Walk or sit quietly for 30 min after meals.[3]

TABLE 2.2
Symptoms of a Dosha Imbalance

Dosha	Mental Symptoms	Behavioral Symptoms	Physical Symptoms
Vata	Worry, anxiety	Inability to relax	Poor appetite
	Overactive mind	Restlessness	Fatigue
	Impatience	Impulsiveness	Constipation
	Poor concentration	Insomnia	Dry or rough skin
	Short attention span		Low stamina
	Depression, psychosis		Loss of energy
			Intestinal gas
			High blood pressure
			Lower back pain
			Menstrual cramps
			Irritable bowel
			Chapped skin, lips
			Intolerance to cold and wind
			Aching or arthritic joints
			Unintentional weight-loss
			Acute pain (especially nerve pain)
			Muscle spasms, seizures
Pitta	Anger	Outbursts of temper	Skin inflammations
	Hostility	Argumentative	Acne
	Self-criticism	Tyrannical	Excessive hunger or thirst
	Irritability	Critical of others	Bad breath
	Impatience	Intolerance of delays	Hot flashes
	Resentment	Addictions	Heartburn, acid stomach
	Jealousy		Ulcers
			Sour body odors
			Rectal burning
			Hemorrhoids
			Patchy, florid complexion
			Intolerance to heat
			Red-rimmed eyes
			Sunburn, sunstroke
Kapha	Dullness	Procrastination	Drowsiness
	Lassitude	Resistance to change	Intolerance to cold and damp
	Stupor	Greed	Sinus congestion
	Depression	Stubbornness	Fluid retention in tissues
	Over-attachment	Possessiveness	Chest congestion
		Oversleeping	Skin pallor
		Lethargy	Loose or aching joints
			High cholesterol
			Heaviness in limbs
			Frequent cold
			Weight gain, obesity
			Allergies, asthma
			Excess phlegm, cough
			Sore throat
			Cysts and other growths
			Diabetes

TABLE 2.3
Restoring Balance

Dosha	Dosha Characteristics	To Restore Balance	Reducing Diet Principles
Vata	Mental alertness, high energy, enthusiastic, imaginative, artistic, and optimistic	Rest adequately Adhere to daily routines Cultivate calmness Cultivate groundedness Moderate to light noncompetitive exercise Meditation Warm weather	Eat sweet, sour, and salty foods Choose warming, moist, lubricating, and heavy foods Eat primarily cooked foods Drink warm beverages Eat adequate amounts of fat and protein Limit dry foods and bitter tastes Eat three scheduled meals Limit bitter, astringent and pungent foods
Pitta	Strong digestion, high energy, keen intellect, bright complexion, goal-oriented, and decisive	Establish clear purpose for lifestyle routines Cultivate serenity Cultivate an even temperament Limit fatty foods Cultivate kindness Avoid competition Moderate, noncompetitive exercise that does not over-heat Exercise for enjoyment Cool weather	Eat sweet, bitter, and astringent foods Choose cooling, heavy, and dry foods Eat plenty of complex carbohydrates Limit spices Cool (not cold) food and drinks Eat three regularly scheduled meals on time Eat substantial size meals Limit sour and pungent foods
Kapha	Calm, rational, good endurance, prudent, compassionate, strong immune system, and dependable	Maintain an attitude of adaptability Stay open to change Vigorous exercise No more than 8 h of sleep Stay active	Eat pungent, bitter, and astringent foods Choose light, dry, stimulating foods Eat one (noon-time meal) or two meals a day Eat a big lunch and small dinner or supper Limit sugar, fat, dairy, and salt Avoid cold foods and drinks Limit sweet, sour, and salty foods

AYURVEDA LIFESTYLE GUIDELINES TAILORED TO EACH DOSHA

Sometimes the psychological or thinking aspect of the individual can manifest as a different quality from the physical body. For example, the physical self can be high in Kapha qualities, but the mind could simultaneously manifest an excess quality of another dosha. When this combination of doshas occurs in an individual, lifestyle recommendations need to take into consideration the qualities of both doshas. Bringing balance to the mind often requires a different approach from the body. For instance, while the Kapha predominant person (both in body and mind) requires stimulation, a Pitta or Vata mind requires a peaceful and quiet environment. Someone with a Kapha body type and a Pitta mind type would need to take

TABLE 2.4
Ayurveda Food List

Food	Vata	Pitta	Kapha
Grains			
Amaranth	↓	↓	↓
Barley	↑	↓	↓
Buckwheat	↑	↑	↓
Corn	↑	↑	↓
Durham flour	↓	↓	↓
Millet	↑	↑	↓
Oat bran	↑	↓	↓
Oats, dry	↑	↑	↓
Oats, cooked	↓	↓	↑
Pancakes, wheat	↓	↓	↑
Pasta, wheat	↑	↓	↑
Quinoa	↓	↑	↑
Rice, basmati	↓	↓	↓
Rice, brown	↓	↑	↑
Rice, sweet	↓	↓	↑
Rice, white	↓	↓	↑
Rye	↑	↑	↓
Seitan, wheat	↓	↓	↓
Spelt	↑	↓	↑
Tapioca	↑	↓	↓
Teff	↑	↑	↓
Wheat	↓	↓	↑
Lentils, red	↑	↓	↓
Lima beans	↑	↓	↓
Mung beans	↓	↓	↓↑
Navy beans	↑	↓	↓
Pinto beans	↑	↓	↓
Soybeans	↑	↓	↑
Split peas		↓	
Toor dhal	↓	↑	↓
Urad dhal	↓	↑	↑
White beans	↑	↓	↓
Soy foods			
Miso	↓	↑	↓
Soy cheese	↓	↑	↑
Soy flour	↑	↓	↑
Soy meat sub.	↓	↑	↑
Soy milk	↓	↑	↑
Soy powder	↑	↓	↑
Soy sauce	↓	↑	↑
Tempeh	↑	↓	↓
Tofu	↑	↓	↑↑
Nuts			
Almond	↓	↑	↑
Brazil	↓	↑	↑
Cashew	↓	↑	↑

↑ Increases dosha; ↓ Reduces dosha; ↑↓ Somewhat increases dosha
To promote balance, primarily choose foods that reduce the predominant dosha.

TABLE 2.4 (Continued)
Ayurveda Food List

Food	Vata	Pitta	Kapha
Coconut	↓	↓	↑
Filberts	↓	↑	↑
Hazelnut	↓	↑	↑
Macadamia	↓	↑	↑
Peanut	↓	↑	↑
Pecan	↓	↑	↑
Pine nut	↓	↑	↑
Walnut	↓	↑	↑
Legumes			
Adzuki	↑	↓	↓
Black-eyed peas	↑	↓	↓
Black beans	↑	↓	↓
Chick Peas	↑	↓	↓
Kidney beans	↓	↓	↑
Lentils, black	↑	↑	↓
Lentils, brown	↑	↑↓	↓
Seeds			
Flax	↓	↑↓	↑↓
Poppy	↓	↑↓	↑↓
Psyllium	↑	↑↓	↑
Pumpkin	↓	↑↓	↑↓
Sesame	↓	↑	↑↓
Sunflower	↓	↑↓	↑↓
Animal foods			
Beef	↓	↑	↑
Chicken, white	↑	↓	↑
Chicken, dark	↓	↑	↑
Duck	↓	↑	↑
Eggs	↓	↑	↑↓
Egg, white	↓	↓	↓
Egg, yolk	↓	↑	↑
Fish, freshwater	↓	↑↓	↑↓
Fish, ocean	↓	↑	↑
Fish salmon	↓	↑	↑
Lamb	↑	↑	↑
Pork	↑	↑	↑
Rabbit	↑	↓	↓
Shellfish	↓	↓	↓
Turkey, white	↑	↓	↓
Turkey, dark	↓	↑	↑
Venison	↑	↓	↓
Yogurt	↓	↑	↑
Vegetables			
Artichoke	↑	↓	↓
Arugula	↑	↓	↓
Asparagus	↓	↓	↓
Beets, greens	↑	↑	↓

↑ Increases dosha; ↓ Reduces dosha; ↑↓ Somewhat increases dosha
To promote balance, primarily choose foods that reduce the predominant dosha.

Continued

TABLE 2.4 (Continued)
Ayurveda Food List

Food	Vata	Pitta	Kapha
Bitter melon	↑	↓	↓
Broccoli	↑	↓	↓
Brussels sprouts	↑	↓	↓
Burdock root	↑	↑	↓
Cabbage	↑	↓	↓
Carrot	↓	↑	↓
Cauliflower	↑	↓	↓
Celery	↑	↓	↓
Chilies	↓	↑	↓
Cilantro	↓	↓↓	↓
Collard greens	↑	↓	↓
Corn, fresh	↑	↑	↓
Cucumber	↓	↓	↑
Daikon radish	↑	↑	↓
Dandelion greens	↑	↓	↓
Eggplant	↑	↑	↓
Endive	↑	↓	↓
Fennel, fresh	↓	↓	↓
Green beans	↓	↓	↓
Kale	↑	↓	↓
Kohlrabi	↑	↓	↓
Leek	↓	↓	↓
Lettuce	↑	↓	↓
Mushroom	↓	↓	↓
Mustard greens	↓	↓	↓
Okra	↑	↓	↓
Olive	↓	↑	↑
Onion	↑	↑	↓
Parsley	↓	↓	↓
Parsnip	↓	↓	↓
Peas	↑	↓	↓
Peppers	↑	↓	↓
Plantain	↑	↓	↓
Potato, sweet	↓	↓	↑
Potato, white	↑	↓	↓
Pumpkin	↑	↓	↑
Radicchio	↑	↓	↓
Radish	↑	↑	↓
Rutabaga	↓	↓	↓
Spinach	↑	↑↓	↓
Sprouts	↑	↓	↓
Squash, winter	↑	↓	↑
Squash, summer	↓	↓	↓
Tomato	↑	↑	↑
Turnip	↑	↓	↓
Zucchini	↓	↓	↑
Fruit			

↑ Increases dosha; ↓ Reduces dosha; ↑↓ Somewhat increases dosha
To promote balance, primarily choose foods that reduce the predominant dosha.

TABLE 2.4 (Continued)
Ayurveda Food List

Food	Vata	Pitta	Kapha
Apple	↑	↓	↓
Avocado	↓	↓	↑
Apricots	↓	↑	↓
Berries, sour	↓	↑	↓
Berries, sweet	↓	↓	↓
Banana, green	↑	↓	↓
Banana, ripe	↓	↑	↑
Cantaloupe	↓	↓	↑
Cherries	↓	↑	↓
Coconut	↓	↓	↑
Cranberries	↑	↑	↓
Dates	↓	↓	↑
Figs	↓	↓	↑
Grapes, green	↓	↑	↑
Grapes, red	↓	↓	↑
Grapefruit	↓	↑	↑
Kiwi	↓	↑	↑
Lemon	↓	↑	↑
Lime	↓	↑	↑
Mango, green	↓	↑	↓
Mango, ripe	↓	↑↓	↑
Melon	↓	↓	↑
Orange	↓	↑	↑
Papaya	↓	↑	↑
Peach	↓	↑	↓
Pear	↑	↓	↓
Persimmon	↑	↑	↓
Pineapple	↓	↑	↑
Plum	↓	↑	↑
Pomegranate	↑	↓	↓
Prunes	↓	↓	↓
Raisins	↓	↓	↓
Rhubarb	↓	↑	↑
Tamarind	↓	↑	↑
Dairy			
Buttermilk	↓	↑	↑
Cheese, hard	↓	↑	↑
Cheese, soft	↓	↓	↑
Cottage cheese	↓	↓	↓
Cow's milk	↓	↓	↑
Ghee	↓	↓	↓
Goat's milk	↓	↓	↓
Ice cream	↓	↓	↑
Sour cream	↓	↑	↑

↑ Increases dosha; ↓ Reduces dosha; ↑↓ Somewhat increases dosha
To promote balance, primarily choose foods that reduce the predominant dosha.

special care to provide both stimulatory and peaceful environments to insure balance. The following are lifestyle recommendations to maintain balance.

Kapha Lifestyle

The Kapha lifestyle thrives on vigorous, competitive exercise, challenging hard work requiring long hours, limited sleep of no more than 6–7 h, travel, and impulsive and spontaneous behavior. A regular change in lifestyle helps to keep Kapha alert. A good pet for Kapha is a bird. For aromatherapy, consider henna, musk, cedar, myrrh, and eucalyptus. Massage should be applied with vigor and deep pressure.

Pitta Lifestyle

The Pitta lifestyle includes moderately vigorous, noncompetitive exercise. Work should include sufficient challenge without a competitive edge. Maintaining a cool and soothing environment and choosing jobs that allow for autonomy are beneficial. Eating regularly scheduled meals offsets irritability stemming from hunger. Planning regular vacations that allow for relaxed and unscheduled time is also beneficial. A good pet for Pitta is a cat. For aromatherapy, consider sandalwood, rose, lavender, and jasmine. Massage therapy should be applied with a deep stroke and in a quiet, meditative environment.

Vata Lifestyle

Gentle, methodical, repetitive, noncompetitive exercise is best for Vata. Work should also have a repetitive quality that promotes routine and discipline. Maintain a warm, calm, and soothing environment both at home and at work. Adequate rest is very important for Vata. Pacing oneself throughout the day is recommended. Limit travel and excitement. A good pet for Vata is a dog, not a show dog but a fun-loving and affectionate dog. For aromatherapy, consider sandalwood, henna, musk, myrrh, and wintergreen. Massage therapy should be applied with gentle, deep, and sensuous strokes.

AYURVEDA CASE STUDIES

Kapha Case Study

A 55-year-old large boned, obese client presents with newly diagnosed type 2 diabetes and a metabolic Syndrome profile that includes hypertension, insulin resistance, and high LDL-cholesterol. She describes herself as a happily married housewife of 30 years. Her physician sent her to you for diabetes education. Her present lifestyle includes no exercise, taking care of grandchildren during the week, skipping meals, and snacking on sugary foods. The Kapha nature is represented by her obesity, large frame, high cholesterol, insulin resistance, diabetes, a preference for sweet foods, and her resistance to exercise. Her mental nature is that of Kapha with her continued role as a caretaker and her desire to stay at home rather than go out into the world. Skipping meals is also part of the Kapha nature.

To reduce Kapha, she will need to change, and Kaphas do not like change. She needs to follow both the Kapha diet and the Kapha-reducing lifestyle that includes avoidance of sweet foods and vigorous exercise. Kaphas need mental and physical stimulation in their lives, and they prefer to be couch potatoes.

PITTA CASE STUDY

A 45-year-old male presents with a long history of gastroesophageal reflux disorder (GERD) and a recent diagnosis of angina. He is 5'10" tall and weighs 180 lbs. He works as a supervisor for a large construction company. He eats on the run, smokes cigarettes, and loves drinking beers with his coworkers after work. He enjoys playing competitive squash in winter and tennis in summer. His wife recently left him, and he is fighting for joint custody of their children. He self-referred himself to you because his GERD has gotten worse and he is having trouble getting to sleep at night.

The Pitta nature is represented in his capacity to work and play hard. He loves the heat of competition, alcohol, and smoking. His GERD is representative of this heat and his poor eating habits. Pitta thrives on stress but it eventually takes its toll as represented by both the GERD and angina. Pittas are independent and will self-refer themselves more than others. This patient also has a mental Vata imbalance due to the anxiety from the divorce. He would need to follow the Pitta diet to reduce the heat in his body while also following a Vata-nurturing lifestyle of routine, rest, and calming activities to reduce the Vata imbalance in the mind.

VATA CASE STUDY

A 55-year-old woman presents with mild osteoporosis, irritable bowel syndrome (IBS), and newly diagnosed chronic fatigue. She is medium boned, 5'6" tall, and weighs 120 lbs. She lives alone and works as a graphic designer in an advertising agency. She found your name in the phone book and is coming to you because she desperately wants you to help her keep working despite her present illness.

The Vata nature is represented by her low body weight, the osteoporosis, IBS, and fatigue. Her creativity and living alone are also suggestive of the Vata nature. However, her mental nature is that of Pitta with her drive to keep on working despite the low energy and her love of the competitive environment of advertising. She needs to follow a Vata diet to reduce the IBS symptoms and to replenish the body. To calm the Pitta mind, she will need to participate in a Pitta-calming lifestyle that includes avoiding competition and participating in an exercise program-like strength training that does not require too much energy. The strength training provides the Pitta mind with a focus point. She needs to be encouraged to take time away from work to participate in fun activities.

REFERENCES

1. Ranade S, Qutab A, Deshpande R. *History and Philosophy of Ayurved*. Pune, India: International Academy of Ayurveda, 1998.
2. Lad V. *Textbook of Ayurveda Fundamental Principles*. Albuquerque, NM: Ayurvedic Press, 2002.
3. Lad V. *Ayurveda: The Science of Self Healing*. Twin Lakes, WI: Lotus Press, 1984.

USEFUL RESOURCES

Chopra D. *Perfect Health*. New York, NY: Harmony Books, 1989.
Chopra D. *Quantum Healing*. New York, NY: Bantam Books, 1989.
Douillard J. *The 3-Season Diet*. New York, NY: Three Rivers Press, 2000.
Frawley D. *Ayurvedic Healing*. Salt Lake City, UT: Passage Press, 1989.
Lad V. *Textbook of Ayurveda Fundamental Principles*. Albuquerque, NM: Ayurvedic Press, 2002.
Lad V. *Ayurveda: The Science of Self Healing*. Twin Lakes, WI: Lotus Press, 1984.
Morningstar A. *Ayurvedic Cooking for Westerners*. Twin Lakes, WI: Lotus Press, 1995.
Tiwari M. *A Life of Balance*. Rochester, VT: Healing Arts Press, 1995.
The Ayurvedic Encyclopedia. Bayville, NY: Ayurveda Holistic Center Press, 1998.

3 Pregnancy and Lactation

Amy A. Drescher, Deborah Pesicka, and Judith Shabert

CONTENTS

Adequate maternal nutrition in pregnancy is important, as it effects fetal and infant development. Dietary nutrients, whether taken directly from maternal diet or indirectly from maternal stores, are the sole source of nutrients to the fetus and the breast milk-only fed infant. Nutritional factors impact a fetus' growth, which is highly correlated with infant mortality and morbidity.[1–3] To optimize fetal health, females of childbearing age would receive preconceptual nutrition education beginning in their early teenage years. Women actively planning a pregnancy would consult their healthcare provider before conceiving so appropriate counseling, based on personal health history, nutritional assessment, family history, physical examination, and laboratory assessment, could be made. This approach would decrease complications during pregnancy and improve the outcome for thousands of infants born annually. In reality, only 50% of women plan their pregnancies and one out of nine pregnancies occur in teenage girls, many of whom are poorly nourished.[4] The number of primagravid women over age 40 is also rising and women in this age group are at increased risk for a number of prenatal and delivery complications.[4] Women may enter pregnancy nutritionally compromised secondary to poor eating habits. Obesity and overweight in America have become epidemic and contribute to increased medical risks during pregnancy.[5] Studies demonstrate that imbalances in maternal nutritional intake can have a deleterious effect on the offspring's health into adulthood.[6,7]

This chapter will focus on the use of conventionally defined nutrients, vitamins, minerals, calories, carbohydrate (CHO), protein, and fat, as well as the use of complementary and alternative medicine (CAM) therapies in pregnancy and lactation. Integrative nutrition therapy (INT) combines both conventional and CAM nutritional therapies. It is necessary to examine the available information regarding INT use in pregnancy and lactation before making recommendations to patients.

PRECONCEPTUAL NUTRITION STATUS AND COUNSELING

Although nutrition education for pregnant women ideally begins years before conception, most young women are unlikely to see a nutritionist until they become pregnant and then only if they are eligible for the Women, Infant, and Children (WIC) program or have a high-risk pregnancy. Nutritional intervention that begins weeks after conception may have little effect in preventing fetal malformations that occur during organogenesis and other fetal and maternal complications. Physicians, nutritionists, and CAM providers should take every opportunity to counsel all women of childbearing age on healthful nutrition guidelines.

An increasing body of data suggests that the mother's health and habits before conception coupled with the *in utero* environment of the fetus influence not only the outcome at delivery but also the health of that individual many years into the future.[8] Godfrey and Barker[7] provide a discussion of fetal nutrition and adult disease. Middle-aged men and women who were low birth weight (LBW) or short at birth had higher rates of coronary heart disease (CHD), hypertension (HTN), high cholesterol levels, and abnormal glucose–insulin metabolism compared to those with normal birth weight and length. The increased risk of disease was regardless of gestational age. Babies with LBW and short length have higher rates of adult HTN, but not CHD. Short babies with relatively normal weight have increased risk of CHD. LBW is associated with insulin resistance syndrome and if coupled with obesity in adulthood, may lead to a high prevalence of type 2 diabetes.[7] Thus, when counseling women, it may be prudent to focus the educational message on the family and on the potential health risk and benefits that a pregnancy entails for the infant's future.

Nutrition therapy in pregnancy should focus on the provision of optimal and adequate nutrients as outlined in conventional nutrition therapy (CNT). Micronutrient deficiencies, including iron and folate, are seen in women of reproductive age. Iron deficiency anemia occurs in 3 to 5% of 16- to 50-year-old women.[8] It is more common in African Americans and Latinos than in Caucasians. Preconceptual folate supplementation of 400 mcg daily is known to reduce the incidence of neural tube defects (NTD).[9,10] From 1996, when folic acid fortification of cereal grain products was mandated, until 2001 the occurrence of NTDs declined by 23%.[11] Folate deficiency may also relate to the occurrence of Down's syndrome.[12–14]

While the typical American diet is rarely deficient in vitamin B-12, the vegan population is at increased risk of B-12 deficiency secondary to it being found only in animal products and B-12 fortified products. A vegan of reproductive age should be encouraged to use B-12 fortified foods or a B-12 supplement. Inadequate vitamin B-12 intake may be related to NTD.[15,16]

More research is needed in both the role of vitamin B-12 in NTD and folate in the etiology of Down's syndrome.

Females with eating disorders are at increased risk for multiple nutritional deficiencies from diets excessively limited in energy and nutrients, anorexia nervosa, or from nutritional deficiencies secondary to bingeing and purging, bulimia nervosa. Erick[17] estimates that there are nearly 40,000 eating-disordered women who become pregnant annually in the United States. Although psychiatric intervention is a key component in the treatment of these women, preconceptual and prenatal nutrition therapy may be of benefit in preventing spontaneous abortions, avoiding small for gestational age (SGA) infants and, possibly, limiting the incidence of postpartum (PP) depression linked to marginal intakes of essential fatty acids and low plasma concentrations of omega-3 fatty acids.[18,19]

Preexisting diseases or disorders may impact a woman's pregnancy. Diabetes mellitus (DM) affects fetal and maternal morbidity and fetal mortality.[20,21] Preexisting DM may be type 1 DM or type 2 DM. Type 1 DM requires exogenous insulin. Women with preexisting DM who conceive with elevated hemoglobin A1c (HA1c) levels have increased risk of fetal anomalies.[22,23] Types 1 and 2 DM each affect $<0.5\%$ of all pregnancies.[20,24] Preconceptual meal planning to normalize glucose and HA1c levels reduces the risk of anomalies to levels approaching those of women without diabetes.[23,25,26]

Chronic HTN exists before pregnancy and increases the risk of preeclampsia. HTN in pregnancy increases the risk of preterm delivery.[27] The dietary approaches to stop hypertension (DASH) diet has been shown to reduce blood pressure in the nonpregnant population.[28] Although the DASH diet has not been tested specifically in pregnancy, its sound nutritional principles make it an ideal eating plan for most pregnant women. (Pregnant women with renal disease may not tolerate the high potassium content of the DASH diet.)

The incidence of overweight and obesity in U.S. adults is 65.1%.[29] Overweight and obese women have increased risks for complications in pregnancy, including type 2 DM, preeclampsia, PP hemorrhage, urinary tract infections (UTI), and intrauterine death.[30] While many weight loss approaches are used to treat overweight and obesity, few have long-term success. Additionally, many weight loss approaches limit specific macro- or micronutrients that may negatively impact nutritional status. Few weight loss approaches have been studied in pregnancy or lactation.

Bariatric surgeries, including gastric banding and gastric bypass, are now performed with increasing frequency, including adolescents.[31] Bariatric surgery patients have significant potential for nutritional deficiencies, including protein, vitamin B-12, folic acid, and iron. Pregnancy increases these risks, as well as increasing the risk for other postoperative complications requiring additional surgery.[32] Close follow-up and nutritional counseling of pregnant women who have undergone bariatric surgery are imperative.

A brief discussion of high-protein, or CHO-modified, diets in the context of pregnancy is warranted as women of reproductive age are likely using them for weight loss, and may be following them before they are aware of a pregnancy. High-protein diets, which are usually high fat and low CHO, originally popular in the 1970s, have seen resurgence in popularity in recent years. Studies demonstrate increased protein intake at the expense of CHO affects offspring into adulthood, with increased blood pressure and cortisol levels, leading to increased risk of the metabolic syndrome.[6,33] In 2003, several studies reported that short-term, the high-protein, low-CHO diets offer greater weight loss and improved lipid values compared to low-fat, high-CHO eating plans, although by 1 year the weight loss was similar between the two groups.[34–36] The recent studies did not include pregnant women. The Motherwell study, reported in Herrick et al.[6] and Sheill et al.,[33] suggest a need for caution in relation to the use of high-protein, low-CHO diets. An unintended, yet conceivable, result of CHO-restricted intakes is the reduced intakes of folate and other nutrients used to fortify refined grain products, perhaps increasing the risk of NTDs. Although there are limited numbers of studies, findings thus far suggest low-CHO diets cannot be recommended for use in pregnancy, and should be avoided by women planning a pregnancy related to the risk of SGA and health issues in the adult offspring.

Preventing or treating nutritional deficiencies and preexisting medical conditions with a nutrition component before conception will help to reduce prenatal risks.

PREGNANCY

The normal physiology of pregnancy anticipates specific physiologic and metabolic changes in organ systems. These changes occur over a continuum, but for ease of discussion they are divided into the three trimesters of pregnancy. Normal alterations in laboratory values and nutrient concentrations occur in pregnancy. Whereas these values would be considered abnormal in a nonpregnant woman, they are the norm in pregnancy. For example, renal blood flow and glomerular filtration rate increase in pregnancy, while the renal threshold for glucose reabsorption decreases. Thus glucosuria in pregnancy may not be indicative of diabetes, as it would be in a nonpregnant female. An increase in the synthesis of estrogen and progesterone leads to significantly elevated cholesterol and triglyceride blood concentrations that are normal in pregnancy.

CNT recommendations in pregnancy are well documented and generally well accepted.[37] The recommended macro- and micronutrient requirements are increased in pregnancy with a few exceptions. Maternal absorption of many nutrients, including calcium, is enhanced in pregnancy, resulting in insignificant changes in the recommended dietary allowances (RDA). While most experts acknowledge the need for supplemental folic acid and iron, there are those who discourage other nutritional supplements during pregnancy, maintaining that adequate maternal and fetal nutrition can be derived from diet.[38] However, physicians commonly prescribe prenatal vitamins (PNVs) and minerals. Epidemiological research suggests that PNV supplementation may have unexpected benefits, such as a decreased incidence of nausea and vomiting of pregnancy (NVP) and neuroblastoma in children whose mother who took PNVs during pregnancy.[39] Table 3.1 highlights the increased nutrient requirements in pregnancy and lactation.

ENERGY

In 2002, for the first time, the Institute of Medicine (IOM) made specific energy and macronutrient recommendations, by trimester, in pregnancy. CHO, protein, fat, and alcohol are the energy-providing macronutrients. Alcohol is not recommended in pregnancy and will not be discussed further. Energy requirements in pregnancy are based on basal energy expenditure (BEE).[40]

The IOM revised the RDA for energy in pregnancy from the original general increase of 300 kcal/day to trimester-specific recommendations. The revision specifies no energy increase in the first trimester and incremental increases in the second and third trimesters. The median energy increases in pregnancy are 340 kcal/day in the second trimester and 452 kcal/day in the third trimester.

Recommended pregnancy weight gain is based on pregravid body mass index (BMI) (see Table 3.2). Inadequate or excessive weight gain indicates a need to assess actual dietary intake. Inadequate weight gain is associated with preterm births and fetal growth restriction.[41] Excessive weight gain in the first trimester, and a continued pattern of gain throughout pregnancy, may contribute to the epidemic of obesity.[42] A 15-year follow-up study was conducted to assess the impact of weight gain during pregnancy on future obesity. Women who gained the most

TABLE 3.1
Increased Daily Nutrient Allowances for Pregnancy

Nutrient	Women (25–50)	Pregnant	Percent Increase
Protein (g)	50	60	20
Iron (mg)	15	30	100
Zinc (mg)	12	15	25
Folic acid (mcg)	400	800	100
Thiamine B_1 (mg)	1.1	1.4	27
Riboflavin B_2 (mg)	1.1	1.4	27
Niacin (mg)	14	18	29
Vitamin B-6 (mg)	1.3	1.9	20
Vitamin B-12 (mg)	2.4	2.6	8
Vitamin C	75	85	13
Magnesium (mg)	320	350	9
DHA	1.1	1.4	27

Sources: Institute of Medicine, Food and Nutrition Board, *Dietary Reference Intakes for Energy, and the Macronutrients, Carbohydrate, Fiber, Fat, Fatty acids, Cholesterol, Protein, and Amino Acids*, National Academy Press, Washington, D.C., 2002.

Institute of Medicine, Food and Nutrition Board, *Dietary Reference Intakes for Vitamin C, Vitamin E, Selenium, and Carotenoids*, National Academy Press, Washington, D.C., 2000.

Institute of Medicine, Food and Nutrition Board, *Dietary Reference Intakes for Vitamin A, Vitamin K, Arsenic, Boron, Chromium, Copper, Iodine, Iron, Manganese, Molybdenum, Nickel, Silicon, Vanadium and Zinc*, National Academy Press, Washington, D.C., 2001.

Institute of Medicine, Food and Nutrition Board, *Dietary Reference Intakes for Thiamin, Riboflavin, Niacin, Vitamin B-6, Folate, Vitamin B-12, Pantothenic Acid, Biotin, and Choline*, National Academy Press, Washington, D.C., 1998. Institute of Medicine, Food and Nutrition Board, *Dietary Reference Intakes for Calcium, Phosphorus, Magnesium, Vitamin D, and Fluoride*, National Academy Press, Washington, D.C., 1997.

weight in pregnancy retained more weight at the 1- and 15-year time points.[43] Another study followed a cohort of 540 women who had their weight recorded early in pregnancy and 6 months PP with long-term follow-up at 5 to 10 years.[42] Women who gained within the recommended amount of weight during pregnancy were 6.5 kg heavier at follow-up whereas those with excessive weight gain in pregnancy were 8.4 kg heavier at follow-up. PP exercise and

TABLE 3.2
Recommended Weight Gain in Pregnancy

Prepregnancy Weight	Total Weight Gain (lb)	Rate of Gain (per Week, in lb)
Normal weight (BMI 19.8–26)	25–35	1
Underweight (BMI < 19.8)	28–40	>1.1
Overweight (BMI 26–29)	15–25	.67
Obese (BMI > 29)	At least 15	

Body mass index $(BMI) = $ weight (kg)/height $(m)^2$.

Sources: From Villar, J. et al., *Am. Soc. Nutr. Sci.*, 133, 1632S, 2003; Institute of Medicine, Committee on Nutrition Status During Pregnancy and Lactation, *Nutrition During Pregnancy, Part 1. Weight Gain*, National Academy Press, Washington, D.C., 1990.

lactation were identified as beneficial in controlling long-term weight retention.[42] More attention by healthcare providers is warranted to encourage weight gain within recommended ranges as well as education on factors that are associated with PP weight loss.

CARBOHYDRATE

Glucose serves as one of the principal fuel sources for the fetus. Estimates of maternal glucose transfer suggest that glucose provides approximately 50 to 70% of the energy for a third trimester fetus.[44] Ketoacids provide the remaining energy. Both glucose and ketoacids are utilized by the fetal brain. It appears that all the glucose transferred from mother to fetus is required for fetal brain metabolism and is not utilized by other fetal tissues.[44] The RDA for CHO in pregnancy is 175 g daily.[44]

No specific recommendations were made for the percentage of CHO as simple CHO or starch, or as refined versus whole grain CHO. This omission is regrettable. The increasing incidence of overweight and obesity, and therefore gestational and type 2 diabetes, in the United States parallels the large increase of refined CHO intake, particularly as added fructose, as high fructose corn syrup, by Americans, suggesting that dietary macronutrient composition may play a major role in this epidemic.[45] More research is needed to provide evidence-based recommendations.

FIBER

Most women in America do not eat sufficient fiber.[46] An adequate intake (AI) of 28 g fiber/day for pregnancy was established.[46] Rapid increase in fiber intake may cause constipation and other recognized physical discomforts. Gradually increasing fiber will generally avoid these. Adequate fluid intake is also important in alleviating constipation. In 2004, an AI was established for total water (to include water from all sources, including foods) in pregnancy of 2.7 l daily.[47]

PROTEIN

Protein requirements increase in pregnancy, although not significantly in the first trimester. The RDA for protein in pregnancy is 1.1 g protein/kg/day or +25 g added protein daily in the second and third trimesters only.[48]

FAT

An AI or estimated average requirement (EAR) of total fat, saturated fat, or monounsaturated fats for adolescents or adults was not set. For the first time, however, a specific AI for the essential fatty acids from the omega-6 and omega-3 families, linoleic acid and alpha-linolenic acid (ALA), respectively, was established.[49] Omega-3 ($n-3$) fatty acids (FA) are one class of polyunsaturated fatty acids (PUFA), omega-6 ($n-6$) are the other. They are metabolized competitively. PUFA influence the composition of cell walls, which in turn determines the type of inflammatory mediator response produced. Omega-6 FA produce aggressive inflammatory response mediators, called cytokines. Conversely, $n-3$ FA produce anti-inflammatory response mediators. The typical American diet provides significantly more $n-6$ FA than diets just a few decades ago and 20 to 40 times more $n-6$ FA than $n-3$ FA.[50] The increase in cytokines from $n-6$ FA is linked to an increased incidence of illness, disease and it affects pregnancy outcome.[51] Omega-3 FA include eicosapentaenoic acid (EPA), ALA, and docosahexaenoic acid (DHA). DHA has an important role in the development of the fetal nervous system and retina and provides the main structural component of brain cell membranes (Textbox 3.1). A DHA deficiency

---

Textbox 3.1   Brief Review: Omega-3 Fatty Acids — Important for Fetal and Maternal Health

Omega-3 FA are one class of polyunsaturated fatty acids (PUFA), $n-6$ are the other. They are metabolized competitively. PUFA influence the composition of cell walls, which in turn determines the type of inflammatory mediator response produced. Omega-6 FA produce aggressive inflammatory response mediators, cytokines. Conversely, $n-3$ FA produce anti-inflammatory response mediators. The typical American diet provides significantly more $n-6$ FA than diets just a few decades ago and 20 to 40 times more $n-6$ FA than $n-3$ FA, compared to the recommended 2 to 4 times more $n-6$ FA than Omega-3 FA.[1] The increase in cytokines from $n-6$ FA is linked to an increased incidence of illness, disease and it affects pregnancy outcome.[2] Omega-3 FA include eicosapentaenoic acid (EPA), alpha-linolenic acid (ALA), and docosahexaenoic acid (DHA). DHA has an important role in the development of the fetal nervous system and retina and provides the main structural component of brain cell membranes. A DHA deficiency during late fetal or early infant development results in impaired learning ability, intelligence, or other aspects of mental functioning.[1] Helland et al. found increased IQ at age 4 years with maternal supplementation of $n-3$ FA.[3] For the first time DRI includes DHA in pregnancy, which is specified at 1.4 g daily and 1.3 g daily in lactation.[4] The main food sources of DHA are cold-water fish, which can meet the DRI if eaten 3 to 4 times per week. However, in December 2003 the FDA drafted a stronger recommendation that pregnant women limit intake of albacore tuna and tuna steaks, and completely avoid other large cold-water fish, due to their mercury content.[5] Alternatively, DHA can be made from linolenic acid, the plant source of $n-3$ FA, but the conversion is not automatic and can be stymied if there is too much $n-6$ FA in the diet or other unknown factors. For example, Francois and coworkers supplemented lactating women with flaxseed oil for 4 weeks but did not see an increase in breast milk DHA.[6] Therefore, it is suggested to get preformed DHA in fatty fish (in accordance with FDA limitations), fortified eggs, or DHA supplements.[7]

Food Sources of Omega-3 Fatty Acids

Sardines	Walnuts
Sword fish*	Flax products
Salmon*	Omega-3 enriched eggs
Albacore tuna*	Canola oil
Herring	Soy oil
Mackerel*	Omega-3 supplements

*See Ref. 5 for limits on certain fish due to mercury exposure.

[1] Weil, A., *Eating Well for Optimum Health: The Essential Guide to Bring Health and Pleasure Back to Eating*, Quill, New York, 2001, p. 88, 262.

[2] Hornstra, G., Essential fatty acids in mothers and their neonates, *Am. J. Clin. Nutr.*, 71, 1262S, 2000.

[3] Helland, I.B. et al., Maternal supplementation with very-long-chain $N-3$ fatty acids during pregnancy and lactation augments children's IQ at 4 years of age, *Pediatrics*, 111, 39, 2003.

[4] Institute of Medicine, Food and Nutrition Board, *Dietary Reference Intakes for Energy, and the Macronutrients, Carbohydrate, Fiber, Fat, Fatty Acids, Cholesterol, Protein, and Amino Acids*, National Academy Press Washington, D.C., 2002.

[5] Draft advice for women who are pregnant, or who might become pregnant, and nursing mothers, about avoiding harm to your baby or young child from mercury in fish and shellfish, U.S. Food and Drug Administration, available at www.fda.gov/oc/opacom/mehgadvisory1208.html, accessed January 27, 2003.

[6] Francois, C.A. et al., Supplementing lactating women with flaxseed oil does not increase docosahexaenoic acid in their milk, *Am. J. Clin. Nutr.*, 77, 226, 2003.

[7] Krause, *Krause's Food Nutrition and Diet Therapy*, W.B. Saunders, Philadelphia, 2004, p. 205.

TABLE 3.3
Food Safety in Pregnancy

Infection/Teratogen	Sources of Infection	Effects
Listeria monocytogenes	Soft cheeses, uncooked cold cuts, raw milk, smoked seafood, garden soil	Spontaneous abortion, fetal newborn meningitis
Toxoplasmosis	Raw meat, unwashed vegetables, cat litter, pet reptiles	Spontaneous abortion, blindness, mental retardation
Salmonella	Raw sprouts, undercooked meat and eggs, raw oysters, cross contamination of food preparation surfaces with raw meat and poultry, pets; cat, dog, and reptile feces	Fever nausea, vomiting meningitis, typhoid fever
Methylmercury	Industrial pollution of water cold-water fish, shark, mackerel, sword fish, albacore tuna	Believed to harm the developing brain *in utero*
Escherichia coli (*E. coli*)	Unpasteurized milk and juices, undercooked meats, unwashed fruits and vegetables	Bloody diarrhea and abdominal cramps

Sources: Adapted from National Center for Disease Control CDC Food related diseases, http://www.cdc.gov/ncidod/diseases/food/index.htm accessed April 2, 2004; Krause, *Krause's Food Nutrition and Diet Therapy*, W.B. Saunders, Philadelphia, 2004, chap. 7; Jones, C. and Hudson, R.A., *Eating for Pregnancy an Essential Guide to Nutrition with Recipes for the Whole Family*, Marlowe and Co., New York, 2003, p. 54, 257, 217.

during late fetal or early infant development results in impaired learning ability, intelligence, or other aspects of mental functioning.[50] Helland et al.[52] found increased IQ at 4 years of age with maternal supplementation of $n - 3$ FA.[52] For the first time dietary reference intakes (DRI) includes DHA in pregnancy, which is set at 1.4 g daily, and 1.3 g in lactation.[49] The main food sources of DHA are cold-water fish, which can meet the DRI if eaten three to four times weekly. However, the Food and Drug Administration (FDA) recommends limits on many fish due to mercury and polychlorinated biphenyls (PCB) contamination[53] (see Table 3.3 and "Food Safety in Pregnancy" section). Alternatively, DHA can be made from linolenic acid, the plant source of $n-3$ FA, but the conversion is not automatic and can be stymied if there is too much $n-6$ FA in the diet or by other unknown factors. For example, Francois et al.[54] supplemented lactating women with flaxseed oil for 4 weeks but did not see an increase in breast milk DHA.[54] Therefore, it is suggested to get preformed DHA in fatty fish, in accordance with FDA limitations, fortified eggs, or DHA supplements.[55]

Trans-fatty acids (tFA) are a specific type of fat formed when liquid oils are made into solid fats such as shortening and hard margarine. However, a small amount of *trans*-fat is naturally occurring, primarily in some animal-based foods.[56] Animal studies suggest that tFA in the diet may displace the essential omega-3 and omega-6 FA in breast milk and in fetal and infant brain.[57,58] The IOM recognizes the deleterious effects that tFA have on blood lipids, stating that an upper tolerable limit (UL) would be zero.[49] However, "because tFA are unavoidable in ordinary diets, achieving a UL would require extraordinary changes in patterns of dietary intake...and unknown and unquantifiable health risk may be introduced by any extreme adjustments in dietary pattern."[49] Effective January 1, 2006, the FDA will require tFA content be listed on the Nutrition Facts food label.[56] Thus, in general, products containing partially hydrogenated fats, the primary source of tFA, should be avoided.

FOOD SAFETY IN PREGNANCY

An estimated 65 to 76 million cases of foodborne illnesses occur annually in the United States. This results in 325,000 hospitalizations and 5,000 to 9,000 deaths.[59] Food safety is of particular concern in pregnancy. Pregnancy alters normal immune system activity, making common foodborne pathogens more deleterious to both mother and fetus.[60] One factor thought to contribute foodborne illness is the overuse of antibiotics in animals for human consumption.[61] Widespread use of antibiotics leads to resistant organisms, making it more difficult to treat human infectious diseases effectively. Certain foods such as some fish, soft cheeses, ready-to-eat meats and poultry, and raw sprouts pose health risks during pregnancy. Undercooked meat, poultry, eggs, and fish can cause infections from listerosis, *Escherichia coli*, salmonellosis, and toxoplasmosis. Informed food choices, adequate cooking, and safe food handling practices can help prevent illnesses.[62]

The infectious agent holding the greatest risk to pregnant women is *Listeria monocytogenes*.[63] Pregnant women are 20 times more likely to become infected with *Listeria* than nonpregnant individuals. Infection with this microorganism requires hospitalization in 88% of the cases with a 30% mortality rate. The United States Department of Agriculture (USDA) suggests that pregnant women should not eat luncheon meats unless they are served steaming hot, or soft cheeses such as Feta, Brie, blue-veined cheeses, and Mexican-style cheeses. They also advise against eating refrigerated pates, smoked seafood, or unpasteurized or raw milk.[63] Other foodborne illnesses and contamination risks are summarized in Table 3.3.

Mercury contamination poses another foodborne risk to pregnant women. Environmental mercury contamination begins when the inorganic mercury effluent is released into waterways from manufacturing plants, primarily paper mills and chemical plants, or by the release of mercury from the earth's crust.[64] Mercury in an aquatic environment is converted to its organic form, methylmercury, by bacteria, which ultimately contaminates fish food sources. State or local advisories alert the public of bodies of water containing contaminated fish species.[65] The National Academy of Sciences estimates 60,000 infants are born annually with excessive mercury exposure.[66] The mercury exposure is neurotoxic and causes irreversible brain function deficits.[67] Chronic low-dose prenatal methylmercury exposure from maternal fish consumption is associated with poor performance on neurobehavioral tests, particularly attention, fine-motor function, language, visual–spatial abilities, and verbal memory.[68]

In 2004, the Food and Drug Administration (FDA) and Environmental Protection Agency (EPA) jointly released a revised consumer advisory on methylmercury in fish to pregnant and lactating women, women of childbearing age, and young children.[53] The following fish are advised to be avoided: shark, tilefish, swordfish, and king mackerel. Fish lower in mercury, such as canned light tuna, salmon, pollock, and catfish, may be safely consumed within limits of 12 oz per week. Fish from local waters, albacore tuna, and tuna steaks are limited to 6 oz per week.

PCBs also present a risk to pregnant women. The stable, nonflammable nature of PCBs made them ideal for use in electrical transformers and capacitors.[69] They were widely used throughout the world but were banned in North America in 1976 when their health risks became known. Because of their long half-life, there are at least 600,000 million pounds of PCBs present in the environment, primarily in rivers, lakes, and coastal areas of a number of states.[69] PCBs are absorbed through the gastrointestinal tract and tend to accumulate in lipid-rich tissues such as adipose tissue and breast milk. The absorption of PCBs from breast milk ranges from 90 to 100%.[70] In animals PCBs have been shown to produce lesions, neurobehavioral effects, decreased birth weight, and infant death. Such effects in humans have been difficult to document due to study limitations such as confounding factors and uncertain exposure estimates. One 16-year longitudinal study of consumption of PCB-contaminated fish in pregnancy demonstrated lower birth weight, smaller head circumference, delays in neuromuscular maturity, and lower intelligent quotient (IQ) when tested at 11 years of age.[71] In a separate study, they report that nearly all adverse effects associated with PCB exposure are related more to prenatal rather than PP, lactation, exposure, and that those effects were stronger in children who are not breast-fed.[72] Women living in areas where the concentration of PCBs is known to be high should be advised not to eat fish taken from local waterways.[65]

SOY

Although soy product use has increased as health benefits of soy consumption have been documented, some evidence suggests potential adverse effects to male fetuses.[73–75] Soy products have been part of a typical Asian diet for centuries, but their introduction in the Western diet is relatively recent. Products made from soybeans include traditional Asian foods such as miso, tempeh, and tofu, as well as more refined soy products such as soy milk, soy protein, and vegetarian meat analogs, consumed mainly in the United States. In addition to the adult intake of soy products, soy infant formula is often substituted when infants are intolerant of milk-based formulas. Franke et al.[76] determined the isoflavone concentration of four different soy formulas. After adjusting for body weight, infant intake was found to be four to six times that of adults consuming soy foods regularly. Whether this relatively high exposure results in beneficial or adverse effects remains to be determined. There are many phytochemicals in soy that may confer health benefits, but the two most extensively investigated are the flavones, genistein and daidzein, which are also sold as individual supplements. These are known as phytoestrogens, but both have estrogenic and antiestrogenic properties. The high intake of soy products by the Japanese is thought to contribute to their low incidence of hormone-dependent cancers such as prostate and breast cancer.[73] It is hypothesized that this effect is due to *in utero* exposure to soy isoflavones or secondary to a lifetime of eating a soy-rich diet. Additionally, some investigators hypothesize breast-feeding by a mother who consumes soy foods may contribute to cancer prevention in infants due to exposure to isoflavones during a critical development period.[76] Researchers have raised concerns about potential adverse effects of estrogen-like compounds on the male fetus.[75] Adverse effects of phytoestrogens on reproduction and sexual development have been demonstrated in livestock and research animals.[77] Worldwide, there is an increased incidence of cryptorchidism (a condition where one or both testes does not descend into the scrotum by 1 year of age) and hypospadias (a birth defect where the urethra is located on the underside of the penis), and a suggested decline in sperm counts.[74] Trends in surveillance studies for the incidence of hypospadias in the United States have been inconclusive, but suggest a progressive increase.[78] Researchers have raised concern that phytoestrogens from increased soy consumption may be a contributing factor.[79] In a prospective cohort of women in England, an increased incidence of hypospadias was found in the male offspring of vegetarians.[80] Of the 7928 males in the study, 51 had hypospadias.[80] However, soy intake was not a statistically significant predictor of hypospadias and less than 3% of the mothers reported regular consumption of soy meat substitutes or soy milk. An alternate explanation for the increased incidence may be that pesticides and fertilizers, which can be estrogenic, may act as endocrine disruptors and are more prevalent in a vegetarian diet.[75] Further, if the association between soy foods and hypospadias was strong, one would expect that historically it would be more common in Japan because of traditionally high intakes of soy. This correlation is not seen. Japan, like other developed countries, is experiencing an increased incidence of hypospadias at time when they are adopting a westernized diet with less soy intake, not more.[80]

Common conditions in pregnancy include constipation, indigestion, leg cramps, and NVP. Common disorders of pregnancy include HTN, preeclampsia, anemia, preterm delivery, obstructed labor or cesarean section (C/S), infection, and altered birth size. We will discuss each, including a summary of relevant CNT and CAM therapies.

OVERVIEW OF COMPLEMENTARY AND ALTERNATIVE MEDICINE IN PREGNANCY

Thirty-six percent of surveyed U.S. adults used some form of CAM therapy, excluding prayer for medical reasons, in the past 12 months.[81] Women use CAM therapies more than men, the majority of them in the reproductive age.[82,83] A survey of the use of CAM practices by multiracial adult females in New York City found that over half used CAM therapies that include not only nutritional supplements but also mind–body approaches and manual manipulation.[84] Tsui et al.[85] found 13% of the women surveyed at an academic medical center used dietary supplements during pregnancy. Hollyer et al.[86] report 62% of callers to an NVP helpline used some sort of CAM. Thurer[87] reports that 36% of 136 PP women used herbs before or during pregnancy. Fugh-Berman and Kronenberg[82] reviewed 45 randomized controlled clinical trials of CAM in pregnancy. They found the most common CAM therapies used in pregnancy to be herbs, specifically ginger, peppermint, raspberry leaf, and chamomile, vitamin B-6, and acupuncture or acupressure for the treatment of NVP or hyperemesis, which are consistent with Hollyer's and Thurber's studies. Comparing CAM studies is difficult as the definition of CAM may vary. Despite this, it is clear that CAM therapies are used in pregnancy and are likely increasing.

Pregnant women seek information about CAM therapies from various sources, but usually *not* their healthcare provider. Tsui's study suggests 25% of CAM users garnered information from their physician or nurse practitioner, while Hollyer's study suggests just 8% received information from their physician or a pharmacist.[85,86] It is promising to note that more pregnant CAM users reported the use to their physicians than nonpregnant users, 59 to 70% versus 40%, respectively, despite the fact that healthcare workers seldom ask about herbal of supplement use.[83,85,87,88] Advice on the use of herbs is readily available on the Internet, and pregnant women frequently utilize the Internet for information.[83,85,87] Morris and Avorn[89] found that 76% of 443 Web sites located on the first page of search results using the five most commonly used search engines sold the herb product or had a direct link to a vendor.[89] The standard, mandatory FDA disclaimer, "This statement has not been evaluated by the Food and Drug Administration. This product is not intended to diagnose, treat, cure, or prevent any disease" was omitted on 52% of the sites. Current regulation of dietary supplements is marginally effective, placing patients at a safety risk.[89] Although as readily available, dietary supplements do not receive the premarket safety or quality control testing that over the counter medications receive. A study was conducted in which herbalists with e-mail addresses available on the Web were asked to provide advice concerning the use of three herbs in pregnancy.[90] Response rate to the 83 e-mail addresses was 51%. The results on the use of three herbs, ginger, raspberry, and juniper, were as follows: 45% of the herbalists recommended ginger, 17% recommended raspberry, and none recommended taking juniper during pregnancy. Twenty-one percent of those surveyed did not mention the potential adverse effects of ginger and 12% did not mention the adverse effects of raspberry leaf.

CAM practitioners recommending herbs and botanicals in pregnancy typically follow self-defined "usage guidelines." These guidelines are not consistent among individual practitioners.[91,92] Frequently shared principles in their guidelines include avoidance of herbs in the first trimester unless a condition exists that may be treatable with herbs, such as NVP, avoidance of internally ingested herbal volatile oils (essential oils), and avoidance of concentrated extracts. There is less agreement among practitioners as to which herbs are safe in pregnancy.[91–95] This lack of consensus is likely related to both the inconsistency and limited amount of studies in the scientific literature. There is also an overwhelming amount of lay information on herb use in pregnancy, which is also notable for numerous inconsistencies. One factor is the lack of consensus regarding this application of herbs may relate to the fact that, in the United States, herbalists are not licensed. Anyone may, with training or not, offer "expert" advice on herbs and botanicals. The American Herbalists Guild, founded in 1989, grants membership only after a five-member review committee ascertains that a candidate has a high degree of proficiency and knowledge in the use of herbs.[96] In the United States, it may be difficult to find a knowledgeable herbalist, even when the attempt is made.

The information available to lay users is generally not coming from conventional sources and often comes from the Internet. It therefore falls, to an arguable extent, to the medical practitioner to complement their medical practice with CAM information.

Herbs and botanicals have been used for centuries, which does not prove safety but it may lend legitimacy for their usefulness.[97] The current paucity of scientific research makes recommending the use of herbs and botanicals in pregnancy difficult. In fact, many conventional medical practitioners have directly recommended avoidance of herbs and botanicals in pregnancy and lactation.[82,98–100] When scientifically sound research becomes available, conventional healthcare providers will more likely accept newly established INT therapies. For now it is important to avoid being judgmental when patients share the use of dietary supplements and to offer guidance as current research allows.

Constipation is a common concern in pregnancy. Factors in its etiology include decreased bowel motility caused by increased progesterone and steroid metabolism, displacement of the intestines by the fetus, and iron supplementation.[101] CNT includes adequate fluid intake, particularly water, adequate fiber intake, especially from whole grains, fruits and vegetables, and physical activity. If iron supplementation is a suspected cause, a different iron formulation may be beneficial. CAM for constipation includes the use of bulk-producing laxatives, such as plantago seed, also known as psyllium seed. When taken with adequate fluid the seeds swell, producing bulk and lubrication. They are safe in pregnancy.[97] Stimulant herbal and botanical laxatives, such as senna, internally ingested aloe, and casarca, should not be used in pregnancy or lactation.[97] They result in overemptying of the bowel and eventual dependency. They may also cause uterine contractions, and are absorbed into the general circulation, and are known to be present in breast milk.[97,102]

Indigestion, a common problem in pregnancy, is likely secondary to stomach displacement by the enlarging uterus, slowed gastric motility, and relaxed esophageal sphincter in response to progesterone.[101] CNT includes avoidance of offending foods, beverages and known gastric irritants, eating small, frequent meals, and sitting upright immediately after eating. Calcium carbonate is commonly used as treatment with the resultant benefit of enhanced calcium intake. The use of sodium bicarbonate (baking soda) and antacids containing it should be avoided as they may lead to electrolyte imbalances.[101] Severe cases of indigestion can be safely treated with prescription antisecretory agents.[101] CAM includes mint,[97] as teas or lozenges, and meadowsweet,[103] as tea or supplement. However, meadowsweet contains salicylates indicating the need for caution in pregnancy.[101]

Gastrocnemius muscle cramping occurs when pressure from the enlarging uterus on pelvic nerves or blood vessels is increased.[101] This condition is more common as the pregnancy progresses. Previous advice to women with leg cramps was to take calcium supplements, but this approach is not supported by the literature. Young and Jewell[104] reviewed five randomized trials involving 352 women to determine which interventions were effective for pregnant women with leg cramps. The only placebo-controlled trial showed no benefit of calcium supplementation. A trial of multivitamins with minerals was effective but the reviewers stated that no conclusions could be made as to which ingredient in the combination was responsible for providing relief. The authors concluded that the best evidence for relief of leg cramps in pregnant women through INT is oral magnesium lactate or citrate. In the study, both magnesium salts reduced next-day persistence of nocturnal leg cramps when compared to control subjects. However, symptoms decreased significantly in both groups.[82]

NUTRITION-RELATED DISORDERS IN PREGNANCY

ANEMIA

Iron demands increase in pregnancy for expanded maternal blood cell mass and fetal needs, these are 500 and 300 mg, respectively, resulting in an increased requirement of 800 mg elemental iron for the duration of the pregnancy. Although iron absorption across the gut increases in pregnancy, up to 50% increased absorption in the third trimester, it is often not sufficient to compensate for the metabolic demands of pregnancy, particularly if maternal dietary intake of iron is inadequate.[105] Target hemoglobin (hgb) of ≥ 11 g/l and hematocrit (hct) levels ≥ 33 g/l are desirable throughout pregnancy.[105] A first trimester ferritin concentration >35 mcg/l suggests that iron status will be adequate throughout pregnancy.[105] Most physicians prescribe routine iron supplementation during the second and third trimesters of pregnancy. A daily PNV with 30 mg iron is sufficient for most pregnant women who are iron replete, providing they have adequate dietary intake.

Women of childbearing age may enter pregnancy with low iron stores and iron deficient anemia, <11 g/l hgb or <12 mcg/l ferritin, because of iron-poor diets or heavy menses. Anemia occurs in 8% of first trimester pregnancies, 12% of second trimester pregnancies, and 29% of third trimester pregnancies.[24] Anemic women are at increased risk for premature and LBW infants, although conflicting associations can be found in the literature.[24] Correction of anemia is recommended and can be achieved with 120 mg/day supplemental elemental iron until hgb concentrations are ≥ 11 g/l.[105] The usual choice of iron supplementation is ferrous sulfate, but other iron salts, such as gluconate, may be advised because they cause less gastric irritation. Daily dosing of iron appears more effective than weekly supplementation in treating anemia.[1,2]

Some authors have expressed concern that iron supplementation will interfere with the absorption of calcium and zinc. Taken on an empty stomach, iron supplementation may interfere with their absorption, but this does not occur when iron supplementation is taken with food.[106] Meals high in calcium, however, may interfere with iron absorption. Iron-rich and calcium-rich foods should be separated by 2 h.[1,2] Interestingly, high hgb levels may be associated with SGA, LBW, and preterm birth perhaps associated with poor maternal plasma expansion.[24]

Low vitamin A stores can also present as apparent iron-deficient anemia because vitamin A is required to mobilize iron from tissue storage sites for heme production.[106] Therefore, PNV supplements typically contain vitamin A, either as preformed vitamin A or beta-carotene. Excessive supplemented vitamin A is known to be teratogenic. Preformed vitamin A is found in most multivitamin supplements and foods, including some meats, eggs, dairy products, and fortified cereals. A 1995 study found that women who took more than 3000 mcg of vitamin A daily, nearly four times the RDA, in the first 2 months of pregnancy had more than twice the risk of birth defects such as cleft lip or palate, hydrocephalus (water on the brain), or heart defects.[107] The RDA for vitamin A in pregnancy is 750 to 770 mcg daily with a UL of 3000 mcg daily.[108] Pregnant women should avoid consuming high vitamin A foods such as beef liver, which may have as much as 9000 mcg in a 3-oz portion.[109]

NAUSEA AND VOMITING OF PREGNANCY

NVP affects 70 to 85% of pregnant women, 13% going beyond 20 weeks gestation.[110,111] Among employed pregnant women, nearly 50%[86] reported reduced work efficiency related NVP, with 25 to 66% requiring time off from work.[86,110,111] NVP appears related to changes in human chorionic gonadatropin and estrogen levels.[110,111]

CNT for NVP is to eat small, bland, low-fat meals frequently to avoid an empty stomach, consuming dry CHO foods, i.e., crackers or toast, before arising and during the night as needed, drink fluids between meals rather than with meals, and avoid caffeine. Other strategies include lighting a scented candle to mask offending or strong odors; consuming liquids in the form of ice chips; using tart, salty, or spicy beverages to increase fluid intake; keep foods that ease stomach discomfort on hand at all times such as chewing gum or hard candies; and eating foods that sound good despite the "rules."[112]

There are also several standard pharmaceutical treatments for NVP with extensive safety data.[113] Despite pharmaceutical interventions, NVP may continue. Previous drug tragedies such as with thalidomide in the 1960s and the perceived advantage of natural herbal and alternative products make CAM therapies attractive to women with NVP.

The three most common CAM therapies for NVP are vitamin B-6, ginger, and acupressure or acupuncture.[82,86,88] Vitamin B-6 acts as an essential coenzyme in the metabolism of macronutrients. Deficiency of this vitamin does not seem to be clinically related to NVP, however, vitamin B-6 in doses of 10 to 25 mg three times daily, shows some evidence for improving NVP.[82,110,113] This dosage, although much greater than the RDA of 1.9 mg/day, appears safe.[113] Investigators have tested the effects of vitamin B-6 alone. A 3-day study, randomized, double-blind, placebo-controlled trial demonstrated that pyridoxine (B-6) was effective in reducing nausea in women with NVP.[114] A 5-day study, also randomized, double-blind, placebo-controlled, provided pyridoxine at 30 mg/day to pregnant women with NVP and demonstrated a significant decrease in nausea in the women who received pyridoxine compared with the placebo group. The reduction in the number of episodes of vomiting was initially less in the pyridoxine group, but was equal in the two groups at the end of 5 days.[115]

Ginger is a commonly used spice. Fulder[116] reports it is traditionally used as a "stimulating carminative," acting to increase gastrointestinal blood flow aiding digestive function and comfort.[116] In traditional Chinese herbal medicine up to 9 g of fresh gingerroot daily is widely recommended.[85] Powdered dried ginger in a dose of 250 mg four times daily appears to be helpful in treating NVP.[82,110,116–118] No evidence of ginger toxicity or adverse effects in pregnant women has been found in the medical literature.[116] Further, the use of ginger was found to be useful and not teratogenic by the conclusions of a 2002 Cochrane Review, which examined ginger and other treatments for NVP.[85]

Despite the research findings thus far regarding the use of ginger for NVP, the German Commission E lists ginger as contraindicated in pregnancy[119] (see Table 3.4 for the Commission's list of contraindicated herbs). The basis of the Commission's decision was studies demonstrating mutagenicity using extremely large doses of purified ginger extracts. The dose and other aspects of the scientific methodology were problematic and led others to question the validity of the studies. In contrast to the mutagenic properties in the isolated in ginger extract, used in the aforementioned study, whole ginger contains powerful antimutigenetic fractions.[116] Especially critical of the results of these studies, the European–American

TABLE 3.4
Herbs Contraindicated in Pregnancy

Aloe	Comfrey root	Mayapple root, resin
Autumn crocus	*Echinacea angustifolia*, herb, root	Mugwort
Basil oil		Nutmeg
Black cohosh root	*Echinacea purpurea*, herb (injectable)	Pallida herb
Bryomia root		Parsley herb, seed, oil, root
Buckthorn bark	Fennel oil	Pasque flower
Buckthorn berry	Fennel seed	Petasites root
California poppy	Gingerroot	Rhubarb root
Cascara sagrada bark	Indian snakeroot	Rue
Chaste tree fruit	Juniper berry	Saffron
Cinchona bark	Kava kava	Sage leaf
Cinnamon bark, flower	Licorice root	Senna leaf
Coltsfoot leaf	Liverwort herb	Tansy flower, herb
Comfrey herb, leaf	Marsh tea	Uva ursi leaf

Source: From The American Botanical Council, *The Complete German Commission E Monographs, Therapeutic Guide to Herbal Medicines,* Blumenthal, M. et al., Eds., American Botanical Council, Austin, 1998.

Phytomedicine Coalition filed a citizen's petition with the FDA for ginger to be reviewed as an over the counter (OTC) medication for NVP.[119]

Research on the use of ginger for NVP is ongoing and a comprehensive work is underway, as ginger is included among 21 botanicals for monograph development by the U.S. Pharmacopeia (USP).[120] One recent study by Portnoi et al.[117] concludes that ginger is not associated with rates of malformations above the expected baseline of 1 to 3% and has a mild beneficial effect in treatment of NVP.[117] To achieve maximum benefit, ginger may need to be taken for several days. Vutyavanich et al.[121] demonstrated that it might have a cumulative effect as women taking ginger had better outcomes after taking it for 3 to 4 days. The study showed significant differences in both nausea scores and vomiting episodes between the treatment group and the placebo group. Only minor adverse events were reported, e.g., headache, abdominal discomfort, heartburn, and diarrhea for 1 day, none of which kept the participants from taking the study "medication." Additionally, the study showed no adverse effects on pregnancy outcome.

Ginger, as tea and in other forms, has long been promoted as a tonic for generalized nausea and vomiting. Its effect on NVP has been demonstrated in at least two small trials in which both nausea and vomiting decreased significantly compared to women receiving a placebo.[122,123] An animal study by Wilkinson[123] used a research protocol that closely mimicked the quantity of ginger tea that a human would consume to alleviate symptoms of nausea. One of the two concentrations of ginger tea, 20 and 50 g/l of water, was provided to pregnant laboratory rats. Embryonic loss (reabsorption of fetal tissue) in the ginger tea group was double that of control animals. This study needs replication, but until further research is conducted, it seems prudent to advise against the use of ginger as a tea in NVP. However, the use of powdered dried ginger in a dose of 250 mg four times daily is supported by numerous trials and there is no evidence of toxicity or serious adverse events in the medical literature. Despite its popular use and mostly positive study results to date, there is a lack of consensus regarding the use of ginger during pregnancy. Those wishing to use ginger should be informed of this status and should only do so with medical supervision.

Acupressure and acupuncture are other CAM therapies commonly used in treating NVP. Fugh-Berman and Kronenberg[82] report "acupuncture point stimulation for NVP should be considered a proven treatment." The technique places pressure at acupuncture point P6, variously known as pericardium 6 or Neiguan acupuncture point, on the volar aspect of the wrist.[111,113] In the review, 10 of 14 studies found significant benefit using acupuncture and acupressure at P6. This technique has been demonstrated to be safe in alleviating NVP.[82,98] Rosen et al.[111] evaluated the effectiveness of acustimulation, or noninvasive electrical stimulation, at P6, in treating NVP. Their study showed a significant reduction in nausea and vomiting and significantly greater weight gain in the study group versus the control group.[111]

HYPEREMESIS GRAVIDARUM

In hyperemesis gravidarum (HG), severe vomiting during pregnancy appearing before 20 weeks gestation and with such severity as to typically require hospitalization, CNT and CAM therapies offer little or no benefit. HG occurs in 0.5 to 3% of pregnancies and can lead to significant weight loss, dehydration, loss of electrolytes, and ketosis.[86,113,124] HG is thought to be multifactorial with hormonal changes, gastrointestinal dysmotility, and possibly *Heliobacter pylori* infection all contributing factors.[125] HG may require intravenous (IV) rehydration with replacement electrolytes. If symptoms persist, hospitalization may be required with the provision of enteral or parenteral nutrition therapy.[124] A number of case studies have reported thiamin deficiency in pregnant women with HG.[126,127] These cases report serious complications of Wernicke's encephalopathy and maternal visual loss. As a precautionary measure, all women with HG should receive thiamin supplementation.[127] Women who are admitted to the hospital for IV rehydration should also receive IV vitamins, a practice that was not undertaken in any of the reported cases. Erick[113] provides a useful management algorithm for NVP. There is resurgence in interest in using hypnosis, including self-hypnosis, as a treatment for HG.[128] A trial including 138 women with HG resulted in 88% of them having resolution of vomiting after one to two sessions of hypnosis.[129] Since this form of therapy has little risk and a potential for benefit, it is an approach worthy of trial.

INT offers several treatment options to women with NVP. Most appear to be safe, although future studies and trials should be undertaken to provide additional efficacy, safety, and outcome data. Alleviating NVP will improve maternal and fetal nutritional status simply by allowing for consumption of an adequate, normal diet.

HYPERTENSION IN PREGNANCY

HTN is the most common medical disorder in pregnancy,[130] occurring in 5 to 8% of pregnancies and accounting for 15% of all preterm births.[27] A number of hypertensive disorders can occur in pregnancy. These can generally be defined as a blood pressure $\geq 140/90$. Infants born to women with HTN during pregnancy have a fivefold increased risk of morbidity and mortality, and tend to be SGA.[27]

Chronic HTN exists before the pregnancy. Pregnancy-induced HTN (PIH) describes a wide spectrum of hypertensive disorders in pregnancy. Preeclampsia is the most common PIH syndrome. Incidence reports vary from 2 to 7% in nulliparous women[130] to 8 to 10% of primiparous women.[131] It occurs more often in twin gestations (14%) and when there is a history of preeclampsia in a previous pregnancy (18%).[130] Preeclampsia is characterized by HTN and proteinuria of ≥ 0.3 g protein in a 24-h urine specimen. Eclampsia is the severest form of PIH and is characterized by preeclampsia with seizures that may progress to coma. Despite decades of research the exact cause, or causes, of preeclampsia and eclampsia remains elusive.

A number of nutritional interventions have been tested as potential treatments or preventative regimes for PIH. Trials have been conducted using supplemental magnesium, zinc, iron, folic acid, balanced energy and protein, and restricted energy and protein to limit weight gain in obese pregnant women. None of these interventions were preventative or have demonstrated improvement in HTN treatment.[1,2] Additionally, sodium restriction is not effective in treating or preventing HTN or preeclampsia, or chronic HTN in pregnancy, except in those few women with documented sodium-sensitive HTN.[1,2] Sodium restriction also did not significantly change caesarean section (C/S) rates.[1,2] Many studies have shown that excessive sodium restriction may be deleterious in pregnancy but it remains, however, a relatively common practice.[1,2] Calcium supplementation reduced the incidence of HTN and preeclampsia in women with low calcium intakes and in those at increased risk for HTN in pregnancy, but no benefit was seen in women with adequate calcium intake.[1,2] Calcium reduced C/S rates in women with an increased risk of HTN.[1,2] Omega-3 FA, particularly those in fatty fishes, demonstrated a protective effect against HTN and preeclampsia in several epidemiological studies.[1,2] In a small study, Chappell et al.[132] found vitamins C and E were effective at reducing preeclampsia in women at risk for the condition. These findings are intriguing and larger trials would be beneficial.

DIABETES

Diabetes occurs in 3 to 5% of all pregnancies.[21] Gestational diabetes mellitus (GDM) is defined as "carbohydrate intolerance of variable severity with onset or first recognition during pregnancy." The name GDM applies whether or not insulin is used as treatment and whether or not preexisting diabetes is suspected, but not diagnosed. GDM is the most common form of diabetes in pregnancy, affecting 3 to 4% of all pregnancies, accounting for ~90% of all diabetes cases in pregnancy. GDM occurs in higher proportions of pregnancies in high-risk populations, including Asian, Black, Hispanic, and Native Americans, and in women with a history of GDM.[21] The incidence of GDM is highest in the Pima Indians of Arizona where it is nearly 40%.[133] GDM should be reclassified PP. Their risk for developing overt diabetes in the 5 to 16 years following a gestational diabetic pregnancy is 17 to 63%.[134]

CNT for diabetes in pregnancy, whether preexisting or gestational, relies primarily on limiting CHO content of the diet, to approximately 35 to 40% of total calories, with emphasis on whole grains, vegetables, and low fat or nonfat dairy products. CHO and energy are distributed in three meals and two to three snacks, less in the morning than later in the day.[133,135] Energy needs are based on pregravida weight.[135,136] Energy, vitamin, and mineral needs do not differ from usual recommended amounts in pregnancy. Nonnutritive sweeteners, including all those approved by the FDA, saccharin, aspartame, acesulfame potassium, and sucralose, are safe in pregnancy and can be used to reduce CHO intake.[136] Patients should receive individual nutrition therapy counseling by a registered dietitian, ideally one with a specialty in diabetes.

Studies have shown that chromium may be helpful in managing glucose levels in diabetes. Jovanovic[137] and Trail[138] reported at an April 2003 symposium, "Chromium in Health and Disease" on studies they had completed on chromium supplementation in pregnancy. Jovanovic[137] reported significantly lower glucose levels in GDM after 8 weeks of treatment with chromium picolinate versus placebo in a control group. Trail[138] reported the possible benefit of chromium picolinate supplementation in reducing the risk of progressing from glucose intolerance to GDM. Chromium picolinate has shown no toxicological basis for setting tolerable upper limits. Additional research is needed before specific recommendations can be made. No references were found specific to herbal use in pregnancies complicated by diabetes.

INFECTION AND PREGNANCY

Pregnant women have an increased risk of UTIs compared to nonpregnant women. Complications of UTIs in pregnancy include premature delivery and increased fetal mortality. The conventional approach for prevention of recurrent infections in pregnant women is long-term suppression with continuous low-dose antibiotics throughout pregnancy. With the high rate of antibiotic-resistant stains of uropathogenic bacteria that often occurs, continuous low-dose suppression may further promote resistant organisms, leading to treatment failures and an increased risk of pyelonephritis. A CAM approach with significantly less risk is the daily consumption of cranberry juice.[139]

Howell and Foxman[140] obtained uropathogenic E. coli isolates from 39 nonpregnant women both before and after the women drank 240 cc cranberry juice cocktail. The bacterial isolates were incubated, harvested, and tested for their ability to adhere to uroepithelial cells, the mechanism whereby they cause infection. The pathogenic bacteria from collections before cranberry juice consumption were able to adhere in all of the uroepithelial cell samples. Adhesion was prevented in 80% of the cell samples from the urine that was collected following cranberry juice ingestion. This group included 79% of the 24 antibiotic-resistant isolates. The additional calories from 240 cc cranberry juice need to be considered, particularly in the pregnant woman with overweight/obesity issues or diabetes. The National Center for Complementary and Alternative Medicines (NCCAM) is currently funding studies investigating the use of cranberry extract in prevention and treatment of UTIs. Cranberry extract would avoid the potential problem of the excess energy and CHO intake from cranberry juice. Echinacea, one of the ten most commonly used herbs,[141] was recently reported in pregnant women by Leigh.[142] Echinacea is considered an immunostimulant, particularly related to upper respiratory infections.[141] The study was the first controlled prospective study of echinacea in pregnancy. The use of echinacea was not associated with increased risk of birth defects. Researchers studied women who had contacted a teratogen information service with question about the safety of echinacea in pregnancy. Of the 412 women surveyed, 206 had taken echinacea, whereas 206 opted not to take it. The two groups were matched for age, alcohol use, cigarette use, and presence of upper respiratory infections during pregnancy. Fifty-four percent of the echinacea group took the herb during the first trimester, 8% took it throughout the pregnancy. There were six major and six minor malformations in the echinacea group and seven major and seven minor malformations in the control group. Of the malformations in the herb group, four major and two minor occurred in women taking the herb in the first trimester. No significant differences were found in delivery method, maternal weight gain, infant birth weight, gestational age, or fetal distress.

One finding not addressed in Leigh's report was their report of nearly twice as many spontaneous abortions in the echinacea group ($n = 13$) than in the control group ($n = 7$). The authors did not discuss the significance of this finding. They conclude "gestational use of echinacea during organogenesis is not associated with an increased risk for major malformations."[142] Additional studies are necessary to establish safety of echinacea in pregnancy.

PRETERM DELIVERY

Preterm delivery, delivery between 20 and 37 weeks gestation, is the number one cause of neonatal mortality.[27] Despite decades of research, preventing premature delivery remains elusive.[143] Its rate is increasing, with 11.9% preterm births in 2000 compared to 9.4% in 1994. Calcium supplementation produces a statistically nonsignificant reduction in preterm delivery.[1,2] In several studies when magnesium was supplemented before 25 weeks gestation, there was a statistically significant reduction in preterm delivery. However, the methodologies of the studies are problematic. In the larger trials and those with stronger scientific merit, there was less of a protective effect seen.[1,2] In three studies, zinc supplementation had an overall protective effect against preterm birth.[1,2] Observational studies suggest omega-3 FA offer a protective benefit against preterm delivery. Of the several studies completed on omega-3 FA supplementation in pregnancy, the overall results are promising, but not definitive. One large study of 5000 participants using fish oil supplementation reported a 20% reduction in preterm delivery, but the trial used alternate treatment allocation and did not blind outcome measurements. Two well-designed studies found no effect of fish oil supplementation on preterm delivery, but the results may have been influenced by the small sample size. Although no complete studies have demonstrated it, theoretically omega-3 FA could increase the risk of hemorrhage as a side effect of their action.[1,2] Reports of increased incidence of hemorrhage in pregnancy are not found in areas where relatively large amounts of omega-3 FA intake are common.

OBSTRUCTED LABOR AND CESAREAN SECTION

Obstructed labor, or failure to progress, is a major complication of delivery.[1,2] It often leads to C/S. C/Ss occur in 21% of pregnancies and are rising. Trials of magnesium and balanced energy and protein supplementation did not affect length of labor. Iron and folic acid supplementation had mixed results in relation to obstructed labor or C/S rates. In three studies, zinc provided a significant reduction in C/S rate.[1,2]

A variety of CAM approaches have been used to facilitate labor and delivery. Medical hypnosis may be the most effective. Martin et al.[144] conducted a randomized trial of pregnant adolescents followed at a county public health department. The intervention group was taught self-hypnosis in addition to receiving prenatal care; the control group received routine prenatal care only. The self-hypnosis group had a significant decrease in lengths of hospital stay, surgical interventions, and birth complications. There was also less anesthesia, Pitocin, and PP medications used in the hypnosis group, although these reductions did not reach statistical significance.[144]

A retrospective, observational study of 108 women reported that 52.8% consumed red raspberry leaf, as an aid to shorten the duration of labor with no major side effects to mothers or infants.[145] These same investigators performed a randomized, double-blind, placebo-controlled trial with 192 women to test the effectiveness of using raspberry leaf from 32 weeks gestation to term to shortening the duration of labor.[146] The second stage of labor was significantly shortened by 9.59 min and there was a significant reduction in the use of forceps in the women who consumed the raspberry leaf during pregnancy.

Other popular CAM approaches are castor oil, perineal massage, and aromatherapy. A prospective trial using castor oil to augment the onset of labor in full-term pregnancies demonstrated a significant difference in the number of women whose labor began within 24 h compared to the women in the group who did not receive castor oil.[147] A survey of women who received perineal massage during pregnancy to augment delivery reported a high degree of satisfaction with this technique.[148] A prospective study of more than 8,000 mothers who delivered at a large British teaching hospital from 1990 to 1998 and received aromatherapy were compared to more than 15,000 mothers, who delivered at the same hospital without aromatherapy.[149] Following the introduction of aromatherapy to the maternity ward, there was a significant decrease in the use of pain medications from 6 to 0.2%.

McFarlin et al.[150] surveyed 500 Certified Nurse-Midwives (CNM) regarding their herbal use to stimulate labor and cervical ripening.[150] Of those who responded, 52% used herbs for this purpose. CNMs who used herbs to induce labor were more likely to deliver in a birthing center or at home. The most commonly cited rationale for herb use in this study was that herbs are "safe and natural." Other reasons for herb use included restricted use of Pitocin or prostaglandins in some of the birthing areas and lower cost of herbs compared to conventional treatments. It is ironic that this healthcare practice group is using herbs and botanicals, which are not inspected to insure safety, purity, effectiveness, or quality of labeled components, with somewhat regularity, while those medications with extensive testing are used less, by choice or mandate. McFarlin's study indicates that a majority of CNMs did not receive formal training in use of herbs and botanicals.

In McFarlin's study, the most common herbs used for labor stimulation and cervical ripening were castor oil (90%), blue cohosh (64%), red raspberry leaf (63%), evening primrose oil (60%), and black cohosh (45%). In subjective grading, the CNMs felt castor oil was the most effective for labor stimulation and evening primrose oil was most effective for cervical ripening.

Adverse events related to herbal use were reported in this study. Twenty-one percent of the CNMs reported complications when herbal products were used to stimulate labor. The complications included precipitous labor, tetanic uterine contractions, nausea, vomiting, and diarrhea, meconium-stained fluid, which is a sign of asphyxial insult to the fetus and thrombosed hemorrhoids.[101]

There are reports that active constituents in blue cohosh, used in labor, resulted in cardiac disturbances, including myocardial infarction, congestive heart failure, and cardiovascular shock in one infant and seizures, kidney damage, and the need for mechanical ventilation in another infant.[100] Castor oil use was related to significantly more cases of meconium passage than controls.[100] A letter reporting severe neonatal hypoxia with neurological impairment following the use of black and blue cohosh at a home delivery has been reported.[119] German Commission E lists black cohosh as contraindicated in pregnancy, but does not address blue cohosh. Its relationship to the development of neonatal hypoxia, however, is not clear.

FETAL WEIGHT STATUS

Studies have examined nutritional interventions to improve fetal weight status. In separate studies, CNT as balanced maternal energy and protein supplementation and maternal magnesium supplementation each resulted in 30% reductions in SGA infants.[1,3] Calcium appears to reduce LBW by prolonging the gestational period. In contrast, high protein supplementation in women without evidence of protein deficiency resulted in increased rates of SGA and neonatal death.[1,3] A restriction of maternal energy and protein in obese pregnant women reduced fetal growth. Zinc supplementation did not affect birth weight, but was associated with increased long bone growth as measured by fetal ultrasonography.[1,2]

POSTPARTUM/LACTATION NUTRITION

Nutritional requirements for lactation and pregnancy are similar. The RDA for energy during lactation is an additional 340 kcal/day for the first 6 months and an additional 400 kcal/day for the second 6 months.[40] Less energy is required in the first 6 months because of readily available energy from maternal adipose tissue stores providing ~170 kcal/day. (The total energy requirement in the first 6 months is ~500 kcal/day.) In the second 6 months of lactation, maternal fat stores make little or no contribution to the energy requirements of lactation.[40] The IOM did not make recommendations for energy needs beyond 12 months lactation.

Vitamin K is provided routinely by injection for infants born in a hospital setting in the United States. This may not occur in home-born infants. Those infants who do not receive vitamin K and who are breast-fed are at high risk for bleeding.[151]

Under specific circumstances vitamin D supplementation may be desirable for breast-fed infants. Although there is evidence that limited sunlight exposure prevents rickets in many breast-fed infants, in light of growing concerns about sunlight and skin cancer and the various factors such as skin color and culturally sensitive clothing that negatively affect sunlight exposure, the American Academy of Pediatrics recommends that all breast-fed infants be given supplemental vitamin D.[152] This recommendation has been met with some controversy as the recommendations for all infants are based on a subset of lactating women who may not provide adequate vitamin D in their breast milk. Case reports describe several children who developed vitamin D deficiency, infantile rickets, or seizures whose mothers fit these characteristics.[153] Additional research is needed to more fully understand the factors underlying the development of vitamin D deficiency and rickets in some breast-fed infants.

With few exceptions, lactation is beneficial to both mother and infant. Breast milk is the ideal food for the human infant and many medical professionals believe it can be the exclusive food for the infants for first 6 months of life.[154] Kramer and Kakuma[154] reviewed 2668 citations of which 20 independent studies were thoroughly investigated to determine the benefits or risks of 6 months or more of exclusive breast-feeding. They concluded that breast-feeding for 6 months or more reduced the risk of gastrointestinal infections and promoted normal growth. The American Academy of Pediatrics[152] recommends breast-feeding as the optimal mode of feeding for the infant's first year. Achieving this duration of lactation is desirable for the mother as well as it is associated with a decreased risk of premenopausal breast cancer.[155]

Women with a history of lactation also have reduced risks for ovarian cancer, decreased PP blood loss, and increased fat mass loss.[156] Benefits to the infant include reduced incidence and severity of infection, asthma and allergies, and enhanced cognitive development.[156] Adolescents who were breast-fed had better lipid profiles compared to adolescents who were formula fed.[157]

Lactation should be avoided in women taking immunosuppressive and mutagenic drugs, such as cyclosporine or methotrexate.[158] Women who are exposed to radioactive compounds during diagnostic testing should refrain from breast-feeding for several days to weeks. Those receiving radioactive iodine for thyroid cancer are advised to permanently stop breast-feeding (consult Ref.[158] for a complete list of drugs and their effect on lactation).

Lactation should also be avoided in women who are HIV-positive. It is estimated that 30 to 40% of maternal-to-child transmission of the HIV infections are through maternal milk although with the advice to HIV-positive mothers not to breast-feed, the rate of transmission of HIV in the PP setting is declining.[159]

There is no scientific evidence that alcoholic beverages benefit breast-feeding, despite cultural beliefs. However, evidence suggests that alcohol in moderate amounts, 0.5 g alcohol/kg/day, equal to ~2.5 oz liquor, 8 oz of wine, or 24 oz of beer, is not harmful to the breast-fed infant.[160] The lactating woman can express breast milk before alcohol intake, then avoid breast-feeding, using the previously expressed milk as needed, for several hours until the alcohol has been eliminated from her body.[161] Clearance time to alcohol-free breast milk varies among individuals. Toddlers whose mothers were "moderate" alcohol drinkers while breast-feeding their infants demonstrated slight but significant impairment on developmental scales.[162] Deficits increased with increasing quantities of alcohol.

The use of pharmacological galactogogues (breast milk stimulators), such as metoclopramide (or Reglan) and domperidone (or Motillium), is not common in the United States.[163]

Breast milk stimulation is a secondary effect of each of the medications. Reglan is readily available in the United States, while Motillium is not. The American Academy of Pediatrics had approved Motillium for use in pregnancy; however, in June 2004 the FDA issued a warning of potential safety concerns and serious adverse effects associated with the use of domperidone to increase lactation.[164]

CAM therapies during lactation are not well documented in the medical literature. Fenugreek is the most commonly used herbal galactogogue.[163,165] Its mechanism of action is not well known.[163] Fenugreek is available as a tea or in capsules, with the capsules being the most effective. A dose of 1000 to 2000 mg three times daily, with a maximum dose of 6000 mg/day, is suggested.[166] It may cause a maple-like odor to maternal sweat and urine, and may increase glucose levels. It is therefore not an appropriate choice for mothers with diabetes. Fenugreek is related to peanuts, so should be avoided if a family history of peanut allergy exists. Fenugreek should not be used in pregnancy, as it is a uterine stimulant. Other herbs suggested as beneficial and safe in lactation include thistle, brewer's yeast, goat's rue, European vervian, fennel, and chaste berries.[94,163,166] Sage and jasmine flowers are historically used as lactation suppressants.[167,168]

POSTPARTUM MOOD DISORDERS

Three types of PP mood disorders are recognized.[169] The first, "baby blues," affects 75 to 85% of primigravidas, beginning 3 days PP and lasting up to 14 days. PP depression (PPD) lasts beyond 2 weeks, is more intense, and affects 10% of primigravidas. The third is psychosis, which affects 1 in 1000 women and is characterized by hallucinations.[169] CAM therapy includes extracts from St John's Wort.[170] Lee et al.[171] studied 30 lactating women taking different strengths of St John's Wort for PPD.[171] Compared to controls, no differences were detected in reported milk supply, infant development, or weight gain in their first year. Adverse infant events were higher, but they were mild and not statistically significant. In a case report a breast-feeding woman was taking St John's Wort three times daily for PPD.[170] Both active components of St John's Wort, hyperforin and hypericin, were excreted in minimal amounts and were undetected in infant plasma. Neither developmental delays nor adverse events were reported in the infant. Both studies suggest that St John's Wort may be safe to treat PPD in lactating women, but the authors are cautious to recommend it without long-term studies of infant outcome.

SUMMARY

Some CAM therapies in pregnancy appear to be safe and beneficial. Fugh-Berman and Kronenberg recommend acupressure or acupuncture point stimulation for NVP. They also suggest that magnesium supplementation decreases leg cramps, and is benign. Several studies on the use of ginger and vitamin B-6 to treat NVP are promising. Table 3.5 lists commonly used herbs and suggested uses in pregnancy. Several scientific studies are currently in progress, examining the use of nutritional interventions in pregnancy (see Web site review).

CONCLUSION

The combination of conventional and CAM therapy will continue to be a part of contemporary medicine. There is a great deal of benefit to be gained for both the public and professionals who serve them by learning about the safe integration of these modalities. In obstetrics where the practitioner has two patients, the mother and fetus, this is particularly

TABLE 3.5
Ten Commonly Used Herbs[1] and Reported Safety Issues in Pregnancy or Lactation

Herb	Action	Safe in Pregnancy
Echinacea	Immunostimulant,[2] prevent or treat upper respiratory infection (URI)[1]	Thought to be safe in pregnancy[3,4] except with ragweed or chrysanthemum allergy
St. John's Wort	Anti-depressant for mild to moderate depression,[1,2] nervousness, sleep disturbances[2]	In lactation only with consultation with physician[4] No data specific to pregnancy[5, p. 318]
Gingko Biloba	Dementia,[1] memory loss[6]	No human data for use in pregnancy or lactation[5, p. 211]
Garlic	Hypercholesterolemia, HTN, atherosclerosis[1,2]	No information specific to pregnancy found
Saw Palmetto	Benign Prostate Hyperplasia[1-7]	Not studied, not marketed for pregnancy or lactating women[5 p. 329]
Panax Ginseng	Adaptogenic-stimulating or sedating depending on body's need[6]	Safety not established in pregnancy and lactation[5 p. 74, 85]
Goldenseal	Common cold, URI	Do not use in pregnancy or lactation[1-7]
Aloe	Orally as laxative	Avoid in pregnancy and lactation[2,7]
Siberian Ginseng	See panax ginseng above	Safety unknown in pregnancy and lactation[5 p. 335]
Valerian	Anxiety and sleep disorders[2]	Do not use in pregnancy or lactation,[5 p. 357-358] FDA lists as GRAS (generally regarded as safe) herb[6 p. 210]

1. Garrard, J. et al., Variations in product choices of frequently purchased herbs, *Arch. Intern. Med.*, 163, 2290, 2003.
2. Tyler, V.E., *Herbs of Choice the Therapeutic Use of Phytomedicinals*, Pharmaceutical Products Press, New York, 1994.
3. Leigh, E., First study on safety of echinacea during pregnancy, *HerbalGram*, 51, 21, 2001.
4. Lawrence, R.A., *Herbs and Breastfeeding*, available at www.breastfeeding.com, accessed January 20, 2004.
5. Rotblatt, M. and Ziment, I., *Evidence Based Herbal Medicine*, Hanley and Belfus, Philadelphia, 2002.
6. Miller, L.G., and Murray, W.J., Eds, *Herbal Medicinals*, Pharmaceutical Products Press, New York, 1998.
7. Hardy, M.L., Women's health series: herbs of special interest to women, *J. Am. Pharm. Assoc.*, 40, 234, 2000.

important. There is promise for integration, if studies such as those using hypnosis to decrease NVP, can be expanded and put into routine clinical practice. It is clear that the popularity of dietary supplements, particularly herbs and botanicals, is rapidly growing in the United States. With women of reproductive age as the largest users of CAM, it is likely that use of herbs and botanicals will grow during pregnancy and lactation also.

INT is a growing field. It offers hope for many new treatment options for promoting and maintaining successful pregnancy and lactation. There is a vast amount of information available related to CAM, but little is specific to pregnancy or lactation and much of it is not scientifically based. Consensus on particular treatments is lacking. Despite historical and anecdotal usefulness of herbs and botanical products, more research, particularly randomized, controlled studies, is needed before definitive recommendations can be determined regarding the efficacy and safety of CAM therapies in pregnancy and lactation.

GLOSSARY

Adequate intake (AI): The recommended average daily intake level based on observed or experimentally determined approximations or estimates of nutrient intake by a group of apparently healthy people that are assumed to be adequate — used when an RDA cannot be determined.

Estimated average requirement (EAR): The average daily nutrient intake level estimated to meet the requirement of half the healthy individuals in a particular life stage and gender group.

Gestational diabetes mellitus (GDM): Diabetes that is first diagnosed during pregnancy.

Low birth weight (LBW): Any neonate, regardless of gestational age, with a birth weight <2500 g.

Neural tube defect (NTD): Congenital anomaly with incomplete closure of the spine.

Phytochemical: The active health-protecting compounds that are found as components of plants.

Preeclampsia: A condition in pregnancy with proteinuria and hypertension (HTN).

Postpartum (PP): After delivery.

Primigravida: A woman who is pregnant for the first time.

Recommended dietary allowance (RDA): The average daily dietary nutrient intake level sufficient to meet the nutrient requirement of nearly all (97 to 98%) healthy individuals in a particular life stage and gender group.

Small for gestational age (SGA): Birth weight <10 percentile for gestational age.

Teratogen: A drug or other agent that causes abnormal prenatal development.

REFERENCES

1. Villar, J. et al., Nutritional interventions during pregnancy for the prevention or treatment of maternal morbidity and preterm delivery: an overview of randomized controlled trials, *Am. Soc. Nutr. Sci.*, 133, 1606S, 2003.
2. Villar, J. et al., Characteristics of randomized controlled trials included in systematic reviews of nutritional interventions reporting maternal morbidity, mortality, preterm delivery, intrauterine growth restriction and small for gestational age and birth weight outcomes, *Am. Soc. Nutr. Sci.*, 133, 1632S, 2003.
3. Merialdi, M. et al., Nutritional interventions during pregnancy for the prevention or treatment of impaired fetal growth: an overview of randomized controlled trials, *Am. Soc. Nutr. Sci.*, 133, 1626S, 2003.
4. Martin, J.A. et al., Births: final data for 2000, *National Vital Statistics Reports*, 50, 1, 2002.
5. Flegal, K.M. et al., Prevalence and trends in obesity among US adults, 1999–2000, *JAMA*, 288, 1723, 2002.
6. Herrick, K. et al., Maternal consumption of a high-meat, low-carbohydrate diet in late pregnancy: relation to adult cortisol concentrations in the offspring, *J. Clin. Endocrinol. Metab.*, 88, 3554, 2003.
7. Godfrey, K.M. and Barker, D.J.P., Fetal nutrition and disease, *Am. J. Clin. Nutr.*, 71 (Suppl.), 1344S, 2000.
8. Looker, A.C. et al., Prevalence of iron deficiency in the United States, *JAMA*, 277, 973, 1997.
9. Fleming, A., The role of folate in the prevention of neural tube defects: human and animal studies, *Nutr. Rev.*, 59, S13, 2001.
10. Lumley, J. et al., Periconceptional supplementation with folate and/or multivitamins for preventing neural tube defects, *Cochrane Database Syst. Rev.*, DC001056, 2001.
11. Mathews, T.J., Honein, M.A., and Erickson, J.D., Spina bifida and anencephaly prevalence — United States, 1991–2001, *MMWR Recomm. Rep.*, 51, 9, 2002.
12. Hobb, C.A. et al., Polymorphisms in genes involved in folate metabolism as maternal risk factors for Down syndrome, *Am. J. Hum. Genet.*, 67, 623, 2000.
13. O'Leary, V.B. et al., MTRR and MTHFR polymorphism: link to Down syndrome? *Am. J. Med. Genet.*, 107, 151, 2002.

14. Hine, R.J. and James, S.J., Down syndrome and folic acid update, *J. Am. Diet. Assoc.*, 100, 1004, 2000.
15. Afman, L.A. et al., Reduced vitamin B 12 binding by transcobalamin II increases the risk of neural tube defects, *Q. J. Med.*, 94, 159, 2001.
16. Kirke, P.N. et al., Maternal plasma folate and vitamin B 12 are independent risk factors for neural tube defects, *Q. J. Med.*, 86, 703, 1993.
17. Erick, M., Eating disorders: a few more thoughts, *J. Am. Diet. Assoc.*, 102, 477, 2002.
18. Franko, D.L. et al., Pregnancy complications and neonatal outcomes in women with eating disorders, *Am. J. Psychiatry*, 158, 1461, 2001.
19. Peet, M. et al., Depletion of omega-3 fatty acid levels in red blood cell membranes of depressive patients, *Bio. Psychiatry*, 43, 315, 1998.
20. Engelgau, M.M. et al., The epidemiology of diabetes and pregnancy in the U.S., 1988, *Diabetes Care*, 18, 1029, 1995.
21. Gabbe, S.G. and Graves, C.R., Management of diabetes mellitus complicating pregnancy, *Obstet. Gynecol.*, 102, 857, 2003.
22. Kitmiller, J.L. et al., Preconception care of diabetes, congenital malformations, and spontaneous abortions (Technical Review), *Diabetes Care*, 19, 514, 1996.
23. Towner, D. et al., Congenital malformations in pregnancies complicated by NIDDM, *Diabetes Care*, 18, 1446, 1995.
24. Scanlon, K.S. et al., High and low hemoglobin levels during pregnancy: differential risks for preterm birth and small for gestational age, *Obstet. Gynecol.*, 96, 741, 2000.
25. Position Statement, American Diabetes Association, Preconception care of women with diabetes, *Diabetes Care*, 25, S50, 2002.
26. Position Statement, American Diabetes Association, Evidence-based nutrition principles and recommendation for the treatment and prevention of diabetes and related complications, *Diabetes Care*, 25, S82, 2002.
27. Goldenberg, R.L. and Rouse, D.J., Prevention of premature birth, *N. Engl. J. Med.*, 339, 313, 1998.
28. Sacks, F.M. et al., Effects on blood pressure of reduced dietary sodium and the Dietary Approaches to Stop Hypertension (DASH) diet, DASH-Sodium Collaborative Research Group, *N. Engl. J. Med.*, 344, 3, 2001.
29. Hedley, A.A. et al., Prevalence of overweight and obesity among US children, adolescents, and adults, 1999–2002, *JAMA*, 291, 2847, 2004.
30. Sebire, N.J. et al., Maternal obesity and pregnancy outcome: a study of 287,213 pregnancies in London, *Int. J. Obes. Relat. Metab. Disord.*, 25, 1175, 2001.
31. Strauss, R.S., Bradley, L.J., and Brolin, R.E., Gastric bypass surgery in adolescents with morbid obesity, *J. Pediatr.*, 138, 499, 2001.
32. Weiss, H.G. et al., Pregnancies after adjustable gastric banding, *Obes. Surg.*, 11, 3003, 2001.
33. Shiell, A.W. et al., High meat low-carbohydrate diet in pregnancy: relation to adult blood pressure in the offspring, *Hypertension*, 38, 1282, 2001.
34. Foster, G.D. et al., A randomized trial of a low-carbohydrate diet for obesity, *N. Engl. J. Med.*, 348, 2082, 2003.
35. Brehm, B.J. et al., A randomized trial comparing a very low carbohydrate diet and a calorie-restricted low fat diet on body weight and cardiovascular risk factors in healthy women, *J. Clin. Endocrinol. Metab.*, 88, 1617, 2003.
36. Stern, L. et al., The effects of low-carbohydrate versus conventional weight loss diets in severely obese adults: one-year follow-up of a randomized trial, *Ann. Int. Med.*, 140, 778, 2004.
37. Institute of Medicine, *Nutrition During Pregnancy*, National Academy Press, Washington. D.C., 1990.
38. Ladipo, O.A., Nutrition in pregnancy: mineral and vitamin supplements, *Am. J. Clin. Nutr.*, 72 (Suppl.), 280S, 2000.
39. Olshan, A.F. et al., Maternal vitamin use and reduced risk of neuroblastoma, *Epidemiology*, 13, 575, 2002.
40. Institute of Medicine, Food and Nutrition Board, Energy in *Dietary Reference Intakes for Energy, Carbohydrates, Fiber, Fat, Protein and Amino Acids (Macronutrients)*, IOM, National Academy Press, Washington, D.C., 2002, chap. 5.

41. Cunningham, F.G., Ed., *Williams Obstetrics*, 21st ed., McGraw-Hill, New York, 2001, available at www.online.statref.com, accessed July 9, 2004.

42. Rooney, B.D. and Schauberger, C.W., Excess pregnancy weight gain and long-term obesity: one decade later, *Obstet. Gynecol.*, 100, 245, 2002.

43. Linne, Y. et al., Long term weight development in women: a 15-year follow up of the effects of pregnancy, *Obes. Res.*, 12, 1166, 2004.

44. Institute of Medicine, Food and Nutrition Board, Carbohydrate in *Dietary Reference Intakes for Energy, Carbohydrates, Fiber, Fat, Protein and Amino Acids (Macronutrients)*, IOM, National Academy Press, Washington, D.C., 2002, chap. 6.

45. Elliot, S.S. et al., Fructose, weight gain, and the insulin resistance syndrome, *Am. J. Clin. Nutr.*, 76, 911, 2002.

46. Institute of Medicine, Food and Nutrition Board, Fiber in *Dietary Reference Intakes for Energy, Carbohydrates, Fiber, Fat, Protein and Amino Acids (Macronutrients)*, IOM, National Academy Press, Washington, D.C., 2002, chap. 7.

47. Institute of Medicine, Food and Nutrition Board, Water in *Dietary Reference Intakes for Water, Potassium, Sodium, Chloride, and Sulfate*, IOM, National Academy Press, Washington, D.C., 2004, Summary.

48. Institute of Medicine, Food and Nutrition Board, Protein in *Dietary Reference Intakes for Energy, Carbohydrates, Fiber, Fat, Protein and Amino Acids (Macronutrients)*, IOM, National Academy Press, Washington, D.C., 2002, chap. 10.

49. Institute of Medicine, Food and Nutrition Board, Fat in *Dietary Reference Intakes for Energy, Carbohydrates, Fiber, Fat, Protein and Amino Acids (Macronutrients)*, IOM, National Academy Press, Washington, D.C., 2002, chap. 8.

50. Weil, A., *Eating Well for Optimum Health: The Essential Guide to Bring Health and Pleasure Back to Eating*, Quill, New York, 2001, p. 88 and 262.

51. Hornstra, G., Essential fatty acids in mothers and their neonates, *Am. J. Clin. Nutr.*, 71, 1262S, 2000.

52. Helland, I.B. et al., Maternal supplementation with very-long-chain $N-3$ fatty acids during pregnancy and lactation augments children's IQ at 4 years of age, *Pediatrics*, 111, 39, 2003.

53. What you need to know about mercury in fish and shellfish, March 2004, Food and Drug Administration, available at www.fda.gov, accessed March 2004.

54. Francois, C.A. et al., Supplementing lactation women with flaxseed oil does not increase docosahexaenoic acid in their milk, *Am. J. Clin. Nutr.*, 77, 226, 2003.

55. Krause, *Krause's Food Nutrition and Diet Therapy*, W.B. Saunders, Philadelphia, 2004, p. 205.

56. FDA announces changes to food label, U.S. Food and Drug Administration, available at www.fda.gov, accessed August 8, 2004.

57. Koletzko, B., Potential adverse effects of *trans* fatty acids in infants and children, *Eur. J. Med. Res.*, 1, 123, 1995.

58. Innis, S.M. and King, D.J., *Trans* fatty acids in human milk are inversely associated with concentrations of essential all-*cis* $n-6$ and $n-3$ fatty acids and determine *trans*, but not $n-6$ and $n-3$ fatty acids in plasma lipids of breast-fed infants, *Am. J. Clin. Nutr.*, 70, 383, 1999.

59. Mead, P.S. et al., Food-related illness and death in the United States, *Emerg. Infect. Dis.*, 5, 606, 1999.

60. Kanellopoulos-Langevin, C. et al., Tolerance of the fetus by the maternal immune system: role of inflammatory mediators at the feto-maternal interface, *Reprod. Biol. Endocrinol.*, 1, 121, 2003.

61. McEwen, S.A. and Fedorka-Cray, P.J., Antimicrobial use and resistance in animals, *CID*, 34 (Suppl. 3), S93, 2002.

62. Foodborne pathogens, *Food Safety*, available at www.FoodSafety.gov, accessed August 2004.

63. News Release: HHS and USDA release Listeria risk assessment and Listeria action plan, United States Department of Agriculture, available at www.usda.gov/new/releases /01/0020.htm.

64. Myers, G.J., Davidson, P.W., and Shamlaye, C.F., A review of methylmercury and child development, *Neurotoxicology*, 19, 313, 1998.

65. Fact Sheet: Update national listing of fish and wildlife advisories, Environmental Protection Agency, available at www.epa.gov/waterscience/fish /advisories/factsheet.pdf.

66. Summary, Mercury in the Environment, Environmental Protection Agency, available at www.epa.gov, accessed July 31, 2004.
67. Mercury, Center for Food Safety and Applied Nutrition, available at www.cfsan.gov, accessed July 31, 2004.
68. Health Effects of Methylmercury, *Toxicological Effects of Methylmercury*, 2000, open book available at www.nap.edu/openbook/030907, accessed July 31, 2004.
69. Ribas-Fito, N. et al., Polychlorinated biphenyls (PCBs) and neurological development in children: a systematic review, *J. Epidemiol. Community Health*, 55, 537, 2001.
70. Fact Sheet: PCBs, Environmental Protection Agency, available at www.epa.gov, accessed July 31, 2004.
71. Jacobson, J.L. and Jacobson, S.W., Intellectual impairment in children exposed to polychlorinated biphenyls *in utero*, *N. Engl. J. Med.*, 335, 783, 1996.
72. Jacobson, J.L. and Jacobson, S.W., Prenatal exposure to polychlorinated biphenyls and attention at school age, *J. Pediatr.*, 143, 780, 2003.
73. Adlercreutz, H. and Mazur, W., Phyto-oestrogens and Western diseases, *Ann. Med.*, 29, 95, 1997.
74. Poulozzi, L.J., International trends in rates of hypospadias and cryptorchidism, *Environ. Health Perspect.*, 107, 297, 1999.
75. Kim, K.S. et al., Induction of hypospadias in a murin model by maternal exposure to synthetic estrogens, *Environ. Res.* 267, 2004.
76. Franke, A.F., Custer, L.J., and Tanaka, Y., Isoflavones in human breast milk and other biological fluids, *Am. J. Clin. Nutr.* Suppl, 68, 1466S, 1998.
77. Sheehan, D.M., Letters: isoflavone content of breast milk and soy formulas: benefits and risks, *Clin. Chem.*, 43, 850, 1997.
78. Thomas, D.F.M., Hypospadiology: science and surgery, *BJU Int.*, 93, 470, 2004.
79. Foster, W.F. et al., Detection of phytoestrogens in sample of second trimester human amniotic fluid, *Toxicol. Lett.*, 3, 199, 2002.
80. North, K., Golding J., and The ALSPAC Team, A maternal vegetarian diet in pregnancy is associated with hypospadias, *BJU Int.*, 85, 107, 2000.
81. Barnes, P.M. et al., Complementary and alternative medicine use among adults: United States, 2002, Advance Data from Vital and Health Statistics, CDC, 343, 2004.
82. Fugh-Berman, A. and Kronenberg, F., Review complementary and alternative medicine (CAM) in reproductive-age women: a review of randomized controlled trials, *Reprod. Toxicol.*, 17, 137, 2003.
83. Eisenberg, D.M. et al., Trends in alternative medicine use in the United States, 1990–1997, *JAMA*, 280, 1569, 1998.
84. Factor-Litvak, P. et al., Use of complementary and alternative medicine among women in New York City: a pilot study, *J. Altern. Complement. Med.*, 7, 659, 2001.
85. Tsui, B., Dennehy, C.E., and Tsourounis, C., A survey of dietary supplement use during pregnancy at an academic medical center, *Am. J. Obstet. Gynecol.*, 185, 433, 2001.
86. Hollyer, T. et al., The use of CAM by women suffering from nausea and vomiting during pregnancy, *BMC Complement. Altern. Med.*, 2, 5, 2002.
87. Thurer, K.A., The use of complementary and alternative medicine: a postpartum survey, *Obstet. Gynecol.*, 101 (Suppl.), 87S, 2003.
88. Rubin, J.D. et al., Use of prescription and non-prescription drugs in pregnancy, *J. Clin. Epidemiol.*, 46, 581, 1993.
89. Morris, D.A. and Avorn, J., Internet marketing of herbal products, *JAMA*, 290, 1505, 2003.
90. Ernst, E. and Schmidt, K., Health risks over the Internet: advice offered by "medical herbalists" to a pregnant woman, *Wein. Med. Wochenschr.*, 152, 190, 2002.
91. Bone, K., Safe use of herbs in pregnancy, *Townsend Letter for Doctors and Patients*, January, 54, 2002.
92. Belew, C., Herbs and the childbearing woman guidelines for midwives, *J. Nurse Midwifery*, 44, 231, 1999.
93. Useful herbs in pregnancy, *Earth Mama*, available at www.earthmama.com, accessed December 19, 2003.

94. Herbs to avoid during pregnancy, *Earth Mama*, available at www.earthmama.com, accessed December 19, 2003.
95. Gentle Expectations, *Earth Mama*, available at www.earthmama.com, accessed December 19, 2003.
96. Herbal Medicine Accrediting Organizations, *Weekly Bulletin*, available at www.DrWeil.com, accessed January 7, 2003.
97. Tyler, V.E., *Herbs of Choice the Therapeutic Use of Phytomedicinals*, Pharmaceutical Products Press, New York, 1994.
98. Ernst, E.E., Complementary/alternative medicine in gynecology: no simple messages please! (Letter to the Editor), *Acta Obstet. Gynecol. Scand.*, 82, 391, 2003.
99. Ernst, E. and Pittler, M.H., Herbal medicine, *Med. Clin. NA*, 86, 149, 2002.
100. Ernst, E., Herbal medicinal products during pregnancy? (Short Communication), *Phytomedicine: Int. J. Phytother. Phytopharmacol.*, 9, 352, 149, 2002.
101. London, M.L. et al., *Maternal-Newborn and Child Nursing*, Prentice Hall, Upper Saddle River, 2003.
102. Hardy, M.L., Women's health series: herbs of special interest to women, *J. Am. Pharm. Assoc.*, 40, 234, 2000.
103. Blementhal, M., *Herbal Medicine: Expanded Commission E Monographs*, American Botanical Council, Austin, 2000.
104. Young, G.L. and Jewell, D., Interventions for leg cramps in pregnancy, *Cochrane Database Syst. Rev.*, CD0000212, 2002.
105. McGanity, W.J., Dawson, E.B., and Van Hook, J.W., Maternal nutrition, in *Modern Nutrition in Health and Disease*, Shils, M.E., Olson, J.A., Shike, M., and Ross, A., Eds., 9th ed., Lea U Febiger, Philadelphia, 1999, chap. 50.
106. Kolesteren, P. et al., Treatment for iron deficiency anemia with a combined supplementation of iron, vitamin A, and zinc in women of Dinajpur, Bangladesh, *Eur. J. Clin. Nutr.*, 53, 102, 1999.
107. Rothman, K.J. et al., Teratogenicity of high vitamin A intake, *N. Engl. J. Med.*, 333, 1369, 1995.
108. Dietary Reference Intakes: Vitamins, Food and Nutrition Information Center, available at www.nal.usda.gov, accessed August 8, 2004.
109. Vitamin A toxicity and foods, *March of Dimes*, available at www.modimes.org, accessed August 28, 2004.
110. Jewell, D. and Young, G., Interventions for nausea and vomiting in early pregnancy, *Cochrane Database of Syst. Rev.*, 3, 2003.
111. Rosen, T. et al., A randomized controlled trial of nerve stimulation for relief of nausea and vomiting in pregnancy, *ACOG*, 102, 129, 2003.
112. Bennet, G., Queasy no more! *Parenting*, 147, 1997.
113. Erick, M., Hyperemesis gravidarum: a practical management strategy, *OBG Management*, 25, 2000.
114. Sahakian, V. et al., Vitamin B-6 is effective therapy for nausea and vomiting of pregnancy: a randomized, double-blind, placebo controlled study, *Obstet. Gynecol.*, 78, 33, 1995.
115. Vutyavanich, T., Wongtrangan, S., and Ruangsri, R., Pyridoxine for nausea and vomiting of pregnancy: a randomized, double-blind, placebo-controlled trial, *Am. J. Obstet. Gynecol.*, 173, 881, 1995.
116. Fulder, S., Ginger as an anti-nausea remedy in pregnancy: the issue of safety, *HerbalGram*, 38, 47, 1996.
117. Portnoi, G. et al., Prospective comparative study of the safety and effectiveness of ginger for the treatment of nausea and vomiting in pregnancy, *Am. J. Obstet. Gynecol.*, 189, 1374, 2003.
118. Brown, D.J., Ginger alleviates nausea and vomiting of pregnancy, *HerbalGram*, 53, 21, 2001.
119. The American Botanical Council, *The Complete German Commission E Monographs, Therapeutic Guide to Herbal Medicines*, Blumenthal, M. et al., Eds., American Botanical Council, Austin, 1998.
120. Brevoort, P., The booming U.S. botanical market: a new overview, *HerbalGram*, 44, 33, 1998.
121. Vutyavanich, T., Kraisarin, T., and Ruangsri, R., Ginger for nausea and vomiting in pregnancy: randomized, double-masked, placebo-controlled trial, *Obstet. Gynecol.*, 97, 577, 2001.
122. Keating, A. and Chez, R.A., Ginger syrup as an antiemetic in early pregnancy, *Altern. Ther. Health Med.*, 8, 89, 2002.

123. Wilkinson, J.M., Effect of ginger tea on the fetal development of Sprague–Dawley rats, *Reprod. Toxicol.*, 14, 507, 2000.

124. Miscellaneous authors, ACOG Practice Bulletin #52. Nausea and vomiting of pregnancy, *Obstet. Gynecol.*, 103, 803, 2004.

125. Eliakim, R., Abulafia, O., and Sherer, D.D., Hyperemesis gravidarum: a current review, *Am. J. Perinatol.*, 17, 207, 2000.

126. Accetta, S.G. et al., Memory loss and ataxia after hyperemesis gravidarum: a case of Wernick–Korsakoff syndrome, *Eur. J. Obstet. Byn. Reprod. Biol.*, 102, 100, 2002.

127. Tesfaye, S. et al., Pregnant, vomiting and going blind, *Lancet*, 352, 1594, 1998.

128. Simon, E.P. and Schwartz, J., Medical hypnosis for hyperemesis gravidarum, *Birth*, 26, 248, 1999.

129. Fuchs, K. et al., Treatment of hyperemesis gravidarum by hypnosis, *Int. J. Clin. Exp. Hypn.*, 28, 323, 1980.

130. Sibai, B.M., Diagnosis and management of gestational hypertension and preeclampsia, *Obstet. Gynecol.*, 102, 181, 2003.

131. Krause, *Krause's Food Nutrition and Diet Therapy*, W.B. Saunders, Philadelphia, 2004, chap. 7.

132. Chappell, L.D. et al., Effect of antioxidants on the occurrence of preeclampsia in women at increased risk: a randomized trial, *Lancet*, 354, 810, 1999.

133. Hicks, P., Gestational diabetes in primary care (Review), *Med. Gen. Med.*, eJournal, 5, 2, 2000.

134. Kjos, S.L. and Buchanan, T.A., Current concepts: gestational diabetes mellitus, *N. Engl. J. Med.*, 341, 1749, 1999.

135. Javonovic, L., Achieving euglycaemia in women with gestational diabetes. Current options for screening, diagnosis, and treatment, *Drugs*, 64, 1401, 2004.

136. American Diabetes Association, Evidence-based nutrition principles and recommendations for the treatment and prevention of diabetes and related complications, *Diabetes Care*, 26 (Suppl. 1), S51, 2003.

137. Jovanovic, L., Chromium and women's health, in *Chromium in Health and Disease*, A Council for the Advancement of Diabetes Research and Education (CADRE) Chromium Summit, Boston, 2003.

138. Trail, P., Chromium and women's health, in *Chromium in Health and Disease*, A Council for the Advancement of Diabetes Research and Education (CADRE) Chromium Summit, Boston, 2003.

139. Avron, J. et al., Reduction of bacteruria and pyruria after ingestion of cranberry juice, *JAMA*, 271, 1571, 1994.

140. Howell, A.B. and Foxman, B., Cranberry juice and adhesion of antibiotic resistant uropathogens, *JAMA*, 287, 3082, 2002.

141. Garrard, J. et al., Variations in product choices of frequently purchased herbs, *Arch. Intern. Med.*, 163, 2290, 2003.

142. Leigh, E., First study on safety of echinacea during pregnancy, *HerbalGram*, 51, 21, 2001.

143. Preterm and low birth weight in the United States, *Peristats, An Interactive Perinatal Data Resource*, available at www.marchofdimes.com/peristats, accessed January 19, 2004.

144. Martin, A. et al., The effects of hypnosis on the labor processes and birth outcomes of pregnant adolescents, *J. Fam. Prac.*, 50, 441, 2001.

145. Parson, M., Simpson, M., and Ponton, T., Raspberry leaf and its effect on labour: safety and efficacy, *Aust. Coll. Midwives Inc. J.*, 12, 20, 1999.

146. Simpson, M. et al., Raspberry leaf in pregnancy: its safety and efficacy in labor, *Midwifery Women's Health*, 46, 51, 2001.

147. Garry, D. et al., Use of castor oil in pregnancies at term, *Altern. Ther. Health Med.*, 6, 77, 2000.

148. Labrecque, M., Eason, E., and Marcous, S., Women's views on the practice of prenatal perineal massage, *BJOG*, 108, 499, 2001.

149. Burn, E.E. et al., An investigation into the use of aromatherapy in intrapartum midwifery practice, *J. Altern. Complement. Med.*, 6, 121, 2000.

150. McFarlin, B.L. et al., A national survey of herbal preparation use by nurse-midwives for labor stimulation. Review of the literature and recommendations for practice, *J. Nutr. Midwifery*, 44, 205, 1999.

151. Zipursky, A., Prevention of vitamin K deficiency bleeding in newborns, *Br. J. Haematol.*, 104, 430, 1999.
152. Position Paper, American Academy of Pediatrics, www.aap.org, accessed August 27, 2004.
153. Pugliese, M.T. et al., Nutritional rickets in suburbia, *J. Am. Coll. Nutr.*, 127, 637, 1998.
154. Kramer, M.S. and Kakuma, R., Optimal duration of exclusive breastfeeding, *Cochrane Database Syst. Rev.*, CD003517, 2002.
155. Newcomb, P.A. et al., Lactation and a reduced risk for premenopausal breast cancer, *N. Engl. J. Med.*, 330, 81, 1994.
156. ACOG issues guidelines on breastfeeding, *American College of Obstetrics January 2002 News Release Online*, available at www.acog.org/from_home/publications/press_releases, accessed January 20, 2004.
157. Owen, C.G. et al., Infant feeding and blood cholesterol: a study in adolescents and a systematic review, *Pediatrics*, 110, 597, 2002.
158. American Academy of Pediatrics, Committee on Drugs, The transfer of drugs and other chemicals into human milk, *Pediatrics*, 108, 776, 2001.
159. van de Perre, P. and Cartoux, M., Retroviral transmission and breast-feeding, *Clin. Microbiol. Infect.*, 1, 6, 1995.
160. *Nutrition during Pregnancy and Lactation: An Implementation Guide*, an open book available at www.nap.edu/openbook/0309047382, accessed July 31, 2004, National Academy of Sciences, 1992.
161. Menella, J., Alcohol's effect on lactation, *Alcohol Res. Health*, 25, 230, 2001.
162. Little, R.E. et al., Alcohol, breastfeeding, and development at 18 months, *Pediatrics*, 109, E72, 2002.
163. Herbal Galactogogue, *Breast Feeding after Reduction*, available at www.bfar.org, accessed January 21, 2004.
164. FDA Talk Paper: FDA warns against women using unapproved drug, domperidone, to increase milk production, June 7, 2004, available at www.fda.gov/bbs/topics, accessed July 15, 2004.
165. Huggins, K.E., Fenugreek: one remedy for low milk production, *Breastfeeding Articles*, available at www.breastfeeding.org, accessed January 21, 2004.
166. Lawrence, R.A., *Herbs and Breastfeeding*, available at www.breastfeeding.com, accessed January 20, 2004.
167. Miller, L.G. et al., Eds., *Herbal Medicinals*, Pharmaceutical Products Press, New York, 1998.
168. Herbs and breastfeeding, *Le Leche League Breastfeeding Abstracts*, available at www.LeLeche League.org, accessed January 20, 2004.
169. Answers to common questions about postpartum depression, *American College of Obstetrics January 2002 News Release Online*, available at www.acog.org/from_home/publications/press_releases, accessed January 17, 2004.
170. Klier, C.M. et al., St John's wort (hypericum perforatum) — is it safe during breastfeeding? *Pharmacopsychiatry*, 35, 29, 2002.
171. Lee, A. et al., The safety of St John's wort (hypericum perforatum) during breast feeding, *J. Clin. Psychiatry*, 64, 966, 2003.

4 Infant and Child Health

Lisbeth Benoit

CONTENTS

INFANT HEALTH

INTRODUCTION

Appropriate nutrition during infancy is critical for optimal growth, development, and future health. Breast milk is the ideal infant food and is recommended by the American Academy of Pediatrics (AAP) and the American Dietetic Association to provide optimal nutrition to infants. Breast milk is a complex food, specifically designed for the human infant. Its complete composition is still under study. Is an infant at risk without breast milk? Epidemiological studies provide compelling evidence that infants who receive human milk as food have decreased incidence or severity of infectious diseases, including bacterial meningitis, bacteremia, diarrhea, respiratory tract infection, otitis, and urinary tract infection.[1] AAP professes that breastfeeding "ensures the best possible health as well as the best developmental and psychosocial outcomes for the infant."[1]

NORMAL NUTRITION

It is generally recommended that an infant receives breast milk for at least the first 6 months of life. Many experts believe that exclusive breastfeeding during this time is the best option (see Table 4.1). There is room for improvement in the United States, which is well below the Healthy People 2010 goal for initiation and duration of breastfeeding.[1]

    The AAP recommends the following practices to enhance breastfeeding and provide the best possible environment for success[1,2]:

- Healthcare professionals should recommend and promote breastfeeding, unless there are contraindications such as a mother with human deficiency virus (HIV)
- Peripartum practices that support breastfeeding
- After delivery, healthy infants should be in direct skin-to-skin contact with the mother until breastfeeding is initiated (usually by the infant). Delay weighing, measuring, bathing, needle sticks, and eye prophylaxis until after the first feeding
- Avoid pacifier use
- Encourage 8–12 feedings per 24-h period for the first weeks after delivery in response to the infant rooting or just showing physical activity. Crying indicates the infant has been hungry for sometime
- The mother can record time and length of feedings as well as urine and stool amounts. If there are problems, this information will be valuable
- Infants should visit their pediatrician when 3–5 days old. If there is more than 7% weight loss, aggressive intervention may be necessary to improve breast milk output or breastfeeding success
- Infants should visit their pediatrician when 2–3 weeks old
- Pregnant and lactating women should avoid peanut consumption to reduce the risk of the infant developing a serious, life-threatening food allergy

TABLE 4.1
Exclusive Breastfeeding

Organizations That Recommend *Exclusive* Breastfeeding (No Supplemental Water, Juice, Formula, Food) for the First 6 Months of Life	Common Reasons Breastfeeding Is Discontinued	Overcoming Challenges
World Health Organization	Lack of prenatal education	Educate mother and father before and after delivery
United Nations Children's Fund	Disruptive hospital practices	If breastfeeding is not possible, expressed milk should be provided
AAP Section on Breastfeeding	Inappropriate disruption of breastfeeding	Provide effective breast pumps
American College of Obstetricians and Gynecologists	Early hospital discharge	Identify local breastfeeding resources (i.e., WIC)
American Academy of Family Physicians	Lack of follow-up care	If a physical challenge exists, determine if it is temporary — pumping can maintain milk production until breastfeeding can be continued
Academy of Breastfeeding Medicine	Maternal employment	Human milk banks in North America must follow strict quality control guidelines and provide a safe source of human milk
And others	Lack of family and community support	Before discontinuing, weigh the risks of depriving an infant of breast milk
	Bottle-feeding portrayed as "normal" by media	
	Commercial promotion of formula — particularly in hospital discharge packs with samples and coupons	

Sources: From Garther, L.M. et al., American Academy of Pediatrics Section on Breastfeeding; *Pediatrics*, 115, 496, 2005; Kramer, M.S and Kakuma, R., *Adv. Exp. Med. Biol.*, 554, 63, 2004.

Some of the observed numerous benefits of human milk include[3–6]:

- Provide optimal nutrition — human milk cannot be duplicated
- Provide immunologic and enzymatic compounds resulting in decreased incidence of ear, respiratory, and gastrointestinal infections in breastfed infants
- Result in leaner body composition at 1 year of age and may be less prone to obesity
- Support brain development resulting in optimal cognitive development
- Possibly fewer food allergies
- Support less incidence of constipation
- Support less risk of overnutrition, which can later lead to obesity, as the infant has control over the quantity of milk received

• Some pediatric experts believe that breastfeeding reduces the incidence of particular degenerative diseases later in life by providing nutritional components that strengthen various organs and body parts such as the joints

Human milk is a secretion of the mammary gland and its composition changes during feeding as well as during the first year of life. The time of day and the mother's diet can also impact milk composition. For example, the fat content increases near the end of feeding to provide satiety.[5] There is no true replacement for breast milk because of the numerous components that cannot be duplicated and the varying composition during feeding.[5,8]

Unfortunately, there are medical situations for which breastfeeding is contraindicated. Infants with galactosemia (galactose 1-phosphate uridyltransferase deficiency) require a medically controlled diet. Mothers with active tuberculosis (or who are human T-cell lymphotropic virus type I or type II positive), human immunodeficiency virus (HIV),* who are receiving or are exposed to radioactive isotopes, receiving chemotherapy drugs, using street drugs or who have herpes simplex lesions on the breast** should not breastfeed.[1]

VITAMIN AND MINERAL SUPPLEMENTATION

Some pediatric nutrition experts recommend iron and vitamin D supplementation (Textbox 4.1) for breastfed infants of 0–12 months (Table 4.2).

Textbox 4.1   Docosahexaenoic Acid

Docosahexaenoic acid (DHA) is a long-chain essential fatty acid (EFA) that plays a role in the optimal development of the brain and eyes.[15–17] Many formulas in the United States are not fortified with DHA. Breast milk supplies ample quantities of this fatty acid — unless the mother is deficient. Studies indicate that a continuous supply of long-chain fatty acids from breast milk may be needed for at least the first 4 months for optimal development, particularly visual acuity. If formula is the sole source of nutrition and lacks DHA, it may be prudent to supplement the infant's diet with DHA. It is essential that a pure source of the oil be used. This oil can be added to the formula. Note that some infant foods now contain DHA and the effects of cumulative sources are unknown. The dose should be based on the infants' weight and other potential dietary sources.

FORMULA FEEDING

If breastfeeding is not an option, an iron-fortified formula is recommended as a sole source of nutrition for the first 4–6 months of life. Standard cow milk formulas are most commonly recommended. They contain altered milk that has had the butterfat removed, vegetable oil and carbohydrate added, and the protein content lowered. Demineralized whey is sometimes the source of protein, which has a whey/casein ratio of 60:40 while a standard cow's milk formula is typically a 20:80 ratio. Human milk ranges from 60:40 in colostrum, the first milk

---

*Unlike the United States, women in certain countries who are HIV positive (i.e., Africa) may be advised to breastfeed. Some research indicates that these exclusively breastfed infants have reduced rates of HIV infection.[1]

**If herpes lesions are present on one breast but not the other, it is safe to breastfeed on the lesion-free breast.[1]

TABLE 4.2
Supplementation during 0–12 Months

Nutrient	Recommended Amount	Comments
Iron	1 mg/kg/day	If an infant is deficient in iron, permanent cognitive and motor impairments may result
	Maximum dose of 15 mg/day by 6 months	
	Iron drops	Supplementation is controversial if iron deficiency symptoms are not present
		Iron bioavailability in human milk is high
		There is clinical evidence that breastfed (term) infants are iron sufficient for 9–12 months[9]
		Other research indicates that iron supplementation in healthy breastfeeding infants from 1 to 6 months of age may have beneficial hematologic and developmental results[10]
		Full-term low birth weight infants appear to benefit from iron supplementation[11,12]
		Note: Usually, infant cereal is fortified with iron
Vitamin D	200–400 IU/day	AAP recommends that all breastfed infants receive daily 200 IU of oral vitamin D drops from 2 months until the infant is consuming vitamin D fortified formula or milk[1,13]
	Drops — usually found in combination with iron	Supplementation is controversial since breast milk should provide complete nutrition. Infants at highest risk for deficiency:
		Live in northern urban areas of the United States, particularly in winter
		Have dark skin
		Are often covered (for cultural or other reasons)
		If nursing mother is deficient, breast milk may be low in vitamin D. Supplementation by nursing mother may be adequate
Fluoride	0.25 mg/day after 6 months if local water has <0.3 ppm fluoride drops	

Source: Adapted from Samour, P.Q., Helm, K.K., and Lang, C.E., Eds., *Handbook of Pediatric Nutrition*, 2nd ed., Aspen Publishers, Inc., Maryland, 2003.

produced, to 55:45 in mature milk. Formulas containing demineralized whey seem to be a better choice but clinical evidence to support this is not available. Protein requirements for infants range from 1.8 to 4.5 g/100 cal.

Many formulas contain the amino acid taurine, which is found in human milk but not cow's milk. Research suggests that taurine supports neurodevelopment. However, it is not currently mandatory to include taurine in formulas.

TABLE 4.3
Vitamin and Mineral Supplementation — Formula-Fed Infants

Nutrient	Dose	Source
Iron	1 mg/kg/day Maximum dose of 15 mg/day by 4 months	Iron-fortified formula
Vitamin D	400 IU/day	Iron-fortified formula
Fluoride	0.25 mg/day after 6 months if local water has <0.3 ppm fluoride	Contained in ready-to-feed formula

Source: Adapted from Samour, P.Q., Helm, K.K., and Lang, C.E., Eds., *Handbook of Pediatric Nutrition*, 2nd ed., Aspen Publishers, Inc., Maryland, 2003.

Iron is a key mineral in formulas but only about 4% of this iron is absorbed. It is therefore important to use the iron-fortified formula (12 mg/qt) and not low iron (1 mg/qt) if formula is the sole source of nutrition.[5,14]

Soy formulas are recommended for infants with suspected milk allergy, galactosemia, or lactose intolerance. Unfortunately, studies show that 50–60% of infants with intolerance to milk protein also have soy intolerance. Milk intolerance caused by lactose intolerance may be caused by acute inflammation of the digestive tract. In this case, temporary use of soy formula could be used while the small intestine repairs itself. Some soy formulas are sucrose- or corn-free. Soy formulas are not recommended for preterm infants because they are not designed or recommended for preterm infants who weigh <1800 g (Table 4.3 and Textbox 4.2).[5]

PROTEIN HYDROLYSATE FORMULA

Formulas that contain a casein hydrolysate with nonantigenic peptides of <1200 Da molecular weight can be successfully used by infants who are allergic to the intact proteins in cow's milk or soy formula. Research suggests that normal growth is supported by these products.[21,22] Protein hydrolysate formulas vary in nutrient composition. The AAP does not recommend protein hydrolysate formula to treat colic, sleeplessness, or irritability because research has not confirmed the connection of these symptoms to sensitivity to cow's milk protein.[5,23]

Textbox 4.2   Isoflavones

Isoflavones, compounds naturally found in soy, have been shown to inhibit the growth of intestinal cells in piglets.[18] Other components of soy such as phytates and manganese may also have negative effects on iron absorption, growth, and brain health.[19] Soy formulas contain high levels of manganese — up to 300 μg/qt. Although the effects of long-term consumption of these levels are not known, it is possible that there could be long-term negative consequences to cognitive development. Elevated manganese in umbilical cord blood, measured at birth, has been correlated to reduced psychomotor scores throughout early childhood.[20]

COW'S MILK IS NOT FOR INFANTS

Infants under the age of 1 year should not be given goat's milk, evaporated milk, whole cow's milk, skim milk, or low-fat milk. An infant's body is not ready for the high-renal solute load in some of these foods and the macronutrient profile is not conducive to infant health.[5] It has been suggested that consumption of cow's milk in infancy may trigger an autoimmune process that leads to the development of insulin-dependent diabetes. This relationship is controversial and recent studies have not supported this hypothesis.[24]

STARTING SOLIDS

Breast milk or formula should be provided for the first year of life. It should be the sole source of nutrition from birth to the first 4–6 months, but it is still a critical source of nutrition when solids are included in the diet.[5,25] Obesity is now a major health concern in the United States and among countries around the world. Overconsumption and unhealthy food choices can start during infancy. Infants should be allowed to play a role in deciding how much they eat.

In the southern States, there are several standard practices that cause problems: giving a baby tea in their bottle (tannins bind the iron) and adding cereal to the formula to help the baby sleep through the night sooner.

While there are general recommendations for feeding solids, each child is unique and feeding recommendations should be tailored to the infant's stage of development. An infant's readiness, not age, should determine when an infant should begin eating solids.

Usually, an infant shows signs of readiness between 4 and 6 months; however, the AAP Section on Breastfeeding recommends exclusive breastfeeding for the first 6 months, if possible.[1] Research suggests that exclusive breastfeeding for at least 6 months reduces the risk of atopic disease.[2]

The following are signs of readiness of solid food[5]:

- No extrusion reflex (the tongue pushes the food out of the mouth). Food can be moved from the front of the mouth with the tongue to the back of the mouth and swallowed. Choking on food indicates an infant is not ready to eat solids. Initially, a gag reflex is normal. Infant can hold head up without support
- Sits independently
- Can balance to remain in sitting position while grasping for objects
- Opens mouth when hungry and turns head away when satiated. Without this action, an infant could be fed beyond satiety, which may lead to a propensity to become overweight

Infants should be provided the opportunity to control their food intake. Prevention of obesity begins in infancy. An infant who is not yet able to communicate that he/she is full may learn to feel stuffed. Also, when an infant cries it should not always be assumed he/she wants to eat. The caretaker should make sure the baby is not seeking comfort but is truly hungry.

If the infants control their food intake, they will greatly reduce the possibility of over-feeding. Ways to encourage infants to control quantity of food and self-feeding include[6]:

- Present soft finger foods for self-feeding
- Encourage infant to sip from cup independently
- Respond when infant indicates hunger by providing self-feeding opportunity

As the infant becomes comfortable with self-feeding, new foods can be introduced regularly. Even if rejected, new foods should be repeatedly offered.

Textbox 4.3   Avoid Cow's Milk

An infant of 0–12 months does not have a mature gastrointestinal lining and consumption of cow's milk can lead to occult blood loss and development of food allergies because large protein molecules are able to cross the intestinal barrier at this stage of development.[5]

FIRST SOLIDS

Single foods need to be introduced independently to identify any allergic reactions to particular foods. Rice cereal has low allergenicity and recommended as the first food. Each food should be fed for at least 2–3 days without introducing any new foods. Signs of intolerance to a food are skin rash, wheezing, diarrhea, and vomiting.[5] General recommendations include[6]:

- Once the infant is eating one third to one half of a cup of rice, cereal, fruits, and vegetables can be independently added to the diet
- Salt, sugar, and fats should not be added to baby food
- Whole cow's milk is not recommended until 1 year of age (Textbox 4.3). Reduced fat milks should not be used for the first 2 years of life as they have insufficient fat and calories

TO JUICE OR NOT TO JUICE

Fruit juice consumption needs to be carefully monitored, especially during the first year. Juice consumption should always be 100% fruit juice (or 100% juice with water added) and should never exceed 4–6 oz/day for infants and children up to 6 years of age. While the sweet taste of fruit juice makes it a preferable taste to the infant, excess juice consumption can lead to excess calorie consumption or the displacement of other calories, such as protein calories, that are essential to growth.[5,26]

Fruit juice contains water and carbohydrates like sucrose, fructose, glucose, and sorbitol whose concentrations range from 11 to 16 g/100 ml. The carbohydrate load is much greater than that of breast milk or formula, which is 7 g/100 ml. Specially prepared infant juices are made without sulfites or added sugars.[26]

Excessive juice consumption by young children can lead to malnutrition, short stature, and obesity.[27] In infants with a high intake of juice — above the recommended amount — malabsorption is more evident with juices such as apple and pear that contain a greater amount fructose than glucose. White grape juice is better tolerated as it has an equal quantity of these two sugars. Only pasteurized juice should be given to an infant. Pathogens such as *Escherichia coli*, *Salmonella*, and *Cryptosporidium* organisms have been found in unpasteurized juice.[26]

The AAP recommends that fruit juice[26] (see Textbox 4.4):

- Not be given to infants less than 6 months old
- Should not replace whole fruit
- Should not be used as a replacement drink with diarrhea
- Excessive consumption can lead to tooth decay, diarrhea, flatulence, and abdominal distension
- Should not be given to infants in a bottle or at bedtime

Textbox 4.4   Juice for Constipation

Fruit juice (100% juice) may be beneficial for infants suffering from constipation. Juice that contains sugars like fructose, glucose, and sorbitol — such as pear and apple juice — may lead to more frequent and comfortable bowel movements for infants. A dietitian or physician should be consulted for specific recommendations.[5]

NUTRITION CHALLENGES IN INFANCY

JAUNDICE

In newborns, the yellow tinge of the skin and eyes is due to elevated bilirubin. Feed infants frequently to stimulate breast milk production and increase infant gut motility, which will decrease bilirubin absorption.[5] The Cholestasis Guideline Committee of North America Society for Pediatric Gastroenterology, Hepatology, and Nutrition recommends that infants that are jaundiced at 2 weeks should be evaluated for cholestasis by measuring total and direct bilirubin. If the infant is breastfed, the committee recommends waiting until 3 weeks if no other abnormalities are present.[28]

DENTAL CARIES

Sadly, many infants develop tooth decay during their first year of life. This is most often due to filling bottles with juice and other sugary drinks and the bottle remaining in the infant's mouth for prolonged periods of time. If infants fall asleep with the bottle in their mouth, the salivary flow decreases and the liquid pools in the mouth, bathing the teeth in sugar. This is called bottle mouth syndrome.

MILK SENSITIVITY

Signs of milk sensitivity usually appear during the first 4 months of infancy. Diarrhea is a common symptom and may be due to an allergy to a protein component in milk or intolerance to the primary sugar in milk, lactose. An allergy to milk protein will also cause diarrhea and can lead to vomiting as well. Other symptoms of milk allergy are skin rashes and respiratory symptoms. In severe cases, anaphylactic shock may occur. Lactose intolerance is due to inadequate lactase enzyme production. Milk allergies may occur because the gastro-intestinal tract is still forming and may allow milk antigens to cross into the bloodstream, leading to an allergic reaction. In this situation, it is optimal to remove cow's milk formula from the diet and reintroduce, with close surveillance, at 2 years of age. If the infant must receive formula, casein hydrolysates are recommended and have been shown to result in normal growth and improvement of allergenic symptoms.[5,22]

ACUTE DIARRHEA

Sudden onset of increased stool frequency, volume, and water content may be caused by viral, bacterial, or parasitic infection. Antibiotics, which disturb the gut bacterial ecology, may also cause diarrhea. Rehydration is essential and, if more than 10% of the body fluid is lost, intravenous rehydration may be required. If the infant is breastfeeding, continued feedings will help with rehydration (Textbox 4.5). This is the recommended method of rehydration for infants and also is preventative.[29] For formula-fed infants, an infant rehydration solution with an osmolality of 250 mOsm/l, 25 g/l sugar, 20 meq/l potassium, and 45 meq/l of sodium is

---

Textbox 4.5   Probiotics

Probiotics may offer additional support to an infant who is suffering from diarrhea or who is given antibiotic therapy. Bifidobacteria supplementation has been researched in infants and children with no adverse effects found. Bifidobacteria are the predominant colonic flora in infants and are the bacteria of choice for supplementation. Not only does bifidobacteria supplementation reduce diarrhea, it also may reduce the incidence of atopy. Beneficial probiotic strains appear to be *Lactobacillus GG*, *Lactobacillus reuteri*, and bifidobacteria and the beneficial yeast *Saccharomyces boulardii*.[31–33]

---

optimal during the first 4–6 h following an acute episode. The AAP recommends that the regular diet be resumed after a brief rehydration period. Beverages with high osmolality, such as juice, broth, and sports rehydration drinks should not be given and will worsen the condition.[5,6,30]

FOOD REFUSAL

Rejection of food is most often due to either stress (negative emotional environment) or illness. Too little sleep due to stress or illness can exacerbate the problem. Examples of stressful situations include aggression or restriction at mealtime, restriction of food exploration, rushing meals, or lack of routine. The prescription for food refusal of an emotional origin is a calm, interactive, and supportive environment.[5,6]

OBESITY

The prevalence of obesity over the past 20 years has become a major concern. Obesity is a growing problem for toddlers and children as well as adults. Overfeeding infants and providing them with sodas, juices, and other sugary drinks, high-fatty foods such as French fries, and lack of physical activity have resulted in higher rates of obesity among infants and toddlers.

In the United States, between 1970 and 2000, preschoolers between the ages of 2 and 5 years and children between the ages of 6 and 11 years have experienced an increase in weight.[33,34] As a result, the risk for adult obesity has increased along with health complications. However, before children reach adulthood, children are faced with an increased incidence of cardiovascular-related diseases, type 2 diabetes, mental health issues, and other diseases (see Textbox 4.6).[35,36]

Prevention of excess adiposity in childhood and adulthood can begin at birth. The following are practices to consider:

- Breastfeed infants for at least 6 months to provide the best nutritional advantage to the infant and give the infant control of his food intake
- Delay feeding solid food until the infant shows signs of readiness and can let the caregiver know when they are satisfied
- Do not always feed the infants when they cry. If the infant was fed recently, determine whether discomfort or a need for attention is the reason for the crying
- Limit juice (never more than 6 oz daily) during the first year
- Play and move with the baby

COLIC

Some parents have found that herbal tea is helpful. The combination of chamomile, fennel, verbena, licorice, and balm mint was found to be effective in one study.[46] Other traditional herbs for colic tea include anise, catnip, caraway, cumin, mint, fennel, dill, and ginger root. Gripe

Textbox 4.6   The Problem of Obesity
Pamela Williams

In the past 10 years, the number of scientific and lay articles has multiplied, many of them expressing the incidence, causes, problems, and solutions associated with obesity. More recently, the literature has focused on the increased incidence of overweight during infancy and childhood. The American Heart Association released a scientific statement revealing that between 1980 and 2000, the prevalence of childhood overweight in the United States has tripled.[37] Among 2–5-year-olds, the prevalence has increased from 7.2 to 10.4% and among 6–11-year-olds, 6.5 to 15.3%.[33,38] The trend of an increased prevalence has not only been noted in the United States but also in other countries such as Australia, Canada, China, France, Germany, Finland, Japan, Mexico, and the United Kingdom.[37,39,40]

A generic definition of obesity has been identified as the result of "an imbalance between energy intake and energy expenditure."[37] Determining the actual definition of obesity has been problematic. Scientists use variations of the body mass index (BMI) to identify obesity. As BMI varies with age in children, using the BMI is difficult. A general guideline is children between the 85th and 95th percentile are considered to be at risk for overweight. Children above the 95th percentile are considered overweight.[37] The incidence of obesity has affected all groups of people but is highest among certain groups — African Americans, native Americans, Hispanics, children in low-income families, and children in the southeastern region of the United States.

The increased incidence of obesity is associated with an increase in several diseases. Primarily, type 2 diabetes has been seen in the older population. This trend is changing. Type 2 diabetes is now on the rise in children and adolescents. If the symptoms associated with diabetes are as complicated as diabetic adults, the difficulty of minimizing complications increases healthcare costs. Other chronic diseases of concern are cardiovascular disease, metabolic syndrome, hypertension, atherosclerosis, depression, nonalcoholic fatty liver disease, obstructive sleep apnea, orthopedic complications, asthma, adult obesity, and others.[37,41–43]

Although genetics play a role in the prevalence of obesity, the increased incidence is directly related to lifestyle choices and habits. With a decrease in consumption of low to moderate calorie foods, an increase in high-calorie foods and beverages, and a decrease in physical activity, obesity has become more prevalent. Today more than ever, children, including babies, consume foods such as potato chips and French fries that are high in fat and drink high-sugar beverages such as sodas. In addition, this population has increased television viewing and other sedentary activities. According to researchers, to reverse this trend will take several strategies. The most effective strategies recommended include changing eating and physical activity habits and involving family members in changing behavior before obesity becomes a problem.[44,45]

Among infants, some but not all studies have shown that breastfeeding may reduce the risk of later overweight. Research reports that only 64% of women breastfeed their infants and this number decreases to 29% by the time the infant is 6 months old. Only 17% of infants are exclusively breastfed until they are 6 months old. Promoting breastfeeding may be a way to help prevent overweight among toddlers and children. The barriers and cultural norms that discourage breastfeeding should be addressed to help encourage women to breastfeed their children.[37]

During the preschool years, a reasonable goal of 2.5 lb/in. of growth has been suggested to help maintain desired weight until 8 or 9 years old but an increase of 5 lb/in. may predict overweight during elementary school years. Getting families involved in establishing eating and physical activities may be an effective approach in maintaining

Continued

Textbox 4.6   The Problem of Obesity (continued)

a desirable weight during these developmental years.[37] Environmental factors at home, school, church, and within the community can help establish behavioral habits that help maintain a healthy lifestyle, which, in turn, help maintain a healthy weight. Programs with educational components such as the Women, Infant & Children Program help parents develop and maintain healthy habits for young children. Encouraging the consumption of five fruits and vegetables a day, fibrous foods, small portions of low-fat products such as milk after a child reaches 2 years old will help establish healthy eating habits. Making these dietary adjustments and engaging in physical activity for at least 60 min a day and minimizing television viewing to 1–2 h a day help children maintain a healthy weight.

   The problem of obesity is complex and so is the solution. Identifying and implementing one approach to resolve the problem is not enough to reverse the trend of weight gain. Effective approaches would take a multiple solution approach. In the future, these approaches could include alternative nutrition therapies that have yet to be developed. Further research will continue to define the matrix of obesity and offer a variety of alternative solutions to make a positive difference in the outcome of the obesity dilemma.

---

water, available in Britain and Canada, is made from dill. These remedies are not produced or regulated in the same standardized ways that medications are regulated. In addition, the use of these herbs has not been studied in children and, therefore, it is not certain that they are safe. Some herbs contain contaminants that may be harmful to an infant. Carefully conducted research is needed to assure that these preparations are safe and effective.[47]

   Oftentimes, people believe that if something is "natural," it is good to include in the diet. "Natural" does not equal "safe" and mothers should be cautioned on using herbal teas and other natural remedies.

CONCLUSION

While many advances have been made to understand the nutritional needs of infants, human milk continues to be and is increasingly valued as the superior source of nutrients during the first years of life. Providing human milk as the sole source of nutrition for most infants during the first 6 months of life appears to allow the greatest potential for optimal health. Advancing science continues to offer choices for infants who are sick or at risk so that natural approaches, such as dietary changes, probiotics, and even herbs, can be utilized as a sole or complementary treatment.

CHILD HEALTH

BASIC NUTRITIONAL NEEDS

Normal, healthy children grow at different rates. After the rapid growth of infancy, the rate of physical growth and appetite will slow and undulate over the years. While children should not be force-fed nutritious foods, they should be offered a variety of healthy foods and have minimized exposure to processed, high-sugar, high-fat foods. Children have a greater probability of developing a preference for healthy foods if they are exposed to only these foods at a young age. Whole grains such as cereals and breads, fresh fruits, cooked and uncooked fresh vegetables, organic dairy products, and select protein foods will provide the greatest potential for maximizing growth and health.

Young eaters usually do best with small pieces of food that can be picked up and does not require major chewing. Small, frequent feedings should be encouraged with snacks that are mini-meals. Protein containing foods, fruits, vegetables, whole grain products, and dairy products should be offered. Making eating fun and pleasurable will promote the consumption of healthy foods.

MACRONUTRIENT REQUIREMENTS

Energy needs are derived from body size, basal energy expenditure, physical activity, and altered states of health. Height is one of the better references for determining energy needs in a child. When a child's appetite increases during a growth spurt, foods of high-nutritional value should be readily available. When growth slows, children should not be pressured to consume a certain quantity of food, as long as they appear healthy. Instead, allow appetite to dictate how much they eat (Textbox 4.7).

The percentage of caloric intake from proteins drops after infancy and increases at puberty. The typical diet in the United States usually contains sufficient, if not excess, protein. However, certain children may have to increase their protein intake due to reduced food intake, food preferences, strict vegetarianism, and food allergies.

Fat choices are especially important to the growing child. So much of the processed food available — including foods targeted for children — contain *trans*-fatty acids. *Trans*-fatty acids are structurally different from naturally occurring unsaturated fats. The chemical structure of unsaturated fatty acids has a bent shape at room temperature due to their double bonds as *cis* isomers (adjacent carbons on the same side of the double bond). *Trans*-fatty acids have carbon atoms adjacent to their double bonds on opposite sides and therefore are straight and solid at room temperature. Extensive metabolic and epidemiological evidences support adverse effects of *trans*-fats — particularly on blood lipid levels.[50] These fats are particularly unhealthful as they incorporate into membrane lipids in the cells and affect the physical properties of the cells and membrane bound enzymes.[51] Omega-3-fatty acids, particularly DHA, are key to optimal neurological and visual development and should be part of the child's food intake. *Trans*-fatty acids should be minimized and eliminated if possible. By 2006, food manufacturers will be required to include the quantity of *trans*-fat on labels. Foods

---

Textbox 4.7 Measuring Nutrient Requirements

The most current reference values that have been published in the United States by the Food and Nutrition Board of the Institute of Medicine (IOM) are dietary reference intakes (DRIs), which include the recommended dietary allowances (RDA), adequate intakes (AI), estimated average requirement (EAR), and the tolerable upper intake level (UL). The EAR represents the nutrient level that is believed to meet the requirements of 50% of healthy individuals in an age and sex group. The RDA is calculated as two standard deviations greater than the EAR and is meant to specify the intake level for a population group that meets the requirements of 97–98% of all persons in that group. RDAs are used to determine dietary goals for individuals in specific groups. DRI values are used as guides to preventing deficiency and promoting health. However, much of the recommended levels for children are extrapolated values and may not represent accurate requirements. In some cases, intakes of less than the DRIs may support healthful growth. For energy, it has been suggested that the RDA may be 25% too high.[48,49]

TABLE 4.4
Dietary Reference Intakes (DRIs): Acceptable Macronutrient Distribution Ranges

	1–3 Years (%)	4–8 Years (%)
Fat[a]		
($n-6$) Polyunsaturated fatty acids (linoleic acid)	5–10	5–10
($n-3$) Polyunsaturated fatty acids (α-linolenic acid)	0.6–1.2	0.6–1.2
Carbohydrate	45–65	45–65
Protein	5–20	10–30

[a]As percent of total calories.

Sources: From IOM Dietary Reference Intakes, http://www.iom.edu/project.asp?id=4574; Food and Nutrition Board, Institute of Medicine, National Academies (2002).

containing partially hydrogenated oils, often found in prepackage professed food and fast food, are the main source of *trans*-fat and should be avoided.

The DRIs for macronutrients and fiber, set by the IOM of the National Academy of Sciences, are presented in Table 4.4 and Table 4.5.

MICRONUTRIENT REQUIREMENTS

The IOM set DRIs for micronutrients for children and are presented in Table 4.6 and Table 4.7. The DRIs are the most up-to-date nutrient recommendations recognized by the U.S. government. Also included in these two tables are the tolerable ULs and refer to the highest level of daily nutrient intake that is likely to pose no risk of adverse health effects to almost all individuals in the general population of the specified age group. As intake increases above the UL, the risk of adverse effects may increase.

MICRONUTRIENTS OF CONCERN

According to dietary intake studies conducted in the United States, the following nutrients are most likely to be deficient in children's diets[52]:

- Calcium
- Zinc
- Vitamin A
- Folic acid
- Vitamin B_6

TABLE 4.5
DRI: Fiber

	AI (a)
1–3 years	19 g
4–8 years	25 g

TABLE 4.6
Dietary Reference Intakes (DRIs): Recommended Intakes for Individuals, Vitamins

Age	Vit A[a]	Vit C	Vit D	Vit E[b]	Vit K	Thiamin	Riboflavin	Niacin	Vit B6	Folate	Vit B12	Pantothenic Acid	Biotin	Choline
1–3 years	RDA	RDA	AI	RDA	AI	RDA	RDA	RDA	RDA	RDA	RDA	AI	AI	AI
	300 µg	15 mg	200 IU	6 mg	30 µg	0.5 mg	0.5 mg	6 mg	0.5 mg	150 µg	0.9 µg	2 mg	8 µg	200 mg
	UL	UL	UL	UL	UL	UL	UL	UL	UL	UL	UL	UL	UL	UL
	600 µg	400 mg	2000 IU	200 mg	NA	ND	ND	10 mg	30 mg	300 µg	ND	ND	ND	1.0 mg
4–8 years	RDA	RDA	AI	RDA	AI	RDA	RDA	RDA	RDA	RDA	RDA	AI	AI	AI
	400 µg	25 mg	200 IU	7 mg	55 µg	0.5 mg	0.6 mg	8 mg	0.6 mg	200 µg	1.2 µg	3 mg	12 µg	250 mg
	UL	UL	UL	UL	UL	UL	UL	UL	UL	UL	UL	UL	UL	UL
	900 µg	650 mg	2000 IU	300 mg	NA	ND	ND	15 mg	40 mg	400 µg	ND	ND	ND	1.0 mg

RDA = Recommended dietary allowance (set to meet needs of 97–98% of group).

AI = Adequate intake (believed to cover needs but lack data regarding percentage of individuals covered).

UL = The maximum level of daily nutrient intake that is likely to pose no risk of adverse effects.

ND = Not determinable due to lack of data.

[a] As retinol activity equivalents (RAEs). 1 RAE = 1 µg retinol, 12 µg β-carotene, 24 µg α-carotene, or 24 µg β-cryptoxanthin. The RAE for dietary provitamin A carotenoids is twofold greater than retinol equivalents (RE), whereas the RAE for preformed vitamin A is the same as RE.

[b] As α-tocopherol. α-Tocopherol includes RRR-α-tocopherol, the only form of α-tocopherol that occurs naturally in foods, and the 2R-stereoisomeric forms of α-tocopherol (RRR-, RSR-, RRS-, and RSS-α-tocopherol) that occur in fortified foods and supplements. It does not include the 2S-stereoisomeric forms of α-tocopherol (SRR-, SSR-, SRS-, and SSS-α-tocopherol), also found in fortified foods and supplements.

Sources: From IOM Dietary Reference Intakes, http://www.iom.edu/project.asp?id=4574; Food and Nutrition Board, Institute of Medicine, National Academies (2004).

TABLE 4.7
Dietary Reference Intakes (DRIs): Recommended Intakes for Individuals, Minerals

Age	Calcium	Chromium	Copper	Fluoride	Iodine	Iron	Magnesium	Manganese	Molybdenum	Phosphorus	Selenium	Zinc	Potassium	Sodium	Chloride
	AI	AI	RDA	AI	RDA	RDA	RDA	AI	RDA	RDA	RDA	RDA	AI	AI	AI
1–3 years	500 mg	11 µg	340 µg	0.7 mg	90 µg	7 mg	80 mg	1.2 mg	17 µg	460 mg	20 µg	3 mg	3 g	1 g	1.5 g
	UL	UL	UL	UL	UL	UL	UL	UL	UL	UL	UL	UL	UL	UL	UL
	2.5 g	ND	1000 µg	1.3 mg	200 µg	40 mg	65 mg from pharmaceutical agent (i.e., laxatives) only	2 mg	300 µg	3 g	90 µg	7 mg	ND	1.5 g	2.3 g
	AI	AI	RDA	AI	RDA	RDA	RDA	AI	RDA	RDA	RDA	RDA	AI	AI	AI
4–8 years	800 mg	15 µg	440 µg	1 mg	90 µg	10 mg	130 mg	1.5 mg	22 µg	500 mg	30 µg	5 mg	3.8 g	1.2 g	1.9 g
	UL	UL	UL	UL	UL	UL	UL	UL	UL	UL	UL	UL	UL	UL	UL
	2.5 g	ND	3000 µg	2.2 mg	300 µg	40 mg	110 mg from pharmaceutical agent (i.e., laxatives) only	3 mg	600 µg	3 g	150 µg	12 mg	ND	1.9 g	2.9 g

Sources: From IOM Dietary Reference Intakes, http://www.iom.edu/project.asp?id=4574; Food and Nutrition Board, Institute of Medicine, National Academies (2004).

Calcium

Rates of growth and the levels of phosphorus, vitamin D, and protein in the diet affect individual calcium requirements. The Food and Nutrition Board recommends daily calcium intakes of 500 mg for 1–3-year-olds, 800 mg for 4–8-year-olds, and 1300 mg for children 9–18 years of age for optimal bone mineralization. Many children are not consuming calcium at these levels. Studies show that children taking calcium supplements have increased bone density.[53] Some calcium supplements may contain lead.[54] It is important to use calcium supplements from a reputable company that tests their calcium supplements for lead content. Supplements should not contain more than 0.15 μg of lead per tablet. See Table 4.8 for suggested food sources of calcium.

Vitamin D is essential for proper utilization of calcium by the body. Adequate vitamin D can be acquired through 10–15 min of direct sunlight daily (without sunscreen). Otherwise, fortified milk and other products may be the only source of vitamin D. If there is minimal sun exposure and fortified products are not part of the diet, vitamin D supplementation (200 IU or 5 μg) is recommended.

Iron

Up to 9% of 1–3-year-olds have iron deficiency anemia associated with poor cognition and delayed psychomotor development.[5] Iron deficiency also increases the risk of lead uptake in the intestine because insufficient iron levels allow other cations, such as lead, to be absorbed from the intestines at a greater rate than when the body is iron sufficient.[55,56] Iron deficiency affects brain function and can lead to abnormal dopaminergic neurotransmission and may contribute to attention-deficit hyperactivity disorder (ADHD).[57] Iron supplementation for a

---

TABLE 4.8
Calcium Sources

Food	Quantity	Amount of Calcium (Average, in mg)
Dried figs	5	258
Blackstrap molasses	1 tablespoon	187
Yogurt	1/2 cup	178
Cheese	1 oz	150
Fortified juice	1/2 cup	150
Salmon with bones	2 oz	150
Whole milk	1/2 cup	145
Cooked greens	1/2 cup	90
Egg	1	90
Legumes	1/2 cup	90
Almond butter	2 tablespoons	86
Ice cream and ice milk	1/2 cup	75
Chicken	2 oz	70
Almonds	2 tablespoons	50
Corn tortilla	1	50
Fortified rice and soy milk	1/2 cup	40–150

Source: From Samour, P.Q., Helm, K.K., and Lang, C.E., Eds., *Handbook of Pediatric Nutrition*, 2nd ed., Aspen Publishers, Inc., Maryland, 2003.

child should include an iron form that is nonirritating to the intestinal tract, such as a chelated form of iron, such as iron glycinate and amino acid-chelated iron. Inorganic forms of iron, such as ferrous sulfate, tend to irritate the gastrointestinal lining and often cause constipation. As the chelated forms are highly absorbable, lower quantities are needed compared with inorganic sources. Consumption of vitamin C foods or dietary supplements with iron-containing plant foods will increase absorption of nonheme, unchelated iron. Heme iron, which is found in animal foods, is highly absorbable and red meat is an excellent source of iron.

Zinc

Zinc plays a key role in cellular metabolism and growth. Adequate zinc status is required for a healthy immune system and intestinal mucosa. In developing countries, supplementation with zinc in children can help prevent pneumonia and diarrhea.[58] In the United States, zinc status is adequate compared to developing countries. This situation is believed to be due to food fortification and a lower intake of phytate-containing plant foods that reduce the absorption of zinc. It has been suggested that up to 25 g/day of dietary fiber and 1 g/day of phytic acid are not likely to affect zinc status.[59]

The 2001 DRIs for children recommend a significantly lower level of zinc than the previous RDA level of 10 mg for ages 1–3 and 4–8 years. The new levels are 3 and 5 mg, respectively. This suggests that earlier studies examining zinc intake among children may not be accurate.[60] Also, the new UL for zinc for children is 12 mg, which is very close to the old RDA levels. Possible effects of excess zinc intake are alterations in lipoprotein metabolism, impaired immune responses (also an effect of inadequate zinc status), and reduced copper and iron and possibly other cation absorption.[60]

Vitamin A

While vitamin A deficiency is a serious public health problem in developing countries, it is less prevalent in the United States. However, vitamin A deficiency has serious consequences and children are especially susceptible so it is worthy of attention. Effects of vitamin A deficiency include night blindness; xerosis of the conjunctiva and cornea; xerophthalmia (causing blindness); keratinization of the gastrointestinal tract, urinary tract, and lung epithelia; growth retardation; and reduced immune function.[61]

According to the third National Health and Nutrition Examination Survey, 16.7–33.9% of children aged 4–8 years had serum vitamin A concentrations <1.05 μmol/l, which is indicative of a potentially suboptimal vitamin A status. There was a higher prevalence in non-Hispanic, black, and Mexican American children than in non-Hispanic white children.[62,63]

Good sources of vitamin A and beta-carotene are dairy products, fish, dark-colored fruits and vegetables, and leafy vegetables. Liver is also an excellent source but should be consumed in limited quantities as excess consumption can lead to vitamin A toxicity.

BUYER BEWARE

Many food products purchased for children are fortified with vitamins and minerals. All packaged food must have nutrition labeling in order for consumers to be aware of nutrients levels contained in a serving of that product. It is important to understand that values used on nutrition labels are different from the DRIs (RDAs) for the specific age groups. A measure called reference daily intake (RDI) is used for nutrition labeling. The RDIs differ from DRIs — sometimes significantly. For example, a product that contains vitamin C may indicate it contains 100% of the daily value (DV) for children less than 4 years of age, which equals

40 mg. However, the current RDA for vitamin C for children ages 1–3 is 15 mg. Also, nutrition labeling considers all children of 4 years and over to have nutrient requirements identical to adults so the adult RDI applies to all children of 4 years of age and above which is important to understand if nutrient intakes are to be closely monitored.[64] See Table 4.9 for a comparison of age-specific RDAs and RDIs.

NUTRITIONAL STRATEGIES FOR THE TREATMENT OF ATTENTION-DEFICIT HYPERACTIVITY DISORDER AND HYPERACTIVITY

ADHD affects up to 2 million children, leading to significant challenges at home, in the classroom, and with life in general. Estimates suggest that up to 12% of school-age children have ADHD, but more boys are diagnosed with the disorder than girls.[65,66]

The criteria set forth in the latest *Diagnostic and Statistical Manual* (American Psychiatric Association, DSM-IV-R, 1994) are used to identify children with ADHD and describes them as having developmentally inappropriate degrees of inattention, impulsiveness, and hyperactivity. Typical characteristics of children with ADHD include mood liability, temper outbursts, and academic underachievement.[67]

The etiology of ADHD is not known at this time but it is most likely multifaceted. Current research suggests a number of possible influences, such as genetic factors, lead toxicity, neurotransmitter imbalances, food sensitivities, EFA deficiencies, hormonal imbalances, chemical sensitivities, and nutritional deficiencies.[65,68–70] Metabolic studies have demonstrated dopamine, norepinephrine, glucose, thyroid, and hypothalamic–pituitary–adrenal axis dysfunction.[67,71] Clinical studies indicate children with ADHD tend to get sick more often than their peers.[69]

Treatment of ADHD usually involves counseling, special education, medication, and occasionally nutritional recommendations. Nutritional approaches may be a first line of treatment for mild cases and may be a complementary treatment in more severe situations. It is possible that younger children may respond more favorably to a nutritional approach because any nutritional balances that exist may be less severe than in older children. Nutritional supplements may significantly reduce symptoms in some young children to a point where medication could be avoided or dosages could be reduced.

ESSENTIAL FATTY ACIDS

For almost two decades, researchers have recognized an association of hyperactivity with EFA deficiency.[65,69] Researchers noted that children with hyperactivity appear to be thirstier than children who are not hyperactive. An increase in thirst is an important indicator of EFA deficiency. Other symptoms associated with EFA deficiency, such as eczema and asthma, have also been seen in hyperactive children and alleviated by EFA supplementation.[65]

In a study that examined 53 young boys (6–12 years) with ADHD and 42 control subjects, researchers found that the boys with ADHD had a significantly greater incidence of asthma (but not other immunological dysfunction), stomachaches, ear infections, and antibiotic use throughout their lives. Additionally, 81% of the control children were breastfed compared with only 43% of those with ADHD. Subjects' plasma fatty acids were measured and the ADHD children had significantly lower concentrations of $20:4n–6$, $20:5n–3$, and $22:6n–3$ and a significantly higher concentration of $18:1$. The mean content of total $(n–3)$ fatty acids was lower in ADHD children. The total mean concentration of $(n–6)$ was the same for both groups and the mean ratio of $(n–6)$ to $(n–3)$ fatty acids was significantly higher in the ADHD group. Other studies have also shown decreased $20:4n–6$ and $22:6n–3$ levels in subjects with hyperactivity.[65]

TABLE 4.9
Reference Daily Intake (RDI) — Comparison to DRI

Age		Vit A	Vit C	Vit D	Vit E[a]	Vit K	Thiamin	Riboflavin	Niacin	Vit B6	Folate	Vit B12	Pantothenic Acid	Biotin	Choline
Under 4 years		RDI 2500 IU (758 µg)	RDI 40 mg	RDI 400 IU	RDI 10 IU	RDI None	RDI 0.7 mg	RDI 0.8 mg	RDI 9 mg	RDI 0.7 mg	RDI 200 µg	RDI 3 µg	RDI 5 mg	RDI 150 µg	RDI None
1–3 years		RDA 300 µg	RDA 15 mg	AI 200 IU	RDA 6 mg	AI 30 µg	RDA 0.5 mg	RDA 0.5 mg	RDA 6 mg	RDA 0.5 mg	RDA 150 µg	RDA 0.9 µg	AI 2 mg	AI 8 µg	AI 200 mg
	UL	600 µg	400 mg	2000 IU	200 mg	NA	ND	ND	10 mg	30 mg	300 µg	ND	ND	ND	1.0 mg
Over 4 years (same as adult)		RDI 5000 IU	RDI 60 mg	RDI 400 IU	RDI 30 IU	RDI 80 µg	RDI 1.5 mg	RDI 1.7 mg	RDI 20 mg	RDI 2 mg	RDI 400 µg	RDI 6 µg	RDI 10 mg	RDI 300 µg	RDI None
4–8 years		RDA 400 µg	RDA 25 mg	AI 200 IU	RDA 7 mg	AI 55 µg	RDA 0.6 mg	RDA 0.6 mg	RDA 8 mg	RDA 0.6 mg	RDA 200 µg	RDA 1.2 µg	AI 3 mg	AI 12 µg	AI 250 mg
	UL	900 µg	650 mg	2000 IU	300 mg	NA	ND	ND	15 mg	40 mg	400 µg	ND	ND	ND	1.0 mg

Age	Calcium	Chromium	Copper	Fluoride	Iodine	Iron	Magnesium	Manganese	Molybdenum	Phosphorus	Selenium	Zinc	Potassium	Sodium	Chloride
Under 4 years	RDI 800 mg	RDI None	RDI 1 mg	RDI None	RDI 70 µg	RDI 10 mg	RDI 200 mg	RDI None	RDI None	RDI 800 mg	RDI None	RDI 8 mg	RDI None	RDI None	RDI None
1–3 years	AI 500 mg / UL 2.5 g	AI 11 µg / UL ND	RDA 340 µg / UL 1000 µg	AI 0.7 mg / UL 1.3 mg	RDA 90 µg / UL 200 µg	RDA 7 mg / UL 40 mg	RDA 80 mg / UL 65 mg from pharmaceutical agent (i.e., laxatives) only	AI 1.2 mg / UL 2 mg	RDA 17 µg / UL 300 µg	RDA 460 mg / UL 3 g	RDA 20 µg / UL 90 µg	RDA 3 mg / UL 7 mg	AI 3 g / UL ND	AI 1 g / UL 1.5 g	AI 1.5 g / UL 2.3 g
Over 4 years (same as adult)	RDI 1 g	RDI 120 µg	RDI 2 mg	RDI None	RDI 150 µg	RDI 18 mg	RDI 400 mg	RDI 2 mg	RDI 75 µg	RDI 1 g	RDI 70 µg	RDI 15 mg	RDI	RDI	RDI 3.4 mg
4–8 years	AI 800 mg / UL 2.5 g	AI 15 µg / UL ND	RDA 440 µg / UL 3000 µg	AI 1 mg / UL 2.2 mg	RDA 90 µg / UL 300 µg	RDA 10 mg / UL 40 mg	RDA 130 mg / UL 110 mg from pharmaceutical agent (i.e., laxatives) only	AI 1.5 mg / UL 3 mg	RDA 22 µg / UL 600 µg	RDA 500 mg / UL 3 g	RDA 30 µg / UL 150 µg	RDA 5 mg / UL 12 mg	AI 3.8 g / UL ND	AI 1.2 g / UL 1.9 g	AI 1.9 g / UL 2.9 g

RDI = Value established by the Food and Drug Administration (FDA) for use in nutrition labeling.

Source: From PDR Health, http://www.pdrhealth.com/drug-info/drug-info/nmdrugprofiles/nutsupdrugs/vit-0260.shtml

In an effort to identify a subgroup of ADHD subjects more likely to have EFA deficiencies, researchers measured seven symptoms of EFA deficiency — thirst, frequent urination, dry hair, dandruff, dry skin, follicular keratoses, and brittle nails.[65] Children with evidence of EFA deficiency had a significantly increased incidence of allergic rhinitis, temper tantrums, and problems getting to sleep. Fluid intake was also much higher for ADHD boys with EFA deficiency symptoms. Medication use was not a factor and food intake did not explain the EFA differences.

Decreased cellular concentrations of $20:4n-6$ and $22:6n-3$ cause physiological changes that can lead to behavioral effects. Eicosanoid production may be decreased with inadequate levels of these fatty acids affecting behavior patterns. A lower level of these polyunsaturated fatty acids (PUFAs) could also change cellular membrane fluidity and transport processes, resulting in a myriad of consequences. The authors proposed that decreased concentrations of $20:4n-6$ and $22:6n-3$ could potentially be due to increased metabolism of these fatty acids to eicosanoids or an impaired systemic or cellular transport system.[65] It has also been suggested that a fatty acid deficiency can lead to impaired thyroid function, resulting in reduced production of norepinephrine and altered brain chemistry.[72]

Researchers have tried supplementing ADHD children with gamma-linolenic acid to alleviate behavior problems thought to be associated with EFA imbalances. Two previous studies with primrose oil, supplying gamma-linolenic acid, did not find significant improvements in behavior in subjects with ADHD.[65,69]

Adequate levels of DHA appear to be essential for the optimal functioning of the central nervous system (CNS). Supplementing with $22:6n-3$ (DHA) may have a more direct effect, particularly for ADHD children identified with potential EFA deficiencies. Many studies are demonstrating the necessity of DHA in brain development in the infant and suggest that DHA in the cerebrum is dependent on dietary intake.[73,74]

DHA, the primary PUFA in the brain and CNS, accumulates principally in phosphatidylserine (PS).[75] Recently, PS, a key component of brain tissue, has been recognized for its role in increasing synaptic efficiency and facilitating neurotransmitter release making it of particular interest for conditions like ADHD.[75,76] DHA appears to be a modulator of PS. Researchers at the National Institutes of Health discovered through animal and *in vitro* experiments that a deficiency in $22:6n-3$ results in a decrease in PS synthesis and that synthesis is increased when cells are supplemented with this fatty acid.[75]

In order to increase the DHA and PS levels in the brain, a continuous source of the omega-3-fatty acids must be supplied in the diet. Researchers in Italy examined 20 healthy men and found that supplementation with EPA and DHA significantly increased these PUFAs in plasma fractions and red blood cells. However, after a 3-month washout, only small differences were detectable between levels obtained during treatment and initial values.[77]

Because PS is essential for cellular signaling and other neural cellular processes, it is an important component to consider when examining the nutritional supplement options for the child with ADHD. The link between DHA and PS is of particular interest because DHA is a dietary component notoriously consumed in less than adequate quantities. There is strong evidence of EFA deficiency in at least a subgroup of children with ADHD.

ZINC LINK

Other research suggests that a fatty acid deficiency in ADHD may be due at least in part to a zinc deficiency. In rats, EFA deficiencies are exasperated by a low-zinc intake, possibly due to reduced $\Delta 6$-desaturase activity. A study with 48 ADHD and 45 control children (boys and girls) found the mean free fatty acid (FFA) level was approximately one third less in the ADHD group and a statistically significant correlation was found between reduced zinc and

FFA levels. Significantly lower levels of both FFA and zinc are found in this group of ADHD children. The authors speculate that aggressive behavior and conduct disorder are associated with reduced melatonin and serotonin levels as a result of zinc deficiency.[68] Melatonin has a direct biochemical action on dopaminergic, noradrenergic, and serotonin functions that may be involved with the development of ADHD.[68,78]

Research in the United Kingdom with 20 hyperactive boys and matched controls found hyperactivity associated with low-zinc status. Zinc was measured in urine, scalp hair, serum, 24-h urine, fingernails, and saliva but saliva did not show a statistically significant difference. These researchers also conducted a double-blind placebo-controlled study of the effect of tartrazine (E102), a chemical additive found in commercial orange beverages, on the zinc status of 10 hyperactive boys and 10 controls. In this study, the children received 200 ml of a commercial tartrazine-containing orange beverage. Tartrazine ingestion led to a reduction in serum and saliva zinc concentrations and an increase in urinary zinc. In the hyperactive children, this reduction is correlated with negative behaviors. The authors speculate that the tartrazine may act as a chelating agent with blood zinc, thereby increasing urinary zinc and exacerbating an already depleted zinc status in hyperactive children.[70]

William J. Walsh and colleagues have been conducting ongoing research examining the connection between metal metabolism and aggression in boys. This group has repeatedly found a strong relationship between violent behavior and abnormal blood levels of zinc and copper. Zinc is believed to modulate neurotransmitter and synapse functioning and low levels could alter neuron activity, potentially affecting behavior. Increased blood copper has been associated with hyperactivity. A study by Walsh[79] examined 153 boys, aged 3–20 years, from 27 states and found a significantly higher copper/zinc ratio for the aggressive boys as compared to nonviolent controls.

LEAD POISONING AND HYPERACTIVITY

Physicians have noticed for many years that lead toxicity results in aggressive behavior.[80] Behaviors such as "impulsivity" and "inability to inhibit inappropriate responding" are shown in experimental animals given lead in their drinking water.[81] Studies with rodents have shown that lead interferes with norepinephrine-mediated inhibitory processes, which could lead to impulsivity.[80]

A retrospective cohort study examined a group of 212 public school students in Pittsburgh, Pennsylvania at 7 years old and again at 11 years old. Bone lead was used to determine body lead status and a number of behavioral and neurological tests were performed. Measuring lead in bone is an accurate measurement of long-term lead exposure because lead has an affinity for bone and replaces calcium over time. Researchers found there was a modest relationship between lead levels and behaviors at age 7, as noted by teachers rather than parents. However, by age 11 those children with high-lead scores tended to have a marked decline in appropriate behavior (aggressiveness and antisocial behavior) noticed at home and at school. Children at 11 years of age who were considered asymptomatic for lead toxicity but had elevated bone lead levels were regarded as more aggressive by both teachers and parents as compared with low-lead level counterparts.[80]

Other research with 277 first grade students in Massachusetts public schools examined hair lead levels and determined the relationship of this measurement to attention-deficit behaviors in the classroom. Hair lead levels reflect metal excretion rates during a 4–5-month period. Blood levels can rise and fall during a brief period of time and may not reflect the lead load in the body. A strong association was found between high-lead concentrations in the hair and negative teacher ratings of attentiveness and impulsiveness. A distinct dose–response relationship became apparent between the lead levels and negative teacher ratings indicating that there is not a safe threshold for lead (i.e., one at which no negative effects are found). Further, when children already diagnosed for ADHD were identified, there was an even stronger correlation between lead and this condition. This study not only reinforces the relationship of ADHD with lead toxicity, but also presents an excellent noninvasive technique for identifying children with high lead levels.[82]

Experts studying the effect of lead in children have determined that blood levels as low as 10 μg/dl, a level once considered safe, can result in detectable physical, psychobehavioral, and cognitive deficits. About 12% of children in the United States (3 million) are estimated to have blood lead levels above 10 μg/dl.[82]

Our modern world offers many opportunities for lead exposure. Sources of lead include lead paint chips and dust; lead glazed plates, cups, and eating utensils; home hobbies; air and soil pollution; and drinking water. Many children are exposed to lead as a fetus and then later in life as their hand to mouth behavior increases. Unfortunately, the bodies of young children do not possess the same clearance mechanisms as adults and lead can build up quickly. Sadly, lead exposure peaks during the most inopportune time, between the second and third year of life, when the pruning back of neuronal fibers takes place. Disruption of this process by lead could lead to changes in the brain that may result in inappropriate behavior (responsiveness).[80]

Nutritional remedies that may reduce lead toxicity include zinc, N-acetyl-L-cysteine (NAC), and proanthocyanidin supplementation. NAC, a form of the amino acid, cysteine, is naturally produced in the body and recognized as a precursor to cellular glutathione (GSH). GSH is the body's main defense against free radicals. In addition to its antioxidant effects, NAC is believed to act as a detoxifying and chelating agent, protecting the liver and kidney as well as enhancing elimination of heavy metals.[83-86] The safety of NAC, even with prolonged administration at high doses, is supported by clinical experience and by research.[83] Proanthocyanidins can act as antioxidants, potent free-radical scavengers, and toxic heavy metal chelators.[87,88] Also, the minerals iron, calcium, and zinc will compete with lead for absorption in the intestinal tract so it is important to have an adequate intake of these nutrients.[72]

MAGNESIUM IMPROVES ATTENTION-DEFICIENT HYPERACTIVITY DISORDER SYMPTOMS

Research suggests that magnesium deficiency can lead to or exacerbate ADHD symptoms, such as excessive fidgeting, anxious restlessness, psychomotor instability, and learning difficulties despite a normal IQ.[90] A study in Poland with 50 children diagnosed with ADHD and deficient in magnesium found that supplementation with 200 mg of magnesium for 6 months led to a significant decrease in hyperactivity.[89] Possible reasons for this effect include magnesium's involvement with enzymes necessary for neurotransmitter release, magnesium's role in protecting cell membranes from excitatory neurotransmitters such as glutamate, and important roles of this mineral in the production of energy in the body.[90] Marret et al.[91] suggest that magnesium improves brain fueling of oxygen and glucose.

IRON TREATMENT

Researchers in Israel hypothesized that iron deficiency may play an important role in the etiology of ADHD because iron is involved in the regulation of dopaminergic activity. Hypoactivity of the brain dopaminergic system may be an important factor in the development of ADHD. Iron supplements (Ferrocal equal to 0.05 mg/kg/daily elemental iron) were given to 14 nonanemic boys with ADHD for 30 days. Significant increases in serum ferritin levels and significant decreases in mean parents' behavior scores, but not teachers' scores, were found. This preliminary study suggests that increases in serum ferritin in nonanemic ADHD children may be beneficial and should be studied further.[92]

B COMPLEX VITAMIN SUPPLEMENTATION

Several researchers have discovered that a subset of children diagnosed with ADHD respond well to supplementation of B vitamins, particularly vitamin B_6 (pyridoxine).[93–96] In a 1982 study, Brenner[93] found that pharmacological doses of thiamin or pyridoxine or niacin produced dramatic improvement in symptoms in a small percentage of the study population. For example, Brenner found that of his sample of 100 children, 18 improved and 16 worsened with pharmacological doses of pyridoxine. It appears that particular biochemical parameters may help predict the success of vitamin pharmacological dosing in children with ADHD. Brenner notes that in the group of pyridoxine-responsive children, low blood serotonin, abnormal zinc levels, and increased kryptopyrole were predictive. He also explains that children with normal serotonin levels also responded to treatment with pyridoxine but those with elevated serotonin levels reacted negatively to the vitamin supplement. Brenner states that "(to) date, the biochemical markers denoting vitamin-dependent behavioral disorders have not been clarified." It appears that well-accepted parameters have not yet been identified 17 years later.

Other biochemical connections noted by Brenner include:

- Abnormal tryptophan excretion and pyridoxine deficiency and dependency
- Abnormal creatinine metabolism with thiamin dependency

Brenner admits that "in most instances it was not possible to differentiate on clinical grounds which therapeutic agent would be beneficial to a specific child, suggesting similar neurotransmitter imbalances due to different deficiency states."[93]

Some scientists have found that children who respond well to pyridoxine supplementation tend to have decreased serotonin levels.[93,95] Pyridoxine has been shown to increase serotonin levels, particularly when given in pharmacologic doses.[93–96] However, supplementation with pyridoxine probably will not be effective without the presence of adequate blood levels of zinc and magnesium, which act as cofactors for pyridoxal kinase.[93] When considering the research findings from pharmacological dosing of specific B vitamins, it becomes apparent that there is a multitude of unexplained etiologies (i.e., biochemical imbalances) that may result in the symptoms identified as ADHD.

SUGAR EFFECTS

Although past research could not prove a relationship of sugar intake to hyperactivity and inattentiveness, newer research is identifying unique effects of sugar consumption in ADHD children. Researchers at Yale University measured the metabolic and behavioral response to glucose ingestion in 11 normal and 17 children with ADHD. Based on previous research, epinephrine levels were measured. Children with ADHD had a significantly lower rise in epinephrine levels following the late postprandial fall in plasma glucose,[97] which may lead to behavioral changes. Other research with a similar number of subjects found that sugar ingestion increased inattention, but not aggressiveness, in children with ADHD but not normal controls.[98] Other limited research suggests that children with ADHD have an improvement in symptoms with a high-protein diet versus a high-carbohydrate diet.[99] Based on the research available, it is wise to encourage a diet low in refined sugar with adequate protein and to avoid long periods of time between meals and snacks.

ELIMINATION DIET SUCCESS

A double-blind, placebo-controlled study with 78 children illustrated that a strict elimination diet can improve behaviors in some children with ADHD. Whereas a small number of children reacted to food additives, most of the children with improvements reacted to common foods (such as wheat or dairy products). Irritability appeared to be the most prevalent behavior change with the elimination diet. The authors comment that although this diet is an effective regime for some children, it places a strain on the entire family. They suggest determining if a less restrictive diet can be as effective.[100] Other research found that eliminating reactive foods, particularly those containing artificial colors, had beneficial effects.[71] Children most likely to respond positively to an elimination diet are atopic, have a family history of migraine headaches, are young, and have a parent who noticed a behavioral response to food.[101]

AMINO ACID SUPPLEMENTATION

Researchers have theorized that supplementation with tyrosine or phenylalanine, precursors of the catecholamines, norepinephrine, and dopamine, would help treat catecholamine deficiencies in children with ADHD. No benefit has been found in the existing research.[99]

WILL NUTRITIONAL MODIFICATION HELP CHILDREN WITH ADHD?

It appears that the cause of ADHD probably varies among individuals and thus the response to particular nutritional treatments would differ as well. For some children, mineral deficiencies may cause or precipitate the condition, and for others (or perhaps even the same children) lead toxicity may explain, at least in part, the etiology of ADHD. Still other children with ADHD may have EFA deficiencies or sensitivities to particular foods or additives. There are also other physiological reasons for the condition in many children that are not completely understood at this time.

Current research suggests that many children with ADHD may have nutrient deficiencies, particularly magnesium, zinc, and EFAs. Also, lead toxicity has been strongly linked to ADHD symptoms. It is important for other research to continue to identify subgroups with the ADHD population that will respond well to pharmacological doses of vitamins. Physicians treating children with ADHD should be aware that pharmacological doses of certain B vitamins may be an option that can help prevent the use of long-term drug therapy for treatment of ADHD.

Although there is only preliminary research examining the use of nutritional therapies for the treatment of ADHD, it seems prudent to test some of the research hypotheses regarding many of these nutritional connections.

CONCLUSION

Today children have greater access to a wide variety of foods than ever before but essential vitamins and minerals may still be consumed at inadequate levels. In addition, children are consuming high-saturated fat, *trans*-fat, high-sugar and low-fiber, and low-fruit and vegetable diets — an inadequate profile of macronutrients. Conversely, caloric intake is increasing, energy expenditure is decreasing, and obesity and the risk of chronic diseases in children are skyrocketing. Childhood health and future wellness depends greatly on balanced micro- and macronutrient intake during the formative years. Modifying micro- and macronutrients may also be a useful way to treat common childhood conditions such as ADHD. Health professionals are challenged with this dilemma as well as interpreting future research to determine what traditional and alternative resources are available to help solve health problems among children. Once the resources have been identified, the key challenge becomes to educate children on how and why to make appropriate health choices which may prevent obesity and chronic diseases and promote health and wellness.

REFERENCES

1. Gartner, L.M. et al., American Academy of Pediatrics Section on Breastfeeding. Breastfeeding and the use of human milk, *Pediatrics*, 115, 496, 2005.
2. Zeiger, R.S., Food allergen avoidance in the prevention of food allergy in infants and children, *Pediatrics*, 111, 1662, 2003.
3. Oddy, W.H., The impact of breast milk on infant and child health, *Breastfeed Rev.*, 10, 18, 2002.
4. Arifeen, A. et al., Exclusive breastfeeding reduces acute respiratory infection and diarrhea death among infants in Dhake slums, *Pediatrics*, 108, E67, 2001.
5. Samour, P.Q., Helm, K.K., and Lang, C.E., Eds., *Handbook of Pediatric Nutrition*, 2nd ed., Aspen Publishers, Inc., Maryland, 2003.
6. Sears, W. and Sears, M., *The Family Nutrition Book*, Little, Brown and Company, Boston, 1999.
7. Kramer, M.S. and Kakuma, R., The optimal duration of exclusive breastfeeding: a systematic review, *Adv. Exp. Med. Biol.*, 554, 63, 2004.
8. Walker, W.A., The dynamic effects of breastfeeding on intestinal development and host defense, *Adv. Exp. Med. Biol.*, 554, 155, 2004.
9. Yurdakok, K. et al., Efficacy of daily and weekly iron supplementation on iron status in exclusively breast-fed infants, *J. Pediatr. Hematol. Oncol.*, 26, 284, 2004.
10. Friel, J.K. et al., A double-masked, randomized control trial of iron supplementation in early infancy in healthy term breast-fed infants, *J. Pediatr.*, 13, 582, 2003.
11. Nagpal, J. et al., A randomized placebo-controlled trial of iron supplementation in breastfed young infants initiated on complementary feeding: effect on haematological status, *J. Health Popul. Nutr.*, 22, 203, 2004.
12. Aggarwal, D. et al., Haematological effect of iron supplementation in breast fed term low birth weight infants, *Arch. Dis. Child.*, 90, 26, 2005.
13. Collier, S., Fulhan, J., and Duggan, C., Nutrition for the pediatric office: update on vitamins, infant feeding and food allergies, *Curr. Opin. Pediatr.*, 16, 314, 2004.
14. Wharton, B.A. et al., Low plasma taurine and later neurodevelopment, *Arch. Dis. Child. Fetal Neonatal Ed.*, 89, F497, 2004.
15. Frits, A.J. et al., Is docosahexaenoic acid (DHA) essential? Lessons from DHA status regulation, our ancient diet, epidemiology and randomized controlled trials, *J. Nutr.*, 134, 183, 2004.
16. Gibson, R.A., Neumann, M.A., and Makrides, M., Effect of dietary docosahexaenoic acid on brain composition and neural function in term infants, *Lipids*, 31, S177, 1996.
17. Birch, E.E. et al., Visual maturation of term infants fed long-chain polyunsaturated fatty acid-supplemented or control formula for 12 mo, *Am. J. Clin. Nutr.*, 81, 871, 2005.
18. Chen, A.C. et al., Genistein inhibits intestinal cell proliferation in piglets, *Pediatr. Res.*, 57, 192, 2005.
19. Davidsson, L. et al., Iron bioavailability studied in infants: the influence of phytic acid and ascorbic acid in infant formulas based on soy isolate, *Pediatr. Res.*, 36(6), 816, 1994.
20. Takser, L. et al., Manganese, monoamine metabolite levels at birth, and child psychomotor development, *Neurotoxicology*, 24, 667, 2003.

21. Savino, F. et al., "Minor" feeding problems during the first months of life: effect of a partially hydrolysed milk formula containing fructo- and galacto-oligosaccharides, *Acta Paediatr. Suppl.*, 91, 86, 2003.

22. Verwimp, J.J. et al., Symptomatology and growth in infants with cow's milk protein intolerance using two different whey-protein hydrolysate based formulas in a primary health care setting, *Eur. J. Clin. Nutr.*, 49, S39, 1995.

23. Giampietro, P.G. et al., Hypoallergenicity of an extensively hydrolyzed whey formula, *Pediatr. Allergy Immunol.*, 12, 83, 2001.

24. Atkinson, M.A. and Ellis, T.M., Infant diets and insulin-dependent diabetes: evaluating the "cow's milk hypothesis" and a role for anti-bovine serum albumin immunity, *J. Am. Coll. Nutr.*, 16, 334, 1997.

25. Kleinman, R.E., American Academy of Pediatrics recommendations for complementary feeding, *Pediatrics*, 106, 1274, 2000.

26. Committee on Nutrition, American Academy of Pediatrics: the use and misuse of fruit juice in pediatrics, *Pediatrics*, 107, 1210, 2001.

27. Dennison, B.A., Rockwell, H.L., and Baker, S.L., Excess fruit juice consumption by preschool-aged children is associated with short stature and obesity, *Pediatrics*, 99, 15, 1997.

28. Moyer, V. et al., North American Society for Pediatric Gastroenterology, Hepatology and Nutrition. Guideline for the evaluation of cholestatic jaundice in infants: recommendations of the North American Society for Pediatric Gastroenterology, Hepatology and Nutrition, *J. Pediatr. Gastroenterol. Nutr.*, 39, 115, 2004.

29. Morrow, A.L. and Rangel, J.M., Human milk protection against infectious diarrhea: implications for prevention and clinical care, *Semin. Pediatr. Infect. Dis.*, 15, 221, 2004.

30. Hugger, J., Harkless, G., and Rentschler, D., Oral rehydration therapy for children with acute diarrhea, *Nurse Pract.*, 23, 52, 1998.

31. Saavedra, J., Probiotic and infectious diarrhea, *Am. J. Gastroenterol.*, 95, S16, 2000.

32. Chouraqui, J.P., Van Egroo, L.D., and Fichot, M.C., Acidified milk formula supplemented with bifidobacterium lactis: impact on infant diarrhea in residential care settings, *J. Pediatr. Gastroenterol. Nutr.*, 38, 288, 2004.

33. Liepke, C. et al., Human milk provides peptides highly stimulating the growth of bifidobacteria, *Eur. J. Biochem.*, 269, 712, 2002.

34. Obden, C.L. et al., Prevalence and trends in overweight among US children and adolescents, 1999–2000. *JAMA*, 288, 1728, 2002.

35. Freedman, D.S. et al., The relation of overweight to cardiovascular risk factors among children and adolescents: The Bogulasa Heart Study, *Pediatrics*, 103, 1175, 1999.

36. Dietz, W.H., Health consequences of obesity in youth: childhood predictors of adult disease, *Pediatrics*, 101, 518, 1998.

37. Daniels, S.R. et al., AHA Scientific Statement. Overweight in children and adolescents: pathophysiology, consequences, prevention, and treatment, *Circulation*, 111, 1999, 2005.

38. Odgen, C.L. et al., Prevalence and trends in overweight among US children and adolescents, 1999–2000, *JAMA*, 288, 1728, 2002.

39. Matsushita, Y. et al., Trends in childhood obesity in Japan over the last 25 years from the National Nutrition Survey, *Obesity Res.*, 12, 205, 2004.

40. del Rio-Navarro, B. et al., The high prevalence of overweight and obesity in Mexican children, *Obesity Res.*, 12, 215, 2004.

41. Strauss, R.S., Childhood obesity and self-esteem, *Pediatrics*, 105, 1, 2000. Available at http://pediatrics.aappublications.org/cgi/content/full/105/1/e15

42. Holcomb, S.S., Obesity in children and adolescents: guidelines for prevention and management, *Nurse Pract.*, 29, 9, 2004.

43. Dietz, W.H., Overweight in childhood and adolescence, *N. Engl. J. Med.*, 350, 855, 2004.

44. Reilly, M.L. et al., Obesity: diagnosis, prevention, and treatment; evidence based answers to common questions, *Arch. Dis. Child.*, 86, 392, 2002.

45. Gidding, S.S. et al., Understanding obesity in youth, *Circulation*, 94, 3383, 1996.

46. Weizman, Z. et al., Efficacy of herbal tea preparation in infantile colic, *J. Pediatr.*, 122, 650, 1993.

47. Lucassen, P.L., Effectiveness of treatments for infantile colic: systematic review, *Br. Med. J.*, 316, 1563, 1998. Taken from http://www.med.umich.edu/1 libr/yourchild/colic.htm

48. Cryan, J. and Johnson, R.K., Should the current recommendations for energy intake in infants and young children be lowered? *Nutr. Today*, 32, 69,1997.

49. IOM Dietary Reference Intakes, http://www.iom.edu/project.asp?id=4574

50. Ascherio, A. et al., *Trans* fatty acids and coronary heart disease, *N. Engl. J. Med.*, 340, 1994, 1999.

51. Mohamedain, M.M. and Kummerow, F.A., Hydrogenated fat high in *trans* monoenes with an adequate level of linoleic acid has no effect on prostaglandin synthesis in rats, *J. Nutr.*, 129, 15, 1999.

52. U.S. Department of Agriculture, Agricultural Research Service, Data tables, results from USDA's 1994–96 continuing survey of food intakes by individuals and 1994–96 diet and health knowledge survey (online), ARS Food Surveys Research Group. Available at http://www.barc.usda.gov/bhnrc/foodsurvey/home.htm

53. Johnston, C.C. et al., Calcium supplementation and increases in bone mineral density in children, *N. Engl. J. Med.*, 327, 82, 1992.

54. Kim, M., Kim, C., and Song, I., Analysis of lead in 55 brands of dietary calcium supplements by graphite furnace atomic absorption spectrometry after microwave digestion, *Food Addit. Contam.*, 20, 149, 2003.

55. Wright, R.O. et al., Association between iron deficiency and blood lead level in a longitudinal analysis of children followed in an urban primary care clinic, *J. Pediatr.*, 142, 9, 2003.

56. Kwong, W.T., Friello, P., and Semba, R.D., Interactions between iron deficiency and lead poisoning: epidemiology and pathogenesis, *Sci. Total Environ.*, 330, 21, 2004.

57. Konofal, E. et al., Iron deficiency in children with attention-deficit/hyperactivity disorder, *Arch. Pediatr. Adolesc. Med.*, 158, 1113, 2004.

58. Bhatnagar, S. and Natchu, U.C., Zinc in child health and disease, *Indian J. Pediatr.*, 71, 991, 2004.

59. Williams, C.L. and Bollella, M., Is a high fiber diet safe for children? *Pediatrics*, 96, 1014S, 1995.

60. Arsenault, J.E. and Brown, K.H., Zinc intake of US preschool children exceeds new dietary reference intakes, *Am. J. Clin. Nutr.*, 78, 1011, 2003.

61. PDR Health, http://www.pdrhealth.com/drug_info/nmdrugprofiles/nutsupdrugs/vit_0260.shtml

62. Ballew, C. et al., Serum retinol distributions in residents of the United States: third National Health and Nutrition Examination Survey, 1988–1994, *Am. J. Clin. Nutr.*, 73, 586, 2001.

63. Stephens, D., Jackson, P.L., and Gutierrez, Y., Subclinical vitamin A deficiency: a potentially unrecognized problem in the United States, *Pediatr. Nurs.*, 22, 377, 1996.

64. Institute of Medicine, *Dietary Reference Intakes: Applications in Dietary Assessment (2000)*, National Academy of Sciences, Washington, D.C., 2000.

65. Stevens, L.J. et al., Essential fatty acid metabolism in boys with attention-deficit hyperactivity disorder, *Am. J. Clin. Nutr.*, 62, 761, 1995.

66. Kozielec, T. and Starobrat-Hermelin, B., Assessment of magnesium levels in children with attention deficit hyperactivity disorder (ADHD), *Magn. Res.*, 10, 143, 1997.

67. Kaneko, M. et al., Hypothalamic–pituitary–adrenal axis function in children with attention deficit hyperactivity disorder, *J. Autism Dev. Disord.*, 23, 59, 1993.

68. Bekaroglu, M. et al., Relationships between serum free fatty acids and zinc, and attention deficit hyperactivity disorder: a research note, *J. Child Psychol. Psychiatry*, 37, 225, 1996.

69. Mitchell, E.A. et al., Clinical characteristics and serum essential fatty acid levels in hyperactive children, *Clin. Pediatr.*, 26, 406, 1987.

70. Ward, N.I. et al., The influence of the chemical additive tartrazine on the zinc status of hyperactive children — a double-blind placebo-controlled study, *J. Nutr. Med.*, 1, 51, 1990.

71. Boris, M. and Mandel, F.S., Foods and additives are common causes of the attention deficit hyperactive disorder in children, *Ann. Allergy*, 72, 462, 1994.

72. Lombard, J. and Germano, C., *The Brain Wellness Plan*, Kensington Publishing Corporation, New York, 1997.

73. Gibson, R.A. et al., Effect of dietary docosahexaenoic acid on brain composition and neural function in term infants, *Lipids*, 31, S177, 1996.

74. Willatts, P. et al., Effect of long-chain polyunsaturated fatty acids in infant formula on problem solving at 10 months of age, *Lancet*, 352, 688, 1998.

75. Garcia, M.C. et al., Effect of docosahexaenoic acid on the synthesis of phosphatidylserine in rat brain microsomes and C6 glioma cells, *J. Neurochem.*, 70, 24, 1998.

76. Rosadini, G. et al., Phosphatidylserine: quantitative EEG effects in healthy volunteers, *Neuropsychobiology*, 24, 42, 1990–91.

77. Prisco, D., Filippini, M., and Francalanci, I., Effect of $n-3$ polyunsaturated fatty acid intake on phospholipid fatty acid composition in plasma and erythrocytes. *Am. J. Clin. Nutr.*, 63, 925, 1996.

78. Sandyk, R., Zinc deficiency in attention-deficit hyperactivity disorder, *Int. J. Neurosci.*, 52, 239, 1990.

79. Walsh, W.J. et al., Elevated blood copper/zinc ratios in assaultive young males, *Physiol. Behav.* 62, 327, 1997.

80. Needleman, H.L. et al., Bone lead levels and delinquent behavior, *JAMA*, 275, 363, 1996.

81. Brockel, B.J. and Cory-Slechta, D.A., The effects of postweaning low-level Pb exposure on sustained attention: a study of target densities, stimulus presentation rate, and stimulus predictability, *Neurotoxicology*, 20, 921, 1999.

82. Tuthill, R.W., Hair lead levels related to children's classroom attention-deficit behavior, *Arch. Environ. Health*, 51, 214, 1996.

83. Faintuch, J., Aguilar, P., and Nadalin, W., Relevance of *N*-acetylcysteine in clinical practice: fact, myth or consequence? *Nutrition*, 15, 177, 1999.

84. Kelly, G.S., Clinical applications of *N*-acetylcysteine, *Altern. Med. Rev.*, 3, 114, 1998.

85. Meyer, A., Buhl, R., and Magnussen, H., The effect of oral *N*-acetylcysteine on lung glutathione levels in idiopathic pulmonary fibrosis, *Eur. Respir. J.*, 7, 431, 1994.

86. Lauterburg, B., Corcoran, G., and Mitchell, J., Mechanism of action of *N*-acetylcysteine in the protection against the hepatotoxicity of acetaminophen in rats *in vivo*, *J. Clin. Invest.*, 71, 980, 1983.

87. Bagchi, D., Garg, A., and Krohn, R., Protective effects of grape seed proanthocyanidins and selected antioxidants against TPA-induced hepatic and brain lipid peroxidation and DNA fragmentation, and peritoneal macrophage activation in mice, *Gen. Pharmacol.*, 30, 771, 1998.

88. Werbach, M.R. and Murray, M.T., *Botanical Influences on Illness*, Third Line Press, Tarzana, CA, 1994.

89. Starobrat-Hermelin, B. and Kozielec, T., The effects of magnesium physiological supplementation on hyperactivity in children with attention deficit hyperactivity disorder (ADHD). Positive response to magnesium oral loading test, *Magn. Res.*, 10, 149, 1997.

90. Shils, M.E. et al., Eds., *Modern Nutrition in Health and Disease*, Lea & Febiger, Philadelphia, 1999.

91. Marret, S. et al., Prevention by magnesium of excitotoxic neuronal death in the developing brain: an animal model for clinical intervention studies, *Dev. Med. Child Neurol.*, 37, 473, 1995.

92. Sever, Y. et al., Iron treatment in children with attention deficit hyperactivity disorder. A preliminary report, *Neuropsychobiology*, 35, 178, 1997.

93. Brenner, A., The effects of megadoses of selected B complex vitamins on children with hyperkinesis: controlled studies with long-term follow-up, *J. Learning Dis.*, 15, 258, 1982.

94. Bernstein, A.L., Vitamin B6 in clinical neurology, *Ann. NY Acad. Sci.*, 585, 250, 1990.

95. Coleman, M. et al., A preliminary study of the effect of pyridoxine administration in a subgroup of hyperkinetic children: a double-blind crossover comparison with methylphenidate, *Biol. Psychiatry*, 14, 741, 1979.

96. Bhagavan, H., Coleman, M., and Coursin, D., The effect of pyridoxine hydrochloride on blood serotonin and pyridoxal phosphate contents in hyperactive children, *Pediatrics*, 55, 437, 1975.

97. Girardi, N.L. et al., Blunted catecholamine responses after glucose ingestion in children with attention deficit disorder, *Pediatr. Res.*, 38, 539, 1995.

98. Wender, E.H., Effects of sugar on aggressive and inattentive behavior in children with attention deficit disorder with hyperactivity and normal children, *Pediatrics*, 88, 960, 1991.
99. Werbach, M., *Nutritional Influences on Mental Illness*, Third Line Press, Tarzana, CA, 1991.
100. Carter, C.M. et al., Effects of a few food diet in attention deficit disorder, *Arch. Dis. Child.*, 69, 564, 1993.
101. Breakey, J., The role of diet and behavior in childhood, *J. Paediatr. Child Health*, 33, 190, 1997.

5 Adolescence

Mary Marian, Richard Wahl, and John D. Mark

CONTENTS

INTRODUCTION

Adolescence, the time period that begins the transition from childhood to adulthood, around age of 11 years, is a time of dramatic change. Physical, developmental, and psychological changes influence the adolescent's lifestyle habits placing this segment of the population at nutritional risk due to a number of reasons. First, nutrient needs are greater than at any other time in the life cycle and inadequate nutrient intake can negatively impact on growth and development. Second, the eating practices of teens tend to result in diets inadequate in many of the key nutrients required not only for normal growth and development, but also for the prevention of chronic disease in adulthood. Lastly, adolescents are increasingly diagnosed with chronic diseases, such as obesity, type 2 diabetes, and hypertension, that were previously uncommon in this population. Other nutritional challenges include teens participating in sports, following vegetarian diets, and using complementary and alternative therapies.

REVIEW OF NORMAL GROWTH AND DEVELOPMENT

GROWTH EXPECTATIONS

Adolescence is a time of rapid growth and development. The rates of gain in both weight and height are second only to that seen in the first year of life. During puberty, adolescents gain 50% of their adult weight, 50% of their skeletal mass and bone mineralization, and 20% of their final adult height.[1] Lean body mass doubles in adolescent boys, while adolescent girls normally have twice the body fat deposition during this time period than do boys (see Table 5.1).[2]

As the growth spurt winds down, boys will be on average 12–13 cm taller than girls. Peak height velocity (PHV) begins 1.5–2.0 years earlier for girls, but averages 2 cm/year less for girls than boys.[2]

Pubertal weight gain accounts for 50% of the ideal adult body weight. Peak weight velocity (PWV) varies greatly, but averages 4.6–10.6 kg/year for girls and 5.7–13.2 kg/year for boys. PWV occurs 6–9 months after PHV in girls, and coincides with PHV in boys.

PHYSIOLOGIC DEVELOPMENT

The trigger for the onset of puberty is not completely understood, but appears to be related to decreased sensitivity of the hypothalamus and pituitary gland to circulating sex hormones, resulting in increased levels of luteinizing hormone (LH) and follicle-stimulating hormone (FSH) in both boys and girls. The presence of increased levels of ovarian and testicular hormones results in rapid growth and secondary sexual development. Tanner (and others) has identified specific stages of sexual maturation, often called Tanner Stages.[3,4] As usually characterized, Stage I in both sexes represents prepubertal development, while Stage V identifies full adult

TABLE 5.1
Prepubertal Growth Rates

First year of life	25 cm/year
Second year	10 cm/year
Third year	8 cm/year
Fourth year	7 cm/year
5–10 years	5–6 cm/year

Pubertal Growth Spurt
Girls 9 cm/year (range 5.4–11.2 cm/year) = 23–28 cm total
Boys 10.3 cm/year (range 5.8–13.1 cm/year) = 26–28 cm total

TABLE 5.2
Body Fat Deposition Based on Pubertal Stage

Pubertal Stage	Body Fat Percentage
Girls: T-I	15.7
II	18.9
III	21.6
IV–V	26.7
Boys: T-I	14.3
II–V	11.2

---

development.[4] In boys, these stages identify changes in pubic hair appearance and genital growth, while in girls these stages identify pubic hair appearance and breast development.[3]

Pubertal growth patterns result in dramatic changes in body composition. Lean body mass increases during growth in both boys and girls, but the combination of greater adipose tissue deposition in girls and the anabolic effects of androgens in boys results in a decrease in relative lean body mass (as a percentage of total body weight) in girls and an increase in boys (see Table 5.2).[2]

PSYCHOLOGICAL/COGNITIVE DEVELOPMENT

Adolescence is commonly divided into three stages: early adolescence (11–14 years), middle adolescence (15–18 years), and late adolescence (19–21+ years), corresponding roughly to junior high or middle school, high school, and post-high school periods.

Early adolescents are usually functioning at the "concrete operational" level, as identified by Piaget.[5] These younger teens will have very concrete or literal thought processes. Discussions with these young adolescents often must be on a literal basis to avoid misunderstanding.

Middle adolescence is a time of transition to Piaget's "formal operational" thought. Older teens are better able to handle abstractions, and take a less concrete or literal approach to understanding the world.

By late adolescence, most young adults have attained formal operational thought, and can understand more difficult abstractions. Many studies have shown, however, that a certain proportion of adults maintain a concrete operational interpretation throughout their lives. Keeping these developmental stages in mind as you discuss nutritional issues with adolescents will help to avoid misunderstanding, such as when a teen takes your more metaphorical statement quite literally.[6]

ADOLESCENT EATING PRACTICES

As a child becomes an adolescent, eating habits and behaviors tend to change as a variety of environmental and social factors influence food choices. Eating habits are characterized by skipping meals, eating on the run, consuming more meals from fast-food establishments, and fad dieting. Greater independence, developing decision-making skills, time pressures, greater involvement in activities away from home, financial independence, peers, body image, and less reliance of parents for transportation and meal are factors that influence their meal times and food choices. Taste and appeal of food are the prime reasons affecting food selections followed by time and convenience.[10] Teens also tend to rebel against the traditional ways of doing things or the norm. This may be of concern when teens should be adhering to special dietary recommendations due to health reasons [e.g., insulin-dependent diabetes mellitus (IDDM), renal disease].

Adolescents are the largest segment of snackers and grazers in the U.S. population, and skipping breakfast is common practice.[11,12] Studies report that between 20% and 40% of adolescents skip breakfast on any given day,[10] resulting in a lower total daily intake for calories, vitamins, and minerals compared with those who eat breakfast.[1–13] Snacks from vending machines, snack bars, and fast-food establishments are frequent targets of choice for eating on the go. Teens spend more than $5.4 billion in fast-food restaurants and more than $9.6 billion on food and snacks yearly.[14,25]

Although adolescents reportedly know the importance of nutrition and what foods they should and should not eat, this knowledge does not readily translate into practice as many studies show adolescents have poor eating habits. The Bogalusa Heart Study analysis reveals that adolescent diets are often deficient in vitamins A, B_6, E, D, and C as well as folic acid.[13] Minerals such as iron, zinc, calcium, and magnesium are also likely to be deficient. Less than 10% of the adolescent population reports taking a daily multivitamin or mineral supplement.[13] Fruit or fruit juice, vegetable, and milk intake steadily decline with an increased intake in sodas from childhood to adolescence.[16]

Fat consumption during adolescence is associated with an increased risk for chronic diseases such as coronary heart disease (CHD) and some cancers in adulthood while a low calcium intake is linked to low bone density and increased risk for osteoporosis. National dietary data shows that only 34% of adolescent females and 27% of adolescent males meet the estimated recommendation for limiting saturated fat intake. Furthermore, only 36% of girls and 30% of boys aged 12–19 years meet recommended national guidelines for total fat intake.[17] National Health and Nutrition Examination Survey (NHANES) III data revealed that adolescent intake of sodium also exceeded recommended guidelines as adolescent boys tend to consume 4000–5000 mg/day while adolescent girls consume about 3000 mg/day compared to the national recommendation of 2400 mg/day.[18] Excessive intakes for saturated fat, total fat, and sodium are similar across all ethnicities and income levels.

Adolescents also fail to meet national recommendations for daily servings of fruits and vegetables. CSFII data reveals that 23% of girls and 22% of boys eat two or more daily servings of fruit while only 38% of girls and 55% of boys consume at least three servings of vegetables daily.[19] This is of concern since fruits and vegetables are low in fat and good sources of various micronutrients, phytonutrients, and fiber, all of which have been tied to a reduced risk for developing CHD, some cancers, and hypertension.

According to NHANES III data, to meet the recommended daily intake levels for fiber (daily fiber requirement = age + 5 = total fiber grams goal), adolescents would need to increase their fiber intake by 25–50%.[17,18] This is also of importance since fiber intake has been inversely associated with risk for CHD and certain types of cancer.

Table 5.3 reflects barriers and promoters of health promotion in the adolescent population. Teens report that time is their biggest barrier to consuming a health diet as they are too busy to think about specifics related to diet and meal planning.[20] Nutrition counseling that will promote dietary changes and promote health through risk reduction should focus on the multitude of factors that impact on their time and food choices. Recommendations for program development are discussed later in this chapter.

ASSESSING GROWTH

Childhood and adolescence are a time of rapid changes in height and weight, and it is important to have access to a longitudinal record of growth for any given teen. Changes in growth rate, either above or below that expected, can signal the beginnings of a significant health problem.

TABLE 5.3
Barriers and Promoters of Health Promotion

Barriers	Promoters
Economic status	Affordable
Social support	Social support
Culture	Culturally appropriate
Education	Education
Information irrelevant	Personally relevant
Poor self-esteem	Self-esteem

Health care providers routinely monitor height and weight during childhood using standard growth charts (see Appendix F). This practice remains very important during the adolescent years, as is the determination of body mass index (BMI).

Teens should be weighed without shoes or heavy clothing, using a balance beam. A useful formula for older adolescents for calculating ideal body weight based on height is:

Males: 5 ft = 106 lb + 6 lb per additional inch

Females: 5 ft = 100 lb + 5 lb per additional inch

Height measurements should be made with the adolescent barefoot, using a wall-mounted stadiometer, with heels pressed against the wall.[2]

The BMI offers the best assessment of weight for height. The formula for calculating the BMI is

$$BMI = \frac{weight\,(kg)}{height^2\,(m^2)}$$

General guidelines for interpreting BMI in older adolescents are noted in Table 5.4.[21]

Adolescents with a weight for height < 5th percentile or BMI less than normal may be undernourished and should receive a comprehensive nutrition assessment and be evaluated for the presence of any medical conditions. Conversely, adolescents with a BMI > 85th percentile are considered at risk for becoming overweight while a BMI > 95th percentile defines the adolescent as overweight.

Nutritional status plays an integral role in growth and thus should be assessed in conjunction with an assessment of growth. The foundation for the provision of optimal

---

TABLE 5.4
Body Mass Index and Ideal Body Weight

BMI	% Ideal Body Mass
17	75
18	85
20–26	Normal
27–35	120–135
35–42	135–200
>42	>200

---

medical nutrition therapy is a comprehensive nutritional assessment, which includes four components: diet history, anthropometric measurements, biochemical evaluation, and evaluation of clinical and physical status. These four components, together with the clinician's expertise, provide direction for development of the nutrition care plan. Nutrition assessment data, along with growth, should be reevaluated on an ongoing basis for monitoring and improving or maintaining nutritional status.

NUTRITIONAL REQUIREMENTS

Except for the first 2 years of life, there is no time when growth and development are as rapid as during the early teen years. Puberty begins at different times for girls (range 8–13 years of age) than for boys (range 9.5–13.5 years of age), as well as varies widely among these ages.[22] These differences in growth influence self-image and identity.

Beginning at about 10 years of age, girls start their growth spurt with PWV occurring about 6–9 months prior to PHV.[23] From ages 10 to 17 years, girls on average gain about 24 kg (~42% of adult weight). The onset of menses occurs once a critical body weight or body fatness is obtained.[24] This is also a peak time of caloric consumption (~2500 kcal/day) for girls.

Nutritional needs increase markedly due to the doubling of body mass. Girls also experience an increase in the width of the hips associated with a broadening pelvic girth and an increase in fat deposition. The size of many of the abdominal organs also increases. Shortly after adult height is reached, muscle mass peaks.

Adolescents with acute and chronic illnesses may experience a decrease in growth and activity during illness. Additional needs for calories and protein may be required to promote catch-up growth and should be included in nutritional goals.

ENERGY

Energy needs for adolescents are substantial in order to meet the need for rapid growth and sexual maturation. This period of rapid growth is only secondary to growth through infancy. Energy needs differ between males and females based on age and individual growth rates. Table 5.5 exhibits various methods available to estimate adolescent energy needs.

The recommended daily allowances (RDAs) for energy of adolescents, as shown in Table 5.5, are commonly used in clinical practice to determine calorie needs. The RDAs are the average daily dietary intake level that is sufficient to meet the nutrient needs of nearly all healthy people (97–98%).[25] Teen energy needs, however, may vary based on growth rates, body composition, physical activity levels, and general overall health. Because it is difficult to know precisely what the energy needs for a teen are, the RDAs are categorized based on chronological age versus maturation. Therefore, the clinician must consider where the teen is in the growth and sexual maturity continuum when applying the RDAs to an individual. Additionally, the RDAs have a safety factor build in; therefore, if an individual's needs are less than or greater than the calculated RDA, this may be acceptable. On the other hand, energy intake for females has been found to correlate with stage of development (prepubescent, rapidly growing, and postpubescent) rather than age. Hence, using height as the preferred index for determining energy needs has also been advocated.[26]

Estimating energy needs for hospitalized adolescents presents a challenge as no consensus currently exists as to which method is the best. Calculating resting energy expenditure (REE) from the World Health Organization (WHO) or utilizing other equations for predicting REE from body weight as shown in Table 5.5 are available.[27]

TABLE 5.5
Methods for Calculating Energy Requirements for Adolescents

Dietary Reference Intakes
Age of females (years)
| | |
9–13   2070 kcal/day
14–18   2370 kcal/day
Age of males (years)
9–13   2280 kcal/day
14–18   3150 kcal/day

Energy needs based on height
Age of females (years)
11–14   14.0 kcal/cm
15–18   13.5 kcal/cm
Age of males (years)
11–14   16.0 kcal/cm
15–18   17.0 kcal/cm

Equations for predicting REE (WHO)
Age of females (years)
10–18 $(12.2 \times \text{wt (kg)}) + 746 = \text{kcal/day}$
Age of males (years)
10–18 $(17.5 \times \text{wt (kg)}) + 651 = \text{kcal/day}$
Harris–Benedict equation (recommended for ages >15 years)
Females: $655.1 + 9.65 \, (\text{wt in kg}) + 1.85 \, (\text{height in cm}) - 4.68 \, (\text{age}) = \text{kcal/day}$
Males: $66.42 + 13.75 \, (\text{wt in kg}) + 5 \, (\text{height in cm}) - 6.78 \, (\text{age}) = \text{kcal/day}$

Source: From National Academy of Sciences, *Recommended Dietary Allowances*, 10th ed., National Academy Press, Washington, D.C., 2002.

PROTEIN

Although protein requirements increase for adolescents to meet the needs for growth, the average protein intake for U.S. teens is reportedly in excess of needs.[28] Using the RDA for protein based on height (see Table 5.6) has been recommended for estimating needs to parallel increased needs related to growth. Protein needs may be further altered by the presence of disease or other medical conditions and should be taken into consideration when estimating protein requirements. Declines in energy consumption, related to inappropriate dieting practices or severe energy restriction, illness or trauma, or food security, may also result in diminished consumption of protein. This in turn may result in loss of lean body mass and declines in growth.

MICRONUTRIENTS

The need for micronutrients parallels that of growth, thereby resulting in an increased requirement for vitamins, minerals, and trace elements, with the exception of vitamin D and iron, for children starting at the age of 9 years. Vitamin D requirements remain unchanged. Various micronutrients have been shown to play a role in the development of chronic diseases such as coronary artery disease, hypertension, osteoporosis, and anemia. Although food consumption increases during adolescence compared to childhood, adolescent diets often exclude foods such as fruits, vegetables, whole grains, and dairy products, providers of various important micronutrients.[13] Consequently, adolescent diets tend to be deficient in vitamins A, B_6, E, D, and C as well as folic acid.[17] Minerals such as iron, zinc, calcium, and magnesium also have been found to be low.[13,17]

TABLE 5.6
Recommended Daily Protein Intake

Age (years)	Based on Weight (g/kg/day)	Based on Height (g/cm)
Females		
9–13	0.95	0.29
14–18	0.85	0.26
Males		
9–13	0.95	0.28
14–18	0.85	0.33

Source: From Institute of Medicine, *Recommended Dietary Allowances*, 10th ed., National Academy Press, Washington, D.C., 2002.

VITAMINS

The requirements for the B vitamins, thiamin, riboflavin, and niacin increase in relation to increase in energy needs while the requirements for the other vitamins (A, C, E, folic acid, B_6, and B_{12}) increase relative to increased demands for cellular synthesis and tissue growth. Because of the important role that folic acid plays in preventing fetal neural tube defects, adolescent girls of childbearing age should be encouraged to consume foods rich in folic acid or consume a daily multivitamin supplement to meet the RDA of 400 μg/day.

In Bogalusa Heart Study, mean intakes of thiamin, riboflavin, niacin, folic acid, vitamins A, C, B_6, and B_{12} were greater for adolescents who consumed ready-to-eat cereals, compared to those not consuming cereals.[13] Additionally, teens eating cereals generally consumed at least two thirds of the RDA for vitamin A, B_6, B_{12}, C, D, thiamin, riboflavin, and folic acid compared to the nonconsumers. Daily use of a general multivitamin–mineral supplement may be indicated if the diet history reveals continued deficits of key vitamins and minerals.

MINERALS

Calcium

Dietary surveillance data consistently shows that teens, especially females, do not consume adequate amounts of calcium. The NHANES III data show a decline in calcium intake when compared with NHANES II data (see Table 5.7).[29] Over 28 million people, 80% women, in the United States reportedly have low bone density or osteoporosis. The economic burden as a result is great as approximately $10 billion is spent annually on related conditions.[30] Since there is no cure, prevention is paramount. Recently new recommendations for adolescents

TABLE 5.7
Adolescent Calcium Intake Data

Age (years)	NHANES II (1976–1980) (mg/day)	NHANES III (1988–1991) (mg/day)
12–15	854	796
16–19	725	822

regarding adequate calcium intake were established at a time when most adolescents were not meeting the old guidelines. Since adolescence is a critical time period for amassing bone density, maintaining adequate calcium nutriture is thought to be critical during this time to maximize bone health. However, in their review of the literature, Lanou et al. found that the majority of controlled trials investigating dairy supplementation or total dietary calcium intake show that increasing dairy or total dietary calcium consumption is not associated with or is a predictor of bone mineral density of fracture.[31] Conversely, other studies have reported a positive effect of an increased intake of either dairy products or calcium supplementation.[32,33] The data is also conflicting whether the gains in bone accretion remain after calcium interventions ceases as some studies report that the benefit is lost when the intervention ends while other studies found the effects were maintained.[34,35]

This disparity in study results is likely due to the fact that other factors such as genetics, vitamin D, magnesium, and other micronutrient intake, and physical activity likely play a role in bone mineralization. Lloyd et al. reported that physical activity (load-bearing activities such as soccer, dance, and running) is more important than calcium intake in the development of bone mass and bone strength, at least in young women.[36]

Calcium intake has also been associated with having antiobesity effects.[37] Although the precise mechanism for this correlation has not been clearly elucidated, it has been observed that as calcium intake increases, cellular calcium content decreases which in turn, influences the metabolism of fat, thereby facilitating weight loss. Children and adolescents who consume greater amounts of calcium have been found to have less body fat, especially with the highest levels of intake.[38] In adults, the impact of calcium on weight loss is greatest when consumed as low-fat dairy products instead of calcium supplements. Increased dairy intake has also been correlated with a reduced risk for insulin resistance syndrome.

The current recommended daily intake for calcium for adolescents aged 11–18 years is 1300 mg/day. NHANES data shows that calcium intake peaks for males during adolescence, while intake for females peaks in childhood and declines during adolescence.[17] Bone deposition reaches a maximum in girls shortly before menarche at which time calcium deposition in the bone is approximately five times that of adulthood with a gradual decline in deposition rate after menarche.[30]

Dairy products are the primary dietary sources of calcium in the U.S. diet. Milk consumption has steadily declined since peaking in the mid-1970s coinciding with an increased consumption of soft drinks (see Textbox 5.1 for further discussion).

Harel et al. report that adolescents are aware of the health benefits associated with calcium, but lack the knowledge regarding calcium requirements and what foods to consume to best meet requirements.[39] Thus nutritional education for adolescents should focus on these issues in order to promote achievement of optimal bone mass.

Iron

The need for iron decreases from 10 mg/day for children aged 4–8 years to 8 mg/day for males and females aged 9–13 years. Iron requirements then increase to 11 mg/day for males 14–18 years of age before dropping back to 8 mg/day for the rest of the life cycle starting at the age of 19 years. Similarly to males, the daily iron requirement for females also decreases to 8 mg/day after the age of 8 years, but then increases to 15 mg/day for females aged 14–18 years. The increase for iron is necessary for expanding the blood volume as well as for sexual maturation in males.[40] Additionally for females, iron requirements increase to replace the iron lost every month through menstruation.

The NHANES III data indicate the prevalence of iron deficiency to be approximately 14.2% for girls aged 15–18 years, and 12.1% for 11–14 year old boys.[18] Dietary surveys reflect an average iron intake of 12.5–14.2 mg/day for girls compared with 13.6–18 mg/day for boys.[18] Iron deficiency anemia may impair immune response, limit growth, cause fatigue, and decrease attention span.[17]

NUTRITIONAL RECOMMENDATIONS

The U.S. Department of Agriculture and the U.S. Department of Health and Human Services nutrition guidelines recommend the following for all Americans over the age of 2 years:

- Consume a variety of foods.
- Balance food intake with physical activity; maintain or improve body weight.
- Consume a diet with plenty of grains, fruits, and vegetables.
- Consume a diet low in fat, saturated fat, and cholesterol.
- Consume a diet moderate in sugar.
- Consume a diet moderate in salt and sodium.[41]

The Food Guide Pyramid (see Appendix G) can also be used as a guide for choosing a healthy diet to promote normal growth and development as well as be used for assessing adequacy of intake.

ADOLESCENT NUTRITIONAL CHALLENGES

A number of nutritional challenges face health care practitioners caring for adolescents. Obesity, altered body image and disordered eating, diabetes, dyslipidemia, and pregnancy are just to name a few. Nutrition during this time of the life cycle is important not only to treat any current existing medical problems but also to implement as primary prevention for the most common diseases such as heart disease, hypertension, cancer, type 2 diabetes, and osteoporosis that commonly afflict adults.

OBESITY

Childhood obesity is becoming an epidemic problem in the United States and around the world and is now considered the most prevalent nutritional disease of children. Current available data indicates that approximately 30% of adolescents are overweight, tripling in the last 3 years, while 15.5% are obese.[42] Overweight adolescents generally remain overweight as adults.[43] This will have a marked impact on future medical needs of these children and adolescents since problems related to childhood obesity include hypertension, type 2 diabetes mellitus, dyslipidemia, left ventricular hypertrophy, nonalcoholic steatohepatitis, obstructive sleep apnea, polycystic ovary disease, orthopedic and psychosocial problems.[44,45] The Harvard Growth Study found that overweight in adolescence was a stronger predictor of mortality risk secondary to CHD than overweight as an adult.[45] Type 2 diabetes is increasing in the adult population with the age of onset with diagnosis in adolescents becoming common.[46] Overweight and obese adolescents also experience stigmatization and discrimination. Expectations for thinness from peers, the media, and even health care professionals put pressure on the overweight adolescent to conform to social expectations for slimness and in many cases, unrealistic thin body shapes. This in turn increases the risk for unhealthy behaviors and adverse psychological, social, and economic outcomes. Mellin et al. found higher levels of unhealthy behaviors such as extreme dieting, skipping meals, and television watching and lower frequencies of psychosocial well-being in overweight adolescents compared with their nonoverweight peers.[47]

Obesity is also associated with psychosocial problems. The Adverse Childhood Experiences Study results showed that adults who had experienced four or more categories of childhood abuse exposures had a 1.4- to 1.6-fold increase in obesity and more sedentary lifestyle.[48] Hence, eliciting information about family dysfunction and history of behavioral disorders is important in order to address issues intertwined with weight.

Although there are many theories as to why children and adolescents are becoming more obese, the exact cause of this rise in obesity is not known. Both genetic and environmental factors are thought to play a role.[49–51] Several genetic mutations that cause obesity have been recently identified. Environmental factors such as food availability, portion sizes and snacking, decreased physical activity, increased television viewing time and playing video games are all factors that have been cited.[52]

Data from the National Heart, Lung, and Blood Institute Growth and Health Study (NGHS) shows that physical activity levels decline between 9 and 19 years. It has been estimated that daily activity levels decline by 35% during this time period.[52]

At present, it remains unclear as to the best way to manage obesity in children and adolescents. Such tests as thyroid function have been done historically, but have had a low yield as have other endocrine causes of obesity. Screening for potential morbid conditions associated with obesity is now becoming more and more common. These include type 2 diabetes, high blood pressure, and hyperlipidemia. There have also been some pharmacologic and surgical treatments of obesity in children including such radical treatments as gastric bypass surgery. This type of surgery and the resultant impact on normal growth is now questioned.

Despite the potential economic, psychosocial, and health consequences of obesity, the treatment for adolescent obesity remains challenging and controversial.[51] Clinical guidelines, however, are available to guide clinicians in treatment. An effective treatment plan has been found to have the following: (1) prevents increased weight gain, (2) causes a 5–10% reduction in initial body weight, and (3) establishes long-term maintenance once weight loss goals are achieved.[47,51]

Additionally, focusing on the dietary glycemic index of foods may also play a role in treating pediatric obesity. The glycemic index describes the impact that specific foods have on the rise of blood glucose levels following a meal. Consumption of refined carbohydrates promotes rapid increases in both blood glucose and insulin levels compared to complex carbohydrates, and most fruit and vegetables, which tend to be low on the glycemic index. Alternatively, diets based on low-fat foods (that also provide a low glycemic load) that produce a low glycemic response may promote greater weight loss as these diets promote satiety, minimize postprandial insulin secretion, and promote insulin sensitivity.[53] The results from several studies investigating this hypothesis show greater weight loss is achieved by subjects consuming an energy-restricted diet based on foods low on the glycemic index compared with diet based on high-glycemic carbohydrates.[53,54]

Furthermore, reestablishing physical education for students in all grades, and assessing the types of foods and beverages available in school cafeterias, snack bars, and vending machines are additional areas that need to be addressed.

The role of health care providers in treating childhood and adolescent obesity is becoming more important. However, there is little data to suggest what type of dietary interventions work and the feeling that "nothing works" is common. It is possible that the dietary and activity intervention used in a toddler would be different than the one used in a 14-year-old. Since dietary and physical activity counseling and behavioral therapy are probably what is needed to treat obesity and since these are very time-consuming, primary care physicians are unlikely to attempt or initiate this therapy in these cost-conscious times. Dietitians along with behavioral therapist may need to be specially trained to deal with childhood and adolescent obesity just like they are for cancer nutrition and smoking cessation respectfully. Standardized guidelines for children at different ages for meaningful diagnosis, clinical evaluation, and treatment need to be established.[52] There is much that can be done including revising physical education in the schools, food provided by public schools, and an increase in opportunities for physical activity by changing even the physical design of schools. Childhood obesity, especially in the adolescent period is widespread, rising to a percentage that some feel is a national crisis. The role of dietary and behavioral treatments needs to be identified and supported by all health care providers and public policies.

Altered Body Image

Adolescents are very self-conscious about their changing bodies and outward appearance. Adolescents are constantly bombarded with societies' adoration of "thinness" through magazine covers and advertisements for a multitude of weight loss diets, slimmer thighs, and bigger muscles. For adolescents who perceive that their body image deviates from the "ideal," self-esteem can be negatively impacted and weight-related disorders such as obesity, anorexia nervosa, bulimia, dieting behaviors, and binge eating disorders can develop. While this influence has traditionally focused on girls, boys have also become a target audience. See Textbox 5.1 on adolescents and body image for a further discussion.

Type 2 Diabetes

Similarly to obesity, type 2 diabetes is increasing rapidly in overweight adolescents of all ethnicities who are overweight. Until recently, type 2 diabetes was rare in the adolescent population. Vinicor et al. found that the risk for type 2 diabetes increased by 4% for every pound of excess body weight.[62] The mean age of newly diagnosed adolescents with type 2 diabetes is 13.5 years, with girls affected more frequently than boys.[63] Furthermore, about 95% of adolescents diagnosed with type 2 diabetes have a BMI >85th percentile for sex and age. Although why excess body fat is associated with an increased risk for this disease is unknown, except that obesity appears to increase the prevalence of insulin resistance syndrome.

Obese teens with type 2 diabetes are also at an increased risk for CHD. Elevated glycohemoglobin levels were associated with a significant threefold excess of raised coronary artery lesions in adolescents.[67] Development of coronary lesions occurred despite a favorable lipoprotein profile.

The rise in type 2 diabetes is likely to place a significant economic burden on the health care system. The costs associated with treating diabetes are estimated at an annual cost of $98 million/year.[18] Since complications related to diabetes commonly occur the longer an individual has the disease, health care costs are expected to rise dramatically for treating diabetes as today's adolescents with type 2 diabetes become adults.

Hyperlipidemia

More Americans die of CHD with it becoming more clear than the origins can begin in childhood and adolescence. Studies indicate that development of atherosclerotic lesions in the vasculature are evident by late adolescence.[14,65,67,68] With the alarming trends in adolescents of increasing obesity, type 2 diabetes, and cigarette smoking, these trends may also result in increased cardiovascular morbidity and morality in adulthood.

Since it is strongly associated with CHD, primary and secondary prevention for CHD have traditionally focused on treatment of hypercholesterolemia. However, attention should

---

Textbox 5.1   Adolescents and Body Image

Concerns about one's body image have been a part of Western civilization for as long as there has been a Western civilization. The Roman poet Terrance wrote a comedy, *Eunuchus*, in 161 BC in which he describes the girls of his day as "having sloping shoulders, a squeezed chest so that they look slim. If one is a little plumper, they say she is a boxer and reduce her diet...so that she will look as thin as a bullrush."[55]

These concerns continue unabated. The 2003 Youth Risk Behavior Survey of U.S. high school students published by the Centers for Disease Control (CDC) revealed the same issues today. While only 9.4% of American girls in their study were significantly overweight (defined as ≥95th percentile for BMI), 36.1% considered themselves to be so. About sixty percent of high school girls reported trying to lose weight during the month before the survey. Sixty-five percent exercised during the month specifically to loose weight, 56.2% restricted their food intake, and 18.3% even fasted for more than 24 hours in an attempt to reduce weight. Even more concerning is that 11.3% used diet pills or powders, and almost 8% used laxatives or vomited a meal trying to lose weight.[56]

These behaviors seem to have their origins well before adolescence. A study of 8-year-old school children from a wide variety of ethnic backgrounds revealed 17% of boys and 35% of girls wanting to lose weight. Twenty-four percent of these young girls had tried to loose weight by dieting, and almost 10% tried to lose weight by fasting.[57,58]

This distortion of body image and resultant attempts to inappropriately control one's weight has lead to an epidemic of disordered eating patterns. Actual eating disorders, such as anorexia nervosa and bulimia nervosa, are becoming increasingly prevalent among adolescent girls. Upwards of 1% of adolescent girls in the United States develop anorexia nervosa, while up to 5% of adolescent girls develop bulimia nervosa.[59,60]

Disordered eating patterns are especially prevalent among high school and college athletes. As many as 60% of college female athletes engage in pathologic eating behaviors which, while not sufficient to be diagnosed as either anorexia nervosa or bulimia nervosa, can still place the athlete at significant health risk. The term "female athlete triad" has been used to describe the combination of disordered eating patterns, amenorrhea, and osteoporosis in these athletes. This association is especially common in activities such as ballet, gymnastics, and skating, which place a major emphasis on an athlete's appearance as well as her performance.[61]

---

also be paid to nonlipid risk factors for CHD such as BMI, systolic and diastolic blood pressure, impaired glucose tolerance, and smoking accelerate atherogenesis in adolescents has been found in spite of favorable lipoprotein levels.[67] Furthermore, nonlipid risk factors were also strongly associated with extent of fatty streaks and fibrous plaques in the aorta and coronary arteries seen during autopsies of adolescents. Hence, a comprehensive assessment of both clinical and lifestyle factors should be evaluated to reduce the risk for developing CHD.

Counseling for adolescents to reduce the risk for CHD in adulthood should focus on addressing diet, physical activity, and tobacco use. Guidelines for screening adolescents at risk and treatment recommendations for diet and lipid-lowering medications are available.

PREGNANCY

Pregnancy may be a risk factor for poor nutrition during adolescence, as adolescence may be a risk factor for poor nutrition during pregnancy. Both the growing adolescent and the

TABLE 5.8
Weight Gain Recommendations for Pregnant Adolescents

Prepregnant Weight	Suggested Total Weight Gain	
	kg	lb
Underweight (BMI < 20)	12.5–18.0	28–40
Normal weight (BMI 20–26)	11.5–16.0	25–35
Overweight (BMI 26–29)	7.0–11.5	15–25
Obese (BMI > 29)	7.0–9.1	15–20

Source: From Institute of Medicine, Subcommittee on Nutritional Status and Weight Gain During Pregnancy, *Nutrition During Pregnancy*, National Academy Press, Washington, D.C., 1990.

growing fetus must compete for what may be limited nutritional resources. The high metabolic needs of a growing fetus, combined with the sometimes poor nutritional choices made by adolescents, can result in some degree of malnutrition in each.

Almost one million adolescent girls become pregnant each year in the United States. Approximately half of these pregnancies result in a live birth, with the other half terminating in either miscarriage or abortion.[69,70]

Infants born to younger mothers (under 15 years of age) are twice as likely to be of low birth weight (under 2500 g) and three times as likely not to survive the neonatal period as infants born to older mothers. Infants born to adolescent mothers (under age 19 years) are more likely to be premature, to have intrauterine growth retardation, and to have developmental disabilities.[71,72]

That the pregnant adolescent herself is often still growing creates nutritional needs that often remain unmet. Pregnant adolescents often themselves grow at a slower rate than their nonpregnant peers. The teen mother is more likely to experience hypertension, anemia, and preterm labor than are older mothers. Pregnant adolescents have twice the mortality rate of nonadolescent mothers-to-be. In addition, these girls are at risk for not returning to school, and are at increased risk of suffering domestic violence.[72,73]

Pregnant teens require an additional 300 cal daily during the second and third trimesters. Pregnant teens under age of 15 years need 200 cal/day above the need of older teens, or 500 cal extra each day. This level of nutritional intake should result in a weight gain for the teenaged mother ranging from 25 lb if already overweight, to 40 lb if underweight (see Table 5.8).[72–74]

Protein requirements increase by 10–15 g daily, bringing the recommended daily protein intake to 60 g daily. Most women in the United States, including those who may be at higher nutritional risk due to either young age or lower socioeconomic status, usually consume at least this much protein.

Vitamin requirements for all vitamins except A and D are increased during pregnancy. A daily prenatal vitamin assures adequate vitamin intake for most teens. Zinc, calcium, and iron needs are also increased, and often need supplementation. Folic acid is now recommended before conception for all women to reduce the risk of neural tube defects in their infants.[72,73]

PHYSICAL ACTIVITY AND PARTICIPATION IN SPORTS

Regular physical activity is associated with many health benefits including promotion of weight control, increased bone density, aerobic endurance, and muscular strength as well as higher levels of self-esteem and lower levels of anxiety and stress.[66] Regular physical activity is also associated with a decreased risk for developing many of the chronic diseases that plaque the American population such as CHD, hypertension, type 2 diabetes, and obesity. Physical activity levels tend to decline from childhood into adolescence.[75] This is of concern since many behaviors practiced as an adult are carried forth from childhood and adolescence. Encouraging maintenance of physical activity is vital throughout the life cycle and must be encouraged and implemented into an adolescent's routine.

The rapid growth experienced during adolescence requires adequate nutritional support, as noted in the above sections. The adolescent athlete places additional demands on their body, and can be placed at risk due to both nutritional deficiencies and excesses.

The first step in counseling adolescent athletes is to assess their current eating patterns and nutrient intake. Information about food preferences, meal timing, fast-food consumption, snacking, nutritional supplement use, alcohol and illicit drug use, and disordered eating patterns are all important in identifying potential problems in nutritional status.

The adolescent who eats a healthy, well-balanced diet that supports normal growth and development will be adequately supported for most athletic endeavors. Some activities, however, place exceptional demands on the young athlete.

Tight weight control is important for activities such as dance, figure skating, gymnastics, and diving, where the athlete's appearance can be as important as their performance.

Pressure by a coach or teacher to achieve a specified weight can coerce an athlete to undertake steps, which may result in rapid weight loss (such as in wrestling) or weight gain (such as in football). Dancers, gymnasts, wrestlers, and distance runners have a very high incidence of disordered eating patterns. These practices, while usually not meeting the full criteria for anorexia nervosa or bulimia nervosa, often include diet restriction and purging behaviors that can place an adolescent athlete at high nutritional risk.[1,15]

The optimal diet for an adolescent athlete provides 60–75% of calories from carbohydrates (500–600 g/day), 15–20% of calories from protein (up to 1.5 g/kg daily), and <20–30% of calories from fat.

Many athletes are increasingly turning to heavily advertised nutritional supplements in an attempt to improve athletic performance, despite the almost total lack of evidence that these supplements actually work. A balanced and varied diet provides adequate protein and nutrition to meet the needs of most athletes.

Adolescent athletes have a proportionally greater water need than do adult athletes. Hydration should begin before strenuous events, and should be carefully monitored during prolonged activities and during hot weather. Athletes should drink one quart of caffeine-free fluids for every 1000 cal consumed, with an additional two cups of water or sports drink 2 h before exercise. For more prolonged exercise, sports drinks that contain 5–8% carbohydrates should provide both for hydration needs and maintenance of glycogen stores. After exercise, each pound of weight lost should be replaced with 16 oz of fluids.[76]

The female athlete can be at increased risk for significant nutritional deficiencies. The female athlete triad is the association of disordered eating patterns, amenorrhea, and loss of bone mineralization in a female athlete. Girls with this disorder are at great risk for significant osteoporosis in later life. The hypometabolic and hypoestrogenic states that result from strenuous exercise and diet restriction are similar to that seen in anorexia nervosa.

Treatment is aimed at reducing the level of exercise and improving nutritional status so that normal menstruation is resumed, as well as assuring that calcium intake meets current recommend.[64]

VEGETARIAN DIETS

Vegetarian diets are becoming more popular with adolescents, particularly young girls. The wish for a not consuming animal products including red meat, chicken, and even fish are many. Often there is the expressed desire to have a "healthier" diet and concern for animals raised for consumption only. Vegetarianism is a complex system usually described by different categories of vegetarianism. A diet excluding any animal products (free of meat and animal related products) is referred to as a vegan diet. Diets that include milk products (lactovegetarian) or eggs (ovovegetarian) tend to be more common. The "semi-vegetarian" diet, which primarily avoids red meat and includes such products as fish and poultry, is probably the most commonly referred diet by adolescents who are "vegetarians."

Recently, it was found in a survey of close to 5000 adolescents students in the Midwest that just over 5% reported as "vegetarian".[77] The most common reason for becoming vegetarian was they were trying to control their weight or were told they had an eating disorder. Their choice was not because of animal welfare or trying to preserve natural resources. It was found that the vegetarians in this study were more likely than their nonvegetarian peers to meet the dietary recommendations of the Healthy People 2010 Objectives. Again, the vegetarians in this study were mostly nonred meat eaters. Their consumption of fast food was less and their consumption of fruit and vegetables were higher than their red meat eating peers. There were some differences in vitamin B_{12}, cholesterol, and fat. The vegetarians actually had a higher iron intake (from fortified cereals). Both groups had a poor intake of dietary calcium and this was considered a major finding since calcium intake during this time often defines the risk for osteoporosis when these adolescents become adults.[78]

USE OF COMPLEMENTARY AND ALTERNATIVE THERAPIES

The use of complementary and alternative therapies by the general population has been increasing throughout the United States and the world over the last decade. The use of these therapies has been well studied in adults, but the use of such therapies in children and adolescents has been only recently published.[79] Adolescents have been reported to use primarily herbal therapies for common problems, which include obesity, weight control, and menstrual irregularities.[80] Ma huang, as an example, is an herbal remedy containing *Ephedra sinica* that has been in many dietary supplements used by adolescents. Ma huang comes in several preparations and also in combinations with other ingredients such as caffeine to help "curb" one's appetite. Despite widely publicized safety concerns, 14% of individuals using nonprescription weight-loss producers in the United States take an ephedra or ephedrine-containing product.[81] The use of Ma huang has also been advertised to "energize" and give one more stamina. It has been reported to have significant side effects including cardiac arrhythmias and even seizures and sudden death. Because of these potential health hazard, dietary supplements containing ephedra are now banned in the U.S.

Adolescents have used complementary and alternative therapies for a variety of problems, especially chronic illness as well as for weight control. Herbal therapies, homeopathic remedies, and mind–body therapies (visualization and guided imagery) have been used for inflammatory bowel disorders (IBD). In one study from multiple centers in the United States and England, the use of complementary medicine in children and young adults with inflammatory bowel disease was 41%.[82] Common therapies were megavitamins, dietary supplements, and herbal medicines. Children and adolescents with cancer have been reported to use high-dose vitamin supplements such as vitamins C and E. Other children with cancer have sought care from alternative practitioners including naturopathic physicians, traditional Chinese medicine practitioners, and homeopathic doctors.[83] In one study of over 1000 children seen in a primary care setting, the use of complementary and alternative therapies was 12%.[79] Therapies most likely to be used in this urban Detroit practice included herb (41%), prayer healing (37%), high-dose vitamin and supplements (34%), folkhome remedies (28%), and manipulative therapies such as massage and chiropractic care (18%).

The use of complementary and alternative therapies in adolescents with asthma was reported by using a questionnaire given to 3800 inner-city high school students in New York city. One hundred and sixty respondents reported having asthma (68% Hispanic and 26% Afro-American) and 33% had weekly symptoms.[84] Overall, 80% of the asthmatic adolescents reported using complementary and alternative therapies. The most common were rubs (74%), herbal teas (39%), prayer (37%), and Jarabe 7 syrup (24%). Over half (59%) felt that these therapies were effective. This use of complementary and alternative therapies in this study population was twice the national average for adults.

Actual research aimed at adolescents and the use of complementary and alternative therapies are few. Researchers have conducted a randomized, double-blind, crossover study examining the use of fish oil in a dietary supplement could reduce the frequency and severity of migraines. The fish oil used in this study was in the form of long-chain $n - 3$ polyunsaturated fatty acids given to 27 adolescents (16 girls and 7 boys) who had had frequent migraines for at least 1 year. They received 2 months of fish oil, followed by a month of washout and then 2 months of a placebo (olive oil). Investigators found a significant reduction in headache frequency. Duration and severity during fish oil treatment and the placebo as compared to prior to starting the study suggest that both fish oil and olive oil may be beneficial in the treatment of migraines in adolescents.[85]

Often the use of complementary and alternative therapies is not disclosed to the child's health care practitioner. The reasons for its use are varied and include dissatisfaction with conventional medicine, fear of conventional medications and their side effects, the "safety" of natural products and the autonomy of treating children and adolescents without first seeing a conventional health care provider. A recent study in England found that 18% of all children had at least once some form of complementary and alternative therapies. The most commonly used therapies included homeopathy, aromatherapy, and herbal medicine. Besides chronic problems such as asthma, inflammatory bowel disease, cancer and arthritis, complementary and alternative therapies were used for problems with the ear, nose, throat, skin, lungs, and emotional or behavioral issues.[86] The most common source for parents using these various therapies was word-of-mouth recommendations through friends or relatives.

There appears to be wide variation in the use of complementary and alternative therapies depending on regional differences and ethnic backgrounds of the families of children and adolescents. In the South, prayer healing is more prevalent than on either coasts of the United States. Homeopathy is more commonly utilized in Europe than in the United States as well as aromatherapy. Chiropractic and massage therapies tend to be used more in the Midwestern United States and among homeless teens, herbal therapies and homeopathic remedies are preferred. The health care practitioner needs to know that the use of complementary and alternative therapies is common and the reasons why they are utilized in order to better treat and help their young patients. The reason is not always dissatisfaction with conventional care, but in the example of asthma, concerns regarding the use of chronic steroids has been an important reason for the high rates of usage in children with asthma (51.7%).[87]

Adolescents tend to have nutritional deficiencies, poor eating habits due to eating snacks between meals, processed foods, "junk foods," and a low intake of fruits and vegetables.

The use of dietary supplements for such things as weight loss, appetite suppression, and menstrual irregularities make addressing these therapies especially important. The use of many over the counter high caffeine and "herbal-fortified" drinks is commonplace by adolescents including even coffee flavored formulations with relatively high fat and sugar content. Not only may these drinks interfere with attempts at establishing a more nutritional diet, but also they may have significant side effects by themselves (nervousness, sleep disruption, high heart rate, and poor appetite). All forms of therapies should be discussed including all teas, supplements, drinks, and alternative health care provider visits at each health care encounter to best advise the adolescent in their nutritional needs.

RECOMMENDATIONS FOR CHANGE

The challenge to nutrition education is to provide programs that motivate adolescents to make long-lasting healthy lifestyle changes while also reducing the barriers associated with these changes (see Table 5.3). Successful nutrition education and intervention programs must consider the changes an adolescent is experiencing as well as understand the complexities of a teenager in today's society.

Adolescents reportedly are aware of their poor eating habits and suggest that greater availability of tasty, convenient, and cheap nutritious foods would help them to improve their eating habits.[88] Encouraging family meals, parental control of access to unhealthy foods, and restricting the sale of soft drinks and foods high in sugar and fat during school hours are strategies that target the environment to influence availability of less nutritious foods. Additionally, numerous nutrition education programs for adolescents targeting outcomes such as knowledge, attitudes, and skills, have been cited in the literature.[88] Based on a review of the literature, Lytle concluded that the following program components contributed to effective interventions: a behavioral focus, incorporation of instructional strategies that are based on appropriate theory, appropriate amount of education needed to promote positive behavioral change, environmental intervention to complement behavioral component, peer and community involvement, and self-reflection and feedback.[88]

The success of a program is determined not only by the program's efficacy but also by the extent to which the population is served.[89] Program success can be limited by lack of dissemination and exposure.

HEALTH PROMOTION PROGRAMS

Health promotion, using appropriate intervention strategies, has been successful in promoting behavior change in adolescents.[89–91] Such programs can be disseminated through a number of avenues such as via health care practitioners, schools, and community programs including summer camps, community center activities, and scouting.

Various opportunities are available for health care practitioners. Health maintenance visits present an opportunity for discussing diet, body image, and physical activity as they relate to health and the prevention of chronic disease. The American Medical Association Guidelines for Adolescent Preventive Services (GAPS) provides recommendations for preventive services and screening.[92] Specific screening recommendations are available for eating disorders, hyperlipidemia, and obesity.

SCHOOL-BASED PROGRAMS

School-based health programs that promote healthy eating and regular physical activity have been shown to have an impact on adolescents when provided as a comprehensive curriculum.

School-based programs also have the advantage of potentially reaching 98% of children in the United States.[89] Coordination of information with the school food service program and school physical education program is recommended to develop an integrated, comprehensive curriculum. A number of nutrition education and health promotion Internet-based programs are also available that allow the use of computer-assisted technology for dissemination of classroom information as well as serving as another option of dissemination of information development of such programs should incorporate features that capture the attention of adolescents such as interactive activities with colorful graphics, use of audio, video, and music clips. Since most schools today have the Internet access availability, this provides a viable option.

Although a number of school-based nutrition education programs have been successful when offered, a review of the literature reveals that less than half of these programs have involved adolescents.[88,89] This may be a result of the decline in availability of health programs to students in grade levels beyond middle school. Approximately 50% of K-8 schools have a state or district requirement for health education, whereas only 40% of schools for 9th and 10th graders and 20% of 11th and 12th graders have such a requirement.[93] This is of concern since by middle school, adolescents have the cognitive and critical thinking skills to make informed choices and adoption of healthy behaviors.

Unfortunately a number of barriers to implementing nutrition education programs such as lack of school funding, lack of teacher interest and knowledge, and competition for curricular time, exist.

COMMUNITY-BASED PROGRAMS

Nutrition education program designed for community dissemination has the advantage of reaching larger audiences. Since adolescents have been found to adopt healthy behaviors when received as consistent messages from a variety of sources, community programs can also provide supplemental information disseminated through the media or school-based programs. Community recreational centers, which tend to offer a number of sporting and other activities, would offer the opportunity of providing information, highlighting the importance of both nutrition and physical activity.

A number of community-based programs have been found to effectively promote behavior change in adolescents[88–91] like the California Project LEAN's food on the run program, which is an evaluation of a high school-based student advocacy nutrition and physical activity program to underserved communities.[94] The mission for this campaign is to improve health and reduce the risk of developing chronic diseases such as CHD, cancer, obesity through healthy eating and physical activity. The Project Lean Food on the Run campaign trains high school students to become promoters of healthy behavior. Nutrition, physical activity, and working with the media are the focus areas for training. The Project Lean campaign successfully resulted in vending machines on the participating high school campuses offering healthier choices, and the high school cafeterias providing more variety of healthy foods. A comparison of pretest and posttest results of a self-report survey, eliciting student information regarding physical activity and dietary intake, showed a significant increase in the knowledge about and positive attitude toward physical activity for student trainers. Nutrition knowledge and positive attitude also significantly increased for student advocates.

Gimme 5: A Fresh Nutrition Concept for Students was a school-based nutrition intervention program designed to increase awareness and positive attitudes for eating at minimum of five servings of fruit and vegetables daily.[93] This 4-year program targeted high school students and high school cafeterias. Five 55-min workshops were also presented that focused on issues important to the students such as assessment of individual eating habits and developing marketing strategies that encourage healthy eating, eating as it relates to appearance and athletic performance, healthy fast-food menu selection, healthy snacks, and microwave cooking techniques. The intervention group significantly increased consumption of daily fruit and vegetable servings by 14%. Knowledge scores and awareness also increased in the intervention group. The researchers concluded that the effectiveness of this program resulted from the use of media marketing as an effective strategy for promoting products and services.

DESIGNING NUTRITION EDUCATION PROGRAMS

Intervention programs that are behavior-based have been found to effectively promote positive dietary behavioral changes that remain over time in adolescents.[94] Programs that have been found to be successful incorporate an environmental component, and offer a sufficient number of sessions or classes that use appropriate, creative, and multiple teaching strategies from a variety of sources.[94]

A number of theoretical frameworks and planning models such as the social cognitive theory (SCT), stages of change, and the PRECEDE model, are available to aid in program design. The SCT model incorporating behavior, personal factors, and environmental influences that continually interact, reportedly has been successful in developing adolescent nutrition education programs.[89]

Altering the environment by changing food selections available either at school or at home is another crucial component of any successful nutrition education program. Many successful programs have involved the school food service administration to alter food accessibility to offer more healthy food choices. Since parental food choices and purchases influence adolescent choices, targeting parents for educational is another component of successful intervention programs. Adolescents who reported having a good relationship with their parents which allows them to discuss their problems have been associated with healthier behaviors, especially among overweight adolescents.[51]

SUMMARY

Adolescence is a time of transition from childhood to adulthood. Eating habits and physical activity practices tend to change to eating a less healthy diet and a more sedentary lifestyle. Obesity is escalating in the adolescent population with the diagnosis of other chronic diseases, previously rare, becoming more common in this segment of the U.S. population. Intervention programs that promote healthy lifestyle habits have been found to successfully change adolescent behaviors. Health care professionals, educators, and parents must be aware of the opportunities to provide adolescents with the knowledge, attitudes, and skills to practice healthy behaviors for optimal growth and development as well as to reduce the risks of developing long-term chronic diseases (Textbox 5.2).

CASE STUDY

Brittney and her mother have an appointment with you to discuss a diet for Brittney that can help her lose weight. Brittney is 15 years old and a sophomore in high school. She is currently 5'3" and weighed 150 lb at her last doctor's appointment. The doctor also encouraged Brittney she should try to lose some weight by eating a healthy diet and becoming over active since her total cholesterol and blood glucose levels are elevated.

Brittney brought a food log that illustrated her intake for the past week. Upon reviewing the information, you notice that she skips breakfast most of the time and taking snacks

---

Textbox 5.2   Liquid Candy: Soda Consumption by U.S. Adolescents

The American population drinks approximately 50 gallons of soda per person per year not including beverages advertised as "fruit" drinks.[95] Since the mid-1960s, milk consumption by children and adolescents has steadily declined as the intake of soft drinks has steadily climbed. Albertson et al. investigated the consumption of milk versus soft drinks in adolescents and found that boys on average consume $2\frac{1}{2}$ 12-oz servings of soft drinks daily compared to only $1\frac{1}{2}$ cups of milk daily.[96] Girls were found to consume $1\frac{3}{4}$ 12-oz servings of soft drinks daily but less than 8 oz of milk daily. Whiting et al. found that substituting milk in the diet with carbonated and other low-nutrient-dense beverages was negatively associated with total body bone mineral content in girls at the time of peak bone mass accrual (mean age, 12.5 years).[97] Bone fractures have been positively associated with consumption of cola beverages, consumption of approximately 0.7 or more of a can or bottle, in girls aged 8 to 16 years.

Whether the consumption of carbonated beverages, especially colas, truly adversely affect bone health is currently the subject of debate. It was previously thought that perhaps it was the caffeine, phosphoric acid, and sugar content of caffeinated beverages that was the likely culprit that influenced the calcium economy as it related to bone health.[98] Caffeine has been found to increase urinary calcium excretion in some observational studies while others have not.[99] The observational study results, which have linked caffeine consumption and risk for osteoporosis, were primarily found in populations where calcium intake was significantly less than established recommendations. It is now known that while caffeine exerts an immediate increase in urinary calcium excretion, this is followed by a decrease in renal calcium clearance, which results in no overall net effect.[98]

The phosphoric acid content of most carbonated beverages is relatively small and thus does not really have an influence on calcium homeostasis.[98] Lastly, given the epidemic of obesity in the U.S. population, the excess consumption of sugar is of concern. However, similarly to caffeine, the sugar intake from soda consumption is essentially negated [98]. Heaney and Rafferty reportedly have found no association between the constituents of carbonated beverages such as soda and bone mineral density.[100] They also concluded that the displacement of milk and other calcium-fortified beverages from the diet is the primary impact of consuming carbonated beverages. However, although consumption of soft drinks reportedly does not impart a negative effect on bone density, sodas contain no nutritional value for health and have been linked to higher energy intakes.[101] Therefore, adolescents should be encouraged to limit their intake of soft drinks and increase their intake of calcium-containing beverages in order to obtain optimal bone mineral densities while also decreasing the risk for obesity.

---

frequently in the late afternoon and after dinner. Most of her food choices are composed of process carbohydrate sources such as commercially prepared breakfast cereals, chips, and ice cream. Brittney would also like to improve her physical fitness because she is taking physical examination this fall and knows that she will be required to run the mile. She currently only swims in the family pool to cool off. Brittney also asks if she should take one of those weight loss supplements that she has seen advertised on TV.

1. What specific nutrition recommendations would you suggest for Brittney to improve her diet?
2. What recommendations would you provide to help Brittney become more physically active?

3. Would you provide any specific suggestions regarding the use of dietary supplements to improve Brittney's diet?
4. How would you address Brittney's question regarding the use of weight loss supplements?

REFERENCES

1. Wald, R.A., Nutrition in the adolescent, *Pediatr. Ann.*, 28, 107, 1999.
2. Neinstein, L., *Adolescent Health Care: A Practical Guide*, 4th ed., Neinstein, L., Ed., Lippincott Williams & Wilkins, Philadelphia, 2002.
3. Marshall, W.A. and Tanner, J.M., Variations in pattern of pubertal changes in girls, *Arch. Dis. Child*, 44, 291, 1969.
4. Wahl, R.A. and Boss, R.D., Adolescent medicine, in *Current Diagnosis & Treatment of Women*, Lemcke, D.P., Cowley, D.S., and Pattison, J., Eds., McGraw-Hill, New York, 2004, chap. 1.
5. Piaget, J., Intellectual evolution from adolescence to adulthood, *Hum. Dev.*, 15, 1, 1972.
6. Orr, D.P., Helping adolescents toward adulthood, *Contemp. Pediatr.*, 15, 55, 1998.
7. Papalia, D., The status of several conservation abilities across the life-span, *Hum. Dev.*, 15, 229, 1972.
8. Papalia, D. and Del Vento, B.D., Cognitive functioning in middle and old age adults: a review of research based on Piaget's theory, *Hum. Dev.*, 17, 424, 1974.
9. Sinnott, J.D., Everyday thinking and Piagetian operativity in adults, *Hum. Dev.*, 18, 430, 1975.
10. Story, M., Neumark-Sztainer, D., and French, S., Individual and environmental influences on adolescent eating behaviors, *J. Am. Diet. Assoc.*, 102, S40, 2002.
11. Lin, B.H., Guthrie, J., and Blaylock, J., *The Diets of America's Children: Influences of Dining Out, Household Characteristics, and Nutrition Knowledge*, U.S. Department of Agriculture, Washington, D.C., 1996. Economic Report Number 746 (AER-746).
12. Dausch, J.G., et al. Correlates of high-fat/low-nutrient-dense snack consumption among adolescents: results from two national health surveys, *Am. J. Health Promot.*, 10, 85, 1995.
13. Nicklas, T.A., et al. Impact of breakfast consumption on nutritional adequacy of the diets of young adults in Bogalusa, Louisiana: ethnic and gender contrasts, *J. Am. Diet. Assoc.*, 98, 1432, 1998.
14. Chapman, G. and MacLean, J., "Junk food" and "healthy food": meanings of food in adolescent women's culture, *J. Nutr. Educ.*, 25, 108, 1993.
15. Gracey, D., et al. Nutritional knowledge, beliefs and behaviors in teenage school students, *Health Educ. Res.*, 11, 187, 1996.
16. Centers for Disease Control and Prevention. DCD Surveillance Summaries. *MMWR*, 49, 1, 2000.
17. Lytle, L.A., Nutritional issues for adolescents, *J. Am. Diet. Assoc.*, 102, S8, 2002.
18. Alaimo, K., et al. Dietary intake of vitamins, minerals, and fiber of persons ages 2 months and over in the United States: Third National Health and Nutrition Examination Survey, Phase 1, 1988–1991, *Adv. Data*, 1, 1994.
19. *Healthy People 2010: Understanding and Improving Health.* U.S. Department of Health and Human Services, Washington, D.C., 2000.
20. Spear, B.A., Adolescent growth and development, *J. Am. Diet. Assoc.*, 102, S23, 2002.
21. Clinical Growth Charts. Available at: www.cdc.gov. Accessed January 2, 2005.
22. Mitchell, M.K., Nutrition during adolescence, in *Nutrition Across the Life Span*, Mitchell, M.K., Ed., W.B. Saunders Company, Philadelphia, 1997, chap. 7.
23. Heald, F.T. and Gong, E.J., *Modern Nutrition in Health and Disease*, 9th ed., Lea & Febiger, Philadelphia, 1998, 52.
24. Merzenich, H., Boeing, H., and Wahrendorf, J., Dietary fat and sports activity as determinants for age at menarche, *Am. J. Epidemiol.*, 138, 217, 1993.
25. Trumbo, P., Schlicker, S., Yates, A.A., and Poos, M., Food and Nutrition Board of the Institute of Medicine, The National Academies. Dietary reference intakes for energy, carbohy-

drate, fiber, fat, fatty acids, cholesterol, protein and amino acids, *J. Am. Diet. Assoc.*, 103, 563, 2003.

26. Wait, B., Blair, R., and Roberts, L.J., Energy intake of well-nourished children and adolescents, *Am. J. Clin. Nutr.*, 22, 1383, 1969.

27. World Health Organization. Energy and protein requirements. WHO Technical Report Series No. 724. World Health Organization, Geneva, Switzerland, 1985.

28. Wait, B., Protein intake of well-nourished children and adolescents, *Am. J. Clin. Nutr.*, 26, 1303, 1973.

29. National Center for Health Statistics (1994) Plan and Operation of the Third National Health and Nutrition Examination Survey, 1988–1994. Vital Health Stat 1 (32) NCHS Hyattsville, MD DHHS Publ No. (PHS) 94–1308.

30. Leonard, M.B. and Zemel, B.S., Current concepts in pediatric bone disease, *Pediatr. Clin. North Am.*, 49, 2002.

31. Lanou, A.J., Berkow, S.E., and Barnard, N.D., Calcium, dairy products, and bone health in children and young adults: a reevaluation of the evidence, *Pediatrics*, 115, 792, 2005.

32. Johnston, C.C., et al. Calcium supplementation and increases in bone mineral density in children, *N. Engl. J. Med.*, 327, 82, 1992.

33. Lloyd, T., et al. Calcium supplementation and bone mineral density in adolescent girls, *J. Am. Med. Assoc.*, 270, 841, 1993.

34. Dibba, B., et al. Bone mineral contents and plasma osteocalcin concentrations of Gambian children 12 and 24 mo after the withdrawal of a calcium supplement, *Am. J. Clin. Nutr.*, 76, 681, 2002.

35. Slemenda, C., et al. Reduced rates of skeletal remodeling are associated with increased bone mineral density during the development of peak bone mass, *J. Bone Miner. Res.*, 12, 676, 1997.

36. Lloyd, T., et al. Lifestyle factors and the development of bone mass and bone strength in young women, *J. Pediatr.*, 144, 776, 2004.

37. Pereira, M.A., et al. Dairy consumption, obesity, and the insulin resistance syndrome in young adults, *JAMA*, 287, 2081, 2002.

38. Carruth, B.R. and Skinner, J.D., The role of dietary calcium and other nutrients in moderating body fat in preschool children, *Int. J. Obes.*, 25, 559, 2001.

39. Harel, Z., et al. Adolescents and calcium: what they do and do not know and how much consume, *J. Adolesc. Health*, 22, 225, 1998.

40. Dallman, P.R., Iron deficiency: does it matter? *J. Intern. Med.*, 226, 367, 1989.

41. *Nutrition and Your Health: Dietary Guidelines for Americans*, 5th ed. Home and Garden Bulletin no. 232. Hyattsville, MD: USDA-DHHS, 2000.

42. Obesity in Youth. American Obesity Association. Available at: www.obesity.org. Accessed March 5, 2005.

43. Serdula, M.K., et al. Do obese children become obese adults? A review of the literature, *Prev. Med.*, 22, 167, 1993.

44. Sorof, J.D., Obesity hypertension in children: a problem of epidemic proportions, *Hypertension*, 40, 441, 2002.

45. Must, A., et al. Long-term morbidity and mortality of overweight adolescents: a follow-up of the Harvard Growth Study of 1922–1935, *N. Engl. J. Med.*, 327, 1350, 1992.

46. Fagot-Campagna, A., et al. Type 2 diabetes among North American children and adolescents: an epidemiologic review and a public health perspective, *J. Pediatr.*, 136, 664, 2000.

47. Mellin, A.E., et al. Unhealthy behaviors and psychosocial difficulties among overweight adolescents: the potential impact of familial factors, *J. Adolesc. Health*, 31, 145, 2002.

48. Felitti, V., et al. Relationship of childhood abuse and household dysfunction to many of the leading causes of death in adults: the Adverse Childhood Experiences Study, *Am. J. Prev. Med.*, 14, 245, 1998.

49. Kimm, S.Y.S., Obesity prevention and macronutrient intake of children in the United States, *Ann. NY Acad. Sci.*, 699, 70, 1993.

50. Trent, M.E. and Ludwig, D.S., Adolescent obesity, a need for greater awareness and improved treatment, *Curr. Opin. Pediatr.*, 11, 297, 1999.

51. Kimm, S.Y.S. and Obarzanek, E., Childhood obesity: a new pandemic of the new millennium, *Pediatrics*, 110, 1003, 2002.

52. Kimm, S.Y.S., et al. Racial divergence in adiposity during adolescence: the NHLBI Growth and Health Study, *Pediatrics*, 107, 34, 2001.

53. Brand-Miller, J.C., et al. Glycemic index and obesity, *Am. J. Clin. Nutr.*, 76, 281S, 2002.

54. Spieth, L.E., et al. A low-glycemic index diet in the treatment of pediatric obesity, *Arch. Pediatr. Adolesc. Med.*, 154, 947, 2000.

55. Chabrol, H., Callahan, S., and O'Halloran, S., The pressure to be thin on adolescent girls in ancient Rome, *J. Am. Acad. Child Adolesc. Psychiatry*, 39, 1345, 2000.

56. Centers for Disease Control and Prevention. Youth Risk Behavior Surveillance — United States, 2001, *MMWR Surveill. Summ.*, 51(SS-4), 2002.

57. Robinson, R.N., et al. Overweight concerns and body dissatisfaction among third-grade children: the impacts of ethnicity and socioeconomic status, *J. Pediatr.*, 138, 181, 2001.

58. Striegel-Moore, R.H., Body image concerns among children, *J. Pediatr.*, 138, 158, 2001.

59. Kreipe, R.E. and Dukarm, C.P., Eating disorders in adolescents and older children, *Pediatr. Rev.*, 20, 410, 1999.

60. Rome, E.S., et al. Children and adolescents with eating disorders: the state of the art, *Pediatrics*, 111, 98, 2003.

61. Sanborn, C.F., et al. Disordered eating and the female athlete triad, *Clin. Sports Med.*, 19, 199, 2000.

62. Vinicor, F., et al. Healthy people 2010: diabetes, *Diabetes Care*, 23, 853, 2000.

63. Dabelea, D., et al. Type 2 diabetes mellitus in minority children and adolescents. An emerging problem, *Endocrinol. Metab. Clin. North. Am.*, 28, 709, 1999.

64. Zieske, A.W., Malcom, G.T., and Strong, J.P., Natural history and risk factors of atherosclerosis in children and youth: the PDAY study, *Pediatr. Pathol. Mol. Med.*, 21, 213, 2002.

65. Strong, J., Coronary atherosclerosis in soldiers: a clue to the natural history of atherosclerosis in the young, *JAMA*, 256, 2863, 1986.

66. Centers for Disease Control and Prevention. National and state-specific pregnancy rates among adolescents — United States, 1995–1997, *MMWR Morb. Mortal. Wkly. Rep.*, 49, 605, 2000.

67. Singh, S. and Darroch, J.E., Adolescent pregnancy and childbearing: levels and trends in developed countries, *Fam. Plan. Perspect.*, 32, 14, 2000.

68. American Academy of Pediatrics Committee on Adolescence. Adolescent pregnancy — current trends and issues: 1998, *Pediatrics*, 103, 516, 1999.

69. Alexander, C.S. and Guyer, B., Adolescent pregnancy: occurrence and consequences, *Pediatr. Ann.*, 22, 85, 1993.

70. Lenders, C.M, McElrath, T.F., and School, T.O., Nutrition in adolescent pregnancy, *Curr. Opin. Pediatr.*, 12, 291, 2000.

71. Gutierrez, Y. and King, J.C., Nutrition during teenage pregnancy, *Pediatr. Ann.*, 22, 99, 1993.

72. Institute of Medicine (U.S.), Subcommittee on Nutritional Status and Weight Gain During Pregnancy. *Nutrition During Pregnancy*, National Academy of Sciences, National Academy Press, Washington, D.C., 1990.

73. Lytle, L., et al. Covariance of adolescent health behaviors: the class of 1989 study, *Health Educ. Res.*, 19, 133, 1995.

74. Kleiner, S.M., Nutrition advisor: eating for peak performance, *Physician Sports Med.*, 25, 123, 1997.

75. Perry, C., et al. Adolescent vegetarian: how well do their dietary patterns meet the Health People 2010 objectives? *Arch. Pediatr. Adolesc. Med.*, 156, 431, 2002.

76. Zlotkin, S., Editorial — Adolescent vegetarians, *Arch. Pediatr. Adolesc. Med.*, 156, 426, 2002.

77. Sawni-Sikand, A., Schubiner, H., and Thomas, R.L., Use of complementary/alternative therapies among children in primary care pediatrics, *Ambul. Pediatr.*, 2, 99, 2002.

78. Gardiner, M.S. and Kemper, K., Herbs in pediatric and adolescent medicine, *Pediatr. Rev.*, 21, 44, 2000.

79. Blanck, H.M., Khan, L.K., and Serdula, M.K., Use of nonprescription weight loss products: results from a multistate survey, *JAMA*, 286, 930, 2001.
80. Heuschkel, R., et al. Complementary medicine use in children and young adults with inflammatory bowel disease, *Am. J. Gastroenterol.*, 97, 382, 2002.
81. Neuhouser, M.L., et al. Use of alternative medicine by children with cancer in Washington state, *Prev. Med.*, 33, 347, 2001.
82. Reznik, M., et al. Use of complementary therapy by adolescents with asthma, *Arch. Pediatr. Adolesc. Med.*, 156, 1042, 2002.
83. Harel, Z., et al. Supplementation with omega-3 polyunsaturated fatty acids in the management of recurrent migraines in adolescents, *J. Adolesc. Health*, 31,154, 2002.
84. Simpson, N. and Roman, K., Complementary medicine use in children: extent and reasons. A population-based study, *Br. J. Gen. Pract.*, 51, 914, 2001.
85. Shenfield, G., Lim, E., and Allen, H., Survey of the use of complementary medicines and therapies in children with asthma, *J. Paediatr. Child Health*, 38, 252, 2002.
86. Lytle, L.A., Nutrition education for school-aged children, *J. Nutr. Educ.*, 27, 298, 1995.
87. Hoelscher, D.M., et al. Designing effective nutrition interventions for adolescents, *J. Am. Diet. Assoc.*, 102, S52, 2002.
88. O'Dea, J., Body basics: a nutrition education program for adolescents about food, nutrition, growth, body image, and weight, *J. Am. Diet. Assoc.*, 102, S68, 2002.
89. Parcel, G.S., et al. Translating theory into practice: intervention strategies for the diffusion of a health promotion innovation, *Fam. Community Health*, 12, 1, 1989.
90. American Medical Association, Department of Adolescent Health, *Guidelines for Adolescent Preventive Services*, American Medical Association, Chicago, 1992.
91. National Center for Education Statistics, Nutrition Education in Public Elementary and Secondary Schools. U.S. Department of Education, Office of Educational Research and Improvement, Washington, D.C., 1996.
92. Agron, P., Takada, E., and Purcell, A., California Project LEAN's food on the run program: an evaluation of a high school-based student advocacy nutrition and physical activity program, *J. Am. Diet. Assoc.*, 102, S102, 2002.
93. O'Neil, C.E. and Nicklas, T.A., Gimme 5: an innovative, school-based nutrition intervention for high school students, *J. Am. Diet. Assoc.*, 102, S93, 2002.
94. Story, M. and Neumark-Sztainer, D., Promoting healthy eating and physical activity in adolescents, *Adolesc. Med.*, 10, 109, 1999.
95. American Beverage Association. Available at: www.nsda.org. Accessed January 2, 2005.
96. Albertson, A.M., Tobelmann, R.C., and Leonard, M., Estimated dietary calcium intake and food sources for adolescent females, 1980–1992, *J. Adolesc. Health Care*, 20, 20, 1997.
97. Whiting, S.J., et al. Relationship between carbonated and other low nutrient dense beverages and bone mineral content of adolescents, *Nutr. Res.*, 21, 1107, 2001.
98. Fitzpatrick, L. and Heaney, R.P. Got Soda? *J. Bone Miner. Res.*, 18, 1570, 2003.
99. Wyshak, G., Teenaged girls, carbonated beverage consumption, and bone fractures, *Arch. Pediatr. Adolesc. Med.*, 154, 610, 2000.
100. Heaney, R.P. and Rafferty, K., Carbonated beverages and urinary calcium excretion, *Am. J. Clin. Nutr.*, 74, 343, 2001.
101. French, S.A. and Story, M., Soda isn't only low in calcium, *J. Bone Miner. Res.*, 19, 870, 2004.

6 Women's Health

Pamela Echeverria and Jyotsna Sahni

CONTENTS

INTRODUCTION

By 2030, a projected 1.2 billion women worldwide will be menopausal or postmenopausal with 47 million additional newcomers annually.[1] Traditionally, reproductive health was the focus of medical care for women. However, similar to their male counterparts, women are susceptible to many chronic diseases and conditions including but not limited to heart disease, hypertension, diabetes, cancer, obesity, and osteoporosis. A major shortcoming of medical care until just recently was that women were treated based on the knowledge of how to treat men. This comes about due to the fact that most clinical studies included only men. Hence, the findings from these studies were applied equally to the medical treatment of women. We now know that women experience unique medical conditions such as premenstrual syndrome (PMS) and menopause that are solely female conditions. We also know that the pathophysiology and the clinical manifestation of disease differ not only by gender but also by ethnicity.[2,3] Until recently, information regarding the medical treatment for various conditions and treatment options for women had been sorely lacking. In 1990, the Women's Health Equity Act was passed and the National Institutes for Health (NIH) established the Office of Research on Women's Health. This resulted in the allocation of research funds for women's health. Subsequently, over the last several years a few large studies focused research on women and women issues including the Women's Health Initiative (WHI). Launched in 1992 with completion scheduled for 2007, WHI includes over 160,000 (including approximately 30,000 minorities) postmenopausal women between the ages of 50 and 79 years, evaluating strategies for preventing heart disease, breast and colorectal cancers, and osteoporosis.[4] Several nutrition aspects are included in the clinical trial component; studying the effect of a low-fat diet in the prevention of breast and colorectal cancers and coronary heart disease, and the role of calcium and vitamin D supplementation in preventing fractures. The results from this study are expected to provide future direction for the healthcare for postmenopausal women on many fronts. Other studies addressing women's health issues have also been initiated and completed. This chapter will present the current recommendations for medical nutrition therapy as well as suggestions for the integration of complimentary therapies based on the best evidence available for disease prevention and intervention and unique issues that impact on women's health.

COMMONLY OCCURRING CONDITIONS AFFECTING WOMEN

PREMENSTRUAL SYNDROME

PMS is defined as a constellation of physical and emotional symptoms that occur during the luteal phase of the menstrual cycle that affects a varying percentage of menstruating women.[5–7] The luteal phase occurs after ovulation and before menstruation. For most women, this is 2 weeks before their periods. Physical symptoms include acne, bloating or weight gain, breast tenderness, fatigue, diarrhea or constipation, headache, muscle or joint pains, and sleep disturbances. Emotional symptoms range from anger, anxiety, crying, depression, food cravings, impulsiveness, irritability, and mood.[8,9]

The precise etiology of PMS is unknown; however, several theories have been proposed. A dysregulation of serotonin and other neurotransmitters in the brain is the favored reason for PMS.[8,10] Hormonal imbalance, either in estrogen or progesterone, fluctuations in calcium homeostasis and parathyroid hormone dysregulation, as well as abnormal levels of other hormones such as prolactin, aldosterone, and gonadotropins are thought to play a significant role.[11] Vitamin deficiencies, light deficiency, thyroid dysfunction, and alterations in glucose metabolism may contribute to some of the symptoms.[9]

A subgroup of women (3–5%) experience extreme symptoms, which can meet the criteria for premenstrual dysphoric disorder (PMDD). This is officially recognized in the Diagnostic and Statistical Manual of Mental Disorders (DSM-IV) as a psychiatric disorder. As numerous other disorders can masquerade as PMS, it is important that a woman with premenstrual symptoms keeps a daily chart of symptoms over the course of three menstrual cycles to ascertain personal cycle. Observation for factors that improve or exacerbate symptoms should be recorded. PMDD can negatively impact daily activities and quality of life. This occurs during the luteal phase of a woman's cycle. Due to severity, it may best be treated with pharmaceutical intervention such as antidepressants, β-blockers, diuretics, oral contraceptives; however, antidepressants in the group of selective serotonin reuptake inhibitors (SSRIs) are the treatment of choice.[12–15]

Recommended Interventions

Once PMS is diagnosed, changes in lifestyle, nutrition intervention, and medical treatment can reduce or alleviate symptoms.[9,10,15–18] Regular aerobic exercise can raise endorphins, which can elevate mood.[11,17,18] PMS can impact the body physiologically and psychologically. Nutrition has been shown to play a role in diminishing symptoms associated with PMS.[17,18]

The nutritional recommendations for PMS follow the same guidelines for proactive disease prevention.

- Limit simple sugars
- Increase fiber
- Eat small frequent meals and snacks
- Avoid caffeine, alcohol, and tobacco
- Limit saturated fats
- Reduce salt

A healthy diet consisting of lean proteins, fruits and vegetables, and complex carbohydrates consumed at regular intervals aid in stabilizing blood sugar levels, which in turn possibly avoid decreases in energy level and hypoglycemia, and increases mental performance.[10,11] Women with PMS can exhibit symptoms similar to glucose intolerance; however, rarely have an abnormal glucose tolerance test.[9,10] For women who suffer from bloating, weight gain, and breast tenderness, avoidance of salt is recommended to decrease fluid retention. Furthermore, consumption of a healthy diet early in life facilitates maintenance of health as well as decreasing the risk for chronic diseases more common in later life.

Dietary Supplements

Symptoms associated with PMS may be correlated with a diet consisting of refined or processed food with subsequently less B vitamins and trace minerals such as zinc, magnesium, and iron consumed. A healthy diet with vegetables, fruits and whole grains, and supplements such as B-complex vitamins, magnesium, and calcium may reduce symptoms.[19–21]

B_6 is an important cofactor for enzymes involved in estrogen conjugation in the liver. B_6 is also involved in the synthesis of several neurotransmitters including dopamine and serotonin. Some evidence suggests that supplement of B_6 in doses up to 100 mg/day is beneficial for alleviating premenstrual depression and premenstrual symptoms.[19,22,23] However, a B-complex is recommended over single B_6-vitamin supplementation due to large doses (>200 mg/day), which can lead to neurological deficits[19,22,23] (see Table 6.1 for symptom management and dosage).

Magnesium aids in the production of prostaglandins, dopamine and serotonin synthesis, as well as estrogen conjugation. Supplementation may lessen PMS symptoms.[20–22] Chocolate cravings may be associated with low magnesium levels.[24] Suggestions for the emotional uplifting properties provided by chocolate could be related to endorphin release in the brain.[23] Sugar and chocolate cravings associated with PMS can lead to overindulgence, which may actually exacerbate symptoms. There is 100 mg of magnesium in 100 g of chocolate. Research is inconsistent as to whether magnesium supplementation is beneficial for reducing PMS symptoms; however, the average daily magnesium intake for U.S. women is less than the reference daily intake (RDI).[20–22] Conversely, calcium supplementation (1000–1300 mg/day) has been associated with lessening symptoms such as irritability, depression, anxiety, and muscle cramps associated with PMS.[20]

Certain herbs have been utilized to help manage PMS. Chaste tree berries (*Vitex agnus-castus*) are mostly used in Europe for the treatment of PMS. Women noted, after using chaste tree berries for three menstrual cycles, an improvement in PMS-related symptoms, specifically, irritability, depression, headaches, and breast tenderness. Black cohosh may help with the mood swings and irritability[25–28] (see "Herbal" section for more details).

Integrative Approach

Integrative approaches such as massage, Reiki, healing touch, meditation, yoga, reflexology, and deep breathing exercise can reduce stress and discomfort during PMS. Acupuncture, which works on energy meridians, may also be helpful. Reduction of stress before the start of the menstrual cycle can reduce PMS symptoms.[29]

Pharmacologic Therapy

Pharmacologic therapy includes a variety of medications such as nonsteroidal anti-inflammatory drugs (NSAIDs), which include ibuprofen and Naprosyn. These are especially helpful for treating menstrual cramps. Occasionally, a mild diuretic is useful in a woman with excessive fluid retention. Birth control pills (BCP) make the menstrual cycle very predictable and allow for planning and management of symptoms. BCP shorten and lighten menstruation as well as reduce cramps. For many women, the pill improves the symptoms of PMS. When anxiety is the predominant disturbance, anti-anxiety drugs such as Xanax® (alprazolam) or Ativan® (lorazepam) can be prescribed.[7] These agents should be taken as directed. The most favored drug therapy at this time targets neurochemical changes, especially in serotonin levels. For this reason, SSRIs are the drug class of choice for PMDD. Both Prozac® (fluoxetine) (Steiner) and Zoloft® (sertraline) have been approved by the FDA for use in PMDD. These medications may be used in a continuous way throughout the month or short term for 1 or 2 weeks during the luteal phase.[12–15]

PREGNANCY

The position of the American Dietetic Association (ADA) on nutrition and pregnancy is that nutrition plays a major role in fetal outcome and is also important in lactation. Optimal nutritional status preconception and through pregnancy ensures adequate gestational growth,

TABLE 6.1
Supplementation Recommendations for PMS Symptoms

Supplement	Recommended Dosage	Food Sources	Symptom Management	Adverse Effects	Upper Limit Level
B$_6$	50–100 mg/day	Fortified cereals, chicken, fish, pork, eggs	Prevents irritability and fatigue	No adverse effects from food. High doses of supplements can lead to neuropathy	Based on age 60–100 mg/day; greater than 20 years: 100 mg/day
Magnesium	300 mg/day	Green leafy veggies, nuts, seeds, unpolished grains, legumes	Prevents menstrual cramps, chocolate and simple sugar cravings	No adverse effects from food. Supplementation that leads to hypermagnesemia can lead to respiratory depression and cardiac arrest	350 mg/day (from supplements only)
Calcium	1200 mg/day	Milk and milk products, sardines, broccoli, kale, collard greens	Reduce menstrual cramps, moodiness and depression	Constipation may inhibit iron and zinc absorption, kidney stones, renal insufficiency	2500 mg/day
Vitamin D	400–800 IU/day	Fish liver oils, flesh of fatty fish, fortified milk, and cereals	Prevent premenstrual acne and oily skin	Elevated plasma 25 (OH) D concentration causing hypercalcemia	Women over 20 years: 50 µg/day
Zinc	25 mg/day	Fortified cereals, meats, seafood	Prevent premenstrual acne and oily skin	Reduced copper status	40 mg/day
Vitamin C	250–500 mg/day	Citrus fruits	Alleviate premenstrual allergies and stress	Gastrointestinal disturbances, kidney stones, excess iron absorption	Women over 20 years: 2000 mg/day

Source: From Bendich, A., *J. Am. Coll. Nutr.*, 19, 3, 2002; Wyatt, K.M. et al., *BMJ*, 381, 1375, 1999; adapted from DRI reports, www.nap.edu, copyright 2001 by The National Academies.

development, and reduction in birth defects.[30] Optimal weight gain, timely vitamin and mineral supplementation, safe food handling, avoidance of tobacco, alcohol, and other harmful substances are paramount for a positive fetal and maternal outcome. Alternative therapies during pregnancy and lactation such as herbals and botanicals are not recommended. Only a few randomized trials have examined efficacy or safety of herbs and botanicals use during pregnancy and lactation. Herbal teas should be limited to 2–8 oz servings per day. Alcohol consumption can lead to fetal alcohol syndrome as well as learning disabilities and birth defects. Caffeine can cross the placenta and should be limited to less than 300 mg/day.[30]

PERIMENOPAUSE

From the age of 35 years, fertility begins to decline. By 45 years, many women enter perimenopause, characterized by intermittent ovarian function and subtle changes in the symptoms, duration, and timing of the menstrual cycle.[31] The average age of menopause is 50 years.[1]

Symptoms, such as hot flashes or flushes, sleep disturbances, skin and vaginal dryness, and decreased libido, associated with menopause for some women can be daunting. About 80% of women going through menopause experience hot flashes. For some, the experience is mild and tolerable, for others, the hot flashes can interfere with activities of daily life. Foods that can warm the body can also exacerbate a hot flash (see Table 6.2 for food sources). For some women, giving up the food may be worst than the hot flash. The goal is not to combine a number of warming foods in one meal. The size of a meal can also contribute to hot flashes. Smaller more frequent meals are recommended versus a large meal that produces more body heat due to the thermal effect of digestion.[32] Sleep disturbances and mood swings are not uncommon. To manage the symptoms, based on severity, medications may be needed. Medications can include several classes of drugs such as hormone replacement medications and antidepressants.[31]

The "natural" approach to perimenopausal symptoms such as exercise, acupuncture, herbals, diet (inclusive of soy), massage, and other integrative approaches may be of benefit; however, efficacy for integrative techniques, supplements, and herbals are still questionable.

MENOPAUSE

Menopause is characterized by low levels of estrogen, progesterone, testosterone, cessation of menstrual periods, and loss of fertility. Ovarian aging is associated with hormonal and subsequent metabolic changes.[31] Many symptoms, similar to the perimenopause experience, such as hot flashes can continue into menopause. Hot flashes can occur from 1 to 5 years and are the most common of the symptoms experienced by women during the transition from perimenopause to menopause.[31] Night sweats, sleep disturbance, vaginal dryness, headaches,

---

TABLE 6.2
Foods Associated with Exacerbating Hot Flashes

Spices	Beverages	Foods	Other
Garlic	Hot drinks	Chocolate	
Onions	Alcohol: wine, beer spirits	Fat	Large meals
Ginger	Caffeine	Acidic foods (orange, tomatoes, etc.)	Hot temperature
Chili: green, red	Alcohol: wine, beer spirits	Sugar	Meals eaten too quickly
Salt			

Source: From Stopler Kasdan T, Menopause and diet, *Idea Today*, 46, 1997.

mood swings, short-term memory loss, and weight gain are additional symptoms that plague women during menopause. Loss of testosterone may contribute to loss of libido, weight gain, less energy, and diminution of pubic and underarm hair growth.[33]

Estrogen was previously recommended as the golden standard for treatment of hot flashes. However, recent research has found that estrogen use by postmenopausal women is associated with an increased risk for heart disease, breast cancer, stroke, and dementia.[34-36] Given the increased risk for many of the chronic diseases, women are now investigating other therapies for the treatment of menopausal symptoms including complementary medicine. The use of soy or other commercially available supplements containing soy or soy derivatives has not been shown in clinical trials to provide any benefits for reducing the incidence or severity of daily hot flashes.[37]

Reportedly, many women find alternative therapies or "natural" forms for treatment of menopausal symptoms beneficial.[38] This may include omega-3 fatty acids or soy isoflavones from foods and herbal formulas (see "Herbal Supplements" section for further discussion). With regard to soy, whole foods are superior over supplements. For example, soy foods in the form of edamame (young soybeans), soy milk, and tofu are preferable to soy pills. The efficacy and safety of taking concentrated pill forms is unknown.[37,39]

Beyond food and supplements, other pursuits for menopausal management can include acupuncture, stress management, or massage.[40]

POSTMENOPAUSE

Postmenopausal women are faced with an increased risk of heart disease, diabetes (especially if overweight), osteoporosis, and various cancers.[4,35,36,41,42] Lower estrogen levels impact on serum lipid levels with increases in total cholesterol and low-density lipoproteins cholesterol (LDL-C) levels while high-density lipoproteins cholesterol (HDL-C) levels decrease. Additionally, decreases in circulating estrogen levels affect bone density where bone resorption is greater than new bone production. Cancers most common at midlife are colon and breast cancer. Additionally, older women in general are more likely to be at nutritional risk when compared to men due to consumption of poorer quality diets.[43]

With aging, losses in lean body mass are commonly increasing the risk for sarcopenia. In general, individuals lose approximately 2–3% of lean tissue after 30 years of age.[44,45] Steady losses of lean body mass contribute to loss of strength, alterations in balance and gait, loss of physical function, and quality of life. Regular physical activity and weight resistance training have been shown to attenuate these losses.[46] Regular physical activity is also associated with decreased mortality and age-related morbidity in older people.[47] The importance of sustained physical activity throughout the life cycle is recommended by the American Heart Association and the American College of Sports Medicine.

The loss of lean body mass results in the loss of metabolically active tissue and a decrease in the metabolic rate of about 15–20% through the aging process.[48] Increases in total body fat often accompany decreases in lean body mass.

FIBROCYSTIC BREAST DISEASE

Breasts are large modified sweat glands that are composed of fat, cysts, and ducts. Breast tissue is organized into 12–20 triangular lobes with a central duct, which branches into smaller collecting ducts that lead to the nipple. Breast tissue is very responsive to hormonal changes, especially in presence of estrogen, during the menstrual cycle. Fibrocystic breast disease is a general term for a variety of breast disorders and is the most common cause of benign breast conditions. In general, it refers to the prominence of the cystic component of breasts that fluctuate over the course of the menstrual cycle, which usually worsens premenstrual. Fibrocystic breast changes occur in one third to one half of all menstruating women. It is most commonly seen in 30- to 50-year-old women. Breast changes can be simply the presence of "lumps" or prominent cysts that are found incidentally on palpation; some cause pain or tenderness that calls attention to the mass. Cysts are usually multiple, which occur in both breasts, and fluctuate in size and tenderness during the menstrual cycle. Increased intake of vegetables and fruits may decrease the incidence of fibrocystic breast disease.[5,49]

When there is a question about a palpated hardened area, the breast lump may represent a simple cyst or something more serious, an ultrasound, needle aspiration or biopsy may be necessary. Mammography use may be less effective for women with dense breasts; however, the use of naval sonar technology can increase breast imaging. This technology was developed by the U.S. Department of Defense.[50]

Treatment targets breast discomfort reduction. Avoidance of caffeine often helps; however, research is anecdotal and the correlation of caffeine avoidance and reduction in breast tenderness is not substantiated in the literature.[51] Some women benefit by salt reduction to limit fluid retention in the breasts. Vitamin E supplementation sometimes suggested to use in the reduction of fibrocystic breast discomfort does not provide much efficacy.[52] Evening primrose oil may alleviate pain, but research for efficacy is not substantiated. Wearing a supportive bra can also make the woman with fibrocystic discomfort more comfortable.[5]

UTERINE FIBROIDS

Fibroids, also called leiomyoma of the uterus, can often lead to a hysterectomy (surgical removal of the uterus). Uterine leiomyomas are a benign neoplasm composed of smooth muscle and connective tissue. In a nonpregnant woman, the fibroid may be asymptomatic; however, heavy or irregular vaginal bleeding can occur and occasionally dysmenorrhea. Symptoms can arise when pressure from the tumor pushes on surrounding organs. Infertility can be caused by a large fibroid that distorts the uterine wall. Due to the usual presentation of heavy bleeding, the woman can also have anemia. Treatment can include pharmaceutical intervention, myomectomy (removal of a muscular tissue tumor), which is preferred for women still in the childbearing years, or hysterectomy. A hysterectomy can put a woman prematurely into menopause, called "surgical menopause." If the fibroid is detected perimenopause, growth stimulation may occur with the use of hormone replacement therapy (HRT). Close observation is recommended for fibroids that tend to shrink after menopause when endogenous estrogen diminishes.[53]

POLYCYSTIC OVARIAN SYNDROME

Polycystic ovarian syndrome (PCOS) (Stein–Leventhal syndrome) is a disorder that has received much recognition recently. Traditionally, it was characterized by enlarged ovaries with multiple cysts, infrequent or absent periods, and infertility. This definition has been expanded to include insulin resistance as well. Obesity, acne, and hirsutism (excess hair growth especially at the mustache, chin, breasts, etc.) are also seen in at least half of women afflicted by PCOS (Textbox 6.1).

CHRONIC DISEASES AND WOMEN'S HEALTH

CORONARY ARTERY DISEASE

Coronary artery disease (CAD) is the number one killer of men and women in the industrialized world and is the leading cause of death among women over the age of 65 years.[58] While

---

Textbox 6.1

Age of onset for PCOS is 15 to 30 years and may be first diagnosed in women who are having difficulty in getting pregnant. Puberty usually progresses normally; however, as adolescence continues, periods may become farther apart. Enlarged ovaries are noted on pelvic exam in about half of the patients. A variety of hormonal abnormalities including high levels of urinary 17-ketosteroids, luteinizing hormone, dehydroepiandrosterone (DHEA), and androstenedione are used for diagnoses. Estrogen and follicle-stimulating hormone (FSH) levels are normal. Ultrasound of the ovaries and laparoscopy may also aid in diagnosis.[5]

Many women with PCOS who are overweight are also insulin-resistant.[54] Diet, exercise, and weight control are the primary nutritional management tools. The diet should be targeted to eating low-glycemic index foods with smaller more frequent meals of lean protein, increased vegetables, fruits, and complex carbohydrates.[55] Exercise should include frequent aerobic activity to enhance insulin sensitivity and promote weight loss.[56]

Medical therapy includes prescribing the BCP if a woman does not desire fertility or Clomid® (clomiphene citrate) if a woman is trying to conceive. Interestingly, a commonly used antidiabetic drug, Glucophage® (metformin), improves fertility rates in some poly-cystic women even if not diabetic. Further research, however, is needed to better elucidate the association between insulin resistance, fertility, and the complex interplay of insulin, glucose, and the female sex hormones.[53,57]

---

women tend to develop their heart disease 5 to 10 years later than men, survival is less.[59] Women may experience symptoms that are different from men's and may be misdiagnosed or mistreated.[60] Women are less likely to receive aggressive treatment after a heart attack and are more likely to die in the hospital.[26] Black women are at even greater disadvantage and are even less likely than men or white women to receive lifesaving therapies for heart attacks.[34] Premenopausal black women are at higher risk for heart attacks than Caucasian women possibly related to a higher saturated fat and cholesterol intake plus higher body mass index (BMI), blood pressure readings, lipoprotein (a), and higher homocysteine levels.[61]

Risk factors for CAD are illustrated in Table 6.3. Lipoprotein (a), a hereditary marker of heart disease, is a specialized LDL molecule that is ten times more likely to lay down cholesterol plaque.[62] Niacin may reduce the risk for this predisposition to heart disease; especially when other modifiable risk factors such as diet and exercise are controlled.

Menopause also affects a woman's heart history.[63] As estrogen levels diminish during the transition to menopause, healthy HDL-C levels may decrease and LDL-C may increase, thereby increasing the risk for CAD. As previously discussed, lifestyle changes such as avoidance of excess weight, physical inactivity, and consumption of a healthy diet are associated with reduced risks and associated morbidity.

Although it would seem prudent to provide supplemental estrogen in light of diminishing levels with menopause, adverse effects from the use of estrogen plus progestin were identified in the WHI with an increased risk of ischemic stroke in relatively healthy postmenopausal women as well.[36]

Lifestyle Recommendations to Reduce Risk

Many of the risk factors for heart disease are amenable to lifestyle modification. For example, avoidance of tobacco abuse and secondhand smoke. The risk for hypertension can be reduced

TABLE 6.3
Risk Factors for Heart Disease

Nonmodifiable risk factors
Family history
Age
Gender
Menopausal status

Modifiable risk factors
Hypertension
Diabetes
Dyslipidemia
Elevated homocysteine levels
Elevated C-reactive protein levels
Elevated fibrinogen levels
Elevated lipoprotein (a) levels
Tobacco abuse
Physical inactivity
Obesity
Poor diet
Stress reduction or avoidance of caffeine and alcohol may be helpful

Source: From Scaefer, E., *Am. J. Clin. Nutr.*, 75, 191, 2002; Hu, B. and Willett, W., *JAMA*, 288, 2569, 2002; Noakes, M. and Clifton, P., *Curr. Opin. Lipidol.*, 15, 31, 2004.

through stress reduction, smoking cessation, regular physical activity, salt and alcohol moderation, maintenance of a healthy weight, and consumption of the dietary approaches to stop hypertension (DASH) diet.[64–67]

Sodium restriction has been an area of controversy with restrictions targeted to those individuals with a salt sensitivity. Observational trials have been inconsistent regarding a universal recommendation for salt restriction for individuals with hypertension.[66] The DASH diet has been shown as a nonpharmacologic strategy for managing hypertension. The diet focuses on increased dietary sources of potassium, magnesium, and calcium.[67]

Serum cholesterol levels (total cholesterol and LDL-C), an independent risk factor for CAD, may be controlled by lowering the intake of both saturated and *trans*-fatty acids and through weight reduction in overweight or obese individuals.[67] Trans isomers when compared to saturated fat are regarded as more atherogenic.[62] High levels of *trans*-fats, labeled as hydrogenated or partially hydrogenated oils, are found in many processed and prepared foods such as crackers, pastries, fried foods, fast foods, and margarine.

The Women's Healthy Lifestyle Project study found that changes in lifestyle such as reducing intake of calories, total fat, saturated fat, and dietary cholesterol, along with increased physical activity resulted in a significantly smaller increase in LDL-C levels during the transition from perimenopause to menopause in the intervention group when compared to the control group where no lifestyle changes were made.[68] Additionally, eating smaller frequent meals per day also contributes to a slight (~3%) decrease in cholesterol levels.[67]

Long-chain omega-3 fatty acids found in cold-water fish (e.g., salmon, sardines, etc.), certain nuts and seeds are beneficial for both primary and secondary prevention of CAD.[38] The benefits associated with omega-3 fatty acids are discussed in "Omega-3 Fatty Acids" section.

An elevated serum triglyceride level is also thought to increase the risk for CAD. Avoidance of excess alcohol consumption (greater than one alcoholic beverage per day), reduction of refined carbohydrates, and less fatty foods can lower triglycerides,[69] while consumption of a diet high in refined carbohydrates, alcohol, and fried foods can increase triglyceride levels. Triglycerides are made up of remnant lipoproteins and lead to elevated LDL level, which can increase the risk for heart disease due to sluggish blood flow (lipemic). Small very low-density lipoproteins (VLDL) are thought to be oxidized quickly and cause more damage to the arteries.[70–72]

Plant sterols are derived from soybeans and corn and are sold in the United States in over-the-counter butter/margarine substitutes known as Benecol and Take Control. Stanols inhibit the absorption of dietary and biliary cholesterol in the intestines. These products are relatively inexpensive, with no interactions to medications and may drop LDL levels by 10–12% if consumed at the recommended dose.[73] However, maintaining a healthy weight by regular exercise and wise food choices is proactive for cardiac disease prevention and required in addition to stanols or "statin"-type drugs.

Which type of diet — high protein, low carbohydrate, high fat, low fat — is the subject of much debate among the experts and confusion for the rest of the population. Decades of research provide agreement among the experts that people should reduce the amount of saturated fat in the diet. The effect of saturated fat on the elevation of LDL is clear: it can increase the risk for heart disease.[74–76]

Very low carbohydrate diet (<60 g/day) appears to be more effective at promoting weight loss over 6 months than a low-fat diet.[77] Study results reveal that these diets also have positive effects on biomarkers of cardiovascular risk as LDL-C and triglycerides levels decrease with weight loss.[78] However, the efficacy and safety of these diets require further long-term follow-up before they can be recommended to the general population.[78]

Consumption of soy protein reportedly lowers total cholesterol (9%), LDL-C (13%), and triglycerides (11%) levels.[79] HDL-C levels have not been shown to be affected. Women who ate a daily diet inclusive of soy had less artery stiffness with the greatest benefit seen in postmenopausal women.[80] Asian women, living in Asia, historically have a lower risk for heart disease, which could be attributed to daily soy intake; however, general lifestyle may also play a key role. Soy provides polyunsaturated fat instead of the saturated fat meat contains. Soy protein ingestion, 25 g/day, can decrease total cholesterol, LDL, and triglyceride levels, but not documented to increase HDL level.[81]

Obesity

Historically, during a cave-dwelling existence, the diet consisted of a complex carbohydrate and a low-fat diet. Dessert was fiber-packed berries. Food processing was simplistic with subsequent slower digestion. Blood glucose was better sustained and prolonged with the diet of the ancient ancestors.[82] Today, Americans are faced with the "supersized," overly processed, and a myriad of simple carbohydrate offerings. As a society, Americans are growing fatter and faced with risk factors for numerous disease states, largely due to obesity. A BMI in excess of 30 sets the stage for heart disease, diabetes, hypertension, and a multitude of cancers. The prevalence of obese adults has more than doubled in the last decade.[83] Sixty-one percent of the American adult population can be classified as overweight or obese in a climate of numerous diet programs, exercise equipment, health clubs, and weight loss spas. The World Health Organization estimates one billion people worldwide tip the scales as overweight or obese.[84] The morbidly obese (BMI > 35 kg/m^2) are a growing population with increasing numbers opting for surgical intervention not only for appearance but also to decrease the incidence of comorbidities.[85]

Obesity is more prevalent among women than men, especially among the Hispanic and African American ethnicities and is increasing rapidly among adolescents.[86] Weight gain during adulthood is also associated with an increased risk for disease. The results of two national epidemiologic studies have found that subjects in the Nurses' Health Study and the Health Professional Follow-up Study, who gained 5.0–9.9 kg (11–22 lb) after the age of 18–20 years, had an increased risk of 1.5 to 3 times for CAD, hypertension, cholelithiasis, and type 2 diabetes compared to their counterparts who had maintained their weights within 2 kg. Obesity has also been shown to affect women's psychosocial status and self-esteem.

With regard to weight loss or weight maintenance, as women progress through the life cycle, small lifestyle changes provide continuity and a long-lasting maintenance regimen. Taking HRT may cause water weight gain. The percentage of body fat (approximately 1 lb/year) has also been shown to increase for many women during the menopause transition without any significant change in body weight.[68,86] Thyroid hormones decrease some, which can lead to a lower metabolic rate. During menopause, estrogen falls about 70% and testosterone about 40%. Less estrogen and presence of circulating testosterone may readily attach to abdominal testosterone receptors, which can lead to the accumulation of central adiposity or "meno-pot."[87,88] The results of the Women's Healthy Lifestyle Project, a randomized clinical trial, showed that a lifestyle intervention that combines dietary changes, reduced intake of calories, and total fat calories as well as a decrease in both saturated fat and increased leisure time physical activity found that weight gain during the transition from perimenopause to menopause could be prevented compared to the control group.[68]

Hypertension

Obesity and metabolic syndrome are associated with a higher incidence of hypertension. Poor-quality diet, especially lacking in potassium and calcium, a stressed existence, and alcohol can lead to elevated systolic and diastolic readings. Poor management of blood pressure can lead to stroke, heart failure, and kidney disease.[65,89] Reducing the alcohol intake to the recommended limit for females (1–2 drinks per day) can reduce blood pressure.[69] Exercise, massage, meditation, chi gong, and a host of other integrative approaches can help to reduce stress. Eating a diet rich in calcium, magnesium, potassium, and fiber such as the DASH diet can have a positive influence of regulating blood pressure. The DASH diet has shown decrease in both systolic and diastolic readings when intervention groups also limited sodium intake to 1,500 mg/day or less. In our fast food, ready to go food, processed food society, adherence may be a challenge.[90]

Do not smoke. Quitting can help enormously in reducing the risk of heart disease and lung cancer. Smoking is the leading cause of lung cancer. According to the American Cancer Society, the number of estimated cancer deaths for 2002 from lung cancer (predominant cause is smoking and a modifiable risk) is 65,700 women.[91] Smoking also increases the risk for vascular problems, discolors the skin, and accelerates facial wrinkles.

Alcohol is a special health dilemma for women. Alcohol in excess of one drink per day can lead to an increased risk of breast cancer and negatively impact on bone health even though it may be good for the heart.[92]

Water is life's elixir and plays an important role all through the life cycle. An average of 60% of a woman's body composition is water. Water is the primary component of blood, tears, and saliva. Water dilutes toxins and helps to regulate body temperature as well as a number of chemical reactions during metabolism. How much water an individual requires is based on weight, the amount of calories burned, climate, and the exercise regimen. Each calorie burned requires 1 ml of water.[93] As women age, fat can replace lean body mass, especially for the postmenopausal woman. Lean body mass and water go together, therefore with more fat mass the body composition of water can decline. A decline in percent of total body water can increase risk for dehydration.[93]

Metabolic Syndrome

Metabolic syndrome, also known as Syndrome X, was coined by Dr. Gerald Reaven in 1988, to describe a group of risk factors. Insulin resistance, Syndrome X, cardiovascular dysmetabolic or metabolic syndromes are synonymous. Insulin resistance can increase the incidence of heart disease, diabetes, and hypertension by the following ways: increased uric acid, blood clotting, oxidative stress, and greater circulating VLDL, plus hyperandrogenicity in women.[94] The role of insulin is to facilitate blood glucose entrance into the cells to be used for metabolic functions. As a result of the body's resistance to insulin, the pancreas must generate increasing amounts of insulin. Hyperinsulinemia compensates for poor glucose utilization, but over time pancreatic beta cell destruction can occur. Insulin resistance can increase circulation of free fatty acids, leading to dyslipidemia.[95] One in five Americans could be labeled as insulin-resistant. As men and women age to the fifth and sixth decades, the incidence on insulin resistance increases 50%.[83] Obesity and insulin resistance are intricately entwined. Due to the increased amount of fat cells, obese individuals are less responsive to insulin. Converting glucose into energy becomes a challenge. The body's response to insulin resistance is to produce more insulin. Not only is the obese state further fueled, but also the comorbidities previously listed. Insulin and several related hormones (growth factors) can expedite cell growth and mutation. The rapid cell reproduction in insulin resistance can negatively impact on colon cells. The risk of colon cancer after the fifth decade is increased in the presence of comorbidities especially obesity and a low-fiber diet.[96–98]

Metabolic syndrome is defined as central adiposity or waist circumference greater than 102 cm in men and 88 cm in women, triglyceride level of >150 mg/dl, HDL <40 mg/dl (in men), and <50 mg/dl (in women), blood pressure of at least 130/85 mmHg, and serum glucose level of 110 mg/dl.[99] In insulin resistance, blood glucose can be at the high end of normal; however, usually the "apple shape" is apparent in conjunction with dyslipidemia.

Prediabetes is synonymous with metabolic syndrome, and is a new term coined by the USDA/HHS and is characterized by a fasting blood glucose level of 110–126 mg/dl. Most individuals screened with prediabetes will be diagnosed with type 2 diabetes within 10 years. An 8 h fasting blood glucose of 126 mg/dl or higher is considered to be diagnostic for type 2 diabetes.[89,100] Type 2 diabetes, also referred to as "adult onset diabetes," or "old age" diabetes, is a rising epidemic in the United States as the population grows older and fatter. As the process of poor glucose control unfolds, cholesterol values change in predicable ways with a rise in triglycerides and decrease in HDL. Women who suffer diabetes are three to five times more likely to get CAD than their nondiabetic cohort.[101,102] Prevention and early treatment of metabolic syndrome and delay of type 2 diabetes are the goal and challenge for health professionals (Textbox 6.2).

Cancer Prevention

Diet, physical activity, and maintenance of a healthy body weight are the key elements for disease prevention and a good quality of life. Over one million people per year are diagnosed with cancer. The prediction is one in three women will develop cancer in their life, mostly in

---

Textbox 6.2

Approximately 25% of the population has insulin resistance.[83] The Pima Indians in Arizona show how genetic predisposition for obesity can be expressed by a sedentary lifestyle and overly processed diet. Presently, 50% of Pima Indians are obese and have type 2 diabetes.[103]

The glycemic index was first coined by David Jenkins back in 1981 to help determine the best food choices for individuals with diabetes. The first published glycemic index list had 62 food values, now the glycemic index lists a multitude of foods. The index is a ranking of foods in response to postprandial blood glucose as compared to an item that provides a quick response such as glucose.[104] The lower glycemic index foods have a gradual rate of digestion. Single foods are the focus of the glycemic index, when most people eat a combination of foods. The glycemic response can be skewed by what foods are combined. Certainly if a myriad of high-glycemic foods are eaten at a meal, the effect on glycemic response and subsequent insulin response will be much greater than a combination of low-glycemic index foods. Choosing low-glycemic index foods can lead to lower level of plasma triglyceride levels postprandially.[105] These foods typically contain more fiber than higher glycemic index foods. A low-glycemic index diet includes greater vegetables, fruits, grains, balanced with lean protein and monounsaturated fat.[95,106]

---

the fifth decade.[107] While HRT may increase the risk of invasive breast cancer, blood clots, gallbladder disease, and ovarian cancer, it is still an option for menopausal management. Long-term therapy is not recommended for most women due to the small increase in risk of breast cancer after 5 years of treatment.[108] Risk factors need to be weighed against the severity of menopausal symptoms on an individual basis.

Breast Cancer

The breast is the most common cancer site in women and behind lung cancer is the leading cause of cancer death of women in the United States. Mortality rates of breast cancer is highest among black women.[109–111] Breast cancer incidence is the lowest among Asian (Korean and Vietnamese) and American Indian women.[109,110] Reduced incidence of breast cancer can be found among women in the Mediterranean, Eastern Europe, and Asia, who are suspected to be reflective of diet. Diets containing soy, fruits and vegetables, or fiber and more specific phytic acid also known as inositol hexaphosphate or IP6 may contribute to cancer prevention.[112] Lifestyle can also be a modifiable factor for cancer risk. Aging, high stress, and atherosclerosis can damage cells by free radicals.[113] Nonmodifiable risk factors include genetic predisposition, tallness, and Jewish heritage. Modifiable risk factors include environment and lifestyle. Several dietary factors have been associated with the decreased risk of breast cancer. However, the role of fat, ratio of omega-3 to omega-6 is not well defined as a protector against breast cancer.[114–116] Benefits of a low-fat diet for breast cancer prevention can be debated; however, the most contributory risk factor is obesity and a matter of weight loss. Obesity leads to increased body fat and subsequent endogenous estrogen, which can increase the risk for breast cancer. Observational studies suggest low-glycemic index foods help control insulin response, provide satiety, and bind with estrogen in the gastrointestinal tract to increase excretion.[55,56,104] Fruits and veggies provide antioxidants, which can decrease cancer risk. Alcohol, even one drink per day may help the heart, but can increase the risk of breast cancer.[92,115]

Reproductive Cancers (Ovarian, Uterine, Cervical)

Uterine and ovarian cancers are considered as hormone-stimulated cancers and account for the fifth and sixth most common cancer deaths in the United States.[117] Etiology of ovarian cancer is not definitive; however, risk factors include first-degree relative with ovarian cancer, greater than 10 years of estrogen replacement therapy, and fertility drugs. Over half of the ovarian cancer diagnosed is in women over the age of 65 years.[118] Hyperinsulinemia and insulin resistance are also hypothesized to be a risk factor for ovarian cancer and in women with polycystic ovary syndrome can be a risk for endometrial cancer.[119,120] Cervical cancer is the second most common cancer diagnosed in women. This can be diagnosed early with the use of a pap smear.[121] Risk factors for cervical cancer include a history of multiple sex partners, incidence of sexually transmitted diseases, smoking, and poor dietary habits.[122]

Daily positive lifestyle and healthy eating habits can reduce risk factors for cancer.[116,123]

- Remain physically active with a healthy weight
- Limit alcohol intake
- Eat a variety of foods with a focus on colorful vegetables and fruits
- Increase vegetables and fruits consumption to 8–10 servings per day
- Consume less fatty foods with a focus to incorporate more omega-3 fats
- Choose whole grains and legumes
- Incorporate daily activities for stress reduction

OSTEOPOROSIS

Aging and bone loss go hand in hand, but not to the point of debilitation except in cases of osteoporosis. In the United States, 15% of the women over 50 years and older are afflicted with osteoporosis.[124] Controllable risk factors for osteoporosis are smoking, alcohol ingestion, poor calcium intake, and lack of exercise. Due to the decline in estrogen during and postmenopause, bone density also declines. Trabecular bone loss leads to porous bones and increases the risk for osteopenia, which can progress to osteoporosis. Bone health is influenced by an adequate intake of key micronutrients associated with bone mineralization (calcium, vitamin D, vitamin K, boron, and magnesium); pharmaceuticals such as bisphosphonates, risedronate, alendronate, and possibly calcitonin are effective tools for hip fracture prevention.[125] Specific recommendations for the maintenance of bone density and treatment of low bone density are discussed in Chapter 8.

DEPRESSION

Depression is a common but much misunderstood illness, affecting millions of American women each year.[126] About one in eight women can expect to develop depression some time during their lives.[126] It affects women two to three times as much as men and occurs most commonly in women aged 25 to 44 years.[127]

Depression is defined by the DSM-IV and refers to either a persistent sad mood or the loss of pleasure in most activities. It is accompanied by at least four additional symptoms: changes in appetite or weight, changes in sleep pattern, fatigue, poor memory and concentration, restlessness or decreased activity, feelings of worthlessness, hopelessness, or inappropriate guilt, and preoccupation with thoughts of death or suicide. If these symptoms persist for two or more weeks and impair usual functioning at work or home, the diagnosis of clinical depression is made. Unfortunately, depression is misdiagnosed or underrecognized in a large number of women.[128]

Risk factors for depression in women include lower socioeconomic status, educational level, and unemployment. These problems in general are seen more often in women than men. Additionally, women who suffer racial or ethnic discrimination, lower educational and economical levels, low status and high-stress work, poor health, larger family size, divorce, and single parenthood are more at risk than Caucasian women.[129] Symptoms relating to depression can vary for different ethnicities; Japanese women have more somatic complaints than American women. Suicide attempts for adolescents also vary based on ethnicities. Hispanic Latino adolescent suicide attempts were significantly higher than African American or Caucasian girls.[130]

Women who have been the victims of sexual and physical abuse are more at risk than other women. Married women have higher rates of depression than unmarried women. Women seem to experience depression somewhat differently from men. Women tend to experience more seasonal depression and unusual symptoms such as extreme sleepiness, extreme hunger especially for carbohydrates, weight gain, a heavy feeling in arms and legs, evening mood exacerbations, and initial insomnia. Seasonal affective disorder (SAD) can present as depressive episodes during the winter months with resolution of symptoms in the summer months. Light therapy can be useful for some individuals who are diagnosed with SAD.[131] Depression in women is also more often associated with anxiety, panic, phobia, eating disorders, and dependent personality. Women also attain higher blood levels of antidepressant medication and therefore require lower dosages.

Careful attention to a woman's depression and the relationship with menstruation, pregnancy, the perinatal period, or the perimenopausal period should be further explored. The role of BCP or HRT can be considered for depression management. In addition, more women than men suffer from hypothyroidism (underfunctioning thyroid gland) and should be ruled out as an organic cause of depression.

Treatment is extremely effective in depression and must be tailored to meet the woman's needs and circumstances. A wide variety of treatment options are available including exercise, light therapy, herbs, appropriate nutrition, psychotherapy, social support, medications, and even electroconvulsive therapy in recalcitrant cases of depression.[131–133] Exercise has been shown to increase endorphin levels, which elevate mood. Exercise also decreases cortisol levels, a stress hormone produced by the adrenal glands, thereby relaxing a patient. In addition, exercise allows a woman to play an active role in her own recovery from depression. Treatment-resistant depression is reported to affect one third of geriatric individuals with depression.[134]

The most common herb used to treat depression is St. John's wort (*Hypericum perforatum*). It is the most commonly prescribed treatment of mild depression in Germany and is used commonly throughout Europe. It works at a receptor site in the brain such as drugs similar to Prozac, and may be equally effective in mild cases of depression. Studies have shown conflicting results, but an NIH trial is currently underway. Since St. John's wort is metabolized through the cytochrome P450 pathway in the liver, it may interfere with the actions of other medications and should be used cautiously.[135]

PHYTOCHEMICAL INTAKE

Health benefits of phytochemicals (plant chemicals) are the integrative approach to cancer, cardiac, and other disease prevention associated with the aging population. Phytochemicals are abundant in fruits, vegetables, grains, nuts, and some herbs. When the diet contains variety, a plethora of antioxidants can be ingested. Common phytochemicals are flavonoids, isoflavones, phytosterols, and carotenoids. The best sources are berries, leafy greens, and cruciferous vegetables.

Flavonoids act as antioxidants, which can reduce the risk of cancer and heart disease. Common sources are citrus fruits, tea, wine, and oregano. Green tea contains flavonoids, epigallocatechin gallate (EGCG), catechin, epicatechin, and epicatechin gallate, which provides antioxidant activity inclusive of a decrease in lipid perioxidation.[136,137] Resveratrol is an antioxidant found in red wine, grapes, and peanuts, which has exhibited anticancer properties. This antioxidant can aid in the uptake of cholesterol, decreases LDL oxidation in the blood, and minimizes platelet aggregation, which can lead to clot formation.[136] With regard to cancer protection, human research has not been consistent. In mice, skin tumors were prevented with the use of green tea. The flavonoid, EGCG, has been documented to stop mitosis and cell division, which mediates anticancer activity.[137]

Carotenoids present in vegetables and fruits, which contain a yellow-orange pigment act as antioxidants to help reduce the risk of numerous cancers.[138] Good food sources are carrots, sweet potatoes, tomatoes, pumpkin, and apricots. To increase phytochemicals in the diet, eat vibrant colored vegetables and fruits.

Phytoestrogens

Soy has increased in popularity over the last decade. Americans have adapted to soy in the diet, consumers report eating a soy product at least one time per week; however, more processed soy foods instead of the whole soy foods or traditional Asian dishes of tofu and tempeh are consumed. Soy milk is the most common source of soy use for Americans.[139] Studies investigating the benefits of soy are predominant in the Asian population as soy is a mainstay of the diet. For non-Asians in the United States, the use of soy is typically not daily.[140]

Isoflavones, a component of soy, are believed to block human-produced estrogen, which can encourage the growth of hormone-sensitive tumors. Isoflavones are heterocyclic phenols and structurally similar to estradiol-17 beta. Isoflavones are selective to estrogen receptor modulators; however, action at the cellular level is dependent on the target tissue receptor sites and the amount of endogenous estrogen available. Estrogenic and antiestrogenic properties have been attributed to isoflavones.[141–143] Soy isoflavones are labeled as genistein, daidzein, and glycitein. Genistein and daidzein are similar in structure to estrogen, but provide weak estrogenic action as compared to endogenous estrogen.[141] Phytoestrogens provided by isoflavones are theorized to bind to the receptor sites of cells and displace endogenous estrogen.[144] Speculated benefit of isoflavones is to inhibit estrogen activity in cells, which may subsequently reduce the risk of ovarian and breast cancer.[142] Presently there is no evidence that isoflavones stimulate endometrium tissue.[145] Cancer is mainly a disease of aging; isoflavones have been suggested to exert anticarcinogenic effects by inactivation of potentially carcinogenic metabolites from the metabolism of estrogen in postmenopausal women.[145–147] The counterpoint to the possible benefits of soy leads to debate. The aura around soy and breast cancer poses the question if the breast tumor is estrogen-dependent would even a weak estrogenic effect induce tumor growth? Does it interfere with Tamoxifen®? These questions require further research. Isoflavone supplementation and chemically extracted soy isolates are not recommended. Supplementation of soy would include isoflavone pills, whose safety or efficacy has not been established[148–150] (Textbox 6.3).

Food sources for isoflavones include legumes and nuts with the richest source in soy. Soy contains many potentially anticarcinogenic compounds including saponins, phytates, protease inhibitors, and isoflavones. The two most studied isoflavones, genistein and daidzein, are believed to contribute to disease prevention.[150] Actions of phytoestrogens may prevent against perimenopausal symptoms, menopausal symptoms, cardiovascular disease, many types of cancers and osteoporosis, obesity, and diabetes. However, the previously mentioned belief

---

Textbox 6.3

The use of soy and a decreased risk for breast cancer is inconclusive. Isoflavone supplementation in postmenopausal women suggests a decrease in breast density, which is a marker for increased risk of breast cancer.[142–146] The opposite is evident in premenopausal women. Other studies show that addition of soy during puberty may decrease estrogen-dependent tumors for postmenopausal women.[148] Isoflavones can bind to estrogen receptors sites and decrease endogenous estrogen action.[145,146] Other actions that isoflavones have demonstrated are nonsteroidal, antioxidant, and antiproliferative. Phytohormones eaten as whole foods may protect breast and uterine tissue from overstimulation of estrogen.[145] However, the efficacy of isoflavones is debated due to conflicting research. Besides the possibility of isoflavones enhancement for good health, the monounsaturated fat, polyunsaturated fat, minerals, fiber, complex carbohydrate, and antioxidants found whole soybean products most likely contribute to reduction in disease states plagued in postmenopausal women (cancer, heart disease, and osteoporosis).[140,145,149,150]

---

that soy can ward off cancer, boost immunity, and guard against diabetes may not be all it is touted to be and subject of much debate in the research. Summation of the literature indicates whole soy foods can be a healthy addition to the diet regardless of the speculated benefits.[150–161]

Cardiovascular Disease Prevention

With regard to cardiovascular prevention, the belief is phytosterols can block the absorption of dietary cholesterol in blood circulation and reduce reabsorption of cholesterol in the liver.[140,145,149,150] Soy supplies quality protein with mostly polyunsaturated fat instead of saturated fat, which is predominant in meat. Addition of soy protein to a diet also rich in legumes and nuts provides soluble fiber and can reduce total cholesterol, LDL, triglycerides, lower insulin requirements, and can aid in weight management.[155,157,158,161,162]

ROLE OF DIETARY FATTY ACIDS IN DISEASE PREVENTION

Essential fatty acids (EFA) are the building blocks of fats omega-3 (alpha-linolenic) and omega-6 (linoleic), which are provided by the diet to the body. The American diet provides greater amounts of omega-6 fatty acids than omega-3 fatty acids whereas the health-related benefits focus on a more even ratio of omega-3 fatty acid to omega-6 fatty acid. The benefits related to consumption of omega-3 fatty acids are the reduced risk of heart disease, reduction in the inflammatory process, and possibly a positive impact on immune function and eye health.[163] Dietary fatty acids are metabolized to one of the two pathways. The metabolism of omega-6 fatty acids results in the production of eicosanoids, prostaglandins, leukotrienes, and their metabolites, which are more inflammation-producing. Conversely, the metabolic pathways of omega-3 fatty acids result in the production of metabolites, which are less inflammatory.[164]

Omega-3 Fatty Acids

Important omega-3 fatty acids are eicosapentaenoic acid (EPA) and docosahexaenoic acid (DHA). DHA plays an important role in vision. Omega-3 fatty acids can decrease inflammation and decrease platelet aggregation, which can reduce the incidence of clots. The best sources of omega-3 fatty acids are fatty fish and flaxseeds. Omega-6 fatty acids are found in vegetables and vegetable oils. To increase omega-3 levels, greater fatty fish consumption of

— two to three times per week (4–6 oz) is recommended; however, wild salmon is preferred over farm-raised salmon due to less chemical contaminants. Flaxseed is a vegetable source that can offer omega-3 fatty acids with a goal of 1–2 tablespoons per day. Flax is a great source of lignans precursor, which converts in the body to a weak antiestrogen. Ground flaxseed or flaxseed oil can be a source of omega-3 for individuals with fish allergies. Omega-3 supplements can be an alternative for individuals who do not eat fish. Cardiovascular protective effects are achieved by combining EPA and DHA, which plays a role in the modulation of the inflammatory process.[165]

Gamma-Linolenic Acid

Gamma-linolenic acid (GLA) is a precursor for anti-inflammatory prostaglandins as the product of transformation of linoleic to eicosanoids. GLA has been used by the Native American Indians for a variety of illnesses such as gynecological problems or gastrointestinal complaints but is limited in the diet except for breast milk. Supplementation can be provided by borage, black currant seed, and primrose oil. However, efficacy for supplemental GLA has not been demonstrated in the literature. Studies have failed to show any benefits with supplementation of GLA for PMS.[166] Other studies investigating the potential benefits associated with GLA and relief of menopausal symptoms have also been inconclusive.[167]

VITAMINS OR MINERALS: SUPPLEMENTS

The role of vitamin and mineral supplements is to "supplement" not to take the place of a well-balanced diet. However, as we age certain nutrients can be helpful in preservation of health. In the case of heart disease, the amount of folic acid, B_{12}, B_6 from the diet may not be adequate to maintain lower homocysteine levels. Supplemental B-vitamins may be warranted to help lower elevated homocysteine levels.[168,169] Folic acid can also reduce the risk of neural tube defects in the developing fetus and possibly reduce the risk for colon and breast cancer.[170–172] The risk for or incidence of strokes may be decreased with adequate potassium (food sources) in the diet especially if prescribed potassium wasting drugs such as diuretics.[173]

The goal for calcium intake for women is 1000–1500 mg/day with variation across the life span and based on bone density. Calcium is important for teenagers for whom bones are still forming and continues to be important throughout the life cycle to maintain bone density. For most women who do not consume dairy products, calcium supplementation should be considered. If the diet falls short of the recommended calcium level, supplementation should also be considered. Supplementation should include vitamin D. Vitamin D is primarily provided by the sun. Vitamin D can be maintained even with the use of sunblock.[174]

In the case of iron, once a woman is postmenopausal, the need for iron is reduced due to the lack of blood loss. Epidemiological studies have suggested an association with increased iron stores and risk for atherogenic potential of LDL; however, through angiographic testing this has since been debated.[175]

HERBAL SUPPLEMENTS COMMONLY RECOMMENDED

IPRIFLAVONE

Ipriflavone is also known as (IP)-7 isopropoxyisoflavone. This product is a derivative of isoflavones. Ipriflavone is used for several types of bone loss disorders such as Paget's disease, diabetes osteopenia (animal data), postmenopausal osteoporosis, osteoporotic pain, renal osteodystrophy.[176–178]

When reviewing this therapy for clinical trials in humans with bone loss disorders, studies found no clinical increase in bone density. As compared to unsupplemented therapy for prevention of bone loss, this supplement seems to help maintain current bone density. It may be an alternative as an adjunct to a healthy diet for bone loss prevention.[176–178]

Side effects and cautions include stomach pain and diarrhea, which can occur with iPriflavone supplementation. It is not recommended to be used in women who have renal dysfunction.[179] Limited safety data are available for treatment of pregnant or lactating women. Ipriflavone has metabolites that are removed from the body through the liver.[179] Caution is suggested for the use of ipriflavone when on the medication theophylline. A few documented cases of individuals who have taken ipriflavone had increased theophylline levels in their blood, leading to theophylline toxicity.[180]

Dehydroepiandrosterone

DHEA is also known as dehydroandrosterone and dehydroisoandrosterone. DHEA is a steroid hormone manufactured in the body's adrenal cortex and under the direction of hypothalamic corticotropin-releasing hormone and the pituitary. Clinical efficacy for DHEA treatment has been conflicting.[181] Human studies indicate benefit for people with low DHEA levels such as anorexia nervosa and infertility from anorexia nervosa or PCOS.[181,182] The effect of DHEA on the immune system has some positive responses reported in elderly patients[183] such as mood and well-being, sexual functioning, cardiovascular effects, and muscle strength.[184] Conflicting data have been reported regarding the benefits of DHEA therapy on memory or cognition, insulin sensitivity, and obesity. Small improvements were seen in a small trial of patients with multi-infarct dementia.[184] DHEA supplementation has improved symptoms of systemic lupus erythematosus (SLE) in several small trials.[185]

During DHEA production, other steroid-like compounds such as androstenedione may contaminate the DHEA supplement; of particular suspect are those DHEA supplements that are marketed for athletic performance.[186] Supplements are not routinely tested by federal or state agencies. The adverse effects of treatment are reported as liver dysfunction, irregular heart rate, acne, or skin rashes.[187] It would be prudent that pregnant or nursing women avoid the use of DHEA.

Black Cohosh

Black cohosh is classified as a hormonal modulator because it is suspected to have weak estrogen-like properties.[188] It is used primarily for the relief of menopausal symptoms including hot flashes, vaginal thinning and dryness, night sweats, sleep disturbances, anxiety, and depression and has been a consideration for use in PMS. Native Americans have used this as a cure for "female problems" for many years.[189]

Human studies have also demonstrated minimal benefit of black cohosh for menopausal symptoms.[190–192]

Adverse effect documented is stomach upset in normal doses, larger doses may lower blood pressure or create dizziness, headache, or tremors. There are also reports of larger doses of this treatment causing nausea and vomiting. The American Herbal Products Association rated black cohosh as class 2b, which identifies not for use during pregnancy and class 2c not for use during nursing. Some studies have shown that black cohosh has weak estrogen-like properties; it should be used with caution in women with tumors that are known to be estrogen-responsive.[191,193]

Chaste Tree Berries (*Vitex agnus-castus*)

Vitex can raise levels of progesterone and estrogen in women with low progesterone levels caused by hyperprolactinemia.[174] Homeopathic preparations of Vitex have been somewhat effective in improving female fertility.[194]

The efficacy of Vitex extract for regulation of menstrual cycle and decreasing excessive bleeding was evaluated. Overall, a perceived improvement of menstrual symptoms was reported, but no change in the duration of the cycle. Adverse effects of extract use included nausea, vomiting, allergic reaction, headaches, and increased menstrual flow for some women.[195]

It is recommended that *Vitex agnus-castus* be avoided for women who are pregnant or nursing. There is a potential interaction with this treatment and the use of dopamine-type drugs.[191,195]

Dong Quai

Dong quai is classified as an anticoagulant and female tonic. In Chinese medicine, dong quai is referred to as "woman's ginseng" because of its proposed benefits as a female tonic. This herb is widely used to treat many gynecological complaints in complimentary practices.[192] Dong quai is used for problems associated with the menses such as irregular or painful bleeding and with a standard dose of 5 g three times daily. Estrogen imbalances that produce fibroid tumors have been treated with dong quai. It is also used to strengthen the uterus and aid patients in supportive functions before pregnancy. As other possible hormone modulators, it should be avoided in pregnancy or when nursing. Adverse effects reported with this treatment include fever, skin sensitivity, and bleeding.[191-194]

Red Clover

Clinical studies for uses of red clover are lacking. Blood vessel flexibility or compliance, an important cardiovascular risk factor, was significantly improved in one small study of women given isoflavones from red clover extract.[196] Chemoprotective and estrogen effects of red clover have been studied in the laboratory and in animals only.[196]

Extracts and teas of red clover flowers are most commonly used to reduce symptoms of menopause and perimenopause. Excessive use should be avoided due to estrogenic constituents in red clover.[191,194]

Wild Yam

Wild yam is sometimes referred to as a phytoestrogen; however, the plant itself contains neither estrogen nor progesterones, yet it has been completely misrepresented in advertising. North American herbalists and practitioners often refer to wild yam as a "female herb" or a herb that contains "female hormone precursors." The rumor comes from the historical use of diosgenin, a constituent of Dioscorea, as a chemical that is used for the industrial synthesis of progesterone.[197,198]

Wild yam is a nerve relaxant useful in painful inflammatory and gastrointestinal conditions due to irritation and spasm. It helps to relieve the cramping pain of smooth muscles like the gallbladder and uterus.[191,194] Wild yam is best given in hot water for pain related to menses. It has shown results with midcycle spotting, premenstrual symptoms, painful menstruation, nausea of pregnancy, and spontaneous abortion due to a spasmodic uterus.

It has been noted that large doses of wild yam can cause nausea and vomiting.[191,194]

SUMMARY

In summary, the health and well-being for women throughout the life cycle is interwoven with lifestyle of healthy eating, exercise, maintenance of a healthy body weight, and stress reduction. Over the last two decades, several studies: PEPI Trial, HERS, HERS 2 looked at HRT as a way to reduce menopausal symptoms and improve disease outcomes.[199–205] The WHI changed the way, and many women think about HRT.[204,206] No longer is HRT recommended for cardiovascular protection or to slow bone loss. Many women left HRT behind in favor of finding alternative remedies for menopausal symptoms and other modalities for cardiovascular and osteoporosis prevention. HRT prescription is still an option for women with low breast cancer risk, but with menopausal symptoms that impede activities of daily life and diminish quality of life. Herbal treatments, vitamin and mineral supplementation, and soy may be helpful for some women to relieve the symptoms of PMS, depression, and perimenopausal symptoms; however, further research in these areas is needed to become standard care for the majority of women. Eating, exercising, reducing stress are daily activities that can be practiced to travel more smoothly from pubescence to postmenses.

CASE STUDY

Vanessa is a 46-year-old woman who lives in Atlanta, Georgia. She has a family history of cardiovascular disease and worries about her own cardiovascular health. She has night sweats, which wake her up at night, leading to insomnia. She has a short temper with her teenage son and daughter and often cries after a battle of wits. Vanessa never had a problem with her weight, but lately she is noticing the scale reads the same, but she is thickening around the middle and her clothes with a waistband fit differently. She is at the peak of her executive career. Instead of enthusiasm, Vanessa is easily distracted and overwhelmed by the numerous duties of her job. She figures a lot of the changes she is experiencing are related to perimenopause and feels her symptoms are not so overwhelming that pharmacological intervention is needed.

1. What could be some diet and lifestyle changes that Vanessa could make to help with her symptoms of perimenopause?
2. What vitamin and mineral supplements if any could be of benefit for prevention of chronic disease?
3. What type of alternative therapies may help with dealing with her teenage children?

REFERENCES

1. Hill, K., The demography of menopause, *Maturitas*, 2, 113, 1996.
2. Sheps, D.S., Kaufmann, P.G., Sheffield, D. et al., Sex differences in chest pain in patients with documented coronary artery disease and exercise-induced ischemia: results from the PIMI study, *Am. Heart J.*, 142, 864, 2001.
3. Doherty, T.M., Tang, W., and Detrano, R.C., Racial differences in the significance of coronary calcium in asymptomatic black and white subjects with coronary risk factors, *J. Am. Coll. Cardiol.*, 34, 787, 1999.
4. Writing Group for the Women's Health Initiative Investigators, Risks and benefits of estrogen plus progestin in healthy postmenopausal women: principal results from the Women's Health Initiative randomized controlled trial, *JAMA*, 288, 321, 2002.
5. DeCherney, A.H. and Pernoll, M.L., Eds., *Current Obstetric and Gynecologic Diagnosis and Treatment*, 8th ed., Appleton & Lange, Norwalk, CT, 1994.

6. Ugarriza, D., Klingner, S., and Obrien, S., Premenstrual syndrome: diagnosis and intervention, *Nurse Pract.*, 23, 49, 1998.

7. Singh, B. et al., Incidence of PMS and remedy usage: national probability sample study, *Altern. Ther. Health Med.*, 3, 75, 1998.

8. Boyle, C., Berkowitz, G., and Kelsey, J., Epidemiology of premenstrual symptoms, *Am. J. Public Health*, 77, 349, 1987.

9. Campbell, E., Premenstrual symptoms in general practice patients: prevalence and treatment, *J. Reprod. Med.*, 42, 637, 1997.

10. Kessel, B., Premenstrual syndrome advances in diagnosis and treatment, *Obstet. Gynecol. Clin. North Am.*, 27, 625, 2000.

11. Deuster, P., Adera, T., and South-Paul, J., Biological, social and behavioral factors associated with premenstrual syndrome, *Arch. Family Med.*, 8, 122, 1999.

12. Frackiewicz, E. and Shiovitz, T., Evaluation and management of premenstrual syndrome and premenstrual dysphoric disorder, *J. Am. Pharmacol. Assoc.*, 41, 437, 2001.

13. Bhatia, S.C. and Bhatia, S.K., Diagnosis/treatment of premenstrual dysphoric disorder, *Am. Family Physician*, 7, 1239, 2002.

14. Berger, C. and Presser, B., Alprazolam in the treatment of two subsamples of patients with late luteal phase dysphoric disorder: a double-blind, placebo-controlled crossover study, *Obstet. Gynecol.*, 84, 379, 1994.

15. Johnson, S.R., Premenstrual syndrome, premenstrual dysphoric disorder and beyond: a clinical primer for practitioners, *Obstet. Gynecol.*, 104, 845, 2004.

16. Massil, H. and O'Brien, P., Approach to the management of premenstrual syndrome, *Clin. Obstet. Gynecol.*, 2, 443, 1987.

17. Dye, L., Lluch, A., and Blundell, J., Macronutrients and mental performance, *Nutrition*, 16, 1021, 2000.

18. London, R., Bradley, L., and Chiamori, N., Effect of a nutritional supplement on premenstrual symptomatology in women with premenstrual syndrome: a double-blind longitudinal study, *J. Am. Coll. Nutr.*, 5, 494, 1991.

19. Wyatt, K. et al., Efficacy of vitamin B_6 in the treatment of premenstrual syndrome review, *BMJ*, 318, 1375, 1999.

20. Bendich, A., The potential for dietary supplements to reduce premenstrual syndrome (PMS) symptoms, *J. Am. Coll. Nutr.*, 19, 3, 2000.

21. Walker, A. et al., Magnesium supplementation alleviates premenstrual symptoms of fluid retention, *J. Women Health*, 9, 1157, 1998.

22. Somer, E., *Essential Guide to Vitamins and Minerals*, Harper Collins, New York, 1995.

23. Daugherty, J., Treatment strategies for premenstrual syndrome, *Am. Family Physician*, 58, 183, 1998.

24. Benton, D. and Donohoe, R.T., *Public Health Nutr.*, 2, 403, 1999.

25. Schellenberg, R., Treatment for the menstrual syndrome with agnus castus fruit extract: prospective, randomized, placebo controlled study, *BMJ*, 322, 134, 2001.

26. Low Dog, T., The use of Vitex for premenstrual syndrome, *Integ. Med. Constr.*, 115, 2000.

27. Berger, D. et al., Efficacy of *Vitex agnus castus* L. extract Ze 440 in patients with pre-menstrual syndrome (PMS), *Arch. Gynecol. Obstet.*, 264, 150, 2000.

28. Tilgner, S., Women's health and women's herbs, *Herbal Transitions*, 4, 7, 1999.

29. Oleson, T. and Flocco, W., Randomized controlled study of premenstrual symptoms treated with ear, hand and foot reflexology, *Obstet. Gynecol.*, 82, 906, 1993.

30. Position paper, Nutrition and pregnancy, *J. Am. Diet. Assoc.*, 102, 1470, 2002.

31. Zapantis, G. and Santoro, N., The menopausal transition: characteristics and management, *Best Pract. Res. Clin. Endocrinol. Metab.*, 17, 33, 2003.

32. Ewies, A.A., A comprehensive approach to menopause: so far one size fits all, *Obstet. Gynecol. Surv.*, 56, 642, 2001.

33. Northrup, C., *Women's Bodies, Women's Wisdom*, Bantam Books, New York, 1998.

34. Gerhard, G. et al., Premenopausal black women are uniquely at risk for coronary heart disease compared to white women, *Prev. Cardiol.*, 3, 105, 2000.

35. Cyr, M., Postmenopausal hormone therapy in the aftermath of the WHI, what patients need to know, *Postgrad. Med.*, 113, 15, 2003.

36. Wassertheil-Smoller, S., Hendrix, S., and Limacher, M., Effect of estrogen plus progestin on stroke in postmenopausal women: the Women's Health Initiative: a randomized trial, *JAMA*, 289, 2673, 2003.

37. Tice, J.A. et al., Phytoestrogen supplements for the treatment of hot flashes: the isoflavone clover extract (ICE) study: a randomized controlled trial, *JAMA*, 290, 207, 2003.

38. Hu, F., Fish and omega-3 fatty acid intake and risk of coronary heart disease in women, *JAMA*, 287, 1815, 2002.

39. Lu, L.J., Tice, J.A., and Bellino, F.L., Phytoestrogens and healthy aging: gaps in knowledge. A workshop report, *Menopause*, 3, 157, 2001.

40. Newton, K. et al., Use of alternative therapies for menopause symptoms: results of a population-based survey, *Obstet. Gynecol.*, 100, 18, 2002.

41. Pradhan, A., Inflammatory biomarkers, hormone replacement therapy, and incident coronary heart disease. Prospective analysis from the Women's Health Initiative observational study, *JAMA*, 288, 980, 2002.

42. Kannel, W.B. et al., Menopause and risk of cardiovascular disease: the Framingham study, *Ann. Intern. Med.*, 85, 447, 1976.

43. Hedikwe, J.K. et al., Dietary patterns of rural older adults are associated with weight and nutritional status, *J. Am. Geriatr. Soc.*, 52, 589, 2004.

44. Dutta, C., Significance of sarcopenia in the elderly, *J. Nutr.*, 127 (Suppl.), 992S, 1997.

45. Volp, E., Nazemi, R., and Fujitas, S., Muscle tissue changes with aging, *Curr. Opin. Clin. Nutr. Metab. Care*, 7, 405, 2004.

46. Hughes, V.A. et al., Longitudinal changes in body composition in older men and women: role of body weight changes and physical activity, *Am. J. Clin. Nutr.*, 76, 473, 2002.

47. Schnohr, P. et al., Changes in leisure-time physical activity and risk of death: an observational study of 7,000 men and women, *Am. J. Epidemiol.*, 158, 639, 2003.

48. Tchernof, A. and Poehlman, E.T., Effects of menopause transition on body fatness and body fat distribution, *Obes. Res.*, 6, 246, 1998.

49. Wu, C. et al., A case–control study of risk factors for fibrocystic breast conditions: Shanghai Nutrition and Breast Disease study, *Am. J. Epidemiol.*, 160, 945, 2004.

50. Wright, T. and McGechan, A., Breast cancer: new technologies for risk assessment and diagnosis, *Mol. Diagn.*, 7, 49, 2003.

51. Boyle, C.A. et al., Caffeine consumption and fibrocystic breast disease: a case controlled epidemiological study, *J. Natl. Cancer Inst.*, 72, 1015, 1984.

52. Ernster, V. et al., Vitamin E and benign breast disease: a double-blind randomized clinical trial, *Surgery*, 97, 490, 1985.

53. Ibanez, L. and de Zeghe, F., Flutamide-metformin plus ethinyl estradiol–drospirenone for lipolysis and antiatherogenesis in young women with ovarian hyperandrogenism: the key role of metformin at the start and after more than one year of therapy, *J. Clin. Endocrinol. Metab.*, 90, 39, 2005.

54. Balen, A. and Rajkowha, M., Polycystic ovary syndrome — a systemic disorder? *Best Pract. Res. Clin. Gynaecol.*, 2, 263, 2003.

55. Brand-Miller, J.C. et al., Glycemic index and obesity, *Am. J. Clin. Nutr.*, 76, 281S, 2002.

56. Bloomgarden, Z.T., Insulin resistance, exercise and obesity, *Diabetes Care*, 22, 517, 1999.

57. Ortega-Gonzales, C. et al., Responses of serum androgen and insulin resistance to metformin and pioglitazone in obese, insulin-resistant women with polycystic ovary syndrome, *J. Clin. Endocrinol. Metab.*, 90, 1360, 2005.

58. Maynard, C., Association of gender and survival in patients with acute myocardial infarction, *Arch. Intern. Med.*, 157, 1379, 1997.

59. Canto, J., Relation of race and sex to the use of reperfusion therapy in Medicare beneficiaries with acute myocardial infarction, *N. Engl. J. Med.*, 342, 1094, 2000.

60. Pope, J., Missed diagnosis of acute cardiac ischemia in the emergency department, *N. Engl. J. Med.*, 342, 1163, 2000.

61. Ruhl, C.E. et al., Serum leptin concentration and body adipose measures in older black and white adults, *Am. J. Clin. Nutr.*, 80, 576, 2004.

62. Lyon, C., Law, R., and Hsueh, W., Minireview: adiposity, inflammation, and atherogenesis, *Endocrinology*, 144, 2195, 2003.

63. Valenzuela, A. and Morgado, N., Trans fatty acid isomers in the human health and in the food industry, *Biol. Res.*, 4, 273, 1999.
64. Zimmerman, E. and Wylie-Rosetti, J., Nutrition therapy for hypertension, *Curr. Diab. Rep.*, 5, 404, 2003.
65. Appel, L.J. et al., A clinical trial of the effects of dietary patterns on blood pressure, *N. Engl. J. Med.*, 336, 1117, 1997.
66. Alderman, M. and Cohen, H., Impact of dietary sodium on cardiovascular disease morbidity and mortality, *Curr. Hypertens. Rep.*, 6, 453, 2002.
67. Appel, L., Nonpharmacologic therapies that reduce blood pressure: a fresh perspective, *Clin. Cardiol.*, SIII, 1, 1999.
68. Kuller, L.H. et al., Women's Healthy Lifestyle Project: a randomized clinical trial, *Circulation*, 103, 32, 2001.
69. Cushman, W.C., Alcohol consumption and hypertension, *J. Clin. Hypertens.*, 3, 16, 2001.
70. Ross, R., Atherosclerosis — an inflammatory disease, *N. Engl. J. Med.*, 340, 115, 1999.
71. Scaefer, E., Lipoproteins, nutrition and heart disease, *Am. J. Clin. Nutr.*, 75, 191, 2002.
72. Stone, N. and Van Horn, L., Therapeutic lifestyle change and Adult Treatment Panel III: evidence then and now, *Curr. Atheroscler. Rep.*, 4, 433, 2002.
73. Law, M., Plant sterols and stanols, margarines and health, *BMJ*, 320, 861, 2000.
74. Hu, B. and Willett, W., Optimal diets for prevention of coronary heart disease, *JAMA*, 288, 2569, 2002.
75. Sacks, F. and Katan, M., Randomized clinical trials on the effects of dietary fat and carbohydrate on plasma lipoproteins and cardiovascular disease, *Am. J. Med.*, 113, 13S, 2002.
76. Aschcrio, A., Epidemiologic studies on dietary fats and coronary heart disease, *Am. J. Med.*, 113, 9B, 2002.
77. Noakes, M. and Clifton, P., Weight loss, diet composition and cardiovascular risk, *Curr. Opin. Lipidol.*, 15, 31, 2004.
78. Acheson, K.J., Carbohydrate and weight control: where do we stand? *Curr. Opin. Clin. Nutr. Metab. Care*, 7, 485, 2004.
79. Andersen, J.W. et al., Meta-analysis of the effects of soy protein intake on serum lipids, *N. Engl. J. Med.*, 333, 276, 1995.
80. Hale, G., Paul-Labrador, M., Dwyer, J., and Merz, C., Isoflavone supplementation and endothelial function in menopausal women, *Clin. Endocrinol.*, 56, 693, 2002.
81. FDA approves new health claim for soy protein and coronary disease, FDA Talk Paper, October, 1999 (www.fda.gov/bbs/topics /ANSWERS/ANS00980.html).
82. Brand-Miller, J. et al. *The Glucose Revolution*, Marlowe & Company, New York, NY, 1999.
83. Keller, K. and Lemberg, L., Obesity and the metabolic syndrome, *Am. J. Crit. Care*, 12, 167, 2003.
84. Ness-Abramof, R. and Apovian, C., An update on medical therapy for obesity, *Nutr. Clin. Pract.*, 18, 145, 2003.
85. Maggard, M.A., Shurgarman, L.R., Suttorp, M. et al., Meta-analysis: surgical treatment of obesity, *Ann. Intern. Med.*, 142, 547, 2005.
86. Hedley, A.A. et al., Prevalence of overweight and obesity among US children, adolescents, and adults, 1999–2002, *JAMA*, 291, 2847, 2004.
87. Ley, C.J. and Stevenson, J.C., Sex and menopause-associated changes in body fat distribution, *Am. J. Clin. Nutr.*, 55, 950, 1992.
88. Mayes, J.S. and Watson, G.H., Direct effects of sex hormones on adipose tissues and obesity, *Obes. Rev.*, 5, 197, 2004.
89. Ludwig, D., The glycemic index physiological mechanisms relating to obesity, diabetes and cardio-vascular disease, *JAMA*, 287, 2414, 2002.
90. Bray, G.A. et al., DASH Collaborative Research Group. A further subgroup analysis of the effects of the DASH diet and three dietary sodium levels on blood pressure: results of the DASH sodium trial, *Am. J. Cardiol.*, 94, 222, 2004.
91. www.cancer.gov. accessed 11/12/02.
92. Tjonneland, A. et al., Lifetime alcohol consumption and post menopausal breast cancer rate in Denmark: a prospective cohort study, *J. Nutr.*, 134, 173, 2004.
93. Rock, C., Nutrition of the older athlete, *Clin. Sports Med.*, 2, 445, 1991.
94. Facchini, F. et al., Relation between insulin resistance and plasma concentrations of lipid hydro-peroxides, carotenoids, and tocopherols, *Am. J. Clin. Nutr.*, 72, 776, 2000.

95. Roberts, K. et al., Syndrome X: medical nutrition therapy, *Nutr. Rev.*, 58, 154, 2000.
96. Michels, K. and Wolk, A., A prospective study of variety of healthy foods and mortality in women, *Int. J. Epidemiol.*, 31, 847, 2002.
97. Martinez, M.E., Primary prevention of colorectal cancer: lifestyle, nutrition, and exercise, *Cancer Res.*, 166, 177, 2005.
98. http:// www.cancer.gov/cancer.2003
99. Ford, E., Giles, W., and Dietz, W., Prevalence of the metabolic syndrome among US adults, *JAMA*, 287, 356, 2002.
100. American Diabetes Association, Diagnosis and classification of diabetes mellitus, *Diabetes Care*, 27 (Suppl. 1), 2004.
101. Orshal, J. and Khalil, R., Gender, sex hormones and vascular tone, *Am. J. Physiol. Regul. Integr. Comp. Physiol.*, 2, 233, 2004.
102. Lichtenstein, A., Dietary fat and cardiovascular disease risk: quantity or quality, *J. Women's Health*, 2, 109, 2003.
103. Baier, L.J. and Hanson, R.L., Genetic studies of the etiology of type 2 diabetes in Pima Indians, *Diabetes*, 53, 1181, 2004.
104. Brand-Miller, J., Glycemic load and chronic disease, *Nutr. Rev.*, 61, S49, 2003.
105. Bouche, C. et al., Five week low glycemic index diet decreases total fat mass and improves plasma lipid profile in moderately overweight non-diabetic men, *Diabetes Care*, 25, 822, 2002.
106. Ludwig, D.S., Dietary glycemic index and the regulation of body weight, *Lipids*, 38, 117, 2003.
107. http://www.cancer.gov/cancer.2003
108. Gass, M., Impact of WHI conclusions and ACOG guidelines on clinical practice, *Int. J. Fertil. Women's Med.*, 48, 106, 2003.
109. Lacey, J., Devesa, S., and Brinton, L., Recent trends in breast cancer incidence and mortality, *Environ. Mol. Mutagen.*, 39, 82, 2002.
110. http://www.cancer.gov/cancer. Breast U.S. racial/ethnic cancer patterns, 2002.
111. http://cancer.gov/U.S. 2000 incidence report.
112. El-Sherbiny, Y., G1 arrest and S phase inhibition of human cancer cell lines by inositol hexaphosphate (IP6), *Anticancer Res.*, 21, 2393, 2001.
113. Mann, J., Diet and risk of coronary heart disease and type 2 diabetes, *Lancet*, 360, 783, 2002.
114. Stein, C. and Colditz, G., Modifiable risk factors for cancer, *Br. J. Cancer*, 90, 299, 2004.
115. Hartman, T.J. et al., Moderate alcohol consumption and levels of antioxidant vitamins and isoprostanes in postmenopausal women, *Eur. J. Clin. Nutr.*, 59, 161, 2005.
116. Duncan, A.M., The role of nutrition in the prevention of breast cancer, *AACN Clin. Issues Adv. Pract. Critical-Care Nurses*, 15, 119, 2004.
117. Greenlee, R. et al., Cancer statistics 2000, *Cancer J. Clin.*, 50, 7, 2000.
118. Amunni, G. et al., The age factor in ovarian cancer, clinical therapeutic and prognostic aspects, *Minerva. Med.*, 89, 65, 1998.
119. Augustin, L.S., Polesel, J., and Bosetti, C., Dietary glycemic index, glycemic load and ovarian cancer risk case–control study in Italy, *Ann. Oncol.*, 14, 78, 2003.
120. Smith, S., Polycystic ovary syndrome, *Postgraduate Obstet. Gynecol.*, 25, 1, 2005.
121. Chingang, L.C. et al., 'Have a Pap smear!'-doctors, their clients and opportunistic cervical cancer screening, *Intl. J. STD AIDS*, 16, 233, 2005.
122. National Cancer Institute, Task force announces new cervical cancer screening guide, http://www.ahrq.gov/clinic/3rduspstf/cervcan/cervical.
123. Ollonen, P., Lehtonen, J., and Eskelinen, M., Stressful and adverse life experiences in patients with breast cancer: a prospective case–control study in Kuopio, Finland, *Anticancer Res.*, 25, 531, 2005.
124. Macdonald, H. et al., Nutritional associations with bone loss during the menopausal transition: evidence of a beneficial effect of calcium, alcohol, and fruit and vegetable nutrients and of detrimental effect of fatty acids, *Am. J. Clin. Nutr.*, 79, 4, 2004.
125. Turkoski, B., Treating osteoporosis without hormones, *Orthop. Nurs.*, 21, 80, 2002.
126. Horton, J., A profile of women's health in the United States, *The Women's Health Data Book*, 2nd ed., Jacobs Institute of Women's Health, Washington, D.C., 1995.

127. National Institute of Mental Health, Unpublished Epidemiological Catchment Area Analyses, 1999.

128. National Institute of Mental Health: "Depression: Treat it. Defeat it." June 1999. Netscape: http://www.Nimh.nih.gov/depression/genpop/gen_fact.htm.

129. Miranda, J. et al., Treating depression in predominantly low-income young minority women: a randomized controlled trial, *JAMA*, 290, 57, 2003.

130. Rew, L. et al., Correlates of recent suicide attempts in a triethnic group of adolescents, *J. Nurs. Scholarsh.*, 33, 361, 2001.

131. Lam, R. et al., Seasonal depression: the dual vulnerability hypothesis revisited, *J. Affect. Disord.*, 63, 123, 2001.

132. Hirschfeld, R. and Russell, J., Assessment and treatment of suicidal patients, *N. Engl. J. Med.*, 337, 910, 1997.

133. Rogers, P., A healthy body, a healthy mind: long-term impact of diet on mood and cognitive function, *Proc. Nutr. Soc.*, 60, 135, 2001.

134. Mulsant, B. and Pollock, B., Treatment-resistant depression in later life, *J. Geriatr. Psychiatry Neurol.*, 11, 186, 1998.

135. Linde, K. et al., St. John's wort for depression: meta analysis of randomized controlled trials, *Br. J. Psychol.*, 186, 99, 2005.

136. Pace-Asciak, C.R. et al., Wines and grape juices as modulators of platelet aggregation in healthy human subjects, *Clin. Chem. Acta*, 246, 163, 1996.

137. Conney, A. et al., Inhibitory effect of green and black tea on tumor growth, *Proc. Soc. Exper. Biol. Med.*, 220, 229, 1999.

138. Lampe, J.W., Health effects of vegetables and fruit: assessing mechanisms of action in human experimental studies, *Am. J. Clin. Nutr.*, 70, 439, 1999.

139. Frankenfeld, C. et al., Validation of a soy food frequency questionnaire with plasma concentrations of isoflavones in US adults, *J. Am. Diet. Assoc.*, 102, 1407, 2002.

140. Messina, M.J., Legumes and soybeans: overview of their nutritional profiles and health effects, *Am. J. Clin. Nutr.*, 70, 439, 1999.

141. Petterson, K., Delaunay, F., and Gustafssson, J.A., Estrogen receptor β acts as a dominant regulator of estrogen signaling, *Oncogene*, 19, 4970, 2000.

142. Zava, D. and Duw, E., Estrogenic and anti-proliferative properties of genistein and other flavonoids in human breast cancer cells *in vitro*, *Nutr. Cancer*, 27, 31, 1997.

143. Lu, L. et al., Decreased ovarian hormones during soya diet: implications for breast cancer prevention, *Cancer Res.*, 60, 4112, 2000.

144. Awad, A. and Fink, C., Phytosterols as anticancer dietary components: evidence and mechanism of action, *J. Nutr.*, 130, 2127, 2000.

145. Dalais, F. et al., Effects of dietary phytoestrogens in postmenopausal women, *Climacteric*, 2, 124, 1998.

146. Xu, X. et al., Soy consumption alters endogenous estrogen metabolism in postmenopausal women, *Cancer Epidemiol. Biomar. Prev.*, 9, 781, 2000.

147. Liener, I., Implications of anti-nutritional components in soybean foods, *Crit. Rev. Food Sci. Nutr.*, 34, 31, 1994.

148. Kumar, N. et al., The specific role of isoflavones on estrogen metabolism in premenopausal women, *Cancer*, 94, 1166, 2002.

149. Kurzer, M.S., Phytoestrogen supplement use by women, *J. Nutr.*, 133, 1983, 2003.

150. Messina, M., Gardner, C., and Barnes, S., Gaining insight into the health effects of soy but a long way to go: Commentary on the Fourth International Symposium on the Role of Soy in Preventing and Treating Chronic Disease, *J. Nutr.*, 132, 547, 2002.

151. Newton, K.M. et al., Use of alternative therapies for menopausal symptoms: results of a population-based survey, *Obstet. Gynecol.*, 100, 18, 2002.

152. Goodman, M.T. et al., Association of soy and fiber consumption with the risk of endometrial cancer, *Am. J. Epidemiol.*, 146, 294, 1997.

153. Albertazzi, P. et al., The effect of dietary soy supplementation on hot flushes, *Obstet. Gynecol.*, 91, 6, 1998.

154. Vincent, A. and Fitzpatrick L., Soy isoflavones: are they useful in menopause? *Mayo Clin. Proc.*, 75, 1174, 2000.

155. Jenkins, D., Effects of high and low isoflavone soy foods on blood lipids, oxidized LDL, homocysteine and blood pressure in hyperlipidemic men and women, *Am. J. Clin. Nutr.*, 76, 365, 2002.
156. Somekawa, Y., Soy intake related to menopausal symptoms, serum lipids, and bone mineral density in postmenopausal Japanese women, *Obstet. Gynecol.*, 97, 109, 2001.
157. Arliss, R., Do soy isoflavones lower cholesterol, inhibit atherosclerosis and play a role in cancer prevention? *Holist. Nurs. Pract.*, 16, 40, 2002.
158. Clarkson, T., Soy, soy estrogens and cardiovascular disease, *J. Nutr.*, 132, 566s, 2002.
159. Bhathena, S. et al., Beneficial role of dietary phytoestrogens in obesity and diabetes, *Am. J. Clin. Nutr.*, 76, 1191, 2002.
160. Harkness L., Soy and bone. Where do we stand? *Orthop. Nurs.*, 23, 12, 2004.
161. Segasothy, M. and Phillips, P., Vegetarian diet: panacea for modern lifestyle diseases? *QJM*, 92, 531, 1999.
162. Rowland, I., Optimal nutrition: fibre and phytochemicals, *Proc. Nutr. Soc.*, 58, 415, 1999.
163. Horrocks, L.A. and Yeo, Y.K., Health benefits of docosahexaenoic acid (DHA), *Pharmacol. Res.*, 40, 211, 1999.
164. Boris, N., Tanja, J., and Hans-Juergen, D., Anti-inflammatory effects of omega-3 fatty acids vary at different stages of inflammation, *Am. J. Physiol. Heart Circ. Physiol.*, 285, 2248, 2003.
165. Mori, T.A. and Beilin, L.J., Omega-3 fatty acids and inflammation, *Curr. Atheroscler. Rep.*, 6, 461, 2004.
166. Budeiri, D., Li, W., and Dornan, J., Is evening primrose oil of value in the treatment of premenstrual syndrome? *Control. Clin. Trials*, 17, 60, 1996.
167. Barre, D., Potential of evening primrose, borage, black currant and fungal oils in human health, *Ann. Nutr. Metab.*, 45, 47, 2001.
168. Rodriquez, J. and Robinson, K., Homocysteine as a cardiovascular risk factor, *Emergency Med.*, 43, 2001.
169. Kushi, L., Dietary antioxidants vitamins and death from coronary heart disease in postmenopausal women, *N. Engl. J. Med.*, 334, 1156, 1996.
170. Kirkham, C., Harris, S., and Grzybowski, S., Evidence-based prenatal care: part 1. General prenatal care and counseling issues, *Am. Family Physician*, 71, 1264, 2005.
171. Han, J. et al., Interaction between genetic variations in DNA repair genes and plasma folate on breast cancer risk, *Cancer Epidemiol. Biomarkers Prevent.*, 13, 520, 2004.
172. Serrano, D., Lazzeroni, M., and Decensi, A., Chemoprevention of colorectal cancer: an update, *Tech. Coloproctol.*, 8 (S), 248, 2004.
173. Sobey, C., Potassium channel function in vascular disease, *Arterioscler. Thrombosis Vasc. Biol.*, 21, 28, 2001.
174. Sollitto, R., Kraemer, K., DiGiovanna, J., Normal vitamin D levels can be maintained despite rigorous photoprotection: six years' experience with Xeroderma pigmentosum. *J. am. Acad. Dermatol.*, 40, 3, 497.
175. Auer, J. et al., Body iron stores and coronary atherosclerosis assessed by coronary angiography, *Nutr. Metabol. Cardiol. Dis.*, 12, 285, 2002.
176. Alexandersen, P. et al., Ipriflavone in the treatment of postmenopausal osteoporosis a randomized controlled trial, *JAMA*, 285, 1482, 2001.
177. Agnusdei, D. et al., Metabolic and clinical effects of ipriflavone in established postmenopausal osteoporosis, *Drugs Exp. Clin. Res.*, 15, 97, 1989.
178. Reginster, J., Ipriflavone: pharmacological properties and usefulness in postmenopausal osteoporosis, *Bone Mineral.*, 23, 223, 1993.
179. Rondelli, I., Acerbi, D., and Ventura, P., Steady-state pharmacokinetics of ipriflavone and its metabolites in patients with renal failure, *Int. J. Clin. Pharmacol. Res.*, 11, 183, 1991.
180. Takahashi, J. et al., Elevation of serum theophylline levels by ipriflavone in a patient with chronic obstructive pulmonary disease, *Eur. J. Clin. Pharmacol.*, 43, 207, 1992.
181. Kirchengast, S. and Huber, J., Body composition characteristics and fat distribution patterns in young infertile women, *Fertil. Steril.*, 81, 539, 2004.
182. Gordon, C. et al., Effects of oral dehydroepiandrosterone on bone density in young women with anorexia nervosa: a randomized trial, *J. Clin. Endocrinol. Metabol.*, 87, 4935, 2002.

183. Dharia, S. and Parker, C.R. Jr., Adrenal androgens and aging, *Semin. Reprod. Med.*, 22, 361, 2004.
184. Dhatariya, K.K. and Nair, K.S., Dehydroepiandrosterone: is there a role for replacement? *Mayo Clin. Proc.*, 78, 1257, 2003.
185. Chen, C.C. and Parker, C.R., Jr., Adrenal androgens and the immune system, *Semin. Reprod. Med.*, 22, 369, 2004.
186. http://www.consumerlab.com/results/dhea.asp
187. Jellin, J.M. et al., *Pharmacist's Letter/Prescriber's Letter Natural Medicines Comprehensive Database*, 3rd ed., Therapeutic Research Facility, Stockton, CA, 2000.
188. Liu, J. et al., Evaluation of estrogenic activity of plant extracts for the potential treatment of menopausal symptoms, *J. Agric. Food Chem.*, 49, 2472, 2001.
189. Mahady, G.B. et al., Black cohosh: an alternative therapy for menopause? *Nutr. Clin. Care*, 5, 283, 2002.
190. Amato, P., Christophe, S., and Mellon, P., Estrogenic activity of herbs and commonly used remedies for menopausal symptoms, *J. North Am. Menopause Soc.*, 9, 145, 2002.
191. Blumenthal, M. et al., *The Complete German Commission E Monographs: Therapeutic Guide to Herbal Medicines*, 1st ed., American Botanical Council, Austin, TX, 1998.
192. Low Dog, T., Riley, D., and Carter, T., An integrative approach to menopause, *Altern. Ther.*, 7, 45, 2001.
193. Huntley, A. and Ernst, E., A systematic review of the safety of black cohosh, *Menopause*, 10, 58, 2003.
194. Tyler, V., The honest herbal, *Sensible Guide to Herbs and Related Remedies*, Pharmaceutical Products Press, New York, 1993.
195. Schellenberg, R., Treatment for the premenstrual syndrome with agnus castus fruit extract: prospective, randomized, placebo controlled study, *BMJ*, 322, 134, 2001.
196. Nestel, P.J. et al., Isoflavones from red clover improves systemic arterial compliance but not plasma lipids in menopausal women, *J. Clin. Endocrinol. Metabol.*, 84, 895, 1999.
197. Chadha, K.L. and Rama, R., Cultivation of wild yam for steroid drug industry, *Indian Hortic.*, 28, 13, 1984.
198. Shoemaker, J., *Dioscorea villosa* — wild yam, *JAMA*, 13, 407, 1998.
199. Hulley, S. et al., Noncardiovascular disease outcomes during 6.8 years of hormone replacement heart and estrogen/progestin replacement study follow-up (HERS II), *JAMA*, 288, 58, 2002.
200. Shah, S. and Alexander, K., Hormone replacement therapy for primary and secondary prevention of heart disease, *Curr. Treat. Opt. Cardiovasc. Med.*, 1, 25, 2003.
201. Grady, D. et al., Cardiovascular disease outcomes during 6.8 years of hormone therapy. Heart and estrogen/progestin replacement study follow-up (HERS II), *JAMA*, 288, 49, 2002.
202. Greendale, G. et al., PEPI safety follow-up study (PSFS) investigators. Bone mass response to discontinuation of long-term hormone replacement therapy: results from the post menopausal estrogen? Progestin interventions PEPI safety follow-up study, *Arch. Int. Med.*, 162, 665, 2002.
203. Derry, P., Time trends in the HERS secondary prevention trial: much to do about nothing? *J. Am. Med. Women's Assoc.*, 4, 215, 2002.
204. Writing Group for the Women's Health Initiative Investigation. Risks and benefits of estrogen plus progestin in healthy postmenopausal women: principal results from the Women's Health Initiative randomized controlled trial, *JAMA*, 288, 321, 2002.
205. Fylstra, D., Postmenopausal hormone therapy: have HERS and WHI given us any new information? *JSC Med. Assoc.*, 8, 299, 2002.
206. Haas, J. et al., Changes in the use of postmenopausal hormone therapy after the publication of clinical trial results, *Ann. Int. Med.*, 140, 184, 2004.
207. Augustin, L.S., Polesel, J., and Bosetti, C., Dietary glycemic index, glycemic load and ovarian cancer risk case–control study in Italy, *Ann. Oncol.*, 14, 78, 2003.
208. Bendich, A., The potential for dietary supplements to reduce premenstrual syndrome (PMS) symptoms, *J. Am. Coll. Nutr.*, 19, 3, 2002.
209. Wyatt, K.M. et al., Efficacy of vitamin B_6 in the treatment of premenstrual syndrome; systematic review, *BMJ*, 381, 1375, 1999.
210. Krebs, E. et al., Phytoestrogens for treatment of menopausal symptoms: a systematic review, *Am. Coll Obstet. Gynecol.*, 104, 824, 2004.
211. Adapted from DRI reports, www.nap.edu, copyright 2001 by The National Academies.
213. Stopler Kasdan, T., Menopause and diet, *Idea Today*, 46, 1997.

7 Men's Health

Aaron W. Crawford

CONTENTS

INTRODUCTION

American men are subject to several grim health statistics. Consider that by the time they reach the age of 65 years, men are twice as likely to die of heart disease than their female counterparts. By this age they are also more likely to have died from cancer, diabetes, kidney, liver, and pulmonary disease. This litany goes on — of the 12 leading causes of death, men post higher mortality rates than women in each category (see Table 7.1).

Given these statistics, it is not surprising that men have significantly lower life expectancy than women and die an average of 5.4 years earlier than women. But why? Is it genetics? Poor planning? Are male tissues more "delicate" than female tissues? Actually, it might have more to do with the male psyche than anything else since men are more likely to be cavalier about their health than women. For example, men are far less likely to have a primary care physician, and can go for years without seeking medical attention or a routine health checkup. This is further compounded by the fact that when they do visit a physician, men are more likely to avoid prescribed treatment or abandon treatment and medication early. In addition, men tend to be more reserved in the presence of doctors than women, and find it

TABLE 7.1

Leading Causes of Death in Men and Women Aged 1–65 Years

Men		Women	
Disease	Number of Deaths/Year	Disease	Number of Deaths/Year
Cancer	90,300	Cancer	82,200
Heart disease	86,800	Heart disease	38,300
Accidental injury	48,500	Accidental injury	17,900
Suicide	19,300	Cerebrovascular disease	9,600
Homicide	12,100	Respiratory disease	8,500
Liver disease	11,900	Diabetes	8,100
Cerebrovascular disease	11,200	Suicide	4,900
HIV	10,500	Liver disease	4,800
Diabetes	10,000	HIV	3,500
Respiratory disease	9,000	Homicide	3,400
Flu/pneumonia	4,000	Septicemia	3,000
Septicemia	3,500	Flu/pneumonia	2,800
	317,100		187,000

Based on 2000 data from the Centers for Disease Control.

difficult to talk about urinary, sexual, and emotional health problems in particular. As a result, physicians may not be privy to important health information about their male patients. Finally, many men tend to ignore warning signs of chronic disease, and avoid seeking medical attention until a crisis erupts. The combination of all these male traits shows that males are indeed difficult patients to diagnose and treat effectively.

MEN AND WOMEN SUFFER FROM MANY OF THE SAME MEDICAL CONDITIONS

Men and women suffer from many of the same physiological problems — for example heart disease is the leading cause of death in both men and women. According to data from the Center for Disease Control, 29.3% of all men die from heart disease, while 29.9% of women succumb to heart-related deaths. Cancer is the next most significant cause of death, accounting for 24.3% of deaths in males and 21.8% in females. The third leading cause of death in both sexes is stroke, accounting for 5.5 and 7.0% of deaths in men and women, respectively. Together, these three diseases account for about 60% of all deaths in men and women.[1]

This data also demonstrates that healthy men and women have very similar health concerns. Not surprisingly, effective preventive measures and treatment for these major medical concerns are similar in males and females. The treatment options for these diseases that are discussed in other chapters are more or less applicable to men and women to the same extent. Overwhelmingly, the best way to reduce the risk of these diseases is to adopt a healthier lifestyle in an attempt to prevent the onset of chronic disease. Excess weight and lack of exercise are major lifestyle factors that dramatically increase the risk of each of chronic diseases such as heart disease and cancer. It is important to note that these are lifestyle factors over which we can exert a large degree of control. For men, it is particularly important to consult a physician for a current medical checkup, and to follow the medical advice that results from these medical consultations. These simple measures may help to erase the 5.4-year disadvantage that men experience in life expectancy.

While some diseases are typically associated with women — such as osteoporosis and breast cancer — men can succumb to these same conditions. For example, the risk of hip fracture in men escalates after the age of 70 years; in one study on bone health, the median age of risk fracture was 67 years, with only 25% occurring prior to 60 years of age.[2] This data suggests that the risk of bone fracture increases as men age, and thus that men are not immune from osteoporosis (although it does occur less frequently than in women).

It has been well established that calcium is essential for bone growth, bone strength, and bone mass density. But calcium alone is not sufficient. A recent study reveals that adequate protein (1.2 g/kg), potassium (>100 mmol/day), and phosphorus (1.7 g/day) benefit bone health in men with adequate calcium intake (1200 mg/day).[3] It should also be noted that a diet rich in vitamin D (400 IU or 10 μg/day) is required for optimal calcium absorption from the gut, and thus is required for good bone health as well. While bone health may not seem life-threatening — consider that pelvic fracture in the elderly dramatically increases mortality despite aggressive treatment.[4] Both men and women increase their risk of death following pelvic bone fractures.

MALE-SPECIFIC HEALTH CONCERNS

In their 20s, men are too strong to see a doctor. In their 30s they are too busy, and in their 40s they are too scared.

— Andrew Kimbrell, cofounder of the Men's Health Network.

While many chronic diseases such as heart disease, hypertension, cancer are nongender-specific, a man presents special healthcare problems (just as a woman opens up another world of special health concerns). Advancing age appears to be the ultimate nemesis since organ and tissue function lose their vim and vigor as time passes by. As men age, they face a very specific set of health concerns in which the core of manhood is threatened. For example, many men experience erectile dysfunction (ED), suffer from hair loss, and begin to notice urinary problems as they exit their youth. All of these ailments may appear in early adulthood, but tend to get progressively common and pronounced as the years pass by. Some degree of ED is reported in about half of all men aged 40–70 years.[5] The statistics for hair loss are just as bleak, where half of the American population is estimated to experience some degree of hair loss by the age of 50 years.[6]

ERECTILE DYSFUNCTION

Normal sexual function in men is comprised of four separate events: libido, erection, ejaculation, and orgasm. Of these, the literature is rich with over-the-counter (OTC) treatments to improve libido and erectile function in general; however, the scientific support for these treatments is often inflated. The appropriate scientific data is weak in many cases — a fact that does not prevent many products from selling.

A number of factors may contribute to ED, and causes can be grouped into roughly seven categories[7]:

- Psychogenic (performance anxiety, stress, depression)
- Neurogenic (stroke, Alzheimer disease, spinal/pelvic injury, surgery, neuropathy)
- Hormonal (hypogonadism, hyperprolactinemia)
- Vasculogenic (atherosclerosis, hypertension, diabetes, Peyronie's disease)
- Drug-induced (antihypertensives, antidepressants, antiandrogens)
- Lifestyle habits (alcohol abuse, cigarette smoking)
- Other diseases (chronic renal failure, coronary heart disease)

Many of these conditions become more frequent or pronounced with advancing age, thus helping to explain that the rate of ED increases steadily and progressively with age.

INT Approaches

Many of the products, especially pharmaceutical agents, aimed at improving ED target the biochemical regulation of smooth muscle relaxation. During an erection, sexual stimulation causes the release of nitric oxide (NO) from endothelial cells in the corpus cavernosum. This gas acts as a chemical hormone, and diffuses to the surrounding smooth muscle cells where it activates guanylate cyclase, and ultimately elevates levels of cyclic guanosine monophosphate (cGMP). As a result, smooth muscle cells relax, blood flows into the penis through the dilated arteries — at the same time that the venous drainage system shuts down — and the penis becomes rigid and erect (see Figure 7.1).

There is a natural biochemical pathway for converting cGMP back into the precursor GMP, a process mediated by phosphodiesterase. Not surprisingly, inactivating this enzyme to keep cGMP levels elevated is a commonly researched approach (for example sildenafil — Viagra®). Another approach is to elevate the level of NO to increase the level of guanylate cyclase activity.

Arginine

Sexual stimulus causes the conversion of the naturally occurring amino acid arginine to NO. Thus, a natural question is whether or not high levels of supplemental arginine can generate high levels of NO to activate increased levels of adenylate cyclase. Early animal experiments suggested that this was indeed the case, where older rats supplemented with arginine experience improved erectile response.[8]

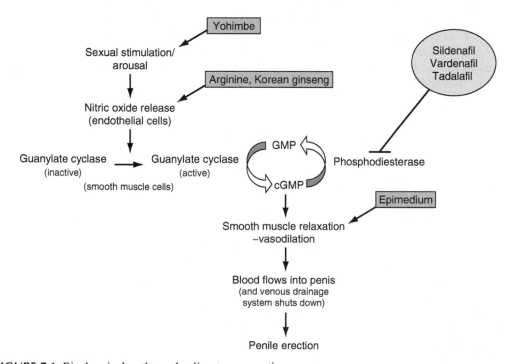

FIGURE 7.1 Biochemical pathway leading to an erection.

Human studies in this area were first conducted in 1994, although the scientific approach was weak and relied on patient self-assessment. Later studies have been conflicting, but it appears that higher doses offer the most benefit. For example, a 1.5 g/day dose was ineffective at improving sexual performance,[9] while a 5 g/day dose yielded a statistically significant response in the treatment group relative to the placebo.[10]

Korean Ginseng

Korean ginseng may also improve the production of NO, however this remains to be validated. Regardless, it may improve male sexual performance. Recent results from a double-blind crossover study suggest that Korean ginseng taken over a short term (8 weeks) improves sexual response, where men report that they are more able to achieve and maintain an erection compared to placebo.[11] These results are similar to an earlier trial, where Korean men who consumed Korean ginseng (Panax ginseng) for a 3-month period reported improved sexual desire and erectile function compared to men receiving a placebo.[12]

Epimedium Sagittatum

If the common name (horny goat weed) is a true indication of function, *Epimedium* is sure to get much research attention. Long used in traditional Chinese medicine, *Epimedium* is used to promote seminal emission and treat impotence. In research animals, *Epimedium* promotes the dilation of blood vessels, a mechanism that may explain its traditional use to treat impotence. Double-blind controlled experiments need to be conducted to verify the benefit of this herbal approach in treating ED.

Yohimbe

The bark of the yohimbe tree has been long hailed as an aphrodisiac, and has traditionally been used to treat impotence. Yohimbe contains a specific compound, yohimbine that may act on the brain to increase sexual arousal. Herbalists contend that the herb works better than the purified compound, although there is no good data to support this, and is usually given in presumed psychogenic ED. To date, only few well-controlled, human studies have been performed with yohimbe. A meta-analysis of these studies, however, concludes that there is a consistent improvement in sexual performance relative to placebo and that this is a reasonable treatment option for ED.[13] On a cautionary note, it is important to note that yohimbe has a very narrow dosing range; low doses may yield no benefit, while high doses may cause significant and serious adverse events.

Interestingly, a few studies have been performed with the combination of yohimbine and arginine, and the results from these studies suggest that there may be a synergistic effect when these two different treatments are combined. In addition, one study suggests that the result is more beneficial in patients with mild-to-moderate ED compared to those individuals with more pronounced sexual dysfunction.[14]

Maca

There is no human data available for this ingredient, but the animal studies are noteworthy for its ability to improve sexual performance. For example, when maca extract was fed to male mice over a 22-day period, it tripled the frequency with which they coupled with females.[15] On a biochemical note, maca contains compounds called macaenes and macamides, specific chemicals that have been shown to improve sexual function in laboratory animals.

Conventional Treatment

Conventional approaches to improving sexual function were rather archaic prior to the introduction of Viagra. For example, vacuum pump devices, penile injections, and penile implants were the primary treatment options at the close of the last century. Vacuum devices employ an airtight tube that is placed around the penis; suction reduces pressure inside the tube, and draws blood into the penis to generate an erection. This mechanical approach, while cumbersome to some, provides satisfactory results to many men who prefer this technique to injection therapy. Also noteworthy is that vacuum devices are noninvasive and thus generate no systemic side effects.

Just as the name implies, penile injections rely on the injection of vasodilators directly into the smooth muscle tissue of the penis. This approach is not applicable for all ED patients, and is generally less successful in patients whose condition derives from vascular complications. While this approach is quick (usually generating an erection within 5 min of injection), and produces a completely normal erection, many men find it an intolerable solution. The success of this approach varies with the individual, but the attrition rate for males electing this alternative is high.[16] In addition, many side effects, including tiny blood clots, burning pain after injection, damage to the urethra, and fibrous tissue build up in the corpus cavernosum may result after frequent injections. Unfortunately, priapism may also be a significant side effect in some. Future delivery systems of vasodilators, for example in the form of a salve that can be applied directly to a flaccid penis, may provide a brighter future for this treatment option. Urethral suppositories, available by prescription only, deliver a smooth muscle relaxant (such as alprostadil) directly to the urethral membrane; an erection generally occurs within 10–15 min, and lasts for 30–60 min.

The most drastic approach to treat ED is a penile implant, a treatment option that requires surgery. This technology has improved dramatically in recent years, and current prostheses are fluid-filled implants that can be regulated by inflatable chambers that are surgically implanted; the control valve, which regulates fluid release is inserted in the scrotum. This approach is reported to completely restore sexual function in impotent men and allow them to lead a normal sex life.

The most popular approach to treat ED is the oral medication sildenafil (Viagra), a phosphodiesterase inhibitor that predominantly inhibits the type V isoenzyme in smooth muscle cells of the corpus cavernosum. Patient satisfaction is generally high with this drug, with clinical efficacy ranging somewhere between 50 and 85%.[17] A recent review of 27 trials — in which 6600 men participated in treatment — concluded that sildenafil nearly triples a man's chance of maintaining an erection and achieving successful intercourse (57 versus 21% in placebo).[18]

It is important to note that this pharmacological approach may lead to transient visual disturbances in some users, such as seeing a bluish tinge or increased sensitivity to light. This mild side effect presumably occurs because sildenafil has a mild inhibitory effect of the type VI isozyme found in the retina.[19] In addition, sildenafil potentiates the effects of nitrates used to treat hypertension, and is strictly contraindicated in patients taking any form of nitrate medication, as it can cause a life-threatening drop in blood pressure. Men with significant heart disease are encouraged to consult with their cardiologist before taking sildenafil (or other recently approved drugs such as vardenafil (Levitra®) and tadalafil (Cialis®) that work by a similar mechanism).

Hair Loss

Androgenetic alopecia (also called male pattern baldness) is a progressive condition that can start as early as late adolescence. The disease can vary in severity, ranging from thinning hair or recession of the hairline to total baldness in its most severe form. Typically the disease becomes more common and more pronounced with age. Androgenetic alopecia is the most common form of hair loss in the United States, and is estimated to affect up to 60 million people to some degree or another (see Figure 7.2). White males are particularly susceptible to

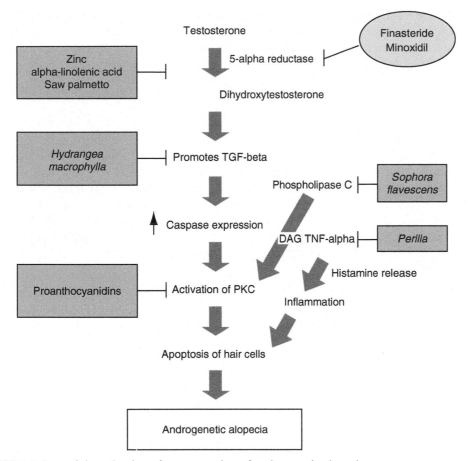

FIGURE 7.2 Potential mechanisms for suppression of androgenetic alopecia.

losing their hair, as it occurs four times more frequently in this population than in black males of similar age.[20]

It is a sad fact that we are born with all of the hair follicles we will ever have, about 100,000 on the scalp.[21] Inactivation or loss of these follicles, through a variety of means such as genetic, biochemical, or inflammatory processes, prevents the growth of terminal hairs and ultimately leads to hair loss and potentially complete baldness. Each follicle experiences multiple cycles of growth (anagen) and rest (telogen) throughout a man's lifetime. It should come as no surprise that current treatments tend to focus on extending or reinitiating anagen, at the expense of telogen, to reenergize hair growth.

Androgenic hormones play an important role in regulating hair growth. Testosterone and its active metabolite dihydroxytestosterone (DHT) act through androgen receptors to either activate or quell hair growth. In puberty, these hormones increase the size of hair follicles in facial, pubic, chest, and axillary regions to stimulate hair growth. Later in life, these same hormones may negatively affect hair follicle activity in the scalp; the result is diminution in hair diameter, leading to fine hair and ultimately loss of hair growth. DHT, and not testosterone itself, appears to be the most significant negative regulator of hair growth, potentially because it has a much higher binding affinity for androgen receptors. Many pharmacological and herbal hair-restoring remedies thus target 5-alpha reductase, the enzyme that converts testosterone to DHT.

To date, there are few documented herbal approaches that reproducibly stem hair loss. Thus, a surfeit of "remedies" are available for hopeful men; but many of these options lack credible scientific merit. The most obvious herbal products are 5-alpha-reductase inhibitors, although the regulation of other enzymes may also have some benefit.

INT Approaches

Saw Palmetto
Since the active ingredient in saw palmetto is a 5-alpha-reductase inhibitor, it has long been postulated that this herbal may be beneficial in treating male pattern baldness. However, direct scientific confirmation of this activity has been lacking. Only recently, a small, short-term trial was performed to suggest that saw palmetto may actually have clinical benefit in this regard. Following a combined treatment of saw palmetto (400 mg/day) and beta-sitosterol (100 mg/day) six of ten men reported a subjective improvement in hair growth after an average treatment period of 4.6 months.[22] Clearly, there was little scientific rigor involved in this trial, and the results obviously need to be substantiated.

OTHER 5-ALPHA-REDUCTASE INHIBITORS

Alpha-linolenic acid, the essential fatty acid, is also a 5-alpha-reductase inhibitor. Many plants are good sources of this fatty acid, and are also rich in other fatty acids that have reductase inhibitory power. Of these, *Boehmeria nipononivea* appears to be the best candidate as a hair restorer, although data to date has been generated only in rat models of hair growth.[23] *Impatiens balsamina* is also a good source of 5-alpha-reductase inhibitory activity, and has a history of folk use to remedy male pattern baldness. It is also interesting to note that zinc sulphate inhibits 5-alpha reductase, an activity that is potentiated by vitamin B6 at low levels of zinc.[24] Significant clinical trials to support the use of any of these agents have not been reported in the scientific or medical literature.

Additional Potential Remedies
A number of enzymes and growth factors may help to regulate hair follicle growth, such as tissue growth factor-beta (TGF-beta), protein kinase C (PKC), tumor necrosis factor-alpha (TNF-alpha), and phospholipase C. Activation of any of these proteins in the hair follicle may trigger a cascade that ultimately leads to apoptosis within the hair follicle and thus cause hair loss. Specific inhibitors to these proteins have been found in a variety of herbs, such as *Hydrangea macrophylla* (inhibits TGF-beta), *Sophora flavescens* (inhibits phospholipase C), *Perilla* (inhibits TNF-alpha), and procyanidins from many different sources (inhibits PKC). Of these potential remedies, only the use of procyanidins (from apples) has been validated by human clinical trials.

Procyanidins
Procyanidins are tannin compounds that exist widely in plants — although predominantly found in apples and grape seed extract — that often inhibit PKC activity. These compounds are thought to inhibit the PKC-mediated pathway that leads to apoptosis of hair follicles, and thus circumvent follicle death that leads to hair loss.

Human trials into procyanidins isolated from apples are promising, yet there is currently no product on the market that contains this ingredient. Six months of topical application of procyanidin B2 isolated from apple juice lead to a significant increase in hair diameter (an increase of 21% over the placebo group) as well as an improvement in total hair density.[25] Indeed, when compared to commercially available treatments such as minoxidil and finasteride, the increase in hair density in response to procyanidin B2 treatment is similar (Textbox 7.1).

Textbox 7.1   Essential Oil Therapy and Hair Loss

Androgenetic alopecia is distinct from alopecia areata. The latter is a hair loss condition that occurs in only 1% of the Caucasian population. Alopecia areata is a common chronic inflammatory disease that typically results in sudden hair loss in a specific region. Its onset is unpredictable, as its sudden resolution.

Essential oil therapy may be beneficial for individuals with alopecia areata. Scalp massage employing essential oil of thyme, rosemary, and other herbs resulted in noticeable improvement in the majority of study patients subjected to this daily treatment for a period of 7 months.[26] The massaging portion of the treatment may play an important role in success, as it improves blood flow to the hair follicles. This may help to support follicle health and thus improve hair growth.

Conventional Treatment

Finasteride (Propecia®) leads to androgen deprivation through inactivation of 5-alpha reductase. This product is taken orally, and prevents additional hair loss in most male patients and promotes hair growth in about half of study subjects.[27] In about one third of patients, hair growth at the vertex is cosmetically important, while new growth at the margins is less pronounced yet statistically significant. Patients are encouraged to take this treatment for 2 years before evaluating the success of the treatment, although new growth may be noticed in as little as 3 months. In addition, treatment should continue indefinitely for continued improvement, as interruption of the treatment will allow balding to recommence. Proscar®, which (finasteride, 5 mg) used to treat benign prostatic hyperplasia (BPH), is the same compound found in Propecia (finasteride, 1 mg), only a lower dose is used to treat hair loss.

Minoxidil (Rogaine®) is a topically applied 5-alpha-reductase inhibitor that helps to restore hair growth in men (and some women). Minoxidil generally yields statistically less significant improvement compared to finasteride in clinical trials. It is interesting to note that combination of minoxidil and finasteride yields superior results than either treatment used alone.[28] In addition, clinical trials indicate that within 3 months of ending treatment of 5-alpha-reductase inhibitors, all regrown hair is lost. Thus continued application is absolutely essential to maintain long-term benefits.

Hair grafts are another option to restore lost hair. Indeed, over the last decade improvements in donor harvesting, graft size, and hairline design have revolutionized this approach to hair restoration. Because this approach results in a natural appearance, it is becoming an increasingly popular approach for many men. However, the substantial price tag — in excess of $10,000 in some cases — is a significant deterrent to a large segment of the population.

BENIGN PROSTATIC HYPERPLASIA

Few men who live a normal life span — about 74 years — will depart this earth unscathed by some sort of prostate ailment, ranging from painful inflammation to benign enlargement to cancer.

— Patrick C. Walsh and Janet Farrar Worthington, *The Prostate: A Guide for Men and the Women Who Love Them*, 1995.

The prostate is a male-specific organ that sits just below the urinary bladder. It is about the size of a walnut in adult males, and produces fluid that ultimately becomes part of the semen. An inescapable fact of being male is that the prostate continues to grow throughout

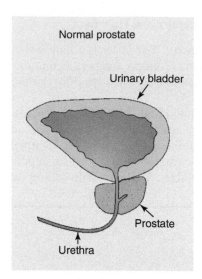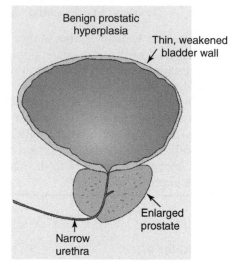

FIGURE 7.3 Prostate gland illustration.

life — often giving rise to an enlarged prostate with advanced age. Prostate enlargement is especially problematic if it occurs in a region called the transition zone (see Figure 7.3). The transition zone is in the center of the prostate, and encircles the urethra — the tube that voids the bladder through the penis. As a result, urine flow from the bladder may become impeded and cause the symptoms typical of BPH, such as nocturia (night time urinations), intermittent urine stream, weak urine flow, hesitancy commencing urine flow, dribbling at the end of urination, and a sense of a full bladder after urination.[29]

In the early stages of BPH, the symptoms may be few and minor. Urine flow may not noticeably change, since the muscular contraction of the bladder may compensate for the narrowing of the urethra. The time of onset of the disease varies with the individual; however, it seems pretty certain that if a man lives long enough, he will begin to experience the symptoms of BPH. Many men experience symptoms in their forties, and the likelihood of experiencing symptoms increases with age. For example, BPH is present in 50% of men over 50 years, and in 80% of men who reach the age of 80 years.

As the prostate ages, it apparently is more sensitive to androgens which encourage cell proliferation, and hence organ enlargement. In addition, smooth muscles within the prostate become more rigid. Together, these events severely restrict the flow of urine through the urethra, and lead to the symptoms associated with BPH.

A number of herbal remedies are available to treat the symptoms of BPH. Among the most common and best known of these is saw palmetto; or more appropriately the ripe berries from the plant known as *Serenoa repens*.

INT Approaches

Saw Palmetto
Several clinical trials support the beneficial use of saw palmetto in relieving the symptoms of BPH. Improvements in the International Prostate Symptoms score rating scale (I-PSS) — which measures urgency, hesitancy, and frequency of urination — and quality of life (QOL) scale are observed following administration of saw palmetto in symptomatic males. Saw palmetto treatment also improves outcomes such as dysuria, nocturia, and urinary flow rate while reducing pain during urination.

Textbox 7.2   Factors to Consider when Choosing Herbal Treatments

In considering the advantages and disadvantages of herbal treatments relative to conventional medications, it is worthwhile to keep in mind several factors. The case of saw palmetto provides a good example with respect to adverse effects, economics, and availability of long-term clinical data. For example, saw palmetto is better tolerated than either finasteride or alpha-blockers. Indeed, some patients report improved erectile function following supplementation with saw palmetto, while ED is a common adverse event of finasteride. Saw palmetto is an economically favorable alternative to pharmacological agents, at one half to one fourth of the cost. However, research for supplements such as saw palmetto is generally less advanced compared to pharmaceutical offerings. Trials are generally shorter and typically enroll fewer patients. Consequently, the ability of saw palmetto to maintain efficacious improvements over the long term has not been investigated, while finasteride is effective at limiting the long-term complications of BPH.

Several head-to-head trials have been performed with saw palmetto compared to pharmacological agents, with favorable results. Similar results were observed for both saw palmetto (320 mg/day) and finasteride (5 mg/day) on I-PSS and QOL scales, as well as urinary flow.[30] Finasteride has a greater impact on reducing prostate size (18% compared to 6% for saw palmetto) and the plasma levels of several hormones in the blood, including testosterone, DHT, luteinizing hormone (LH), follicle-stimulating hormone (FSH). Given patient responses, however, these physiological changes apparently do not translate into symptomatic improvements beyond that obtained for saw palmetto. To underscore the benefit of saw palmetto, it is worthwhile to consider that a recent meta-analysis concluded that this herb produced similar improvements in urinary symptoms and peak urine flow to finasteride.[31] Moreover, the herbal approach was associated with fewer adverse treatment events (Textbox 7.2).

Compared to alfuzosin — an alpha-blocker — saw palmetto is less effective with respect to peak urinary flow (other parameters were either not measured or reported); alfuzosin (7.5 mg / day) increased peak urinary flow by 72% compared to 48% for saw palmetto (320 mg/day) over a 3-week period.[32] Given the quick-acting nature of this type of pharmacological agent, this short period trial may not yield the most accurate results since 1–2 months of treatment with saw palmetto are required for clinically significant results. For example, when compared to a similar drug, prazosin, over a 3-month period, saw palmetto is nearly as beneficial for relieving the irrative symptoms of BPH.[33] In addition, a 1-year trial that compared saw palmetto to yet another alpha-blocker — tamsulosin — demonstrated that the two treatments are equivalent in the treatment of BPH lower urinary tract symptoms over the length of the trial.[34]

Pygeum

The bark from Pygeum (*Pygeum africanum* or *Prunus africana*), also known as the African plum tree, has long been used to treat the symptoms of BPH and urinary complications. The bark contains a variety of biologically active ingredients, including fatty acids, long chain fatty alcohols, and phytosterols. The effectiveness of this herb suggests that pygeum initiates a multipronged approach to improve urinary complications associated with BPH. Among the potential mechanisms are reduction of prostate fibroblast proliferation, increased bladder muscle contraction, and decreased androgen levels.

Open-label studies with pygeum have provided positive results, while double-blind, placebo-controlled trials yield more conflicting results. Nonetheless, recent clinical trials suggest a clear benefit of pygeum compared to placebo. For example, most controlled trials demonstrate that pygeum significantly improves measurable trial outcomes such as nocturia, daytime frequency, peak flow rate, I-PPS, and QOL. One double-blind trial demonstrated that 50 mg pygeum dose twice a day yielded equivalent results as a single 100 mg daily dose, where QOL improved by 28% and I-PSS scores improved 35–38% over a 2-month treatment period.[35] A second study, which had an open-label design, produced similar results, where I-PSS improved by 40%, QOL improved by 31% and nocturnal frequency decreased by 32%.[36] To date, there are no direct head-to-head trials with conventional treatments, thus making it difficult to put these results in perspective relative to other treatments.

Nettle Root

The root of *Urtica dioica radix*, but not the aerial parts of the plant, has long been used for urination disorders deriving from BPH. Nettle root contains a number of compounds, including beta-sitosterol, polysaccharides, and lectins, believed to promote improved urine flow through regulation of metabolism, proliferation, and inflammation in prostate tissue.

Double-blind, placebo-controlled trials with nettle root extract (600 mg/day for 4–6 weeks) have a positive impact on urine flow compared to placebo.[37] Likely the beta-sitosterol is responsible for this improvement, as additional clinical trials which focus on this single compound demonstrate that beta-sitosterol improves peak urinary flow rate, post-void residual urinary volume and also improves I-PSS and QOL scores. An 18-month follow-up study demonstrates that benefits are maintained throughout the administration of nettle root[38] (Textbox 7.3).

Pumpkin Seed

Pumpkin seeds, as well as pumpkin seed oil, contain beta-sitosterols. Not surprisingly, these herbs have also been used to treat the symptoms of BPH, although the scientific substantiation for this approach is less robust than for other treatments listed above. Nonetheless, several clinical trials in Europe indicate that this is an effective approach to relieving the discomfort associated with BPH as measured by I-PSS and QOL scores.[39,40]

Combination Herbal Therapy

Given that these herbal approaches may target different aspects of BPH, a natural question is whether they would work synergistically or additively if used in combination. Few clinical trials have been performed with combination products, although the results of these suggest that indeed a combination approach is effective[41]; of particular benefit appears to be the combination of saw palmetto and nettle root.[42] However, confirmation of these limited scientific studies is needed before the merits of this approach can be seriously considered.

Textbox 7.3 Why Do Ingredients in Herbal Formulations Differ?

As is the case with research on many herbal ingredients, the results with nettle root are not consistent in the scientific literature. There are a variety of ways in which to explain this — differences in trial design and execution, as well as different doses, outcome measures, patient populations, and trial lengths. All have great impact on the final result — and may cause one trial to show a significant response while another yields no benefit. But the most important factor is the herb itself — the level of active ingredients in herbs varies based on season, location, growing conditions, time of harvest, and portion of herb used. Consequently, the herbs used in one trial to the next may differ dramatically in terms of active ingredients. In many instances, the active ingredients in herbs have not even been identified, which makes the process of herbal standardization even that much more challenging. Taking all of these differences into consideration, it is not surprising that similar clinical trials often yield very different outcomes.

Along this line, the combination of two pharmacological agents that inhibit different bio-chemical pathways — finasteride and terazosin — provides greater therapeutic advantage than either of these treatments alone.[43]

Conventional Treatment

5-Alpha-Reductase Inhibitors — Finasteride (Proscar), Dutasteride (Avodart®)
Treatment with Proscar for a period of 2 years results in shrinking the size of the prostate by an average of 25%. While this is an impressive biological result, the improvement in urine flow is much less than achieved through the TUR approach described below. Seventy-one percent of men report an improvement in symptoms overall, but only 31% report a significant improvement in urine flow following this pharmacological treatment.[29] For men with min-imal symptoms, significant gains may be barely noticeable; the most benefit is derived from those with the most extreme symptoms. Because of the time of onset — Proscar may take up to 6 months to register an effect — men with minimal symptoms may be the best candidates to initiate 5-alpha-reductase inhibitor therapy. Patients with extreme symptoms may require more immediate results, offered by options reviewed below.

A therapy similar to finasteride is the newer compound called dutasteride (Avodart). This drug invokes a dual inhibitory action, limiting the activity of both type 1 and type 2 5-alpha reductase, and demonstrates sustained efficacy in BPH patients over a 4-year intervention period. In one trial, prostate volume decreased by 26%, and system scores decreased by 6.1% and peak urinary flow rate increased by 2.8 ml/s.[44] Because of the dual inhibitory action of this compound, it suppresses DHT serum levels more effectively than inhibitors such as finasteride that inhibit only type 2 5-alpha-reductase isoenzymes. For example, over a 24-week intervention, the level of DHT in those taking dutasteride was 94–98% compared to 70% in those taking finasteride.[45]

Because 5-alpha-reductase inhibitors also reduce serum prostate-specific antigen (PSA) levels, these therapies may find application in reducing the risk of prostate cancer in high-risk patients. Limited data to date suggests that dutasteride may be useful in the early treatment or prevention of prostate cancer, since intraprostatic DHT levels are similarly reduced — by up to 97% — and may be responsible for the increased apoptosis in the tissue. Short-term administration (45 days) led to significant decrease in benign epithelial cell width compared to placebo.[46] Indeed the results of this treatment offer sufficient promise to test it in a clinical setting; the REDUCE trial (Reduction by Dutasteride of Prostate Cancer Events) will enroll 8000 high-risk men and observe the conversion rate to prostate cancer over a 4-year period.[47]

Research Note

Finasteride is sold as two distinct prescriptions, and is referred to as either Proscar or Propecia, based on the condition it is designed to treat. Finasteride was first approved by the Food and Drug Administration (FDA) in 1997 to treat male pattern baldness in a low-dose (1 mg) form. The next year it was approved for "reducing the need for prostate surgery" at a dose of 5 mg.[48]

LH–RH Agonists — Leuprolide Acetate (Lupron®), Goserelin (Zoladex®)
Luteinizing hormone–releasing hormone (LH–RH) is made in the hypothalamus of the brain, and signals the nearby pituitary gland to make and release LH (the hormone that signals the production of testosterone in the testes). LH–RH agonists inhibit the synthesis of LH, and thus limit the production of testosterone — a process that has been described as "chemical

castration." While this option does indeed reduce the size of the prostate, it also causes impotence, hot flashes, weight gain, breast swelling, and tenderness. Consequently, this treatment is a viable option only for a very select group of BPH sufferers.

Alpha-Blockers (Terazosin, Prazosin, Alfuzosin, Tamsulosin)
The advantage of this class of drugs is that it works almost immediately by reducing smooth muscle contraction in the prostate gland. These agents block alpha-I adrenoreceptors — particularly abundant in the base of the bladder and the prostate — which mediate the involuntary contraction of smooth muscle cells and thus cause tightening around the urethra to restrict urine flow. A recent meta-analysis of nine clinical trials concludes that terazosin is a useful treatment for BPH, as it improves symptom scores (although only modestly, by 2.2 points over placebo) and increases peak flow rate.[49] In one recent clinical comparison of pharmaceutical options, it was determined that terazosin was more effective than finasteride; terazosin increased peak flow by 2.7 ml/s, while finasteride was similar to placebo (1.6 and 1.4, respectively). Likewise, only terazosin showed a significant improvement in symptom scores (6.1 points versus 2.6 for placebo and 3.2 for finasteride).[50] Side effects, such as dizziness and orthostatic hypotension, are less of a problem if the drug is taken at night, the time when symptoms of BPH are most problematic.

Newer generation alpha-blockers — such as tamsulosin and alfuzosin — appear to be as effective at treating BPH symptoms with less systemic impact. Alpha-1-blockers were initially introduced to manage hypertension; new versions are more "uroselective" and have a decreased risk for adverse cardiovascular effects, such as orthostatic hypotension or other blood pressure — related effects in normotensive patients.[51] A recent review on this topic suggests that tamsulosin has efficacy similar to terazosin and doxazosin, yet is associated with fewer side effects. Likewise, alfuzosin has good efficacy with minimal side effects, in particular, minimizing hypotension.[52]

Research Note

A recent four-arm trial compared the benefit of placebo, doxazosin, finasteride, or the combination in over 3000 men with a follow-up period of 4.5 years. Symptom scores to record clinical progression of BPH were reduced by 39% with doxazosin; 36% with finasteride; and 66% with the combination of doxazosin and finasteride.[53] These results underscore the benefit of combination therapy in treating diseases that can be addressed by inhibiting multiple biochemical pathways.

Surgical Options — Prostatectomy
The most common surgical option for treating BPH by far — accounting for nearly 95% of prostatectomies historically — is transurethral resection of the prostate (TURP). In this procedure, a resectoscope is threaded through the urethra and allows surgeons access to the prostate gland that occludes the bladder. A cutting loop composed of an electrosurgical cautery is attached to the end, and allows the surgeon to cut away excess prostate tissue that blocks the exit of urine from the bladder.

No form of prostatectomy eliminates BPH completely. The TURP approach treats the disease that is present, but may need to be repeated depending on how fast the tissue grows back. TURP improves the symptoms in 93% of men with severe symptoms, and in 70% of men with moderate problems.[29] In those experiencing improvement in urine flow, the benefits last longer than 7 years in most men.

In some cases, a more invasive approach is warranted, wherein surgery is required to access the prostate through an incision in the abdomen. This procedure is called an open prostatectomy, and in some men may provide more complete relief from the symptoms of BPH. Typically, only the overgrown prostate tissue surrounding the urethra is removed in this procedure, leaving the rest of the organ intact. Radical prostatectomies, in which the entire prostate is removed, are generally reserved as a treatment method for prostate cancer.

Transurethral microwave thermotherapy (TUMT) — a minimally invasive technique — is now used with increased frequency to treat the symptoms of BPH. This approach typically leads to symptom improvement of between 9 and 11 points, with increased peak urine flow of 3–5 ml/s.[54] An alternative low-invasive approach in transurethral needle ablation (TUNA) also yields good results. A meta-analysis of this approach indicates that there is a significant improvement in symptoms scores, and peak flow rate increases by about 70%; improvements generally persist for at least 5 years.[55] To put surgical options into perspective, a group of researchers concludes that TURP is still the gold standard of treatment — achieving the highest decrease in prostate volume and the highest increase in peak urinary flow rate — yet acknowledge that this treatment may not be preferred by all men.[56] Some patients may prefer less invasive approaches, pharmaceutical options or herbal remedies; and choice of treatment should consider each patient's performance status, symptoms, invasiveness, cost, risk, convenience, and duration of results.

Prostate Cancer

After skin cancer, prostate cancer is the most common cancer reported in men in the United States, and approximately one in six American men will be diagnosed with prostate cancer during his lifetime.[57] After lung cancer, it is the second leading cause of death from cancer, and is estimated to be responsible for over 30,000 deaths in 2002. In the same year, the American Cancer Society estimates that 189,000 new cases of prostate cancer will be diagnosed.[58] Just a few years ago, the average age of diagnosis for prostate cancer was 72 years, while the average age at death from the disease was 77 years. More reassuring news comes from the Prostate Cancer Foundation, which reveals that the survival rate for prostate cancer is improving with better and earlier diagnosis. For example, of the cases diagnosed in the local and regional stages, the 5-year survival rate is nearly 100%; the 10-year survival rate is 86%; and the 15-year survival rate is 56%.[59]

Improved and routine diagnostic techniques, such as monitoring PSA levels and frequent digital rectal examinations, allow diagnosis of prostate cancer much earlier and lead to early and potentially aggressive treatment (such as radiation therapy or prostatectomy) to rid the body of cancer and improved survivability. There are no early warning signs of prostate cancer that men can diagnose by themselves; by the time men notice signs of this disease it is likely too late to cure it. That is why early diagnosis and preventive measures are important.

INT Approach

Is there any alternative or complementary medical approach that can decrease the risk of prostate cancer? As with all cancers, prevention is the best protocol. But how does one go about preventing prostate cancer? The best approach appears to be through a healthy diet, active lifestyle, and adequate sun exposure.

Vitamin D
UV radiation appears to be important as it helps the body to synthesize vitamin D, an essential nutrient that may play an important role in limiting prostate cell proliferation.

Interestingly, males who live in the northern United States — the geographic location that receives the least UV radiation — are more likely to die of prostate cancer than men who reside in the southern climate.[60] Recent research demonstrates that vitamin D induces apoptosis in prostate cancer cells,[61] a result that suggests vitamin D therapy may be an effective approach to limit prostate cancer in some men. Along this line, it is important to note that phase I studies with vitamin D have been completed with promising results,[62] although more advanced studies are required to determine the precise benefit of this nutritional intervention therapy. A phase II study is currently under way to determine whether calcifediol (a potent form of vitamin D) will delay or prevent the progression of the disease.[63]

Diet

A recent global investigation into the role of diet in cancer prevention suggests the following possible relationship between different food groups and prostate cancer risk.[64] Red meat increases risk of prostate cancer significantly,[65] while a diet rich in vegetables appears to reduce the risk considerably. The World Cancer Research Fund suggests that moderate protection is provided by frequent consumption of tomatoes, carrots, cabbage, and spinach; however, other studies suggest no correlation from these foods. Tomatoes have nabbed the spotlight in part because of their high levels of the carotenoid lycopene. Indeed, there is much evidence to suggest that tomatoes and tomato-based products offer significant protection against future prostate cancer.[66]

In addition to a vegetable-rich diet, omega-3-rich foods may also stem the risk of prostate cancer. Epidemiological studies suggest that high fish diets rich in omega-3 fatty acids decrease the risk of prostate cancer,[67] a result that is consistent with the fact that individuals with prostate cancer typically have reduced omega-3 fatty acid serum levels.[68] Omega-3 fatty acids such as EPA and DHA help cells to regulate prostaglandin synthesis, and decrease proinflammatory cytokines such as COX-2. In addition, both DHA and EPA have inhibited androgen-mediated cell proliferation in prostate cancer cells grown in culture. These mechanisms suggest that omega-3 fatty acids found in fish oils may help to reduce the risk of cancer, although direct scientific evidence from clinical trials is not yet available.

With respect to specific supplemental intervention trials, three nutritional treatments stand out: vitamin E, selenium, and lycopene. One of the most compelling studies on prostate cancer prevention comes from the results of double-blind study involving nearly 30,000 smokers. These patients were given vitamin E (50 mg/day) for a period of 5–8 years, and reported a 32% decrease in the incidence of prostate cancer and a 41% decline in death from prostate cancer.[69] While these results sound impressive, it is important to consider the results from a similar study, which suggest that supplemental vitamin E is beneficial only for smokers or men who have recently quit smoking — and may not translate to the male population as a whole.[70]

The benefit of selenium in prostate cancer was found accidentally, stemming from a trial designed to investigate the benefit of selenium supplementation (200 μg/day for about 2.8 years) in skin cancer. While there was no benefit with respect to skin cancer, selenium reduced the risk of lung cancer (~40%), colon cancer (~50%), and prostate cancer (~66%) in the study population.[71] Because the outcome measures for this trial were not designed to analyze this particular result, additional clinical investigations need to be designed and conducted to validate these findings.

The findings for both selenium and vitamin E are very tantalizing, and because these dietary interventions are both convenient and economical, they represent an ideal approach to prevent prostate cancer. Not surprisingly, these approaches are currently the subject of major clinical trials. SELECT (the Selenium and Vitamin E Cancer Prevention Trial) is a phase III study aiming to enroll 32,000 male patients with prostate cancer and monitor their progress for 7–12 years. A smaller trial is focusing only on selenium and will enroll over 1,000 patients for a 3-year treatment period followed by a 5-year follow-up period. These trials are designed specifically to determine the benefit of dietary supplementation with either selenium or vitamin E, and will provide much needed data in this research area.[63]

Lycopene

Lycopene is a carotenoid responsible for the deep red hues of red-fleshed fruits such as tomatoes, watermelons, and guava. In the body, it accumulates in the prostate gland at much higher concentrations than found in other organs of the body, and may act as an important antioxidant to protect prostate cells against free radical damage. In support of this potential function, researchers have demonstrated that prostate cancer victims have lower levels of plasma and prostate tissue lycopene than individuals without prostate cancer.[72] The most comprehensive of these studies followed dietary habits of nearly 48,000 male health professionals for 6 years, and found that the highest dietary intake of lycopene reduced the risk of prostate cancer in this cohort by 21%.[73] These results are supported by the finding that men with elevated levels of lycopene in their plasma have a lower risk of prostate cancer.[74]

Epidemiological data on this topic is interesting as well. For example, men over the age of 65 years with no apparent family history of prostate cancer were significantly less likely to develop prostate cancer if they had high blood levels of lycopene. For men under the age of 65 years, high blood levels of beta-carotene significantly decreased the likelihood of future prostate cancer. This data suggests that different compounds may offer different protection during the development of this particular cancer.[75]

This data is very provocative, but it leaves unanswered the question of whether or not lycopene can reduce the risk of prostate cancer. The results of a short-term, high-dose lycopene clinical trial are promising in this regard.[76] A small group of men ($n = 15$) who were scheduled to undergo radical prostatectomy consumed 30 mg/day lycopene for 3 weeks prior to surgery. Men who received lycopene decreased their PSA level, and were less likely to have cancerous cells found outside the prostate tissue (27%) compared to those who received no supplementation (82%). Whether lycopene can work over the long term to decrease the risk of prostate cancer has not yet been determined, but trials are in progress to address this very point.

Soy

Because prostate cancer is mediated by androgen sensitivity, plant compounds that mimic androgens may play an important role in reducing the risk of the disease. Given that the age-standardized incidence of prostate cancer is only one tenth of the rate in the United States, the traditional Japanese diet — rich in soy and fermented soy products — may offer cellular protection to promote normal cell growth. Indeed a recent case-controlled study indicates that increasing amounts of soy products, especially natto (fermented soy beans) may protect against prostate cancer in Japanese men.[77] Men diagnosed with prostate cancer and fed a high-soy diet (50 g soy/day, containing 117 mg genistein, daidzein, glycitein in aglycone form) favorably improve their PSA levels and free/total PSA ratio during a 3–4-week intervention.[78]

Compounds such as isoflavones found in soy products may inhibit the catabolism of vitamin D in prostate cancer cells, and in this way may minimize the risk of prostate cancer.[79] Additional evidence suggests that a specific isoflavone, genistein, induces expression of glutathione peroxidase in prostate cell lines, and thus may limit carcinogenic damage to reduce the risk of prostate cancer.[80] A clinical trial is currently recruiting patients with prostate cancer to determine the benefit of dietary isoflavones in treating these patients.

PC-SPES

Laboratory studies indicate that the multiherb mixture — known as PC-SPES — decreases prostate cancer cell growth by 72–80% at the same time that it reduces expression of PSA.[81] Clinical data reveals that PSA is significantly reduced in all men with prostate cancer, although the effect is more pronounced in men with androgen-dependent prostate cancer.[82] The duration of this response and whether it increases survivability of prostate cancer patients has not yet been determined. Researchers note that this treatment results in common side effects such as gynecomastia, nipple soreness, lower libido, and impotence.[83]

Research Note

PC-SPES is a commercial product that recently generated substantial media attention. It is a mixture of eight Chinese herbs, the most abundant of which is saw palmetto, which effectively lowers PSA levels in men with prostate cancer. However, controversy arose when it was determined that the samples contained prescription drugs — most notably warfarin and alprazolam. Accordingly, the FDA instituted a recall of this product, warning that it could cause serious health problems when taken outside of medical supervision.[84] Further analysis of several different lots of the product manufactured between 1996 and 2000 indicated substantial variation in both synthetic agents (such as indomethacin, warfarin, and diethylstilbestrol) and natural products (such as lichochalcone A and baicalin). Certainly, this serves as a cautionary note to the dietary supplement industry — and should encourage this industry to provide reliable and consistent analytical quality assurance. PC-SPES was recalled and withdrawn from the market because certain batches were contaminated with FDA. Subsequently PC-SPES is no longer manufactured.

Conventional Treatment

Prostate cancer is a complex disease that manifests itself at a different rate and different form in different men. The heterogeneity of disease progression makes it sometimes difficult to determine which course of treatment is best for an individual patient. However, one positive similarity about this disease is that it tends to grow very slowly, which makes a variety of different options available.

Conventional treatment for prostate cancer depends on the stage of the disease and the age and general health of the patient. Depending on these individual factors, treatment options may involve a course of hormonal, radiation, or chemical therapy, surgery to remove the cancerous cells, a combination of these approaches, or no intervention at all. Because the symptoms of prostate cancer are not apparent until the disease is very advanced, routine screening is encouraged for men around the age of 50 years, or earlier if they are in the high-risk category.

If the diagnosis is localized or locally advanced prostate cancer, there are typically three treatment options available: "watchful waiting," surgery, or radiation. If the cancer is diagnosed at an advanced stage (i.e., it has spread beyond the prostate), or has returned after surgery or radiation, then hormonal treatment to reduce testosterone levels (or block testosterone activity) is generally initiated. In some cases, such as metastasis or aggressive cancers, chemotherapy may provide the best treatment option.

BPH CASE STUDY

N.C. is a 69-year-old African American male who presented 3 months ago for further evaluation of voiding difficulties. He first sought help 5 years ago when he first began having significant symptoms.

At that time he described a definite decrease in the force of his urinary stream with a longer time to initiate voiding, having to get up to urinate three times on most nights, and he had a feeling that his bladder did not empty to completion. He denied any burning or blood in his urine, and there had not been any prior episode of urinary tract infection. His prostate symptom score at that time was 16. There was no history of prostate cancer in his family.

Examination at that time revealed a smooth feeling prostate gland that was moderately enlarged at 30 g. His PSA at the time was 2.9.

Not fond of pharmaceuticals, he requested treatment with natural remedies if possible. He was started on saw palmetto extract at a dose of 320 mg daily.

Over the next 4.5 years, he did well, with improvement of his symptom score to 8. He was satisfied with this control of his symptoms.

About 6 months ago he began having worsening symptoms again. He had continued on the saw palmetto but his symptom score was back up to 17. Fortunately, he still had had no episodes of urinary tract infection or urinary retention.

His digital rectal exam, and serum PSA, which had been done annually had not changed significantly over the 5 years.

The potential for an operative procedure was discussed with him. He now wanted to try another type of medical therapy before considering surgery. He was started on tamsulosin 0.4 mg daily 3 months ago.

Currently he reports that his symptoms are moderately improved, with his prostate symptom score back down to 10, and he is satisfied for now, but understands that his symptoms might progress, and that he may require invasive treatment.

DISCUSSION

Growth of the prostate gland is a natural result of aging in the typical male. The prostate gland is stimulated by the male hormone testosterone. While all men will have growth of the prostate, not all will have significant symptoms from it. As a result of the growth of the gland, the urethra is squeezed, making emptying of the bladder difficult. The symptoms that result are an effect of this constriction. The force of the urinary stream diminishes, and initiation of the stream is more difficult. The patient will often feel the need to void more frequently and will feel as if the bladder is not completely empty after voiding. He will invariably find himself having to get up at night more to empty his bladder multiple times. This is the most frequent symptom that bring men to be evaluated for prostate problems. These symptoms can be quantified using the AUA BPH Symptom Index.

As prostate cancer is the number one male cancer, screening for prostate cancer is something that should be discussed with every patient. Those in high-risk populations (those with a family history of prostate cancer or African Americans) should begin having yearly PSA blood tests and digital rectal examinations, so if present, the cancer can be detected and treated early.

Benign prostatic disease, as evidenced by the above-mentioned lower urinary tract symptoms, is generally treated medically or surgically. Medical treatment is based either on affecting the hormonal stimulation to the prostate, which, in general, is the method of action for saw palmetto, finasteride, and dutasteride. Alpha-adrenergic blockers, which include prazosin, terazosin, doxazosin, tamsulosin, and alfuzosin, work by relaxing the smooth muscle in the prostate and at the opening of the bladder.

As a rule, BPH is not a medically dangerous problem. Most men are treated because they do not want to deal with the symptoms any further. However, in more significant cases, medical intervention is required. Urinary retention, acute renal failure, recurrent urinary tract infection, intractable bleeding, or the presence of stones in the bladder are indications for medical intervention. Often the acute problem may be addressed and then the patient can be treated medically.

When medical treatment is unsuccessful, surgical treatment is indicated. There are a number of surgical options all designed to remove the enlarged, constricting portion of the prostate. Once performed, the patient's symptoms are relieved and in most cases resumes a normal lifestyle.

REFERENCES

1. Center for Disease Control statistics, http://webapp.cdc.gov/sasweb/ncipc/leadcaus10.html
2. Owusu, W., et al., Calcium intake and the incidence of forearm and hip fractures among men, *J. Nutr.*, 127, 1782, 1997.
3. Whiting, S.J., et al., Dietary protein, phosphorus and potassium are beneficial to bone mineral density in adult men consuming adequate dietary calcium, *J. Am. Coll. Nutr.*, 21, 402, 2002.
4. O'brien, D.P., et al., Pelvic fracture in the elderly is associated with increased mortality, *Surgery*, 132, 710, 2002.
5. Kantor, J., et al., Prevalence of erectile dysfunction and active depression: an analytic cross-sectional study of general medical patients, *Am. J. Epidemiol.*, 156, 1035, 2002.
6. Price, V.H., Treatment of hair loss, *N. Engl. J. Med.*, 341, 964, 1999.
7. Lue, T.F., Erectile dysfunction, *N. Engl. J. Med.*, 342, 1802, 2000.
8. Moody, J.A., et al., Effects of long-term oral administration of L-arginine on the rat erectile response, *J. Urol.*, 158, 942, 1997.
9. Klotz, T., et al., Effectiveness of oral L-arginine in first-line treatment of erectile dysfunction in a controlled crossover study, *Urol. Int.*, 63, 220, 1999.
10. Chen, J., et al., Effect of oral administration of high-dose nitric oxide donor L-arginine in men with organic erectile dysfunction: results of a double blind, randomized, placebo-controlled crossover study, *BJU Int.*, 83, 269, 1999.
11. Hong, B., et al., A double-blind crossover study evaluating the efficacy of Korean red ginseng in patients with erectile dysfunction: a preliminary report, *J. Urol.*, 168, 2070, 2002.
12. Choi, H.K., Seong, D.H., and Rha, K.H., Clinical efficacy of Korean red ginseng for erectile dysfunction, *Int. J. Impot. Res.*, 7, 181, 1995.
13. Ernst, E., and Pittler, M.H., Yohimbine for erectile dysfunction: a systematic review and meta-analysis of randomized clinical trials, *J. Urol.*, 159, 433, 1998.
14. Lebert, T., et al., Efficacy and safety of a novel combination of L-arginine glutamate and yohimbine hydrochoride: a new oral therapy for erectile dysfunction, *Eur. Urol.*, 41, 608, 2002.
15. Zheng, B.L., et al., Effect of a lipidic extract from *Lepidium meyenii* on sexual behavior in mice and rats, *Urology*, 55, 598, 2000.
16. Purvis, K., Egdetveit, K., and Christiansen, E., Intracavernosal therapy for erectile failure — impact of treatment and reasons for drop-out and dissatisfaction, *Int. J. Impot. Res.*, 11, 287, 1999.
17. Morgenthaler, A., Male impotence, *Lancet*, 354, 17713, 1999.
18. Fink, H.A., et al., Sildenafil for male erective dysfunction: a systematic review and meta-analysis, *Arch. Intern. Med.*, 162, 1349, 2002.
19. Gonzalez, C.M., et al., Sildenafil causes a dose- and time-dependent downregulation of phosphodiesterase type 6 expresssion in the rat retina, *Int. J. Impot. Res.*, 11 (suppl 1), S9, 1999.

20. Setty, L.R., Hair patterns of the scalp of white and Negro males, *Am. J. Phys. Anthropol.*, 33, 49, 1970.
21. Price, V.H., Treatment of hair loss, *N. Engl. J. Med.*, 341, 664, 1999.
22. Prager, N., et al., A randomized, double-blind, placebo-controlled trial to determine the effectiveness of botanically derived inhibitiors of 5-alpha-reductase in the treatment of androgenetic alopecia, *J. Altern. Complement. Med.*, 8, 143, 2002.
23. Shimizu, K., et al., Steriod 5 alpha-reductase inhibitory activity and hair regrowth effects of an extract from *Boehmeria nipononivea*, *Biosci. Biotechnol. Biochem.*, 64, 875, 2000.
24. Stamatiadis, D., Bulteau-Portois, M.C., and Mowszowicz, I., Inhibition of 5 alpha reductase activity in human skin by zinc and azelaic acid, *Br. J. Dermatol.* 119, 627, 1988.
25. Kamimura, A., Takahashi, T., and Watanabe, Y., Investigation of topical application of procyanidin B-2 from apple to identify its potential use as a hair growing agent, *Phytomedicine*, 7, 529, 2000.
26. Hay, I.C., Jamieson, M., and Ormerod, A.D., Randomized trial of aromatherapy: successful treatment for alopecia areata, *Arch. Dermatol.*, 134, 1349, 1988.
27. Foley, P.A., Recent advances: dermatology, *BMJ*, 320, 870, 2000.
28. Khandpur, S., Suman, M., and Reddy, B.S., Comparative efficacy of various treatment regimens for androgenetic alopecia in men, *J. Dermatol.*, 29, 489, 2002.
29. Walsh, P.C., and Worthington, J.F., *The Prostate: A Guide for Men and the Women Who Love Them*, Johns Hopkins University Press, Baltimore, 1995.
30. Strauch, G., et al., Comparison of finasteride (Proscar) and *Serenoa repens* (Permixon) in the inhibition of 5-alpha reductase in healthy male volunteers, *Eur. Urol.*, 26, 247, 1994.
31. Wilt, T., Ishani, A., and MacDonald, R., *Serenoa repens* for benign prostatic hyperplasia, *Cochrane Database Syst. Rev.* (3), CD001423, 2002.
32. Grasso, M., et al., Comparative effects of alfuzosin versus *Serenoa repens* in the treatment of symptomatic benign prostatic hyperplasia, *Arch. Esp. Urol.*, 48, 97, 1995.
33. Adriazola Semino, M., et al., Symptomatic treatment of benign hypertrophy of the prostate, Comparative study of prazosin and *Serenoa repens*, Spanish, *Arch. Esp. Urol.*, 45, 211, 1992.
34. Debruyne, R., et al., Comparison of a phytotherapeutic agent (Permixon) with an alpha-blocker (Tamulosin) in the treatment of benign prostatic hyperplasia: a 1-year randomized international study, *Eur. Urol.*, 41, 497, 2002.
35. Chatelain, C., Autet, W., and Brackman, F., Comparison of once and twice daily dosage forms of *Pygeum africanum* extract in patients with benign prostatic hyperplasia: a randomized, double-blind study, with long-term open label extension, *Urology*, 54, 473, 1999.
36. Breza, J., et al., Efficacy and acceptability of Tadenan (*Pygeum africanum* extract) in the treatment of benign prostatic hyperplasia (BPH): a multicentre trial in central Europe, *Curr. Med. Res. Opin.*, 14, 127, 1998.
37. Dathe, G., and Schmid, H., Phytotherpie der benignen Prostatahyperplasie (BPH). Doppelblindstudie mit extractum Radicis Uricae (ERU), *Urologie*, 27, 223, 1987.
38. Berges, R.R., Kassen, A., and Senge, T., Treatment of symptomatic benign prostatic hyperplasia with beta-sitosterol: an 18-month follow-up, *BJU Int.*, 85, 482, 2000.
39. Freiderich, M., Theurer, C., and Schiebel-Schlosser, G., Porsta Fink Forte capsules in the treatment of benign prostatic hyperplasia. Multicentric surveillance study in 2245 patients, *Forsch Komplementarmed Klass Naturheilkd*, 7, 200, 2000.
40. Carbin, B.E., Larsson, B., and Lindahl, O., Treatment of benign prostatic hyperplasia with phytosterols, *Br. J. Urol.*, 66, 639, 1990.
41. Dvorkin, L., and Song, K.Y., Herbs for benign prostatic hyperplasia, *Ann. Pharmacother.*, 36, 1443, 2002.
42. Sokeland, J., Combined sabal and urtica extract compared with finastereide in men with benign prostatic hyperplasia: analysis of prostate volume and therapeutic outcome, *BJU Int.*, 86, 439, 2000.
43. Savage, S.J., et al., Combination medical therapy for symptomatic benign prostatic hyperplasia, *Can. J. Urol.*, 5, 578, 1998.
44. Roehrborn, C.G., et al., Efficacy and safety of dutasteride in the four-year treatment of men with benign prostatic hyperplasia, *Urology*, 63, 709, 2004.
45. Clark, R.V., et al., Marked suppression of dihydrostestosterone in men with benign prostatic hyperplasia by dutastride, a dual 5 alpha-reductase inhibitor, *J. Clin. Endocrinol. Metab.*, 89, 2179, 2004.

46. Andriole, G.L., et al., Effect of the dual 5 alpha-reductase inhibitor dutasteride on markers of tumor regression in prostate cancer, *J. Urol.*, 172, 915, 2004.

47. Andriole, G., et al., Chemoprevention of prostate cancer in men at high risk: rationale and design of the reduction by dutasteride of prostate cancer events (REDUCE) trial, *J. Urol.*, 172, 1314, 2004.

48. www.centerwatch.com/patient/drugs

49. Boyle, P., et al., Meta-analysis of randomized trials of terazosin in the treatment of benign prostatic hyperplasia, *Urology*, 58, 717, 2001.

50. Lepor, H., et al., The efficacy of terazosin, finasteride, or both in benign prostatic hyperplasia. Veterans Affairs Cooperative Studies Benign Prostatic Hyperplasia Study Group, *N. Engl. J. Med.*, 335, 533, 1996.

51. Lowe, F.C., Role of the newer alpha 1-adrenergic-receptor antagonists in the treatment of benign prostatic hypeprplasia-related lower urinary tract symptoms, *Clin. Ther.*, 26, 1701, 2004.

52. Roehrborn, C.G., and Schwinn, D.A., Alpha1-adrenergic receptors and their inhibitors in lower urinary tract symptoms and benign prostatic hyperplasia, *J. Urol.*, 171, 1029, 2004.

53. McConnell, J.D., et al., The long-term effect of doxasozin, finasteride, and combination therapy on the clinical progression of benign prostatic hyperplasia, *N. Engl. J. Med.*, 349, 2387, 2003.

54. Walmsley, K., and Kaplan, S.A., Thrasurethral microwave thermotherapy for benign prostate hyperplasia: separating truth from marketing hype, *J. Urol.*, 172, 1249, 2004.

55. Boyle, P., et al., A meta-analysis of trials of transurethral needle ablation for treating symptomatic benign prostatic hyperplasia, *BJU Int.*, 94, 83, 2004.

56. Minardi, D., et al., Transurethral resection versus minimally invasive treatments of benign prostatic hyperplasia: results of treatments. Our experience, *Arch. Ital. Urol. Androl.*, 76, 11, 2004.

57. Greenwald, P., Clinical trials in cancer prevention: current results and perspectives for the future, *J. Nutr.*, 134, 3507S, 2004.

58. http://www.cdc.gov/cancer/prostate/prostate.htm#public

59. www.prostatecancerfoundation.org

60. Hanchette, C.L., and Schwartz, G.G., Geographic patterns of prostate cancer mortality. Evidence for a protective effect of ultraviolet radiation, *Cancer*, 70, 2861, 1992.

61. Guzey, M., Kitada, S., and Reed, J.C., Apoptosis induction by 1 alpha, 25-dihydroxyvitamin D3 in prostate cancer, *Mol. Cancer Ther.*, 1, 667, 2002.

62. Liu, G., et al., Phase I trial of 1 alpha-hydroxyvitamin d(2) in patients with hormone refreactory prostate cancer, *Clin. Cancer Res.*, 8, 2820, 2002.

63. NIH. www.clinicaltrials.gov

64. World Cancer Research Fund and American Institute for Cancer Research. Food, nutrition and the prevention of cancer: a global perspective, BANTA Book Group, Menasha, WI. pp. 310–323, 1997.

65. Le Marchand, L., et al., Animal fat consumption and prostate cancer: a prospective study in Hawaii, *Epidemiology*, 5, 276, 1994.

66. Giovannucci, E., Tomatoes, tomato-based products, lycopene, and cancer: review of the epidemiologic literature, *J. Natl. Cancer Inst.*, 91, 317, 1999.

67. Terry, P., et al., Fatty fish consumption and risk of prostate cancer, *Lancet*, 358, 1367, 2001.

68. Yang, Y.J., et al., Comparison of fatty acids profiles in the serum of patients with prostate cancer and benign prostatic hyperplasia, *Clin. Biochem.*, 32, 405, 1999.

69. Heinonen, O.P., et al., Prostate cancer and supplementation with alpha-tocopherol and beta-carotene: incidence and mortality in a controlled trial, *J. Natl. Cancer Inst.*, 90, 440, 1998.

70. Chan, J.M., et al., Supplemental vitamin E intake and prostate cancer risk in a large cohort of men in the United States, *Cancer Epidemiol. Biomarkers Prev.*, 8, 893, 1999.

71. Clark, L.C., et al., Effects of selenium supplementation for cancer prevention in patients with carcinoma of the skin. A randomized controlled trial. Nutritional Prevention of Cancer Study Group, *JAMA*, 276, 1957, 1996.

72. Rao, A.V., Fleshner, N., and Agarwal, S., Serum and tissue lycopene and biomarkers of oxidation in prostate cancer patients: a case–control study, *Nutr. Cancer*, 33, 159, 1999.

73. Giovannucci, E.L., et al., Intake of carotenoids and retinol in relationship to risk of prostate cancer, *J. Natl. Cancer Inst.*, 87, 1767, 1995.

74. Gann, P.H., et al., Lower prostate cancer risk in men with elevated plasma lycopene levels: results of a prospective analysis, *Cancer Res.*, 59, 1225, 1999.

75. Wu, K., et al., Plasma and dietary carotenoids, and the risk of prostate cancer: a nested case-control study, *Cancer Epdemiol. Biomarkers Prev.*, 13, 260, 2004.

76. Kucuk, O., et al., Phase II randomized clinical trial of lycopene supplementation before radical prostatectomy, *Cancer Epidemiol. Biomarkers Prev.*, 10, 861, 2001.

77. Sonoda, T., et al., A case control study of diet and prostate cancer in Japan: possible protective effect of traditional Japanese diet, *Cancer Sci.*, 95, 238, 2004.

78. Dalais, F.S., et al., Effects of a diet rich in phytoestrogens on prostate-specific antigen and sex hormones in men diagnosed with prostate cancer, *Urology*, 64, 510, 2004.

79. Farhan, H., et al., Isoflavonoids inhibit catabolism of vitamin D in prostate cancer cells, *J. Chromatogr. B. Analyt. Technol. Biomed. Life Sci.*, 777, 261, 2002.

80. Suzuki, K., et al., Genistein, a soy isoflavone, induces glutathione peroxidase in the human prostate cancer cell lines LNCaP and PC-3, *Int. J. Cancer*, 99, 846, 2002.

81. Hsieh, T.C., and Wu, J.M., Mechanism of action of herbal supplement PC-SPES: elucidation of effects of individual herbs of PC-SPES on proliferation and prostate specific gene expression in androgen-dependent LNCaP cells, *Int. J. Oncol.*, 20, 583, 2002.

82. Small, E.J., et al., Prospective trial of the herbal supplement PC-SPES in patients with progressive prostate cancer, *J. Clin. Oncol.*, 18, 3595, 2000.

83. Marks, L.S., et al., PC-SPES: herbal formulation for prostate cancer, *Urology*, 60, 369, 2002.

84. http://www.fda.gov/medwatch/SAFETY/2002/spes_press1.htm

8 Skeletal System and Joint Health

Lisa High, Melanie Hingle, Renee M. Kishbaugh, and Michael Buchwald

CONTENTS

SKELETAL SYSTEM

INTRODUCTION

The skeleton provides structure for the body's musculature, protects vital organs, and provides a ready reserve of many nutrients, which the body can tap into for functional needs when necessary. Bone mineral density (BMD) increases throughout childhood and adolescence, peaking in the early adulthood, typically by age of 30 years, with progressive declines thereafter. Achievement of optimal peak bone mass is believed to reduce the risk of osteoporosis later in life. Women begin with less and have less bone mass than men at all ages. Bone mass losses are approximately 1% per year after the age of 30 years with a significant increase in loss for women early in the postmenopausal period. Losses over the life cycle may reach 30 to 40% of peak bone mass for females and 20 to 30% in males.[1] Lifestyle factors such as diet, exercise, some medications, smoking cigarettes, and excess alcohol consumption have been shown to influence bone health. Genetic predisposition, hormonal status, and general overall health are important nonnutritional influences on bone density.

Fractures are the most serious effect on the bone, especially hip fractures, which are associated with an increase in morbidity and mortality as well as a potential decrease in quality of life. A mortality rate of 15% is associated with osteoporotic hip fractures in the elderly.[2]

PATHOPHYSIOLOGY

Bone is comprised of both living and nonliving components. Living tissue makes up 2 to 5% of bone while nonliving components contribute 95 to 98%.[3] Bone is comprised primarily of collagen and calcium phosphate, which together makes bone flexible but also provides strength to withstand stress. Approximately 99% of the body's calcium is found in the bones and teeth.[3]

Bone is made up of two major types of bone tissues, trabecular and cortical. Cortical bone constitutes about 80% of the skeleton primarily the body's long bones. Trabecular bone makes up the remaining 20%, which is found at the knobby ends of the long bones.[4] Trabecular bone is less dense than cortical bone, and is also called spongy bone or spongiosa. The trabecular bone also adds support to the cortical bone outer casing of the long bones. Bones of the pelvis, sternum, shoulder, and vertebrae have a thin outer ring of cortical bone filled with an uneven mixture of trabecular bone. Loss of trabecular bone over a lifetime is primarily responsible for bone fractures later in life.[5]

The end of long bones is comprised of segments called epiphyses while the shaft of long bones are called diaphyses.[3] The fanned portion that precedes the epiphysis segments is called the metaphysis.

The surface at the end of the bones is covered with a layer of cartilage. When two bones come together, this forms a joint (further information on joints follows in this chapter). In healthy individuals, the cartilage is well hydrated and lubricated by synovial fluid held in the joint sac. This allows the joint to move smoothly and freely.

The nonliving component of bone is composed of a mineral-encrusted protein matrix also called the osteoid.[3] Buried in the bone matrix are cells called osteocytes. Osteocytes lie in channels called canaliculi, which allow for cellular communications. Osteoblasts and osteoclasts are the two types of cells primarily responsible for production and resorption of bone, respectively. Osteocytes and bone-lining cells, derived from osteoblasts, are two additional cell types that contribute to bone health. A continuity of remodeling exists whereby bone resorption by osteoclasts and bone formation by osteoblasts are modulated by mechanical and hormonal factors such as serum calcium and phosphorus levels; circulating levels of parathyroid hormone (PTH), thyroid hormone, vitamin D, cortisol, and sex hormones, and mechanical strain throughout the life cycle.[2]

Bone modeling is the process that describes skeletal growth as we achieve adult height. During this process bones are elongated and widened. To allow for growth, most bones have one or more plates, called growth plates, of cartilage perpendicular to the main axis of growth.[3] The cartilage cells in the growth plates multiply rapidly pushing the produced bone away from the shafts. Blood vessels invade the cartilage cells initiating calcification. The ends of the bone continue to be pushed away, thus allowing the cycle to continue down the metaphysis from the epiphyses.[3] Once ossification meets the formation of new cartilage edge, growth stops as bony bridges build across the growth plate. High levels of estrogen associated with puberty also facilitate growth plate closure in both males and females. Growth is typically completed by 18 years of age.[3] After obtaining adult height, bone growth continues by a process known as bone consolidation. Continuous bone remodeling is promoted by patterns of strain and dietary intake. Bone is built and maintained efficiently until around the age of 30 years.[3] Thereafter, as an individual ages, the balance between new bone production and bone resorption is altered, favoring bone resorption.

Loss of bone begins in both sexes around the age of 40 years as bone breakdown begins to exceed formation.[3] The reasons for this are unknown. However, it is often more pronounced in females. The specific causes of age-related bone loss are unknown. As previously discussed, osteoblastic and osteoclastic activity is influenced by a number of factors, which impact on bone formation and resorption. This process of bone loss leads to increased risk for fractures.

CALCIUM HOMEOSTASIS

Homeostatic function of bone is controlled by the (a) bone-remodeling process and (b) two calcium-regulating hormones: PTH and 1,25-dihydroxyvitamin D (calcitriol). PTH is the primary determinant of how much bone remodeling occurs while the pattern of strain is a principal determinant of where bone is remodeled.[3] PTH secretion is influenced by the body's need for calcium. With inadequate calcium consumption, portions of the bone are reabsorbed and the released calcium is used for the body's various needs, especially the maintenance of serum calcium levels. In addition to PTH, calcitriol promotes increased absorption of calcium when the calcium intake is suboptimal.[3] However, homeostasis becomes somewhat unbalanced as we age and there is an increase in bone loss. As we age, PTH levels, which contribute directly to bone loss, tend to increase. Furthermore, urinary calcium losses increase in women during the 1 to 5 years of menopause while calcium absorption from the gastrointestinal (GI) tract does not increase to accommodate for increased losses.[4]

Bone resorption helps meet the body's needs for various minerals, primarily calcium and phosphorus, as it allows minerals to be released into the circulation system. When calcium intake is inadequate, serum calcium homeostasis is facilitated by resorption of bone. Bone sites where resorption occurred are repaired later as the site siphons off minerals passing by from the blood (Figure 8.1).[3,6]

NUTRITIONAL INFLUENCES

It is apparent that good bone health is necessary for preventing bone fractures. Nutritional status influences bone health just as it affects overall health. The primary impact of inadequate nutrition is on bone that is remodeled. Bone strength is influenced by the bone amassed during the period of bone building up through young adulthood. Adequate nutrition intake is necessary for creating the bone matrix as well as for normal bone cellular process. Dietary components such as calcium, phosphorous, magnesium, vitamin D, vitamin K, vitamin C, boron, copper, protein, and sodium have been shown to play a vital role in maintaining bone density. Nutritional influences generally affect only currently formed bone and therefore do not generally impact on current bone strength but on future bone health.[7]

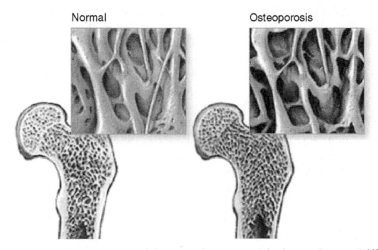

Normal   Osteoporosis

FIGURE 8.1 Difference between normal bone and osteoporotic bone. (From Difference Between Normal Bone and Osteoporosis, All Refer.com Health web site, http://health.allref.com/pictures-images.osteoporsis.html. Accessed June 10, 2005.)

Body weight is also associated with bone mass; the greater the body weight, the greater the bone mass. Low body weights are associated with lower bone mass. Weight loss through dieting also promoted bone loss. An increased body weight facilitates greater bone density as weight places a greater load on the various skeletal sites.

CALCIUM

Adequate calcium intake is essential for bone health, and is especially important during periods of growth as the skeleton develops. Peak bone mass is achieved around the age of 30 years, subsequently bone maintenance and prevention of bone loss become the foci for attaining healthy bone tissue. Without adequate calcium intake, bone growth and mainten-ance are not possible, as 99% of the amount of absorbed calcium is stored in the bones and teeth.[5] Calcium intakes within the recommended range of intakes are associated with im-proved bone density during the growing years, reduced bone loss in older adults, and reduced bone fracture risk.[7] Fifteen randomized, controlled trials have found that when the diet is supplemented with calcium, greater bone mass gains are seen in children and adolescents.[7] Twenty major calcium trials have found significantly less bone loss in postmenopausal women when adequate calcium is present in the diet.[8] Therefore, research has demonstrated that adequate calcium intake helps ensure healthy bones throughout the life cycle.

The recommended adequate intake for calcium is 1000 mg/day for adults 19 to 51 years of age and 1200 mg/day for adults over 51 years of age. Postmenopausal women over 65 years of age, not taking estrogen should also consume 1500 mg/day.[9] Some of the best calcium sources include milk, yogurt, sardines, kale, mustard greens, broccoli, tofu (processed with a calcium salt), and calcium-fortified foods, such as instant oatmeal and calcium-fortified orange juice.

VITAMIN D

Vitamin D is essential for intestinal calcium absorption and utilization. Sunlight exposure of about 15 min on the hands, arms, and face weekly is usually adequate for the body to produce enough vitamin D. The dietary reference intake (DRI) recommended is 400 IU/day for ages 18 to 70 years and 600 IU/day for individuals over 70 years of age. Deficiency of vitamin D is seen in the elderly and in people who do not get adequate sunlight exposure. Supplementation with vitamin D and calcium has been found to significantly improve BMD and reduce the rate of hip fractures.[10,11] This might be due, in part, to a drop in the body's ability to convert vitamin D into its active form as people age. Therefore, supplementation can be beneficial for reduction of fracture risk in individuals who do not consume adequate dietary vitamin D or when exposure to sunlight is limited.[10] Good food sources of vitamin D include cold-water fish, cod-liver oil, egg yolks, and fortified milk (including soy, rice, and almond milks).

MAGNESIUM

Approximately 60% of the body's magnesium levels are found in the bones, with the rest distributed to the muscles and other soft tissues, plasma, and extracellular fluids.[5] Magnesium can affect bone health through its effects on PTH secretion, which helps maintain calcium balance.[12] It can mimic calcium by binding to the same receptors as calcium to induce the proper physiologic responses.[12] Research supports that magnesium intake is associated with higher bone density.[13,14] But evidence is not clear whether or not magnesium *directly* influ-ences BMD.[15] Good food sources of magnesium include nuts, seeds, legumes, whole grains, and dark green vegetables. Refined grains are poor sources of magnesium since this mineral is lost during the processing and is not added as part of the enrichment of food products, such as breads and cereals.[5] The recommended dietary intakes for magnesium are 310 mg/day for women, 420 mg/day for men of age 19 to 70 years, 350–400 mg/day for pregnant women, and 310–360 mg/day for lactating women.[5] Magnesium may be depleted from body stores in diabetics, individuals under chronic high stress levels, and individuals who are on calorie-restricted diets. People with gluten-sensitive enteropathy or other malabsorption syndromes often have magnesium deficiencies, and develop osteoporosis.[16]

PHOSPHORUS

Phosphorus, in the form of phosphate, is part of the bone structure and essential for proper bone mineralization. Next to calcium, it is the second most abundant mineral in the body. The richest food sources include eggs, fish, poultry, meat, dairy, legumes, cereal grains, and vegetables. It is widely available in the diet, and the normal diet usually supplies more than enough to meet daily needs. Many commercial products contain phosphorus additives such as breads and sodas. Eighty percent of the phosphorus in the body is found in the skeleton.[5] Some research in animal models has shown that high phosphorus intakes can lead to bone loss, and when coupled with low calcium intakes, may alter calcium-regulating hormones, such as PTH and possibly vitamin D synthesis as well.[12,17] Average phosphorus intake by U.S. adults is around 1300 mg/day for men and 1000 mg/day for women.[5] The recommended daily intake (RDI) for phosphorus is 1000 mg/day.

VITAMIN K

Vitamin K, though best known for its effects on blood clotting, is also a vital component in the calcium-binding process, which facilitates the binding of calcium ions to specific proteins to increase BMD.[18] Dietary sources of vitamin K are green vegetables such as spinach, broccoli, cabbage, and green beans. Frozen vegetables are not good sources of vitamin K as the freezing can render this vitamin inactive.

ZINC

Zinc aids in the deposition of calcium into the bones and teeth, which help to build strong bones. It acts as a cofactor in several enzymes that are necessary for bone mineralization and development of collagenous bone structure.[18] Zinc is found in red meat, poultry, fish, eggs, legumes, whole grains, and milk.[19] Zinc picolinate is one of the forms that is best absorbed.[20]

VITAMIN C

Vitamin C is an essential cofactor for hydroxylation of proline and hydroxyproline residues in the developing of collagen, which is most important for the development of bone matrix. The RDI is 75 mg/day for females and 90 mg/day for males. Smokers are recommended to consume an additional 35 mg/day of vitamin C to these levels. Some food sources for vitamin C include green peppers, broccoli, strawberries, oranges, and leafy greens. Supplemental vitamin C is best absorbed in smaller dosages (500 mg or less at one time) and the presence of bioflavonoids may help increase the absorption and utilization of vitamin C.

COPPER

Copper is essential for normal bone metabolism and may be effective in preventing bone loss. Research has demonstrated that BMD was greater in postmenopausal women who had dietary calcium and serum copper levels above the median.[21] Copper is needed for collagen cross-linking (as a cofactor for lysyl oxidase), therefore affecting bone strength. It may even affect certain enzymes involved in bone structuring. Further research is needed to determine the role copper plays in bone health.

IRON

It is believed that iron plays a key role in bone health. Iron works as a cofactor for enzymes involved in collagen synthesis and is important in bone formation.[17] It may be prudent to avoid consuming iron- and calcium-rich foods in the same meal due to the inhibitory effort of calcium on iron absorption. Rich food sources of iron include red meat, poultry, spinach, legumes, and whole, unprocessed, or fortified grains. The DRI is 18 mg/day for menstruating women and 8 mg/day for men.

FIBER

The impact of fiber intake on calcium absorption is variable, and at best, very limited. Fiber found in green leafy vegetables and foods with nondigestible oligosaccharides, reportedly increase calcium absorption.[22] Conversely, the fiber in wheat bran decreases the absorption of coingested calcium when measured by single-meal tests.[22] However, except in cases of high-fiber consumption, the impact of this reduction in absorption is nonsignificant. Even when consumed at levels of 40–50 g/day, as seen in many vegans, dietary fiber still has only a modest inhibitory effect on calcium absorption.[5]

CAFFEINE

Caffeine has been shown to increase urinary excretion of calcium, however, studies have yielded conflicting results. Decreased BMD and an increased risk for hip fractures have been associated with caffeine consumption while other studies have found no overall association between BMD, fracture rate, or calcium metabolism, and caffeine intake.[23,24] Caffeine intakes of >300 mg/day have been recently associated with a higher rate of bone loss in postmenopausal elderly (aged 66 to 77 years) women in the hip region, proximal femur, and significantly in the spine.[24] This association continued after adjustment for smoking status, calcium and alcohol intake, medication usage, and age. The researchers also concluded that genotype influenced rate of bone loss as related to caffeine intake. Subjects with the *tt* genetic variant of vitamin D receptor gene (VDR) experienced bone losses twice the rate of women in *TT* genotype group with a high caffeine intake, although this difference was only significant for bone loss in the spinal region.

SODIUM

Sodium-induced calciuria has been well documented and supports a role for the physiological basis for the association between sodium intake and bone loss.[7] However, earlier studies used acute salt loading while the results of subsequent investigations utilizing bone markers for assessment were less conclusive.[7] Evidence also exists that large variations in an individual's salt intake may impact on bone balance, especially in individuals with a reduced capacity to compensate for sodium-induced calcium losses. Therefore, individuals should be counseled to follow the dietary guidelines that recommend avoidance of excessive sodium intake.

PROTEIN

Most epidemiological studies have found a positive association between BMD and protein intake.[17] However, high-protein intakes (2.1 g protein/kg) have been associated with an increase in bone resorption through alterations in calcium metabolism. There is growing evidence that less intakes than the RDA of protein (0.8 g protein/kg) may have a negative effect on bone density by reducing intestinal calcium absorption and lead to secondary hyperparathyroidism. A moderate protein intake (0.9 to 1.0 g protein/kg) may be best for individuals who are concerned about their bone health.[17] This suggests that there may be a narrow window of optimal protein intake to support good bone health.

ALCOHOL AND SMOKING

Excessive alcohol intake and cigarette smoking increase the risk for bone loss and developing osteoporosis, although modest amounts of alcohol have been associated with less lumbar spine bone loss. The mechanism is likely due to toxic effects on osteoblast activity. While occasional alcohol consumption (less than two drinks per day) has not been associated with low bone density, alcohol intake in excess of two drinks per day could cause problems. Excess alcohol consumption occurring over time can lead to greater bone loss. Calcium is resorbed from the skeleton in an attempt to buffer the acidic state alcohol creates in the body.[26] Smoking also appears to negatively affect bone remodeling, favoring bone turnover.[5] In a study in twins, bone densities in those twins who smoked were found to be 0.9 to 2.0% lower for every 10 pack-years of smoking.[27] The authors concluded that women who smoke one pack of cigarettes per day can expect approximately 5 to 10% lower bone densities. Other studies have found that the more a woman smokes, the greater the risk for bone fracture.[27,28] It is likely that alcohol and tobacco affect men in a similar way.

NONNUTRITIONAL INFLUENCES

Nonnutritional factors that influence bone health include genetics, weight-bearing physical activity, physical activity that places torsional strain on bones, hormonal status, ethnicity, smoking history, use of some medications, acid–base balance in the body, and general overall health. Genetics is thought to play a primary role in bone growth and mineralization in that genetic studies show that 60 to 70% of the variability in bone mineral mass can be accounted for by genetic variation.[5] Premenopausal women were found to have lower bone mass when their mothers had osteoporosis.[29] Ethnicity is also associated with peak bone mass. African American and Hispanic populations accrue greater bone mass than Caucasians or Asians.[5]

MEDICATIONS

A number of medications contribute to the development of low bone mass, increasing the risks for developing osteoporosis, by interfering with bone remodeling or by decreasing calcium absorption (Table 8.1).

EXERCISE

Several studies have revealed that resistance exercise, such as weight lifting, or load bearing physical activity such as jogging or running has a significant osteogenic impact on the skeleton throughout the life cycle. Independent of body size, physical activity has been associated with increased bone strength.[30] This may be an important protective factor for older individuals in decreasing the risk of falling since reportedly 90% of hip fractures are diagnosed in older people after falling on their hip.[31] A well-balanced strength training program may be the most sensible approach to improving BMD.[8] Cummings et al.[32] found that specific weight-lifting exercises correlated with gains in BMD and the quantity of weight lifted by accelerating BMD.

TABLE 8.1
Medications Associated with Increased Risk for Osteoporosis

Anticonvulsants
Cytotoxic drugs
Glucocorticosteroid
Adrenocorticotropic
Gonadotropin-releasing hormone agonists
Heparin
Lithium
Tamoxifen (premenopausal use)

Source: From Heaney, R.P., Bone biology in health and disease, in Shills, M.E., Olson, J.A., and Russ, A.C., Eds., *Modern Nutrition in Health Disease*, Lippincott, Williams & Wilkins, Philadelphia, PA, 1999, pp. 1327–1338.

SEX HORMONES

Given that the incidence of osteoporosis significantly affects postmenopausal women, there appears to be a strong link with estrogen levels. Clinical states associated with declining or low levels of estrogen, such as surgical or natural menopause, or hypogonadotropic states, have been associated with loss of bone density.[33] Recent observational studies report that postmenopausal estrogen replacement therapy (ERT) decreases spinal and nonspinal fracture rates in individuals currently using or have taken estrogen within 5 years of the onset of menopause.[34,35] Progestins, commonly used as adjunct therapy to estrogen (together commonly known as hormone replacement therapy (HRT)) for preventing uterine cancer, have been shown to neither affect nor enhance estrogen's beneficial impact on bone density.[36] Lower-than-conventional doses of estrogen therapy have been shown to improve bone density while also suppressing bone turnover.[2] However, the impact of lower doses on fracture rates is currently unknown. Recently, concerns have arisen regarding the long-term use of HRT because the risk for breast cancer increases after using HRT for over 5 years.[37] Since other medications are available for both prevention and treatment of osteoporosis, the benefits and risks should be carefully weighted by individuals considering HRT.

OSTEOPOROSIS

Osteoporosis, or porous bone, is a disease that has been defined as a systemic skeletal disease, characterized by low bone mass and microarchitectural deterioration of bone tissue, with a consequent increase in bone fragility and susceptibility to fracture.[1] Osteopenia occurs when the BMD becomes so low that the skeleton is unable to sustain ordinary strains.[5] Osteoporosis is considered a silent disease, because there are no symptoms and frequently is not typically diagnosed unless a fracture occurs or collapsed vertebrae result in severe back pain, loss of height, or spinal deformities such as kyphosis.[38] Osteoporosis is a major public health problem worldwide that occurs late in life but that can be prevented with adequate nutrient intake, physical activity, and healthy lifestyle choices throughout the life cycle. Postmenopausal Caucasian and Asian females who are thin, petite, and have a family history are at greatest risk of developing osteoporosis than African American or Hispanic individuals.[1] Age, falls, and previous fractures are additional risk factors independent of bone density. See Table 8.1 and Table 8.2 for the risk factors associated with the development of low bone density.

TABLE 8.2
Risk Factors for Osteoporosis

Nonmodifiable	Modifiable
Age	**Diet**
Gender	Low body mass index
Age at menopause	Eating disorders
Petite frame size	Excessive alcohol intake
Family history	Sedentary lifestyle or bedridden
Ethnicity	History of bone fractures
	Age at menopause
	Current or previous smoking
	Absence of normal menstrual cycles
	Low testosterone in men
	Medications (see Table 8.1)
Medical conditions that are associated with an increased risk	
Adrenal atrophy and Addison's disease	Oophorectomy before the age of 45 years
Chronic obstructive pulmonary disease	
Gastrectomy	
Hemochromatosis	
Hyperparathyroidism	
Insulin-dependent diabetes	
Lymphoma, leukemia, multiple myeloma	
Malabsorptive syndromes	
Nutritional disorders	
Osteogenesis imperfecta	
Rheumatoid arthritis	
Sarcoidosis	
Severe liver disease	

PREVALENCE

While osteoporosis is a preventable disease, the health burden associated with this disease is enormous. Osteoporosis afflicts an estimated 44 million Americans, of which 80% are females, although the prevalence of osteoporosis is increasing in men. By 2020, the National Osteoporosis Foundation (NOF) estimates that this number will increase to 61 million.[38] One out of every two women and one in eight men over 50 years will have an osteoporosis-related fracture in their lifetime.[38]

Osteoporosis contributes to 1.5 million fractures annually with 300,000 hip fractures, 700,000 vertebral fractures, 250,000 wrist fractures, and 300,000 fractures at other sites.[38] The estimated direct costs of osteoporotic and associated fractures was about $17 billion in 2001 with costs predicted to continue to rise as aging population grows.[38] Osteoporosis is also associated with a high mortality as one in five patients with an osteoporotic fracture dies within 1 year of sustaining the fracture.[39] Prevalence and fracture risk varies by gender and ethnicity. Although both men and women experience bone loss with aging, Caucasian post-menopausal women experience almost 75% of all hip fractures and have the highest age-adjusted fracture incidence.[40] Additionally, several groups of children and adolescents are at greater risk for osteoporosis than the general population. Glucocorticoids are commonly used to treat a variety of common childhood inflammatory diseases. With the chronic use of high-dose steroids (daily dose of 7.5 mg prednisolone or greater) for many of these conditions, the impact on bone health must be considered.[41] The long-term effects of intermittent courses of systemic steroids or chronic use of inhaled steroids on bone health currently is not known.

Although the benefits of weight-bearing physical activity on bone density are well established in all populations, a growing concern is the increasing number of stress fractures seen in extremely active women. Women of all ages (often professional, collegiate, or elite athletes) who exercise excessively appear to be very susceptible to what is referred to as the "female athlete triad," a coexistence of three separate medical conditions: disordered eating, amenorrhea, and osteoporosis.[42] These conditions are related to one another, in that amenorrhea has been associated with low body weight (specifically low body fat), stress, excessive physical training, undernutrition, and disordered eating behavior. Most researchers consider the combination of excessive activity and inadequate intake to be the primary cause of amenorrhea, where a chronic energy deficit affects hormonal status, reducing levels of lutenizing hormone, and effectively preventing ovulation.[42] The short- and long-term effects of the triad include infertility, irreversible bone loss, and osteoporosis.

SCREENING AND DIAGNOSIS

Osteoporosis or low bone mass can be detected through a number of technological modalities. Dual energy x-ray absorptiometry (DEXA) is considered the gold standard since it is the most widely validated test for measuring BMD.[43] BMD is highly correlated with or related to fracture risk. DEXA measurements of BMD should be made using the same type of instrument because there are systematic differences in measurements among systems. The DEXA BMD measurements are very precise and reliable within a system. DEXA is a noninvasive measure that takes about 5 min to complete and is associated with a very low radiation exposure. When DEXA machines from different manufacturers have been compared, the variance in diagnosing osteoporosis was 6 to 15%.[43]

A variety of other technologies are also available for measuring bone density (see Table 8.3 for a summary). Several machines measure bone density in the hip, spine, and total body whereas peripheral machines measure density in the finger, wrist, kneecap, shinbone, and heel. Several

---

TABLE 8.3
Types of Tests for Determining Bone Mass Density

Dual energy x-ray absorptiometry (DEXA)
DEXA can be used to measure the bone density of the spine, hip, and total body
DEXA scans can be completed within a few minutes with very low-radiation exposure
Peripheral dual energy x-ray absorptiometry (pDEXA)
Measures the bone density of the wrist, heel, or finger
Single energy x-ray absorptiometry (SXA)
Measures the bone density of the wrist or heel
Quantitative ultrasound (QUS)
Measures bone density with sound waves at the heel, shinbone, and kneecap
Quantitative computed tomography (QCT)
Most commonly used to measure bone density in the spine but can measure density at other sites
Peripheral quantitative computed tomography (pQCT)
Measures bone density in the wrist
Radiographic absorptiometry (RA)
Bone density is calculated from an x-ray of the hand and a small metal wedge

Source: From National Osteoporosis Foundation, *Physicians Guide to Prevention and Treatment of Osteoporosis*, Exerpta Medica Inc., Belle Meade, NJ, 1999; Heaney, R.P., Bone biology in health and disease, in Shills, M.E., Olson, J.A., and Russ, A.C., Eds., *Modern Nutrition in Health Disease*, Lippincott, Williams & Wilkins, Philadelphia, PA, 1999, pp. 1327–1338.

TABLE 8.4
Defining Osteoporosis by Bone Mineral Density

The World Health Organization has established the following definitions based on bone density measurement at any skeletal site in Caucasian women as:

Normal: BMD is within 1 SD of a "young normal" adult (*T*-score above −1)

Low bone mass (osteopenia): BMD is between 1 and 2.5 SD below that of a "young normal" adult (*T*-score between −1 and −2.5)

Osteoporosis: BMD is 2.5 SD or more below that of a "young normal" adult (*T*-score at or below −2.5). Women in this group who have already experienced one or more fractures are deemed to have severe or "established" osteoporosis

The National Osteoporosis Foundation suggests that while these definitions are necessary to establish the prevalence of osteoporosis, they should not be used as the sole determinant of treatment decisions.

Source: From NIH, Osteoporosis Prevention, Diagnosis and Treatment Consensus Statement, March 27–29, 17(1), 2000, pp.1–36

---

studies show that the diagnosis of osteoporosis depends on the choice of test and the number of sites tested.[43] Testing in the forearm, hip, spine, or heel generally identifies different groups of patients. Although test results at any site are associated to some degree with risk for fractures at other sites, it may be difficult to use a low *T*-score (see Table 8.4 for definition) from the forearm to determine if an appreciable amount of bone has been lost at other sites as well.

The U.S. Preventive Services Task Force states that bone density measured by DEXA at the femoral neck is the best predictor of hip fracture and is comparable to forearm measurements for predicting fractures at other sites.[43] Heel ultrasonography and other peripheral bone density tests, however, can also predict short-term fracture risk.

The World Health Organization (WHO) defines osteoporosis based on the DEXA scan results of the hip and spine. Bone density is reported as a *T*-score, which is a marker for the number of standard deviations from the mean bone density in sex- and race-matched young normal adults.[2] Table 8.4 provides recommendations for interpreting *T*-scores. The NOF recommends initiating treatment to reduce fracture risk in postmenopausal women with *T*-scores below −2 with no other risk factors and with *T*-scores below −1.5 when other risk factors are present.

The NOF recommends screening for osteoporosis for all women over the age of 65 years and for women of age 50 to 65 years who have one or more risk factors (see Table 8.2).[38] Although national screening guidelines do not advocate routine screening for osteoporosis in premenopausal women, osteoporosis can exist. Therefore, screening females with several risk factors and a strong family history of compromised bone mass should be considered. Secondary causes that increase risk such as medication use should also be assessed. In conjunction with BMD test results, biochemical testing for assessment of serum thyrotropin, protein electrophoresis, PTH, vitamin D, urine calcium, or cortisol may be required to determine the optimal therapeutic intervention.

PREVENTION

As the population ages, and longevity increases, the prevention of osteoporosis is critical in not only reducing the health burden but also in maintaining quality of life. Optimizing bone density before the age of 30 years can be one of the most important defenses in preventing loss of bone mass. Minimizing bone loss in later years is also crucial. Women in general have lower bone densities than men; thereby placing them at greater risk for developing low bone density. Osteoporosis also afflicts African American and Hispanic populations less since the individuals of these ethnicities tend to have greater bone density compared with individuals of Caucasian and Asian descent.

During puberty, bone increases in density during the growth spurt and then slows until peak bone mass is obtained, sometime between 20 and 30 years of age.[44] Approximately 50% of maximal peak bone mass is obtained during puberty in healthy individuals who consume adequate amounts of calcium (1300 mg/day) and vitamin D (400 IU/day).[39] Participation in weight-bearing or resistance activities, producing normal amounts of the sex hormones, androgen and estrogen and growth hormone, limiting caffeine intake and excess alcohol consumption, and not smoking are additional factors that contribute to achieving optimal bone density. The magnitude of which an individual achieves peak bone density determines the risk for future development of osteopenia and osteoporosis.

For women, within the first 1 to 5 years after menopause, bone loss increases by two to six times greater than premenopausal levels with a gradual return to about 1% loss annually around the 10th year of menopause.[3] Until recently, osteoporosis was not commonly associated with men. However, recent studies indicated that declines in bone density in men over the age of 50 years are similar in magnitude to decreases seen in women after 10 years of menopause.[3]

Americans should be educated on fall prevention. Following the guidelines for screening as established by several national health organizations such as the NOF and the U.S. Preventive Services Task Force for diagnosis or identification of individuals at high risk, several studies have shown that it is never too late to prevent or decrease the risk for bone loss.

The previous recommendations for achieving optimal bone health through consumption of a healthy diet also decrease the risk for osteoporosis. Medical nutrition therapy for reducing the risks for osteoporosis based on the results of clinical studies includes consumption of adequate amounts of all essential nutrients, especially calcium during childhood and preferably before the onset of puberty and other nutrients that have roles in building and maintaining healthy bones as previously discussed. Avoidance of unhealthy lifestyle habits such as smoking and consumption of excessive alcohol, sodium and for some, caffeine are also recommended interventions. Regular participation in weight-bearing physical activity also promotes obtaining optimal bone density.

EXERCISE

Regular weight-bearing and resistance exercise has been shown to decrease the risk for hip fractures in both lean and heavy middle aged and older women. Results from the Nurses Health study show that for every hour of walking or equivalent activity, the risk for hip fracture is decreased by 6% for women aged 40 to 77 years.[45] There is also evidence of a positive linear relationship between BMD change and total and exercise-specific weight lifted in postmenopausal women, where a progressive strength training program not only prevented loss, but accelerated regional bone density gain in this population.[32] From these data, it appears a well-balanced strength training program in addition to regular aerobic exercise (including walking) provides a cost-effective approach to the prevention of osteoporosis, with beneficial side effects of improved strength and balance.

PHARMACOLOGIC MANAGEMENT

A number of commonly prescribed medications are used in the pharmacologic management of osteoporosis, which include bisphosphates, selective estrogen receptor modulators (SERMs), and hormones. Table 8.5 and Textbox 8.1 discuss the various pharmacologic interventions available and when intervention may be warranted. Pharmacologic intervention reportedly can stabilize or increase bone density in most patients as well as reduce fracture risk by approximately 50%.

TABLE 8.5
Drug Options for Postmenopausal Women with Osteoporosis

Drug Name	What It Does	Side Effects
Calcitonin	Increases bone density and decreases pain	Nausea and flushing
Alendronate	Increases bone density	Stomach pain and nausea
Estrogens (controversial)	Treatment for estrogen-deficiency osteoporosis (bone softening from calcium loss) restores estrogen levels in tissues	Stomach cramps, appetite loss and nausea

In addition to taking the drug, weight-bearing exercise and adequate dietary intake of calcium and vitamin D are essential in preventing bone loss.

Source: From Griffigh, H.W. and Moore, S.W., *Complete Guide to Prescription and Nonprescription Drugs*, Berkley Publishing Group, New York, NY, 2001.

Textbox 8.1   Bone Health — When the Diet Is Not Enough

Medications may be prescribed to promote optimal bone health when the *T*-score is indicative of low bone density. The Food and Drug Administration has approved the following medications for the prevention or treatment of osteoporosis:

Bisphosphates

Bisphosphates (alendronate, risedronate sodium), which act on the osteoclasts to decrease absorptive activity, have been shown to decrease the risk for fractures by 50% in individuals with low bone mass and patients with previous fractures.[93] Bone density has been found to continue accruing into treatment of 6 to 7 years and bone density is maintained for at least 2 years after cessation of medication.[94] However, bisphosphates have not been known to be of any benefit for individuals without risk factors for low bone mass (Sayegh). Dysphagia, esophageal erosions or ulcers, abdominal pain, and constipation or diarrhea are reported side effects. The results of the Fracture Intervention Trial (FIT) using alendronate suggest that women with several risk factors for fracture, such as age, very low bone density, or previous vertebral fractures, derived the greatest benefit from use of alendronate. However, there was no reduction in risk for fractures seen in study participants with *T*-scores between −1.6 and −2.5 (FIT). Risedronate reduced hip fractures by 40% in women 70 to 79 years of age with severe osteoporosis.

Selective Estrogen Receptor Modulators

Raloxifene is a SERM that acts as an estrogen on bone tissue by slowing bone turnover to rates similar to premenopausal women and has been shown to increase bone density in the spine and hip by 2 to 3%. Raloxifene has antiestrogen properties when acting on other tissues such as found in the breast. Thus raloxifene may decrease the risk for breast cancer while promoting optimal bone density.

Calcitonin

The hormone, calcitonin taken as a nasal spray or by injection, is used to prevent osteoclastic bone resorption by blocking the stimulatory effects of PTH. While calcitonin has been found to be beneficial in preserving bone mass in treating osteoporosis, recent studies indicate the benefit may be very small and calcitonin has not been approved for use in preventing osteoporosis.

SUMMARY

As discussed, skeletal health and obtaining optimal bone density is influenced by a multitude of factors. The current understanding of what the precise mechanisms regarding the bone mineral accrual process and what specific factors influence these mechanisms is far from complete. Further studies are needed to better elucidate the specific genes associated with the regulation of bone mass acquisition and how to best identify individuals at risk. Based on the evidence available thus far, however, it is clear that individuals at risk for developing low bone density should adopt a healthy lifestyle including adequate calcium intake, avoidance of excessive alcohol, and smoking as well as participate in regular weight-bearing physical activity to reduce the risks. To obtain optimal bone density, these interventions should be practiced in childhood and preferably before the onset of puberty.[8] Additionally, regular assessment of bone density is recommended to identify individuals who may benefit from pharmacologic intervention.

JOINT HEALTH

There are many important factors involved in preserving or maintaining good joint health. Some of these factors include, but are not limited to (a) using proper biomechanics during physical activity and activities of daily living, (b) allowing adequate rest and recovery following strenuous activities or after an injury has occurred, and (c) eating properly to ensure optimal nutrient needs are met. These various aspects of good health should not be overlooked when discussing joint health. The best strategy to use when trying to optimize joint health is to take measures that prevent injury or illness from occurring in the first place. However, mainstream medical approaches are often focused on treating problems after they arise, rather than on prevention. For most of the conditions discussed in this chapter, the mainstream medical treatments include use of nonsteroidal anti-inflammatory drugs (NSAIDs), use of orthopedic devices, or surgery. Nutrition unfortunately is usually disregarded and is, therefore, not often considered a valuable adjunct to these therapies. However, proper nutrition does play a very prominent role in protecting joints from injury and preventing illness, as well as help to relieve the pain and inflammation (a common symptom to each of the conditions discussed herein) of joint injury or disease. Specific nutrition recommendations are discussed later in this chapter.

Risk factors for joint problems can include genetic susceptibility to degenerative joints or joint injuries, increasing age, and poor biomechanics during exercise or activities of daily living.

While many of the following joint health issues have not been directly associated with any specific nutrient requirement or inadequacy, it stands to reason that in order to achieve optimal joint health, maximizing good nutrition principles is a necessity. Most joint conditions discussed herein have not been directly linked with specific nutritional interventions, yet they all share common characteristics of inflammation, pain, and free radical production. Nutrition will be discussed at length for a select few joint conditions where greater research is available to support its impact. Otherwise, refer to recommendations for "The Anti-Inflammatory Diet" as discussed later in the chapter.

- Tennis elbow or lateral epicondylitis
- Shoulder impingement or subacromial bursitis
- General muscle sprain or strain

It should be noted that many of the unconventional nutritional recommendations for the following conditions have not been well researched. While well-controlled studies are important, it is not to discredit the use of nutritional strategies that support optimal health, despite the lack of studies that may link directly with one or more of these joint issues. It is also important to note that poor health habits and malnutrition not only compromise health status in general, but also increase the likelihood of injury and other joint troubles, as malnutrition is often associated with increased rates of disease, fatigue, and altered immune system function.

OVERVIEW OF JOINTS

NORMAL JOINT ANATOMY

A joint is made up of two bones, which are held together by ligaments. Joints include a joint capsule that holds the lubricating synovial fluid. The synovium is the inner lining of the capsule that secretes this fluid that lubricates and nourishes the chondrocytes in the cartilage.[46] This cartilage is called articular cartilage and covers the ends of bones acting as a cushion. Articular cartilage resembles hyaline cartilage elsewhere in the body, but has no perichondrium, which is a dense, irregular connective tissue membrane surrounding most cartilages. The matrix, the foundation of cartilage, also contains more water than other types of cartilage. The surface of articular cartilage is slick and smooth under normal conditions.[46] Proper synovial function can continue only if the articular cartilage retains its normal structure. If an articular cartilage is damaged, the matrix may begin to break down, and the exposed surface will change from a slick, smooth, gliding surface to a rough feltwork of bristly collagen fibers.[46] Tendons attach the muscles to the joint, which facilitates stabilization of the joint, and by contracting, provide motion to the joint. Many joints have small fluid-filled pockets that provide additional cushion while protection from friction called bursae.

TYPES OF JOINTS

There are three major classifications of joints based on the range of motion permitted. These functional categories are then subdivided on the basis of anatomical structure or the range of motion permitted.[46] This chapter will be discussing the major category of synovial joints (diarthrosis) and its subdivisions. These subdivisions include:

- Gliding joints: carpals and articular facets of the spinal vertebrae
- Hinge joints: elbow, knee, and interphalangeal joints
- Pivot joints: atlas or axis vertebrae, radial head, and ulna
- Ellipsoidal joints: phalanges of metatarsals and metacarpals
- Saddle joints: carpal metacarpal joints at base of thumb
- Ball and socket: shoulder and hip

BIOMECHANICS OF A NORMAL JOINT

The biomechanics of a normal joint have gross movement, flexion, and extension along with more subtle movements. These subtle movements include the two components, rock and slide. One bone of the moving joint rolls along the opposite articular surface, like a car tire rolling down a street, at the same time it slides across the same articular surface, like the same tire sliding along on ice. These motions that are used simultaneously reduce the stress on the articular cartilage.[47] Articular cartilage is avascular and aneural, which puts this tissue at a disadvantage nutritionally. It receives its nutrients by diffusion inhibition of synovial fluid. Movements of these joints, along with weight-bearing force, distribute the synovial fluid along the cartilage.[46] The synovial fluid circulates whenever the joint moves and the compression and reexpansion of the articular cartilage pumps synovial fluid into and out of the cartilage matrix.[46]

ABNORMAL JOINTS

An immobilized joint or a joint with abnormal function disrupts the scheme previously described. This could lead to malnutrition, or lack of blood-supplying nutrients to the articular cartilage, leading to cartilage damage and joint disease. Inflammation is the body's natural response to tissue damage or to overuse of a diseased joint. It is important to respect these symptoms (swelling, warmth, redness, pain, and loss of function) as they are the body's way of protecting itself from *further* use and injury until it has had time to heal. Caution must be practiced when masking these signals with prescription or over-the-counter pain relief medications. Some medications work to reduce inflammation as well as pain, so they hold an important place as catalysts in the recovery process. But use of analgesics to simply mask symptoms may lead to further disease and dysfunction down the road if not used properly.

ARTHRITIDES

OSTEOARTHRITIS OR DEGENERATIVE JOINT DISEASE

Osteoarthritis (OA) is the second leading cause of disability in the United States.[49] Diarthrodial or synovial joints are the joints affected, most commonly the hip and the knee. These joints are prone to degeneration of the articular cartilage, resulting in the formation of new bone at the joint margins. Pain and stiffness occur due to this new bone formation and the damage or degeneration of the cartilage. OA can have a primary or secondary cause. Primary causes are usually due to a genetic link while secondary causes are either due to direct injury or trauma, joint laxity, joint surgery, infection, or metabolic imbalances due to chronic use of medications.

The age of onset for primary OA is usually 45 years and over. Women are affected symptomatically more than men but both are at risk. Secondary OA is associated with a history of trauma and occurs before the age of 40 years. The signs and symptoms of both types are stiffness; usually in the morning, decreased range of motion, tenderness to palpation, pain with passive motion of joints, joint crepitus, and swelling. There is impairment of gait when hip or knee is involved.[49] OA is a slow progressive condition, which affects the weight-bearing joints including knees, hips, low back, and fingers. Approximately, 70 to 80% of the population over the age of 55 years struggle with OA.[49]

To confirm the diagnosis, x-rays are required. Radiographs reveal nonuniform loss of joint spaces. A patient with advanced OA will show bone spurs (osteophytes), subchondral cysts, and sclerosis of subchondral bone. A CT scan or MRI can be performed to determine the extent of damage.[46] Laboratory values are usually normal but may show a mildly elevated erythrocyte sedimentation rate (ESR) and C-reactive protein, a marker found in the blood that identifies nonspecific systemic inflammation.

Most healthcare practitioners recommend decreasing excess body weight, thereby reducing the absolute load placed on the affected joints, while also increasing physical activity, muscle strength, balance and coordination, and range of motion in the joint area. Low-impact exercises such as swimming and biking are ideal. To decrease pain, deep heat using ultrasound or topical creams may also be of short-term value.[49] Drug management includes prescribing acetaminophen up to 4000 mg for pain control. Commonly prescribed are NSAIDs, which should be used cautiously due to the side effects on the GI mucosa and kidneys with long-term use (see Table 8.6).

TABLE 8.6
Over-the-Counter and Prescription Drug Dangers

Drug	Treatment of Joint Conditions	Potential Side Effects	Drug-Induced Nutrient Depletion	Potential Depletion Problems
Salicylate — aspirin	All	Gastritis, heartburn, vomiting, nausea, fatigue, rash, muscle weakness, hemolytic anemia tinnitus, diminished hearing, duodenal ulcer and hemorrhage (especially in the elderly), dizziness, compromised renal function, hepatotoxicity. Avoid 1 week before surgery due to effects on diminished blood clotting, and possibility of postoperative bleeding	Vitamin C — consumption of foods high in vitamin C may reduce analgesic effect, causing increased urinary excretion of aspirin	Altered immune system, bruising, poor wound healing
NSAIDs — ibuprofen, naproxen, sulindac, celecoxib, indomethacin, diclofenac, diflunisal	All	GI irritation, GI bleeding, elevated liver enzymes, renal toxicity, headache, confusion, worsening of hypertension, edema, liver damage, reduced gastric blood flow, reduced cell repair and replication. Long-term use may contribute to progression of osteoarthritis	Folic acid	Macrocytic anemia, birth defects, cardiovascular disease, cervical dysplasia
			Iron	Anemia, weakness, fatigue, hair loss, brittle nails
			Potassium	Irregular heartbeat, muscle weakness, fatigue, edema
			Sodium	Hypernatremia, muscle weakness, dehydration, loss of appetite, poor concentration
Corticosteroids — cortisone, prednisone, hydrocortisone, sulfasalazine	OA, RA	Muscle weakness, osteoporosis, insomnia, nervousness, increased appetite, indigestion, hirsutism, diabetes mellitus, cataracts, glaucoma, arthralgia, dizziness, headache, vomiting, diarrhea	Folic acid	Macrocytic anemia, birth defects, cardiovascular disease, cervical dysplasia
			Iron	Anemia, weakness, fatigue, hair loss, brittle nails
			Calcium	Osteoporosis, heart and blood pressure irregularities, tooth decay, loss of lean body mass

Drug	Condition	Side Effects	Nutrient	Depletion Effects
			Vitamin D	Osteoporosis, muscle weakness, hearing loss
			Potassium	Irregular heartbeat, muscle weakness, fatigue, edema
			Vitamin C	Altered immune system, bruising, poor wound healing
			Folic acid	Macrocytic anemia, birth defects, cardiovascular disease, cervical dysplasia
			Zinc	Impaired wound healing, loss of sense of taste and smell, altered immune system
			Selenium	Altered immune system, reduced antioxidant protection
			Magnesium	Cardiovascular problems, asthma, osteoporosis, muscle cramps and twitching, Premenstrual syndrome
Hypouricemic — colchicine	Gout	Nausea, vomiting, and abdominal pain. Long-term use — hair loss, numbness and tingling in hands and feet	Vitamin B_{12}	Anemia, fatigue, weakness, increased cardiovascular disease risk
			Sodium	Muscle weakness, dehydration, appetite loss, poor concentration
			Potassium	Irregular heartbeat, muscle weakness, fatigue, edema
			Beta-carotene	Lower immunity, reduced antibiotic protection
Antirheumatic — azathioprine, chloroquine, leflunomide, meloxicam	RA, AS	Rapid heart rate, sudden fever, muscle or joint pain, cough, shortness of breath, appetite loss, nausea, vomiting, headache, indigestion, and heartburn. Long-term use — permanent damage to retina or nerve deafness	No known drug-induced nutrient depletions	
Cytotoxic — methotrexate	RA	Sore throat, fever, mouth sores, chills, abdominal pain, nausea, vomiting, bloody stools, or bloody vomit	Folic acid	Birth defects, cervical dysplasia, anemia, cardiovascular disease

Source: From Pelton, R. et al., *Drug-Induced Nutrient Depletion Handbook. 1999–2000,* American Pharmaceutical Association, Lexi-Comp, Inc. and Natural Health Resources, Inc., Cincinnati, OH, 1999.

Newer drugs used are cyclooxygenase-2 (COX-2) inhibitors, and COX-1 helps protect the stomach lining, thus preventing ulcers. Celebrex and Vioxx are types of these drugs. The disadvantage of using prescription drugs is that symptoms may be masked while the disease still progresses. Recent studies have revealed that these types of pain medications may increase one's risk for heart problems and should be used with caution and only under physician supervision. A topical cream capsaicin, the active ingredient in peppers, aids in pain relief. Topicals require consistent use, usually three to four times per day, to be effective. Corticosteroid injections may bring relief but repeated doses can delay the cartilage repair process. Hyaluronic acid is a naturally occurring substance found in synovial fluid and cartilage, which acts to lubricate the joint. Hyaluronic acid may be injected into the joint as hylaruronan.[49] In severe cases of OA, surgery such as a total knee or hip replacement may be an option.

Diet has been shown to influence OA symptom severity through the ingestion of anti-inflammatory foods, which help to reduce pain and stiffness (refer to the section on "The Anti-Inflammatory Diet"). A healthy diet that incorporates a wide variety of plant-based foods is important for achieving and maintaining a healthy weight, as well as providing the body with a necessary supply of essential vitamins, minerals, and antioxidants to keep the body functioning as optimally as possible.

More than $1 billion each year is spent by Americans on alternative treatments for arthritis, including therapies such as acupuncture, massage, and ingestion of dietary supplements such as glucosamine and chondroitin and omega-3 fatty acids.[50] Table 8.7 describes a list of supplements marketed toward the treatment of OA and its symptoms.

Weight reduction will help to reduce the amount of weight bearing down on the joints for individuals who are overweight, thereby helping to alleviate some of the pain. Extra weight puts extra pressure on already weakened joints, aggravating symptoms of the disease. Smaller, lighter bodies (relatively speaking) may also find it easier to move around, increasing the likelihood of incorporating and sticking with an exercise program versus becoming or remaining sedentary.

While it is a good idea to rest when plagued by the fatigue that often accompanies arthritis conditions, too much rest can lead to muscle and joint stiffness and increased pain. Participating in physical activities may also help to improve one's sense of well-being and may even help reduce inflammation in some joints.

Joint mobilization, performed by Doctors of Osteopath (D.O.) and Doctors of Chiropractic (D.C.), can increase range of motion (ROM) and potentially decrease the pain. In one study, acupuncture and therapeutic touch have been found to decrease pain when used along with conventional therapy.[46]

Recommendations for treatment of OA include range of motion exercises (stretching, dance, Pilates, yoga); strengthening exercise (strength training, yoga); aerobic or endurance exercise (walking, bike riding, swimming laps); assistive devices and supports including canes, braces, walkers; and nutritional and behavioral counseling.

RHEUMATOID ARTHRITIS

Rheumatoid arthritis (RA) is an inflammatory autoimmune disorder. It acts systemically, affecting many joints and connective tissues. It usually begins in the proximal interphalangeal (PIP) and metacarpophalangeal (MCP) joints of the hand. Other joints affected include the wrists, knees, ankle, and toes.

While both sexes can be affected, RA is two to three times more common in females.[51] Although it can strike at any age, it most commonly occurs between the ages of 25 and 50 years. When afflicted with the disease, the joints will appear swollen and feel warm and tender in the

TABLE 8.7
Supplement Review for Osteoarthritis

Supplement Name	What It Is	Use or Advantages	Disadvantages or Concerns	Rx Advice
S-adenosyl methionine (SAM-e)	SAM-e is made from methionine (an amino acid found in protein) and most well-nourished individuals seem to make enough	Shown to be superior to placebo and as effective as NSAIDs in reducing OA symptoms	*Side effects*: nausea, bloating, flatulence, diarrhea, headache	200 mg, three times per day may relieve symptoms of OA
			Trouble is primarily due to lack of supplement industry regulations to ensure quality and potency. Consumers for Science in the Public Interest reported (March 2001 Nutrition Action Newsletter) 3 out of 23 brands tested last year contained no SAM-e at all. And up to 50% of all supplements containing SAM-e contain less than their label states	
	Prevalent in every cell in the body; involved in the formation of DNA and neurotransmitters	Available in Europe by prescription for past 20 years without any major side effects noted. Available over-the-counter in the U.S. Studies up to 2 years duration demonstrate safety		400–1600 mg/day are used to treat depression
		SAM-e production can be increased naturally in the body through increased ingestion of folic acid via dark, leafy green vegetables or supplementation		

Continued

TABLE 8.7 (Continued)
Supplement Review for Osteoarthritis

Supplement Name	What It Is	Use or Advantages	Disadvantages or Concerns	Rx Advice
Methylsulfonylmethane (MSM)	Compound occurs naturally in plants and animals	Treats OA pain	*Side effects*: nausea, diarrhea, headaches	1000–3000 mg, three times per day
		Because it can contribute sulfur to the body, it can be used to make certain amino acids (building blocks of protein) and act as an antioxidant		
	Its biological role is unknown and its mechanism of action is not well understood		Limited research to back up claims	Optimal doses are unknown due to lack of well-designed and controlled clinical studies. The most commonly advised dosage is 2 g daily
			Consumer Lab Web site tested 17 different MSM supplements in February and March 2001. Two failed testing due to low levels of MSM, containing only 85 to 88% of label-stated claims. A listing of supplements that passed can be found on their Web site at www.consumerlab.com	
	An odorless, white, crystalline powder easily contaminated by DMSO, which has a faint sulfur odor (cooked egg smell) to it. If contaminated, may smell like garlic. If MSM is pure, it will not smell			

	Generally considered safe	Has not been evaluated for safety for pregnant or nursing women, children Has been shown to have an aspirin-like effect (thinning the blood) and should not be used by those on other blood-thinning medications unless under medical supervision	
Dimethyl sulfoxide (DMSO)	A chemical solvent	Used primarily for treatment of pain due to osteoarthritis	No longer approved as a supplement and can only be used under medical supervision Was found to be a cause for a wide array of adverse reactions
Glucosamine	A stimulant for proteoglycan synthesis (the starting materials from which cartilage is made that determine the strength and hardness of connective tissue). Prevents proteoglycan degradation	Believed to promote cartilage formation and repair and relieve OA symptoms. May even halt progression of the disease. (Setnikar, I., Antireactive properties of chondroprotective drugs, *Int. J. Tissue React.*, 14 (5), 253–261, 1992.) As effective in relieving OA pain and inflammation as NSAIDs improvements were more progressively consistent in significantly lowering the subjects' pain scores that were measured at the end of an 8-week study period comparing glucosamine sulfate to ibuprofen	*Side effects:* nausea, dyspepsia, headache 500 mg, three times per day for a minimum of 6 weeks

Continued

TABLE 8.7 (Continued)
Supplement Review for Osteoarthritis

Supplement Name	What It Is	Use or Advantages	Disadvantages or Concerns	Rx Advice
			Takes longer than NSAIDs to take effect. May take up to 12 weeks for full benefits to be achieved	Comes in many forms, (such as glucosamine hydrochloride (HCl), N-acetylglucosamine (NAG), glucosamine sulfate) none believed to be better than another. May also contain potassium chloride or sodium chloride salt
Chondroitin	With glucosamine as a requirement for formation of connective tissue substances referred to as proteoglycans, chondroitin is the primary proteoglycan found in cartilage	Believed to inhibit the enzymes that cause cartilage breakdown and promote cartilage elasticity Together with glucosamine, it helps to support healthy joint matrix formation and cartilage structure	Side effects: dyspepsia, nausea, headache Expensive to produce and many mixed products that contain both glucosamine and chondroitin fail to meet chondroitin levels stated on the labels	400 mg, three times per day for a minimum of 6 weeks. Sold as chondroitin sulfate

Source: From Healthy Roads, What is a Sprain/Strain Injury, www.healthyroads.com. Accessed October 2002; The Natural Pharmacist web site, http://www.naturalpharmacist.com. Accessed October 13, 2002; D'Ambrosio, É. et al., *Pharmatherapemutica*, 2, 504, 1981; Vaz, A.L., *Curr. Med. Res. Opin.*, 8, 145, 1982; Pujaste, J.M. et al., *Curr. Med. Res. Opin.*, 7, 110, 1980; Bradley, J.K. et al., *J. Rhenumatol.*, 21, 905, 1994.

morning, usually taking about an hour to achieve full ROM. In the beginning stages, the sites of pain are usually the fingers and wrists. There is often a complaint of fatigue and possible weight loss. A genetic marker has been identified that predisposes a person to the development of RA. This genetic risk factor is the presence of the class II human leukocyte antigen (HLA).[47]

The cause of RA is an autoimmune reaction that results in a synovial inflammatory process that results in a destructive pattern.[47]

Normally, there is a symmetrical involvement of the joints so both hands would be involved. Early changes noticed are soft-tissue swelling, juxta-articular demineralization, uniform loss of joint space, and joint erosions. Flexor contractors and ulnar deviation of the fingers and feet are usually later changes. Instability of the transverse ligament of the C2 vertebrae should be a concern when evaluating for RA. Laboratory findings include a positive rheumatoid factor (IgM antibody found in 75% of patients), and increased ESR, C-reactive protein, and sometimes an associated anemia (hypochromic and normocytic).[47] To confirm the diagnosis, radiographic studies are taken. In the early stages, findings are absent. The early changes seen on x-ray are juxta-articular demineralization and soft-tissue swelling. Advanced stages of x-ray show joint erosions and uniform loss of joint space.

When treating RA, the practitioner should remember that patients with active RA have periods of exacerbation that are usually unpredictable. During acute RA episodes, aspirin, NSAIDs, methotrexate, and corticosteroids are prescribed for pain relief. Corticosteroid treatment and other prescribed medications will improve the symptoms but they will not change the course of RA. Gold therapy for mild to moderate RA is available as oral and injectable forms (auranofin, oral; gold sodium thiomalate and aurothioglucose, injectable). Oral forms are less toxic, but less effective than injectable.[51]

While there is no definite answer as to which dietary strategies are the best to treat RA, some studies have found that diets free of food allergens and nightshade vegetables (peppers, potatoes, eggplant, and tomatoes) are helpful. Fasting for 7 to 10 days, followed by a gluten-free, vegetarian or vegan diet that positively changed fecal flora resulted in significant improvements in the disease course.[52–55]

Probiotics are believed to inhibit intestinal inflammation and have a positive effect on inflammatory disorders such as RA.[56] It is important to note that not everyone who followed this type of diet in these studies saw improvements. Additionally, adverse side effects (nausea, diarrhea) caused some study participants to cease following the diet prematurely. But those individuals who were diet responders saw significant beneficial results. Other studies have found a low-fat, vegan diet can result in similar improvements, as fatty acid intakes may not be as influential in disease course outcomes.[57] This is interesting to note since essential fatty acid (EFA) intakes can influence the body's production of inflammatory mediators.[58] Based on these study results, a lactobacilli-rich vegan or lactovegetarian diet may be a useful adjunct to RA treatments and may even reduce or eliminate the need for gold, methotrexate, or steroid medications in some individuals. Oral digestive enzyme therapy, such as the use of bromelain or papain, active protein substances found naturally in foods, has also shown to be useful, especially when combined with other conventional treatments.[59] Research has found that oral digestive enzymes help to reduce transforming growth factor-beta1 (TGF-beta1), a multifunctional cytokine linked to RA and other diseases, by binding and inactivating it irreversibly.[60] Oral digestive enzymes have an analgesic, anti-inflammatory effect, and should be taken on an empty stomach between meals.[61] Further dietary advice given in the section, "The Anti-Inflammatory Diet" may also be of some use for RA patients.

In summary, nutrition management recommendations for patients with RA include supplementation of diet with probiotics (such as fructooligosaccharides and lignans), avoidance of animal protein sources, identification and elimination of food allergies and sensitivities, and balancing their dietary EFA intakes while eliminating *trans-* or hydrogenated fats.[62]

The following supplement guidelines are recommended for RA to help reduce pain, inflammation, and oxidative damage to joints:

Fructooligosaccharides (FOS): It can be used to help naturally produce healthy bacteria in the gut with 1–4 g/day

Vitamin C: 1000–3000 mg/day in divided doses (less than or equal to 500 mg) along with bioflavonoids

Vitamin E: 100–800 IU/day from 100% natural D-alpha tocopherol with other mixed tocopherols

Coenzyme Q10: 30 mg b.i.d., or 60 mg q.d. in oil soft-gel form

Oral digestive enzymes (bromelain, papain, trypsin, chymotrypsin): Take with meals as per package directions

Omega-3 fatty acids: 2–10 g/day (lower end of the range for fish oil, higher end of the range for plant sources of omega-3s, such as flax oil)

Joint mobilization could aggravate RA patients during periods of inflammation so caution should be taken when choosing this.

Areas for Future Research

The National Institute of Arthritis and Musculoskeletal and Skin Diseases (NIAMS) and the North American Rheumatoid Arthritis Consortium are conducting a study involving 1000 siblings with RA to investigate possible genetic components that may identify individuals at risk for developing RA, looking for genetic material to identify which parts of the DNA are involved in the disease.

ANKYLOSING SPONDYLITIS OR MARIE–STRUMPELL DISEASE

Ankylosing spondylitis (AS) is an inflammatory autoimmune disorder that affects the spine. AS most commonly affects males under 30 years of age at a rate three times greater than females.[48] It causes increasing pain and stiffness due to extra bone growth, resulting in partial or complete fusion of the vertebrae, creating a radiographic sign referred to as bamboo spine. AS is more progressive, with an earlier onset in life. In extreme and chronic cases, the patient stoops forward and surgery may be required to straighten the spine. With severe chronic cases, the rib cage can be affected, causing difficulty in breathing. The heart may also be affected causing atrioventricular (AV) conduction defects.[48] Other joints commonly affected are the hips, knees, and shoulders. There is no known cause but it is suspected to have a genetic link. AS is associated with bowel disorders. In patients with Crohn's disease or ulcerative colitis, an AS-like arthritis develops in about 10 to 20% of patients.[62]

Males are most affected and present with stiffness and low back pain, which may radiate into the buttocks and thighs. Additional early signs and symptoms include low-grade fever, fatigue, anorexia, weight loss, and anemia.[48] The stiffness in the spine progresses as the disease progresses and inflammation occurs at the ligament insertion sites.

As stated earlier, the most common symptoms are chronic low back pain and stiffness with decreased lumbopelvic ROM. Chest expansion can be decreased with long-standing AS. The ESR and HLA-B27 are elevated in laboratory tests but are not diagnostic because these tests are nonspecific. Radiographic studies are diagnostic for AS. X-rays show sclerosis, erosions, and pseudowidening in the sacroiliac joints in the earlier stages. In the spine, marginal sclerosis and erosions of the vertebral bodies, presenting as squaring, are seen. The spinal ligaments and annulus fibrosis calcify showing a "bamboo spine" appearance on x-ray. The tendon and ligament insertion points of the Achilles, plantar fascia, and iliac crests may be involved.[48]

Response to medical intervention is unpredictable. Unfortunately, no cure has been found. Current medications and treatments have not been found to halt spinal symptoms of disease progression. Nonsteroidal anti-inflammatory drugs are usually given to decrease inflammation but should be avoided long term due to the possible gastric and renal consequences. Corticosteroids are also given but with caution due to the adverse side effects, including osteoporosis of the stiff spine.[48] With chronic, severe cases, cardiac and pulmonary involvement should be monitored. Postural and breathing exercises as well as stretching and keeping the spine flexible are part of the management. The patient should be instructed to sleep in a supine position on a firm mattress and should not use a pillow. The drug etanercept is useful in alleviating the pain and stiffness associated with AS. Etanercept was found to work faster than other drug therapies (such as NSAIDs, oral corticosteroids, and antirheumatic drugs) and slowed the disease process.[63] It is referred to as a "biologic agent" drug, designed to disrupt the disease process by blocking tumor necrosis factor (TNF), a protein naturally occurring in the body, which contributes to inflammation. High-dose salicylate therapy often does not control the pain, but other NSAIDs may be helpful. Indomethacin is the one used most often. Methotrexate and sulfasalazine may also be of some benefit. Range of motion and breathing exercises to keep the spine and rib cage moving and flexible are recommended.

GOUT

Gout is a metabolic disorder characterized by recurrent episodes of extremely painful, acute (or chronic) arthritis attacks. This results from deposition of macroscopic crystals (tophi) in or around joints and tissues. The tophi are needle-like, producing fierce pain in the joints and causing swelling, redness, heat, and stiffness. Gout is classified as a rheumatic disease, accounting for approximately 5% of all arthritis cases.[63]

Uric acid is the by-product of purine metabolism, found in all human tissues and many foods. Uric acid normally dissolves in the blood passing through the kidneys and subsequently excreted in the urine. Crystallization of serum uric acid occurs asymptomatically, resulting in sudden, unbearable outbreaks of pain once deposited in tissues and joints. Most first-time attacks are followed by a second attack within 1 year (*The Merck Manual*, p. 490, Ref. 52) while only about 7% of patients never have a second attack.[64] Despite the harsh symptoms, gout is very treatable and even preventable.

Of the two major categories of gout, referred to as primary and secondary, primary gout accounts for 90% of all cases and is likely a result of a genetic defect in a specific enzyme involved in uric acid metabolism (xanthine oxidase).[64] However, this does not account for all cases. Regardless, serum uric acid levels rise too high due to increased uric acid synthesis (only about 10% of cases) or decreased ability to excrete uric acid (90% of cases).[62] In secondary gout (10% of all cases), some other factor is at fault.[64] It could be caused by excessive cell breakdown due to cytotoxic drugs used to treat cancer, for example, kidney disease or insulin resistance. Diuretic therapy used to treat high blood pressure (thiazides) and low-dose aspirin therapy are both possible causes for secondary gout as well since both lead to reduced uric acid excretion.

Uric acid crystals are highly insoluble molecules. The most common site is the first joint of the big toe.[65] In about 50% of first-time cases, it affects the big toe. As the attack progresses, fever and chills will follow. If left untreated, gout can lead to joint breakdown. The first attack most commonly occurs at night secondary to

- High dietary intakes of purine-rich foods
- Certain diuretics
- High dosages of niacin

Gout affects men more commonly than women, and when it does strike women, it usually occurs after menopause.[66] In premenopausal women, there is usually a family history of gout.[66] Genetic predisposition to defective purine metabolism can explain the reasons for this change in physiology.[67] Predisposition for gout includes obesity, high-purine diet, and excessive alcohol consumption.

A painful, swollen big toe is due to tophi, most commonly deposited in the first toe but also the knee, olecranon bursal area, and behind the ears. Tophi causes inflammation and eventual bone destruction after repeated attacks. During the acute stage the joint is swollen, very tender, and red. The patient may complain of fever, chills, and malaise. Laboratory values may demonstrate a high uric acid level (>7.5 mg/dl). Early radiographic changes may not be visible but later x-ray changes may show punched out areas of the bone. For definitive diagnosis, identification of urate crystals in joint fluid or tophi is used.[68]

NSAIDs are most effective during an acute attack of gout for pain control. Relief usually occurs within 24 h after ingestion. Symptoms will often subside in 3 days, at which time NSAIDs use can be discontinued. People with gout are at a higher risk for developing kidney stones. Approximately 90% of people with gout suffer from some degree of kidney dysfunction due to the uric acid deposits.[64] Some medications such as allopurinol reduce uric acid formation by blocking xanthine oxidase and are used for preventing further attacks. It is especially helpful in patients with renal calculi since its mechanism of action does not work through kidney function. Allopurinol blocks uric acid production by interfering with the metabolic pathway that produces xanthine oxidase. Aspirin has been found to inhibit renal excretion of uric acid and should be avoided, as well as salicylates and salicylate-containing foods such as dried plums, raisins, and licorice. For a list of additional foods that contain salicylates, refer to "The Anti-Inflammatory Diet," discussed later. For treating acute gout, the anti-inflammatory drug, colchicine is useful. Its effectiveness comes from inhibiting white blood cell migration to sites of inflammation. Almost all patients given colchicine develop GI toxicity, so this treatment is not normally the first therapy recommended. For treating acute gout of large joints, withdrawing synovial fluid and injecting a long-lasting steroid, such as triamcinolone can be quite effective.[66] This is especially helpful for those people unable to tolerate NSAIDs or colchicines.

Diet is a helpful tool in the management of gout. Some of the most beneficial treatments and preventive strategies include:

1. *Adequate hydration*
Fluid aids purine excretion while eliminating other toxins from the body as well. Avoid overhydration as this can lead to hyponatremia (water toxicity) and in acute gout attacks may worsen the effects of the inflammation.

2. *Low-purine diet*
Certain foods may predispose one to an attack. Restriction of purine-rich foods can help control serum urate levels, but even with a purine-free diet, one is not immune to gout attacks.[69] The typical diet provides 600–1000 mg of purines each day.[5] In severe cases of gout, it is advised that purine content in the diet be limited to 100–150 mg/day.[5] With the advent of gout medications, there is less of a need for strict dietary action. Yet given this, and the fact that the diet only contributes about 10 to 20% to the total uric acid level found in the blood, it is still good advice to limit the level of purine-rich foods to minimize crystal formation.[64]

- High-purine content foods (100–1000 mg purines/100 g food) — avoid: organ meats, shellfish, yeast (brewer's and baker's), consommé and broth, herring, sardines, mackerel, and anchovies

- Moderate purine content foods (9–100 mg purine/100 g food) — use in moderation at 2–3 oz daily: meat, fish (other than those listed above), poultry, asparagus, dried beans, lentils, mushroom, and spinach
- Negligible purine content foods — use daily: fruits, herbs and spices, eggs, nuts, seeds, oils, rice, dairy, and vegetables (except for those listed above)

3. *Folic acid supplementation*

Folic acid supplements in high doses have been recommended for gout over the past 20 years. However, the research is contradictory.[65] Some research studies show folic acid may reduce uric acid formation via its inhibitory effect on xanthine oxidase, the same enzyme that the drug allopurinol works on.[70] The recommended range is 10–40 mg/day. While this is significantly higher than the recommended dietary allowance (the amount recommended to prevent folic acid deficiency), it has not shown to produce any toxic side effects, and may be safer than drugs. Physician supervision is necessary with such high doses due to folic acid's ability to mask a vitamin B_{12} deficiency.

4. *Bromelain*

Bromelain is an enzyme found naturally in raw pineapple and exerts anti-inflammatory effects. It can be taken as a supplement at 500 mg, three times per day for 7 days and then 250 mg, three times per day for the next 2 months.[71] Six ounces of raw pineapple daily can have similar benefits.[71]

5. *Omega-3 fatty acids*

These EFAs have a positive influence on reducing pain and inflammation (refer to "The Anti-Inflammatory Diet"). Good food sources include milled flaxseed, flax oil, canola oil, and walnuts. Fatty fish are excellent sources as well, but due to its higher purine content, fish consumption should be limited to not more than 2–3 oz daily.[5] With reduced intake of fish, eicosapentaenoic acid (EPA) or docosahexaenoic acid (DHA) supplementation may be necessary to meet EFA requirements. Dosage recommendations are 3–6 g/day.[71]

6. *Avoid excess vitamin C and niacin*

These two nutrients are not considered a problem when ingested naturally through the diet. However, the use of supplements should be discouraged. Both increase production and crystallization of uric acid. Good sources of vitamin C include citrus fruits, strawberries, broccoli, bell peppers, and kiwi fruit. Good sources of niacin include whole grains, peanuts, and fortified bread products. Meat and poultry are also excellent sources, but consumption should be limited to 2–3 oz daily.

7. *Vitamin E and selenium*

Vitamin E is a potent antioxidant, which inhibits the production of inflammatory leukotrienes. A dose of 100–400 IU/day as the all-natural, D-alpha tocopherol form containing other mixed tocopherols. Selenium is a mineral that functions synergistically with vitamin E to provide additional antioxidant protection, in doses of 50–200 mcg/day.

Other beneficial dietary recommendations include avoiding a ketogenic diet (as excessive protein and fat intake can lead to ketone production, causing increased uric acid production), avoiding excessive alcohol intake (as this could lead to dehydration and increased uric acid production, as well as reduced uric acid excretion), and maintenance of a healthy weight (as excess weight has a higher association with gout and weight loss in obese individuals can significantly reduce uric acid levels).

ANTI-INFLAMMATORY DIET

The dietary recommendations below are recommended for anyone with an inflammatory condition. The anti-inflammatory diet is rich in antioxidants, immune-enhancing nutrients, inflammatory inhibitors, and nutrients that support wound healing. This diet can be especially helpful for the inflammatory conditions discussed earlier in this chapter: tennis elbow, carpal tunnel syndrome, shoulder impingement or subacromial bursitis, general muscle sprain or strain, OA, AS, and RA. Dietary recommendations are made both for food sources and dietary supplements. However, reference to that condition's section would be advised to cross-check any contraindications or more specific recommendations.

ESSENTIAL FATTY ACIDS

Much research relating to reducing pain and inflammation revolves around consumption of dietary fats, specifically the omega-6 ($n-6$) and omega-3 ($n-3$) polyunsaturated fatty acids. Current dietary intake for Americans heavily favors the intake of saturated fats and ($n-6$) fatty acids. This is due primarily to the excess consumption of animal products (high-fat meats, cheese, milk), and the use of vegetable oils (such as corn, safflower, and sunflower oils) and hydrogenated vegetable oils (primarily soybean and cottonseed oils) in prepared foods. The intake of essential ($n-3$) fatty acids is negligible in many Americans.

High-saturated fat intakes can promote biosynthesis of inflammatory substances in the body via supply and production of arachidonic acid. Arachidonic acid is an inflammatory substance in and of itself, yet is also responsible for the production of inflammatory eicosanoids. Beef fat and egg yolks are the primary dietary suppliers of arachidonic acid. Omega-6 fatty acids can also promote more inflammatory states, as they are precursors to arachidonic acid production, a known inflammatory agent. However, ($n-3$) fatty acids tend to exert anti-inflammatory effects through their metabolism into anti-inflammatory eicosanoids. Table 8.8 exhibits the different pathways for omega-6 versus omega-3 metabolism. With the high dietary intakes of ($n-6$)- and saturated fats, along with deficient intakes of ($n-3$) fatty acids, a significant imbalance is created, thereby promoting a proinflammatory reaction. The balance between the two EFAs is crucial since they direct immune function, intercellular communication, gene expression, and inflammatory responses. The ideal ratio of ($n-6$) to ($n-3$) fatty acids is between 1:1 and 2:1, but today's diet supplies between 10:1 and 25:1.[72]

Omega-3 fatty acids, as alpha-linolenic acid (ALA), are found in canola oil, soybean oil, and milled flaxseed. Soybean oil should be limited since it also contains high amounts of

---

TABLE 8.8
Essential Fatty Acid Metabolism

Omega-3 fatty acids	Omega-6 fatty acids
↓ ← ← **Delta-6 desaturase enzyme** → →	↓
Alpha-linolenic acid (ALA)	**Linoleic acid (LA)**
↓	↓
Stearidonic acid	**Gamma-Linolenic acid (GLA)** → Series 1 prostanoids and series 3 leukotrienes
↓	↓
Eicosapentaenoic acid → Series 3	**Dihomo-gamma-linolenic acid (D-GLA)** Prostanoids and series 5 leukotrienes
↓	↓
Docosahexaenoic acid	**Arachidonic acid** → Series 2 prostanoids and series 4 leukotrienes

($n-6$) fatty acids. Flaxseed oil should be kept refrigerated and stored no longer than 6 months unopened, or 3 months opened. It should not be used as cooking oil, but rather used in cold preparation foods (salad dressings, fruit smoothies) or moderate temperature baking (muffins, breads). Omega-3 fatty acids, such as EPA and DHA, are found in fish, especially cold-water fish such as salmon, albacore tuna, mackerel, and sardines. The body converts ALA into EPA and DHA in healthy individuals, although the conversion may be limited. Only about 10% of ALA is converted into EPA or DHA. Conversion is even less when the diet is unbalanced with too many ($n-6$)-rich foods. Furthermore, in individuals with insulin resistance (metabolic syndrome), diabetes mellitus, or those under chronic stress states, this conversion is impaired. However, ALA may still be the best choice of obtaining ($n-3$) fatty acids for individuals not consuming other dietary sources of EPA or DHA, such as fish or marine oils. Some individuals may also have a delta-6 desaturase enzyme defect or deficiency (the enzyme involved in the first step of fatty acid metabolism). In such individuals, they are unable to metabolize plant sources of omega-3 fatty acids into EPA, DHA, or gamma-linolenic acid (GLA), a metabolite of the essential omega-6 fatty acids. These individuals, therefore, require supplementation with EPA, DHA, and GLA. GLA production may be reduced with excessive alcohol intake, diabetes mellitus, eczema, excessive saturated fat intake, or elevated blood cholesterol levels in the elderly. Supplements may be helpful. Borage seed, evening primrose, and black currant oils are good sources of GLA. These oils, though they are ($n-6$) derivatives, exert anti-inflammatory properties and can be useful in treating inflammatory conditions. Excessive alcohol ingestion, diabetes mellitus, and chronic stress can shift the delta-6 desaturase enzyme toward the more proinflammatory pathway. Some health professionals warn against the use of borage seed for a source of EFAs. Parts of the borage plant contain carcinogenic compounds (pyrrolidine alkaloids) and are potentially toxic to the liver. Significant amounts are not likely to be found in the borage seed oil since the toxins are found in the plant's leaves and roots. However, there is the possibility of contamination and other forms may be safer for longer-term use. The most beneficial effects may arise from the combination of GLA with fish oil (($n-3$) fatty acids), but research is limited and often very weak. Also, GLA supplementation over an extended period of time may have a greater proinflammatory effect via its effects on arachidonic acid production.

Supplements such as EFAs or fish oils discussed earlier may be beneficial, but food sources should be emphasized first, as they contain not only the EFAs, but also dozens of other essential nutrients and antioxidants. Supplements also pose a problem since there are no federal or state regulations governing the freshness or potency of dietary supplements, and ($n-3$) fatty acids may be rancid. This can lead to GI distress and production of harmful by-products such as peroxides and aldehydes that damage the body's cells. Rancid supplements often have an "off" smell or taste, but it may be hard to discern between the natural odor of the supplement even when it is fresh. Other potential health concerns with ingesting EPA and DHA supplements include the potential heavy metal contamination. Side effects noted while using ($n-3$) or ($n-6$) supplements may include mild nausea and diarrhea. Taking smaller doses throughout the day may help minimize these effects. Side effects will be worse if the supplement has turned rancid. Best to store it in a cool, dry, dark place to minimize potential for rancidity. Look for supplements that specifically state the amount of GLA and ALA on the label and which do not try to confuse the consumer with terminology such as "GLA complex" or ALA and GLA blend. GLA and ALA can also act as blood thinners. They should not be used by individuals who have blood clotting disorders and are on Coumadin, unless under medical supervision. Hemophiliacs also need to take extra precaution when supplementing their diets with them. Those expecting to undergo surgery should stop the use of these supplements before any procedure. Other blood thinners include vitamin E, garlic supplements, ginkgo biloba, and aspirin. Recommended dosages are as follows:

- *Gamma-linolenic acid (GLA)*: 360 mg to 2–3 g and can take up to 6 months or more to have an effect. Best to take in divided dosages throughout the day rather than all at once.
- *Omega-3 fatty acids:* 2–10 g/day.

The overall focus should be on rebalancing the EFAs. The best strategy is not just to increase $(n-3)$ intake, but also to simultaneously decrease $(n-6)$ intakes. This is because $(n-3)$ and $(n-6)$ fatty acids compete for the same enzyme, delta-6 desaturase, for their metabolism.[73] An oversupply of $(n-6)$ fatty acids will lead to less enzyme availability to metabolize $(n-3)$ fatty acids. Vitamins such as niacin, B_6, and C, along with the minerals zinc and magnesium, are required for proper delta-6 desaturase function.[73] Inadequate or suboptimal levels of these nutrients may render greater $(n-3)$ intakes ineffective. The body's requirement for EFAs is 1 to 2% of total daily calories from linoleic acid $(n-6)$ and 0.5% from linolenic acid $(n-3)$.[5] This is based on the level needed to prevent deficiency symptoms. For example, a 2000-cal diet, with 1 to 2% of total daily calories contributed by linoleic acid, results in an optimal intake of 2–4 g daily, and 1 g of linolenic acid daily (at 0.5% of total daily calories). However, higher amounts may be required for optimal health.

Below are a list of foods with high-$(n-3)$ and -$(n-6)$ fatty acid contents:

Omega-3 fatty acid-rich foods	*Omega-6 fatty acid-rich foods*
Fatty fish (salmon, mackerel, sardines)	Soybean oil
Flaxseeds or flax oil	Sunflower seeds and oil
Canola oil	Safflower oil
Soybeans — whole, cooked	Corn oil
Pumpkin seeds	Mayonnaise made with soybean oil
Dark leafy green vegetables	
Hemp oil	

Whole food choices should be emphasized as much as possible rather than oils (i.e., walnuts versus walnut oil, flaxseeds versus flax oil) as oxidative damage is more likely to occur in the oils. This is also true of oil soft-gel dietary supplements. Consider concurrent supplementation with vitamin E (10–100 IU/day) if a supplement is not already taken for extra antioxidant protection.

EICOSANOID PRODUCTION

Series 1 and 2 prostaglandins, prostacyclins, leukotrienes, and thromboxanes are eicosanoids (physiologically and pharmacologically active compounds made by the body) derived from $(n-6)$ fatty acids. Series 2 comes from arachidonic acid and are considered proinflammatory.[74] Series 1 eicosanoids are metabolized through a different pathway and are considered anti-inflammatory. Series 3 eicosanoids are derived from $(n-3)$ fatty acids and are also anti-inflammatory. They get metabolized into GLA, a unique anti-inflammatory $(n-6)$ fatty acid. These three eicosanoid series appear to be the primary mediators in the body's inflammation process.[74] Prostaglandins are commonly classified by their effects on blood platelets, such as proaggregatory or antiaggregatory, and blood vessel dilation or constriction. This is important for joint health as increased blood flow to areas of injury and ability to deliver nutrients to injured sites are critical for the body to repair itself. A brief summary of the eicosanoid effects are listed below:

Series 1 and 3 eicosanoids	*Series 2 and 4 eicosanoids*
Vasodilation	Vasoconstriction
Antiaggregatory	Proaggregatory
Anti-inflammatory	Proinflammatory

Series 4 leukotrienes are proinflammatory and can be inhibited by the following nutrients[73]:

N-Acetyl-cysteine (NAC): 20–1000 mg/day

Selenium: 50–300 mcg/day

Turmeric: 250–500 mg/day

Onion: 500–1000 mg, dried root or unlimited dietary intake

Garlic: 500–1000 mg/day, dried root or one bulb raw garlic daily

Boswellia: 250–500 mg/day

Series 4 leukotriene inhibition is how the drug sulfasalazine exerts its effects.

PHOSPHOLIPASE A_2 ENZYME INHIBITION

Arachidonic acid is metabolized from $(n-6)$ fatty acids into the series 2 eicosanoids via the enzyme phospholipase A_2 (PL-A_2). Vitamin E and the flavonoid quercetin have been found to block this enzyme's activity.[73] Licorice (*Glycyrrhiza glabra*) and turmeric also block PL-A_2 activity.[73] The recommended daily dosages for these supplements are as follows[73]:

Vitamin E: 100–1000 IU in oil soft-gel form, from all-natural D-alpha tocopherol and other mixed tocopherols

Quercetin: 100–500 mg

Licorice: 500–1000 mg, dried root

Turmeric: 250–500 mg, capsule form

This PL-A_2 inhibition is how corticosteroids impact the inflammatory process.

COX-1 AND COX-2 ENZYME INHIBITION

Other nutrients can have anti-inflammatory effects via their action on COX-1 and COX-2 enzymes. These enzymes produce the series 2 eicosanoids. The list given below have been shown to inhibit these enzymes[73]:

Ginger: 1–4 g, dried root

Black willow: 50–200 mg, dried bark

Wintergreen: 1–3 enterically coated oil capsule, 0.2 ml each

Omega-3 fatty acids: 2–10 g

Turmeric: 250–500 mg, capsule form

Inhibition of COX-1 and COX-2 enzymes are how NSAIDs exert their effects.

FOOD ALLERGIES AND LECTINS

Food allergens and lectins can cause greater systematic inflammation via their effects on mast cell activity. These mast cells line the gut mucosa as well as connective tissues, and serve important functions in the immune response. Mast cells contain histamine, proteases, glycosamine glycans, and chemotactic agents, which are released when the mast cell is triggered. This leads to inflammation and also triggers PL-A_2 enzyme activity, resulting in greater synthesis of proinflammatory eicosanoids. This is what happens in an IgE (anaphylactic) food allergy reaction. The most common food allergies seen in the United States include wheat, dairy, corn, peanuts, shellfish, strawberries, and eggs.[75]

Lectins may trigger this response and are thus the basis of the Lewis antigen blood type recommendations. Lectin-based dietary recommendations based on one's blood type may reduce inflammatory responses. However, this needs further research to identify which food–blood type interactions are detrimental.

DIETARY SALICYLATES AND AMINES

A multitude of treatments for fighting the pain associated with inflammation have been used for thousands of years. The earliest therapies used herbal concoctions, plants, or leaves. Most, if not all, contained salicylates.[76] Salicylate-rich foods are natural pain relievers. The highest salicylate-containing foods and spices include paprika, curry powder, mustard powder, oregano, rosemary, sage, tarragon, turmeric, thyme, honey, garam masala, cinnamon, fenugreek powder, dill powder, and Worcestershire sauce. These all contain 10 mg salicylates/100 g or more. Other salicylate-rich foods include raisins, prunes, raspberries, licorice, mint (fresh), black pepper, and pickles.[77] But caution must be used in individuals who are sensitive to aspirin as salicylate is an aspirin-like substance and can cause adverse reactions, such as asthma and urticaria.[78]

Diets high in amines may also cause mast cell degeneration as can imbalances of gut microflora, which can cause increased bioproduction of amines. Amine-rich foods include red wines, aged cheese, chocolate, and smoked meats.[73] Other additives that may cause adverse reactions are sulfites, food dyes, nitrites and nitrates, benzoates, preservatives such as butylated hydroxyanisole (BHA), and butylated hydroxytoluene (BHT).[78]

ARTIFICIAL SWEETENERS AND MONOSODIUM GLUTAMATE

Excessive intakes of individual amino acids can upset the body's natural balance. High glutamic or aspartic acid intakes can lead to greater mast cell destruction. Overuse of artificial sweeteners, especially aspartame, should be avoided. Aspartame is a dipeptide composed of the two amino acids, aspartic acid and phenylalanine. This can contribute too much aspartic acid to the diet and cause detrimental effects. MSG can supply excessive amounts of glutamic acid, leading to greater mast cell degradation. Artificial sweetener use and MSG intake should be discouraged.

NUCLEAR FACTOR-KAPPA B

DNA gene expression that promotes inflammation can be influenced by NF-κB, a protein that has been found to induce chronic inflammatory diseases.[79] Supplementation with alpha-lipoic acid, vitamin C, flavonoids, and vitamin E has been shown to help inhibit NF-κB activity, therefore reducing inflammation and also gene expression that leads to greater synthesis of mediators involved in the proinflammatory response.[80]

OXIDATIVE STRESS

Polyunsaturated fats, including the EFAs $(n-6)$ and $(n-3)$ fatty acids, are highly susceptible to oxidation. This can lead to rancidity of these fats and oils. When ingested, often unknowingly, it can lead to greater oxidative stress and damage in the body. Other likely contributors to oxidative damage are air pollution, cigarette smoke, household cleaning agent exposure, chronic stress, and excessive exercise. Antioxidants are helpful in preventing oxidative damage by counteracting these reactive oxygen species (ROS) molecules, which are highly unstable and lead to free radical production. This can potentially lead to a greater risk for cancer development and heart disease, as well as joint inflammation and autoimmune disorders, such as RA. When adequate antioxidants are ingested, the body can manage oxidative stress quite well. But if antioxidant consumption is inadequate, or the body is constantly bombarded with oxidative stress situations, an imbalance is created that shifts the body into a higher stress state.

Cellular antioxidant protection is best achieved through consumption of a healthy, balanced diet, full of a variety of unprocessed, unrefined plant-based foods. Supplementation may be necessary when the diet is inadequate. Key antioxidants that help prevent cellular damage include vitamin C, vitamin E, alpha-lipoic acid, coenzyme Q10, beta-carotene and other carotenoids, quercetin (rutin), selenium, citrus and noncitrus flavonoids, and other plant phytochemicals. Grape seed extract, a flavonoid source, has been shown to reduce inflammation and stabilize collagen structures.[64] Oral enzyme therapy may also be of some benefit due to its positive effects on reducing pain and swelling.[58]

It is also best to limit the intake of processed foods, especially those that are processed *and refined,* as this removes many of the antioxidants (the free-radical squelching molecules that help protect cells from damage) naturally found in unprocessed plant foods. Good examples of unprocessed foods include whole grains, such as oats, brown and wild rice, bulgar, and millet; legumes, such as black, kidney, and soybeans, chickpeas, and black-eyed peas; vegetables, including starchy vegetables; fruit, and nuts and seeds, all of which have anti-inflammatory properties. If foods are processed (such as whole grains processed into breads, cereals, or crackers), it is still better to limit or avoid the refined (white, enriched products). There are also several herbal remedies that have been found to be helpful for joint-related conditions (see Table 8.10).

TWENTY STRATEGIES FOR A HEALTHY DIET

1. Identify and eliminate food allergies and sensitivities, as well as any environmental sensitivities. Salicylate and amine-rich foods may need to be avoided
2. Eliminate use of artificial sweeteners and MSG-containing foods
3. Choose clean, wholesome foods that are unrefined, unprocessed, such as whole grain rice, oats, corn, legumes, and nuts and seeds. If processed, use in moderation, such as breads, crackers, processed meats, and juices
3. Consume 8–10 servings of vegetables and fruit daily, emphasizing vegetables
4. Eliminate hydrogenated fats, also referred to as *trans*-fats. Read food label ingredient lists to identify them. They will be labeled as: partially or fully hydrogenated vegetable oils, or vegetable shortening
5. Choose foods daily that contain omega-3 fatty acids while simultaneously reducing omega-6-rich foods. When choosing fish as an omega-3 source, avoid those with heavy metal or microbial contamination, or those that are considered endangered species
6. Limit consumption of foods high in saturated fats, choosing low-fat or nonfat meat and dairy
7. Limit alcohol to one drink per day for women and two drinks per day for men. A drink is considered 5 oz of wine, 12 oz of beer, or one jigger of 80-proof spirits
8. Buy cold-pressed or expeller-pressed oils. Store them in the refrigerator for no longer than 4 months once opened, or 6 months unopened
9. Buy organic fruits, vegetables, meat, poultry, eggs, and dairy whenever possible. Wash fruit and vegetables well in soapy water with a soft scrub brush
10. Use a variety of herbs and spices to flavor food and add extra antioxidants
11. Eat a wide variety of foods. Avoid overeating any certain food to the exclusion of other nutrient-rich foods
12. Eat a fiber-rich diet. This should naturally be accomplished if one's diet is based on consumption of whole grains, legumes, fruits, and vegetables
13. Avoid foods that contain nitrites and nitrates, food dyes, additives, or preservatives (other than natural antioxidants)
14. Avoid canned, processed foods. Buy fresh or frozen instead
15. Stay adequately hydrated. Consume four cups of fluid for every 1000 cal ingested, or 6–8 oz cups of fluid for most healthy individuals. Remember, fluid-rich foods can help

meet these goals, such as fruits, vegetables, soups, yogurt, and milk. Other good fluid choices include water, herbal teas, mineral water, and fruit juices (in limited amounts). Avoid overconsumption of caffeinated beverages as these may cause fluid losses, leading to dehydration

17. Practice safe food handling techniques. Wash hands and foods well, cook meats to their proper temperature (without overcooking), and store protein-rich foods below 40°F. Avoid leaving food out at room temperature for longer than 2 h. Reheat leftovers to an internal temperature of 165°F

18. If considering using dietary supplements to improve health, work closely with a knowledgeable healthcare practitioner who can guide you on safety and potency issues

19. Become conscious and mindful of hunger and appetite. Avoid overeating or under eating. Try not to become overly hungry. Stop eating when about 80% full

20. The three keys to optimal health include variety, balance, and moderation. Put these into practice daily

The following areas may also be considered as nutritional intervention strategies to help manage chronic inflammation:

- Liver detoxification support
- Mitochondrial support
- Management of dysglycemia

However, finding a holistic or naturopathic healthcare practitioner would be most beneficial as these strategies are complicated and need to be assessed more thoroughly than can be done here.

SPORTS INJURIES

TENNIS ELBOW OR LATERAL EPICONDYLITIS

Tennis elbow has become the accepted standard diagnosis of epicondylar pain and tenderness with related disability. The onset can be sudden or gradual in nature.[81]

Tennis has been implicated in at least half of the reported cases. The other half is reported by individuals with repetitive activities stressing the area.[81] Typically, the patient is middle aged (30 to 50 years) and involved in racquet sports. They also exhibit poor stroke mechanics especially with their backhand.[82] Point tenderness at the lateral epicondyle, the origin of the extensor carpi radialis brevis, usually occurs.[81] The patient will often complain of pain in the extremity with activities of daily living such as turning a doorknob, lifting a milk carton, or opening a jar.[83]

History usually reveals repetitive flexion–extension on pronation or supination activities with overuse. When tennis players are classified by skill level, the higher the skill level the less incidence of lateral epicondylitis, supporting the theory that faulty mechanics are involved.[81]

Two orthopedic tests commonly used to evaluate tennis elbow are Cozens and Mills maneuver. Both tests when positive will elicit pain at the lateral epicondyle. Gardner described the chain test where the patient is asked to lift a chair with one hand, which is pronated. Severe pain confirms the diagnosis. The "coffee cup test," as described by Coonrad, which involves picking up a full cup of coffee with the affected arm, is pathognomonic for lateral epicondylitis.[81]

Initial treatment of acute epicondylitis includes rest from provocative movements, ice, and NSAIDs. The patient must be educated that this is an overuse syndrome. If symptoms persist, are severe, and affect function, steroid injections are often done, but understanding that repeated steroid injections may cause other complications is essential.[83]

Once symptoms abate, rehabilitation should be initiated, emphasizing strength and flexibility of the flexors and extensors of the forearm.[83]

Carpal Tunnel

Carpal tunnel syndrome (CTS) is defined as compression of the median nerve at the wrist as it passes through the carpal tunnel. CTS is the most common upper extremity compression syndrome.[83] It is a common and often disabling condition that affects individuals who engage in repetitive hand motion. It also occurs frequently in individuals with RA, diabetes, hypothyroidism, and women during pregnancy. It is caused by aggravation to ligaments and tendons that pass through the wrist, called the carpal tunnel. Repetitive hand motions may cause these tissues to swell, leading to compression of the medial nerve. Tingling and numbness in the thumb, index, middle, and sometimes half of the ring finger are common signs. The pain and discomfort associated with the condition may disrupt sleep and make it difficult to grasp small objects.

Paresthesias of the thumb, index, middle, and radial half of the ring finger are the patient's usual complaint. It strikes women more often than men. There may also be activity, aggravated weakness on clumsiness of the hand. Athletic activities, driving a car, or any activity with prolonged or repetitive wrist flexion or extension may exacerbate the condition and cause the affected hand to "fall asleep." Aching and discomfort of the arm or forearm with distal numbness is often a presenting complaint. Many patients will complain of nocturnal discomfort of the forearm and hand.[81]

The patient is at a higher risk for median nerve compression or CTS if exposed to repetitive blunt trauma or repetitive motion to the wrist due to occupation or hobby. Both will cause inflammation within the carpal tunnel causing pressure on the median nerve.[83] Use of the wrist is a biomechanically stressful condition, which may also cause swelling and lead to CTS.

Two of the leading tests for CTS are Phalens, consisting of wrist flexion, and Tinnels tapping test.[81] Both tests if positive will increase the patient's symptoms or create tingling or electric shock sensation somewhere along the course of median nerve distribution. Patients with chronic CTS may exhibit thenar atrophy, decreased two-point discrimination and motor weakness.

Conservative treatment consists of ice, NSAIDs, and extension splinting during the day when doing repetitive strain activities, as well as at night during sleep. The patient should be instructed to correct or eliminate any motions or activities that could exacerbate the CTS. Steroid injection may be used, but is minimally successful and remains controversial.[83] If these methods fail to alleviate symptoms, surgery may be necessary, which involves cutting the median nerve at the base of the wrist to free it from the pressure.

In 1976, researchers found that people with CTS were more likely to be deficient in B_6.[62,71] Vitamin B_6 (pyridoxine) and B_2 (riboflavin) function together to convert B_6 into its active form of pyridoxal 5-phosphate (P-5-P). Supplements of P-5-P are available in 25–50 mg, and should be taken three times per day. Do not exceed 1 g/lb body weight for extended periods of time. It is also advised that foods containing the yellow dye, tartrazine, (FD&C yellow #5) be avoided, as this dye can interfere with vitamin B_6 metabolism in the body. High-protein intake can lead to a shortage of vitamin B_6 since it is involved in protein metabolism. Since vitamin B_6 is also involved in the metabolism of carbohydrates, a high-sugar intake, or high intakes of refined, unenriched foods, can increase B_6 needs. Birth control pills increase the body's need for vitamin B_6.[62] The recommended riboflavin dosage is 10 mg daily.

Bromelain, the enzyme found in pineapple that has been shown to reduce inflammation, may be useful in CTS treatment. Studies show that taking bromelain before surgery and afterwards to aid recovery and reduce swelling, bruising, and pain.[62] For best results, start taking it 3 days before surgery and for a minimum of 2 weeks postsurgery.[62] Supplementation at 250–750 mg two times per day between meals is advised.

Alternative care includes prevention, proper ergonomics, taking breaks to rest hands and wrists along with using wrist splints daily. Acupuncture and herbals such as white willow bark can be helpful. Massage may alleviate tension in the upper extremities of affected wrists, possibly relieving the strain surrounding the carpal tunnel. Direct massage to the inflamed areas should be avoided.

SHOULDER IMPINGEMENT OR SUBACROMIAL BURSITIS

Impingement is defined as compromise of the space between the coracoacromial arch and the proximal humerus.[65] Pain develops with laterally raising the arm. The pain may radiate to the insertion of the deltoid muscle on the humerus, or affected side, and increases the closer to 90° the patient raises his arm. Usually the earlier in the ROM arc the patient notices pain, the more chronic or severe the condition. Pain may also be experienced in the shoulder doing activities of daily living such as combing their hair or putting on a jacket.

Shoulder impingement in athletes is the most common shoulder injury due to throwing. It results from constant and long-term irritation of the anterior shoulder structure.[83] Impingement due to subacromial bursitis is common in patients with occupations or hobbies that increase stress within the glenohumeral joint. Sleeping on one side with the arm abducted to 180° has been known to create subacromial bursitis and subsequent impingement syndrome.

History and examination is performed noting any areas of inflammation and tenderness. Active and passive ROM arcs should be performed in each shoulder and the presence of any impingement signs noted. A positive impingement sign is if pain is produced in the last 10° to 15° of maximum passive forward flexion of the shoulder.[81] Also it is positive if pain is increased with forward flexion with internal rotation.[83]

Conservative treatment includes ice, active rest, NSAIDs, and rehabilitative exercises, concentrating on flexibility and correcting any muscular imbalances that might perpetuate the condition. The patient can normally return to normal activities, when the symptoms resolve and range of motion is full and pain-free.[83] In severe cases surgical intervention may be required.

Alternative care may include any single or combination therapies consisting of massage, yoga, manipulation, or acupuncture.

GENERAL MUSCLE SPRAIN OR STRAIN

A sprain is an injury to a ligament and can occur with or without tearing of the ligament. The amount of damage to the ligament in question determines the grade of the sprain. A strain is an injury to a tendon or muscle that occurs the same as a sprain. Some patients will have both, depending on the severity of the injury. A traumatic incident usually precedes the problem with localized inflammation around the area of injury that begins within hours of the trauma. Many times within days, the injured area will exhibit ecchymosis (redness). The amount of pain associated with the sprain or strain is not a good indication of the severity of the injury. In the event of a grade 3 sprain, the ligamentous fibers may be ruptured and are no longer intact to be stressed and cause pain.[84]

Sprains or strains are most likely caused by trauma or a breakdown in body mechanics. Sprains can be attributed to a traumatic twisting of a joint resulting in the stretching of the ligaments that stabilize the joint.[84]

Classically many tests are done to determine sprain versus strain test and the reaction to passive and active range of motion. Both sprain and strain may be painful with active movement due to the stress put on the tissues during movement. Ligamentous sprain will be painful during passive movements as well where strains will not elicit as much if any pain during passive movement due to the fact that the examiner is moving the affected area not the patient's muscles. The sprain or strain is assessed using Table 8.9.

With sprain or strain injuries, the protocol of rest, ice, compression, elevation (RICE) is used. Ice should be used intermittently with 30 min rest in between icing sessions. Ice should be kept on the affected area through all four phases of cold therapies: cold, burning, achy, and numb and then removal for 30 min before repeating. Elevation should be above the heart.

Chiropractic and osteopathic manipulation can be used to keep the affected joint in alignment during the healing process. If the joint is unstable and misaligned, the joint must be adjusted to the correct position in order for it to heal correctly.[83] Table 8.10 also summarizes the variety of herbal supplements that can be used to support pain relief and reduce inflammation for a number of inflammatory conditions.

TABLE 8.9
Assessment of Sprains

Classification	Type of Sprain	Signs and Symptoms
Grade 1	Mild or minimal sprain with no ligamentous tear	Mild tenderness with some swelling
Grade 2	Moderate sprain consisting of incomplete or partial rupture	Obvious swelling, ecchymosis (bruising), difficulty with movement
Grade 3	Complete ligamentous tear	Swelling, hemorrhage, ankle instability, inability to move affected limb

Source: From Beers, M.H. and Berkow, R., *The Merck Manual*, 17th ed., Merck & Co., Whitehouse Station, NJ, 1999.

TABLE 8.10
Herbs That Support Pain Relief and Reduced Inflammation

Anti-inflammatory herbs
  Arnica
  White willow bark
  Chamomile and yarrow
  St. John's wort
  Cayenne
  Turmeric
  Ginger
  Rosemary
Herbs for arthritis
  Butcher's broom
  Devil's claw
  Eucalyptus
  Licorice
  Chamomile
  Turmeric
  White willow bark
  Meadowsweet

Herbs to boost immune system function
  Astragalus
  Echinacea
  Garlic
  Shitake and reishi mushroom
Herbs to reduce joint and muscle pain
  Arnica
  Eucalyptus
  Mustard
  White willow bark
References: 91, 92

Herbals listed above include only those that have been shown to be effective and safe for healthy individuals. Those with questionable efficacy and safety are not listed.

SUMMARY

As discussed in this chapter, osteopenia and osteoporosis are highly preventable diseases. However, prevention must begin with optimizing BMD during adolescence and early adulthood. Postmenopausal women and other individuals with risk factors for developing osteoporosis should be screened according to established national guidelines. Furthermore, nutritional intake for the various nutrients discussed should be assessed to reduce risk. Proper nutritional intake is also vital in protecting joints from injury and in helping them heal. Nutrition is a preventive as well as a useful adjunct to treatment for many diseases that attack both the joints and bones. It should be noted that the standard allopathic approach has been the same for years, with many mainstream treatments coming relatively recently: NSAIDs, orthopedic devices, and surgery. The benefits of nutrition are only beginning to be appreciated, but will hopefully take a stronghold on mainstream medicine as an equally important aspect in disease prevention and treatment plans. Ideally, one should not place greater emphasis on any one particular aspect of health, but rather focus on achieving balance between all. Nutrition is vitally important, but alone does not lead to complete health. Finding balance between eating healthfully, leading an active lifestyle with regular physical activity, getting adequate sleep, and managing stress are also essential for preserving good overall health, including that of the bones and joints.

REFERENCES

1. NIH, Osteoporosis Prevention, Diagnosis and Treatment Consensus statement, March 27–29, 17 (1), 2000, pp. 1–36.
2. Sayegh, R.A. and Stubblefield, P.H., Bone metabolism and the perimenopause: overview, risk factors, screening, and osteoporosis preventive measure, *Obstet. Gynceol. Clin.*, 29, 495, 2002.
3. Heaney, R.P., Bone biology in health and disease, in Shills, M.E., Olson, J.A., and Russ, A.C., Eds., *Modern Nutrition in Health and Disease*, Lippincott, Williams & Wilkins, Philadelphia, PA, 1999, pp. 1327–1338.
4. Anderson, J.J.B., Nutrition for bone health, in Mahon, K.L. and Escott-Stump, S., Eds., *Krause's Food, Nutrition and Diet Therapy*, 10th ed., W.B. Saunders Company, Philadelphia, PA, 2000.
5. Mahon, K.L. and Escott-Stump, S., *Krause's Food, Nutrition and Diet Therapy*, 10th ed., W.B. Saunders Company, Philadelphia, PA, 2000.
6. Difference Between Normal Bone and Osteoporosis, All Refer.com Health web site, http://health.allref.com/pictures-images.osteoporosis.html. Accessed June 10, 2005.
7. Heaney, R.P., Calcium, dairy products and osteoporosis, *J. Am. Coll. Nutr.*, 19 (Suppl. 2), 83S, 2000.
8. Nordin, B.E., Calcium and osteoporosis, *Nutrition*, 12, 664, 1997.
9. Mora, S. and Gilsanz, V., Establishment of peak bone mass, *Endocrinol. Metab. Clin. North Am.*, 32, 39, 2003.
10. Dawson-Hughs, B. et al., Effect of calcium and vitamin D supplementation on bone density in men and women 65 years of age or older, *N. Engl. J. Med.*, 337, 670, 1997.
11. Chapuy, M. et al., Vitamin D and calcium to prevent hip fractures in elderly women, *N. Engl. J. Med.*, 327, 1637, 1992.
12. Groff, J.L. and Gropper, S.S., *Advanced Nutrition and Human Metabolism*, 3rd ed., Wadsworth Thomas Learning, Australia, 2000.
13. Tucker, K.L. et al., Potassium, magnesium, and fruit and vegetable intakes are associated with greater bone mineral density in elderly men and women, *Am. J. Clin. Nutr.*, 69, 727, 1999.
14. Tranquilli, A.L. et al., Calcium, phosphorus and magnesium intakes correlate with bone mineral content in postmenopausal women, *Gynecol. Endocrinol.*, 8, 55, 1994.
15. Martini, L.A., Magnesium supplementation and bone turnover, *Nutr. Rev.*, 57, 227, 1999.
16. Rude, R.K. and Olerich, M., Magnesium deficiency: possible role in osteoporosis associated with gluten-sensitive enteropathy, *Osteoporos. Int.*, 6, 453, 1996.

17. Calvo, M.S. and Park, Y.K., Changing phosphorus content of the U.S. diet: potential for adverse effects of bone, *J. Nutr.*, 126 (Suppl.), 1168S, 1996.
18. Marcic, M. and Gluck, O., Update in the management of osteoporosis, *J. Musculoskel. Med.*, 18, 407, 2002.
19. Nieves, J.W., Osteoporosis: the role of micronutrients, *Am. J. Clin. Nutr.*, 81, 1232S, 2005.
20. Nielson, F.H. et al., Boron enhances and mimics some effects of estrogen therapy in postmenopausal women, *J. Trace Elements Exp. Med.*, 5, 23, 1992.
21. Barrie, S.A. et al., Comparative absorption of zinc picolinate, zinc citrate and zinc gluconate in humans, *Agents Actions*, 21, 223, 1987.
22. Howard, G. et al., Low serum copper, a risk factor additional to low dietary calcium in postmenopausal bone loss, *J. Trace Elements Exp. Med.*, 91, 23, 1992.
23. Lau, E.M. and Woo, J., Nutrition and osteoporosis, *Curr. Opin. Rheumatol.*, 10, 368, 1998.
24. Kiel, D.P. et al., Caffeine and the risk of hip fracture: the Framingham Study, *Am. J. Epidemiol.*, 60, 132, 1990.
25. Rapuri, P.B. et al., Caffeine intake increases the rate of bone loss in elderly women and interacts with vitamin D receptor genotypes, *Am. J. Clin. Nutr.*, 74, 694, 2001.
26. Devine, A. et al., A longitudinal study of the effect of sodium and calcium intakes on regional bone density in postmenopausal women, *Am. J. Clin. Nutr.*, 62, 740, 1995.
27. Hopper, J. and Seeman, E., The bone density of female twins discordant for tobacco use, *N. Engl. J. Med.*, 330, 387, 1994.
28. Law, M.R. and Hackshaw, A.K., A meta-analysis of smoking, bone mineral density, and risk of hip fracture: Recognition of a major effect, *BMJ*, 315, 841, 1997.
29. Chamberlain, L. and Wernick, H., *The Seven Silver Bullets. A Consumer's Guide to Vital Health and Longevity, Webfoot press*, 2000, pp. 40–42.
30. Fitzpatrick, L.A., Secondary causes of osteoporosis, *Mayo. Clin. Proc.*, 77, 453, 2002.
31. Lloyd, T. et al., Modifiable determinants of bone status in young women, *Bone*, 30, 416, 2002.
32. Cummings, S.R. et al., Risk factors for hip fractures in white women. Study of Osteoporotic Fractures Research Group, *N. Engl. J. Med.*, 332, 767, 1995.
33. Cussler, E.C. et al., Weight lifted in strength training predicts bone change in postmenopausal women, *Med. Sci. Sports Exerc.*, 35, 10, 2003.
34. Miller, K.K. and Klibanski, A., Clinical review 106: amenorrheic bone loss, *J. Clin. Endocrinol. Metab.*, 84, 1755, 1999.
35. Cauley, J.A. et al., Estrogen replacement therapy and fractures in older women. Study of Osteoporotic Fractures Research Group, *Ann. Intern. Med.*, 122, 9, 1995.
36. Kiel, D.P. et al., Hip fracture and the use of estrogens in postmenopsausal women. The Framingham Study, *N. Engl. J. Med.*, 317, 1160, 1987.
37. Genant, H.K., Baylink, D.J., and Gallagher, J.C., Estrogens in the prevention of osteoporosis in postmenopausal women, *Am. J. Obstet. Gynecol.*, 161, 1842, 1989.
38. Dick, S.E., DeWitt, D.E., and Anawalt, B.D., Postmenopausal hormone replacement therapy and major clinical outcomes: a focus on cardiovascular disease, osteoporosis, dementia, and breast and endometrial neoplasia, *Am. J. Manag. Care*, 8, 95, 2002.
39. National Osteoporosis Foundation, *Physicians Guide to Prevention and Treatment of Osteoporosis*, Exerpta Medica Inc., Belle Meade, NJ, 1999.
40. Kkulak, C.A. and Bilezikian, J.P., Osteoporosis: preventive strategies, *Int. J. Fertil. Womens Med.*, 43, 56, 1998.
41. Lewis, R.D. and Moolesky, C.M., Nutrition, physical activity, and bone health in women, *Int. J. Sport Nutr.*, 8, 250, 1998.
42. Blake, G.M. and Fogelman, I., Bone densitometry, steroids and osteoporosis, *Curr. Opin. Nephrol. Hypertens.*, 11, 641, 2002.
43. Lo, B.P., Hebert, C., and McClean, A., The female athlete triad — no pain, no gain? *Clin. Pediatr.*, 42, 573, 2003.
44. Lentle, B.C. and Prior, J.C., Osteoporosis: what a clinician expects to learn from a patient's bone density examination, *Radiology*, 228, 620, 2003.

45. Cromer, B. and Harel, Z., Adolescents: at increased risk for osteoporosis? *Clin. Pediatr.*, 39, 565, 2000.
46. Feskanich, D., Willett, W., and Colditz, G., Walking and leisure-time activity and risk of hip fracture in postmenopausal women, *JAMA*, 288, 2300, 2002.
47. Theodosakis, T., Edderly, B., and Fox, B., *The Arthritis Cure*, 1st ed., St. Martin's Press, New York, 1997, chap.2.
48. Souza, T.A., *Differential Diagnosis for the Chiropractor*, Aspen Publications, Gaithersburg, MD, 1998.
49. Martini, F.H., *Fundamentals of Anatomy and physiology*, 3rd ed., Englewood cliffs, New Jersey, 1995.
50. Birchfield, P., Osteoarthritis overview, *Geriatric. Nurs.*, 22, 124, 2001.
51. Mayo Clinic Health Letter, *Arthritis Medical Essay* (*Supplement to Mayo Clinic Health Letter*), Mayo Foundation for Medical Education and Research, Rochester, MN, 2001.
52. Beers, M.H. and Berkow, R., *The Merck Manual*, 17th ed., Merck & Co., Whitehouse Station, NJ, 1999.
53. Peltonen, K. et al., Faecal microbial flora and disease activity in rheumatoid arthritis during a vegan diet, *Br. J. Rheumatol.*, 36, 64, 1997.
54. Kjeldsen-Kragh, K. et al., Controlled trial of fasting and one-year vegetarian diet in rheumatoid arthritis, *Lancet*, 338, 89, 1991.
55. D'Angelo, G. et al., Probiotics in childhood, *Minerva Pediatr.*, 50, 163, 1998.
56. McDougall, J. et al., Effects of a very low-fat, vegan diet in subjects with rheumatoid arthritis, *J. Altern. Complement Med.*, 8, 71, 2002.
57. Haugen, M.A. et al., Changes in plasma phospholipid fatty acids and their relationship to disease activity in rheumatoid arthritis patients treated with a vegetarian diet, *Br. J. Nutr.*, 72, 555, 1994.
58. Rovenska, E. et al., Inhibitory effect of enzyme therapy and combination therapy with cyclosporin A on collagen-induced arthritis, *Clin. Exp. Rheumatol.*, 19, 303, 2001.
59. Desser, L. et al., Oral therapy with proteolytic enzymes decreases excessive TGF-beta levels in human blood, *Cancer Chemother. Pharmacol.*, 47, S10, 2001.
60. Pelton, R. et al., *Drug-Induced Nutrient Depletion Handbook, 1999–2000*, American Pharmaceutical Association, Lexi-Comp, Inc. and Natural Health Resources, Inc., Cincinnati, OH, 1999.
61. Physician's Desk Reference, *The PDR Pocket Guide to Prescription Drugs*, 3rd ed., Simon & Schuster, Inc., New York, NY, 1998.
62. Vickerstaff Joneja, J., *Managing Food Allergy and Intolerance: A Practical Guide*, McQuaid Consulting Group, Inc., Canada, 1995.
63. Murray, M. and Pizzorno, J., *Encyclopedia of Natural Medicine*, 2nd ed., Prima Publishing, Rocklin, CA, 1998.
64. Consumer Lab web site, http://www.consumerlab.com. Accessed December 3, 2002.
65. Meiner, S.E., Gouty arthritis: not just a big toe problem, *Geriatric. Nurs.*, 22, 132, 2001.
66. Abrams, W.B., Beers, M.H., and Berkow, R., Eds., *The Merck Manual of Geriatrics*, 2nd ed., Merck & Co, Inc., Whitehouse Station, NJ, 1995.
67. Ewald, G.A. and McKenzie, C.R., Eds., *Manual of Medical Therapeutics*, 28th ed., Little, Brown and Company, Boston, MA, 1995.
68. Seegmiller, J.E., Loaster, L., and Howell, R.R., Biochemistry of uric acid and its relations to gout, *N. Engl. J. Med.*, 168, 712, 1963.
69. National Institute of Arthritis and Musculoskeletal and Skin Diseases (NIAMS) web site, http://www.niams.nih.gov. Accessed October 13, 2002.
70. DeLee, J.C. and Drez, D., *Orthopaedic Sports Medicine Principals and Practice*, W.B. Saunders company 1994, pp. 524, 558, 863, 998.
71. Ilrich, J. and Kerstetter, J.E., Nutrition in bone health revisited: a story beyond calcium, *J. Am. Coll. Nutr.*, 6, 715, 2000.
72. Rakel, D., Ed., *Integrative Medicine*, Elsevier Science, Philadelphia, PA, 2003.
73. Murray, R.K. et al., *Harper's Biochemistry*, 23rd ed., Appleton & Lange, Norwalk, CT, 1993.
74. The Institute for Functional Medicine, *Nutritional Management of Inflammatory Disorders*, HealthComm International, Inc., Washington, D.C., 1998.
75. Beauparlant, P. and Hiscott, J. Biological and biochemical inhibitors of the NF-kappa B/Rel proteins and cytokine synthesis, *Cytokine Growth Factor Rev.*, 7, 175, 1996.

76. Chudwin, D.S. et al., Sensitivity to non-acetylated salicylates in a patient with asthma, nasal polyps, and rheumatoid arthritis, *Ann. Allergy*, 57, 133, 1986.
77. Lewis, A.S. et al., Inhibition of mammalian xanthine oxidase by folate compounds and amethopterin, *J. Biol. Chem.*, 259, 12, 1984.
78. Vane, J.R., The fight against rheumatism: from willow bark to cox-1 sparing drugs, *J. Physiol. Pharmacol.*, 51, 573, 2000.
79. Metcalfe, D.D. et al., *Adverse Reactions to Foods and Food Additives*, Blackwell Scientific Publication, Oxford, London, 1991.
80. Kjeldsen-Kragh, J., Rheumatoid arthritis treated with vegetarian diets, *Am. J. Clin. Nutr.*, 70, 594S, 1999.
81. Nenomen, J. et al., Uncooked, lactobacilli-rich, vegan food and rheumatoid arthritis, *Br. J. Rheumatol.*, 37, 274, 1998.
82. Kessler, R. and Hertling, D., *Management of Common Musculoskeletal Disorders*, Harper & Row, Philadelphia, PA, 1983, p. 487.
83. Fu, F.H. and Stone, D.A., *Sports Injuries — Mechanics, Prevention, Treatment*, 1994, pp. 195, 931, 946, 995.
84. Magri, G., Strains vs. Sprains, www.coloradostorm.com/healthsouth, 1–3. Accessed October 2002.
85. Healthy Roads, What is a Sprain/Strain Injury, www.healthyroads.com. Accessed October 2002.
86. The Natural Pharmacist web site, http://www.naturalpharmacist.com. Accessed October 13, 2002.
87. D'Ambrosio, E. et al., Glucosamine sulfate: a controlled clinical investigation in arthrosis, *Pharmatherapeutica*, 2, 504, 1981.
88. Vaz, A.L., Double-blind clinical evaluation of the relative efficacy of glucosamine sulphate in the management of osteoarthritis of the knee in out-patients, *Curr. Med. Res. Opin.*, 8, 145, 1982.
89. Pujalte, J.M. et al., Double-blind clinical evaluation of oral glucosamine sulphate in the basic treatment of osteoarthritis, *Curr. Med. Res. Opin.*, 7, 110, 1980.
90. Bradley, J.K. et al., A randomized, double-blind, placebo controlled trial of intravenous loading with *S*-adenosyl methionine (SAM) followed by oral SAM therapy in patients with knee osteoarthritis, *J. Rheumatol.*, 21, 905, 1994.
91. Klein, G. and Kullich, W., Reducing pain by oral enzyme therapy in rheumatic diseases, *Wien. Med. Wochenschr.*, 149, 577, 1999.
92. Tyler, V.E. and Robbers, J.E., *Herbs of Choice: The Therapeutic Use of Phytomedicinals*, Haworth Herbal Press, Binghamton, NY, 1999.
93. Black, D. M. and Thompson, D.E., The effect of alendronate therapy on osteoporotic fracture in the vertebral fracture arm of the Fracture Intervention Trial, *Int. J. Clin. Pract. Suppl.*, 101: 46, 1999.
94. Tonino, R.P. et al., Skeletal benefits of alendronate: 7-year treatment of postmenopausal osteoporotic women. Phase III Osteoporosis Treatment Study Group, *J. Clin. Endocrinol. metab.*, 85(9): 3109, 2000.

Ellen Augur and Mary Atkinson

CONTENTS

INTRODUCTION

Cardiovascular disease (CVD) is the leading cause of morbidity and mortality in the United States, responsible for about one in three deaths per year.[1] These findings are not limited to the United States, however, as it is also the leading cause of death in other developed nations.[2] CVD accounts for approximately 50% more deaths than all cancers combined.[1] With over 500,000 deaths and 1 million myocardial infarctions (MI) occurring every year as a result of CVD, early detection of modifiable risk factors and appropriate interventions are crucial to the reduction of this potentially fatal disease.[3,4] These findings suggest that early detection of modifiable risk factors and appropriate interventions are essential. Numerous observational and prevention studies have identified many such risk factors, of which dyslipidemia is the most significant.

The relationship between lowering low-density lipoprotein cholesterol (LDL-C) levels and the reduction in the rates of coronary events has been well established. The dietary approaches to stop hypertension (DASH) trial showed marked improvement in blood pressure, independent of sodium intake, with the intake of a plant-based, high-fiber diet. The Scandinavian Simvastatin Survival Study (4S) was one of the first major trials to demonstrate the effect of lowering LDL-C on CVD.[5,6] The National Cholesterol Education Program (NCEP) has used this overwhelming trial evidence to recommend two methods for correcting dyslipidemia as well as reducing other CVD risk factors. Therapeutic lifestyle changes (TLC) are recommended as a method of primary and secondary prevention. This approach to diet therapy relies on the inclusion of many cardioprotective foods.[5] Drug therapies are generally recommended as secondary prevention for individuals who have been unable to correct dyslipidemia with TLC, or for those with multiple risk factors and LDL-C >130 mg/dl.[7]

EPIDEMIOLOGY

Researchers have identified risk factors that are highly correlated to the development of CVD. These can be separated into modifiable and nonmodifiable risk factors. Modifiable factors include hypertension, cigarette smoking, diabetes, obesity, physical inactivity, and an atherogenic diet. Nonmodifiable factors include age, sex, and family history.[7]

Age is highly correlated to CVD. With 85% of CVD mortalities occurring in individuals over 65 years of age, this group should be treated with primary prevention strategies regardless of symptoms.[6] Although CVD accounts for approximately 30% of all fatalities among women, men continue to be at greater risk for the development of CVD.[6] The reasons for this are still not fully understood, but may be linked to the development of dyslipidemias and hypertension at an earlier age. Premature development of CVD appears to be familial.[7] For these individuals, as well as for patients with hyperlipidemia not responding to TLC or drug therapies, LDL apheresis is a new and effective means of reducing elevated LDL-C levels. LDL apheresis will be discussed further later in the chapter.[8]

Cigarette smoking and physical inactivity have been identified as risk factors because of their influence on high-density lipoprotein cholesterol (HDL-C) levels.[9] Smoking cessation may produce a 30% increase in HDL-C within a short period after quitting. Increasing physical activity also increases HDL-C,[3] and is correlated to a reduction in blood pressure as well.[10]

Approximately 22% of the U.S. population is affected by metabolic syndrome.[4] It is characterized by the following group of metabolic risk factors, abdominal obesity, hypertension, dyslipidemia, and type 2 diabetes. Obesity for this purpose is defined as a body mass index (BMI) ≥30, hypertension is defined as ≥130/85 mmHg, and dyslipidemia is defined as triglycerides (TG) $\geq$150 and HDL-C <40 for males and HDL-C <50 for females.[4] This syndrome is associated with insulin resistance that in turn is associated with an increased production of very low-density lipoprotein cholesterol (VLDL-C).[3,9] The recommended treatment for this syndrome is resolution of the underlying causes, such as obesity and dyslipidemia, through the treatment of the risk factors, such as increasing HDL-C levels or improving glycemic control.[3]

Obesity, whether an independent risk factor or linked with others as in metabolic syndrome, is one of the most influential and modifiable risk factors. Obesity is a function of inappropriate dietary intake, physical inactivity, and genetics. The Centers of Disease Control and Prevention (CDC) estimate that 60% of adults are not regularly physically active and that 30% of the U.S. population is obese (BMI over 30 kg/m^2).[11,12] Evidence indicates that increased physical activity may positively affect weight and that weight loss of only 5–10% can positively affect glycemic control, blood pressure, and lipid levels. Therefore diet therapy and increased physical activity are appropriate primary intervention for addressing this health issue.[13]

A HISTORICAL PERSPECTIVE OF CARDIOVASCULAR DISEASE

LDL-C has long been identified as the primary atherogenic lipoprotein that leads to CVD.[3] Under normal conditions LDL-C binds to plasma membranes. When plasma levels exceed normal, LDL-C particles become oxidized and are picked up by macrophages which, through the release of various substances, begin the formation of atheromas.[14] Numerous studies over the past decade indicate that lipid-lowering therapies, both pharmacological and non-pharmacological, are effective means of reducing cardiovascular events. Although recommendations have always focused on the reduction of total cholesterol (TC), guidelines published in May 2001 place a greater emphasis on reducing LDL-C through the inclusion of cardioprotective foods versus the exclusion of harmful foods and food groups.[5]

In 1985, the National Institutes of Health (NIH) created the NCEP to address the increasing problem of hypercholesterolemia. The NCEP published its first set of guidelines in 1988[3] that merely focused on optimal lipid levels, but provided no specific recommendations on how to achieve them. In 1993, the NCEP released its new guidelines for the treatment of dyslipidemia in the form of the Step I and Step II diets[3] that were endorsed by the American Heart Association (AHA). The goal of the Step I and II diets was to reduce both TC and LDL-C based on studies that indicated a decrease in CVD with an improvement in lipid profiles. Step I was recommended for patients with elevated cholesterol as a primary prevention. Step II was recommended as a secondary prevention for patients with a history of MI, as a primary prevention for patients with TC $\geq$240 mg/dl, or when Step I failed to produce the lipid-lowering results desired.[15]

Both diets recommended the reduction of total fat and cholesterol intake. With Step I, total fat intake was to be less than 30% of total calories, saturated fat less than 10% of total calories, and cholesterol intake was to be less than 300 mg/day. Step II further restricted the intake of total fat, saturated fat, and cholesterol to less than 25%, 7%, and 200 mg/day, respectively.[15] The guidelines were accompanied by the recommendations to avoid foods high in total fat and saturated fats, and to limit the intake of salt and simple or processed carbohydrates.

Despite the NCEP's recommendations to decrease fat intake, dyslipidemias, obesity, and CVD-related morbidity and mortality continued to be a major health concern for the American population. Observational studies, such as the National Health and Nutritional Examination Survey III (NHANES III), completed after the NCEP released its second set of guidelines, indicated that the American population had indeed decreased their fat intake from

40% in the 1960s to less than 35% in the 1990s.[5] However, people were now consuming a greater amount of total calories in the form of simple and processed carbohydrates. A decrease in physical activity accompanied this increased caloric intake. These two factors combined to produce a population with increasing rates of hypertriglyceridemia, low-HDL-C levels, and obesity. It became evident that the recommendations to restrict or eliminate foods, which often leaves the patient feeling deprived, were not without drawbacks. Questionable patient compliance was one of the major drawbacks of these diet therapies. With more than a dozen studies indicating the positive effects of altering even one of these indicators, NCEP strove to develop more effective guidelines for the treatment of CVD.

CURRENT RECOMMENDATIONS FOR THE TREATMENT OF CARDIOVASCULAR DISEASE

Early detection and intervention are essential components in the control of CVD morbidity and mortality. Recent trials have produced enough epidemiologic evidence to clearly establish risk factors that are linked to its development. Determining an individual's risk category will help clinicians develop the most appropriate treatment methodologies for patients. The three risk categories as defined by the NCEP Adult Treatment Panel (ATP) III are established CVD or CVD equivalent, multiple risk factors, and 0–1 risk factors.[7]

NCEP ATP III recommends beginning with an evaluation of an individual's independent risk factors followed by an assessment of 10-year risk as necessary.[7] The independent risk factors include:

- Cigarette smoking
- Hypertension (BP $\geq$ 140/90)
- HDL-C < 40 mg/dl (HDL-C $\geq$ 60 mg/dl counts as a negative risk factor)
- Family history (CVD in males <55 years; CVD in females <65 years)
- Age ($\geq$45 males; $\geq$55 females)

If an individual has 0–1 risk factors, evaluation of their LDL-C is necessary to determine appropriate treatment. If their LDL-C < 160, TLC is recommended as primary prevention. For individuals, an LDL-C > 160, drug therapy, in addition to TLC, is recommended. If an individual possesses more than two independent risk factors, a 10-year risk score should be calculated using the Framingham risk score.[7]

The Framingham 10-year risk assessment was developed for individuals with multiple risk factors to further assess their risk for development of CVD. It was developed by The Framingham Heart Study, an observational study launched in 1943, designed to identify similar characteristics across a sample population that developed CVD.[16] It identified a correlation between lipid levels, age, sex, blood pressure, cigarette smoking, and CVD. From the study came a comprehensive scoring mechanism that was able to estimate an individual's 10-year risk for the development of a CVD-related event. Table 9.1 shows the Framingham point scores for both males and females. The Framingham score takes into account an individual's age, TC, HDL-C level, smoking status, and systolic blood pressure. An individual with a 10-year risk of less than 10% is considered to be at low to moderate risk, while a 10-year risk score of 10–20% is considered high risk. Individuals with a 10-year risk score more than 20% are at the highest risk, equal to those patients with CVD. This is termed a CVD risk equivalent.[4] Other CVD risk equivalents include type 2 diabetes and noncoronary atherosclerosis. The same treatments should be applied to individuals with CVD risk equivalents as those with CVD.[7]

TABLE 9.1
Framingham Risk Assessment (10-Year Risk)

Age	Points Men	Points Women	Age	Points Men	Points Women
20–34	−9	−7	55–59	8	8
35–39	−4	−3	60–64	10	10
40–44	0	0	65–69	11	12
45–49	3	3	70–74	12	14
50–54	6	6	75–79	13	16

Total Cholesterol	Points at Ages 20–39		Points at Ages 40–49		Points at Ages 50–59		Points at Ages 60–69		Points at Ages 70–79	
	Men	Women	Men	Women	Men	Women	Men	Women	Men	Women
<160	0	0	0	0	0	0	0	0	0	0
160–199	4	4	3	3	2	2	1	1	0	1
200–239	7	8	5	6	3	4	1	2	0	1
240–279	9	11	6	8	4	5	2	3	1	2
≥280	11	13	8	10	5	7	3	4	1	2

	Points at Ages 20–39		Points at Ages 40–49		Points at Ages 50–59		Points at Ages 60–69		Points at Ages 70–79	
	Men	Women	Men	Women	Men	Women	Men	Women	Men	Women
Nonsmoker	0	0	0	0	0	0	0	0	0	0
Smoker	8	9	5	7	3	4	1	2	1	1

Continued

TABLE 9.1 (Continued)
Framingham Risk Assessment (10-Year Risk)

HDL	Points	
	Men	Women
≥60	−1	−1
50–59	0	0
40–49	1	1
<40	2	2

Systolic BP	If Untreated		If Treated	
	Men	Women	Men	Women
<120	0	0	0	0
120–129	0	1	1	3
130–139	1	2	2	4
140–159	1	3	2	5
≥160	2	4	3	6

Point Total		10-Year Risk (%)	
Men	Women	Men	Women
<0	<9	<1	<1
1	9	1	1
2	10	1	1
3	11	1	1
4	12	1	1
5	13	2	2
6	14	2	2
7	15	3	3
8	16	4	4
9	17	5	5
10	18	6	6
11	19	8	8
12	20	10	11
13	21	12	14
14	22	16	17
15	23	20	22
16	24	25	27
≥17	≥25	≥30	≥30

The NCEP ATP III has used evidence-based information to develop new lipid level guidelines to aid in the treatment of CVD. Evidence from studies such as the 4S, the West of Scotland Coronary Prevention Study (WOSCOPS), and the Air Force/Texas Coronary Atherosclerosis Prevention Study (AFCAPS/TexCAPS) demonstrating the positive reduction in coronary events with the reduction in LDL-C led the ATP III to its current LDL-C recommendations, which are separated by risk category. LDL-C for individuals with 0–1 risk factor should be less than 160 mg/dl; LDL-C for those with multiple risk factors should be less than 130 mg/dl; while LDL-C for people with CVD or a CVD equivalent should be less than 100 mg/dl.[6,7] HDL-C, often referred to as the "good" cholesterol, is considered a negative risk factor because of its anti-inflammatory and antiatherogenic properties.[6] Studies such as the Helsinki Heart Study revealed that CVD could be positively affected by increasing HDL-C. More specifically, an increase in HDL-C of 1 mg/dl may equate to as much as a 2–3% decrease in CVD.[6] ATP III concurs with these findings and recommends HDL-C levels be more than 40 mg/dl for the greatest reduction in CVD risk.[9] Whether or not TG levels should be considered an independent risk factor for CVD remains unclear. It appears that there may be some triglyceride-rich lipoproteins that lead to atherosclerosis, including VLDL-C and intermediate-density lipoprotein (IDL-C). For this reason, the ATP III recommends that TG levels less than 150 mg/dl are optimal.[7] Table 9.2 summarizes the ATP III's recommendation for lipid levels.

The NCEP and the AHA continue to support the Step I diet for the general public, however, for those people with CVD or with CVD risk factors, the NCEP ATP III recommends the TLC diet.[15] ATP III recommends primarily focusing on the reduction of LDL-C, but does acknowledge the positive impact of lowering TG and raising HDL-C to desired ranges. In general, the TLC diet recommends correcting lipid levels through the increased consumption of plant-based nutrient-rich foods.[7]

Based on the new lipid level guidelines, NCEP developed a new and innovative approach to diet therapy. NCEP ATP III recommends the TLC diet as a primary prevention as well as a part of all secondary interventions. The TLC diet includes foods that have been shown to improve cardiovascular health rather than merely excluding those that increase the risk of CVD. The TLC diet is based on the Mediterranean diet that includes considerably more plant-based foods than are traditionally included in the American diet. It also provides recommendations regarding vitamins and minerals, herbal supplementation, weight loss, physical activity, smoking, and alcohol intake.

TABLE 9.2
Optimal Lipid Profile

Lipid Constituent	Optimal Level
Total cholesterol	<200 mg/dl
LDL-C	<160 mg/dl (0–1 risk factors)
	<130 mg/dl (multiple risk factors)
	<100 mg/dl (CHD or CHD equivalent)
HDL-C	>40 mg/dl
TG	<150 mg/dl

Source: From National Cholesterol Education Program, Third report of the expert panel on detection, evaluation, and treatment of high blood cholesterol in adults (Adult Treatment Panel III), NIH Pub. No.02-5215, National Heart, Lung, and Blood Institute, Bethesda, MD, 2002.

The recommendation to limit the intake of saturated fats remains constant, but the methodology to achieve this goal is dramatically different. ATP III has somewhat liberalized its recommendation for the intake of fat to 25–35% of total calories and places an emphasis on the increased intake of monounsaturated and polyunsaturated fats,[5] up to 20% of total calories may come from monounsaturated fats, and up to 10% of total calories may come from polyunsaturated fats.[7] Because diets high in saturated fats and cholesterol are linked to the development of CVD, ATP III continues to recommend limiting saturated fat to less than 7% of total calories and cholesterol to less than 200 mg/day.[3] By emphasizing the intake of a more cardioprotective macronutrient, an acceptable fat alternative is offered. *Trans*-fatty acids have no specific recommendations but should be considered as a saturated fat and their intake should be limited.[5]

Fiber acts as a lipid-lowering agent through its ability to inhibit the absorption of bile acid in the intestines. The American Dietetic Association (ADA) recommends 15 g of fiber per 1000 calories.[17] ATP III recommends fiber intake in daily terms, equating to 20–30 g of fiber per day. Plant sterols and stanols have similar cholesterol-lowering effects and ATP III recommends foods such as peanuts and soybeans, which are good sources of these nutrients, in order to achieve an intake of 2 g/day.[3]

Carbohydrate intake exceeding 60% of total daily calories has been linked to the development of hypertriglyceridemia.[7] Therefore, ATP III recommends that the percentage of daily calories from carbohydrate be less than 60%. There has been a great deal of debate over low-carbohydrate diets. While the discussion about fad diets is to follow, ATP III, as well as the ADA and AHA, take the position that low-carbohydrate diets are of no benefit to CVD.[7] Regarding protein intake, ATP III does recommend the replacement of animal proteins with soy protein sources up to 25 g/day and to increase the consumption of fish rich in omega-3 fatty acids to two to three servings per week.[7]

Vitamin and mineral supplementation continues to be of great interest and is the subject of recent studies. Folate, vitamin B-6, and vitamin B-12 seem to be inversely related to homocysteine levels.[2] The relationship between elevated homocysteine levels and CVD will be discussed in greater detail later in this chapter. Despite the seemingly strong correlation between folate, homocysteine, and CVD-related events, ATP III recommends adhering to the recommended dietary allowances (RDAs) of 400 µg/day. The same recommendation is true for vitamin C and vitamin E, which are often recommended in higher doses because of their antioxidant properties. Herbal supplementation of any type is not recommended by the ATP III.[7]

The current guidelines for alcohol and sodium intake remain exclusionary. ATP III continues to encourage limiting sodium intake to less than 2.4 g/day.[7] However, with the inclusion of more plant-based foods in order to meet the fiber recommendations, the reduction of high sodium foods should follow. There is evidence that moderate consumption of alcohol can have a positive effect on CVD. While the mechanism remains unclear, quantity is the key factor. Individuals who currently do not consume alcohol are not encouraged to begin drinking alcohol, but for those who consume alcohol, it is recommended to limit intake to one drink per day for women, and two drinks per day for men. A drink is the equivalent of 12 oz of beer, 5 oz of wine, or 1 oz to 1.5 oz of liquor.

Recommendations for weight loss and increased physical activity are also essential parts of the TLC program. Weight loss is encouraged to achieve a desirable weight defined as a BMI <25 kg/m^2, and daily physical activity is encouraged for improved health and well-being. The Surgeon General and CDC recommend moderate-intensity physical activity for 30 min or more most days of the week.[12] Increased physical activity combined with weight loss positively affects a number of risk factors associated with CVD. While increased physical activity results in improved HDL-C levels, improved blood pressure, and weight loss, the loss of excess weight produces a decrease in LDL-C and TG levels, improved glycemic control, and a lowered blood pressure. When viewed as a causal relationship, it becomes very clear why the ATP III has selected weight loss and increased physical activity as important components of TLC aimed at reducing the occurrence of CVD-related events.

The risk categories and lipid guidelines developed by the NCEP ATP III assist clinicians in the assessment of patients and in the development of appropriate treatment plans. The two treatment methods, the TLC diet and drug therapy, have both been shown to be efficacious in the treatment of CVD. The new inclusionary approach to diet therapy is aimed at improving patient compliance while reducing the incidences of CVD-related morbidity and mortality.

FOODS AND THEIR EFFECTS ON CARDIOVASCULAR DISEASE

Of particular interest is the role of foods and specific properties of foods in chronic disease prevention and treatment. Significant research has been devoted to diet and nutrition and their relation to disease risk. Both epidemiological and clinical studies have shown the impact of diet and nutrition on chronic disease. As mentioned previously, treatment and prevention of CVD begins with nutritional interventions. TLC emphasizes the importance of diet and nutrition as the first-line treatment for most patients with CVD.

FAT

Fat is of particular importance to CVD prevention and treatment. Saturated fats, monounsaturated fats, and polyunsaturated fats have differing effects on serum lipid levels and atherosclerosis.

SATURATED FATTY ACIDS

Saturated fatty acids are those with single bonds between carbons on the fatty acid chain. Predominate saturated fats are palmitic, stearic, myristic, and lauric. Stearic acid has little effect on serum cholesterol levels, while myristic and palmitic have the greatest effects on lipoprotein concentrations.[18] Sources of saturated fatty acids in the U.S. diet are dairy products, meats, palm and coconut oils, palm kernel oil, and shortening. Studies evaluating the effects of saturated fat on the risk of coronary artery disease estimate that replacement of 5% of total caloric intake from saturated fat with polyunsaturated fat would reduce risk for the disease by 42%.[19] For every 1% increase in calories from saturated fat, LDL-C may increase 2% and vice versa.[7] Saturated fat may work to increase LDL-C concentrations by decreasing LDL-C receptor-mediated catabolism.[18] Studies in vascular function using flow-mediated vasodilation have also shown that saturated fats impair vascular function.[5]

TRANS-FATTY ACIDS

Trans-fatty acids are produced from naturally occurring fatty acids in the *cis*-configuration by hydrogenating carbon–carbon double bonds to create a semisolid product such as margarine or vegetable shortening. Elaidic acid is the most common *trans*-fatty acid in the U.S. diet, with major sources being baked products, processed foods, and margarines rich in hydrogenated fats or oils.[18]

Trans-fatty acid is the latest culprit in blood lipid alteration. New evidence has surfaced that these fatty acids more negatively affect blood lipid levels and CVD risk when replacing saturated fats in the diet. *Trans*-fatty acids increase LDL-C while reducing protective HDL-C. When replacing 10% of total caloric intake from saturated fats with *trans*-fatty acids,

HDL-C decreased 15%.[9] Substituting *trans*-fatty acids with *cis*-unsaturated fatty acids is associated with a 50% risk reduction for CVD.[20] Importantly, *trans*-fatty acids have been shown to increase lipoprotein(a), an apolipoprotein that doubles the risk of CVD when elevated above normal blood levels.[18]

MONOUNSATURATED FATTY ACIDS

Monounsaturated fatty acids are those in which there is only one double bond between carbons on the fatty acid chain. Oleic acid is the most common of these acids present in olive and canola oils, nuts, and avocados.[7] Oleic acid makes up approximately 13% of energy of average U.S. diets.[18] Unfortunately, monounsaturated fatty acids are present in a large number of food products that are also high in saturated fat. Therefore, research and diet intervention results can be confounded when increasing sources of both monounsaturated and saturated fats. In fact, there are no controlled clinical trials comparing monounsaturated and saturated fatty acids with cardiovascular end points.[7]

When substituted for saturated fats, monounsaturated fats have a cholesterol-lowering effect on both LDL-C and HDL-C levels. These hypocholesterolemic effects are not as potent as the effects of polyunsaturated fatty acids (PUFA). Replacing saturated fats with monounsaturated fats in epidemiological studies has shown a 30% reduction in coronary heart disease (CHD) risk, which is three times more effective than replacing saturated fats with carbohydrates.[20] This may be important when developing diet interventions for cardiovascular patients, especially when considering alternate choices for foods high in saturated fat.

POLYUNSATURATED FATTY ACIDS

Research has been largely devoted to the effects of polyunsaturated fats on CVD and atherosclerosis. Both epidemiological and nutrition intervention studies evidence cardioprotective effects of these fats. Taken as a whole, PUFAs decrease LDL-C when replacing saturated fatty acids.[7] As mentioned previously, polyunsaturated fats have a greater effect in decreasing serum lipid levels than monounsaturated fats. Polyunsaturated fats are divided into two categories: omega-3 (linolenic acid) and omega-6 (linoleic acid). The difference between the two is in the placement of the double bond from the end of the carbon chain. The optimal dietary ratio between omega-6 fatty acids and omega-3 fatty acids for CVD prevention is roughly four to one.[18] The DASH diet resulted in the conclusion that replacing saturated fat with polyunsaturated fats can decrease LDL-C by 18 mg/dl.[9]

OMEGA-3 FATTY ACIDS

Alpha-linolenic acid is the most prevalent omega-3 fatty acid. Alpha-linolenic acid is an essential fatty acid not biologically synthesized in the body. This fat is a precursor for eicosapentaenoic acid and docosahexaenoic acid. The major source of omega-3 fatty acids is fish and fish oils. Other sources of alpha-linolenic acid, important to individuals refusing to consume fish or fish oil, are seeds, nuts, or vegetable oils such as soybean, canola, or flaxseed.[21]

Epidemiological and interventional studies have repeatedly shown a significant, inverse relationship between alpha-linolenic acid and CVD. Alpha-linolenic acid is cardioprotective for reasons beyond lipid-altering properties. Omega-3 fatty acids decrease platelet aggregation and inflammatory markers in atherosclerotic processes, improve cardiac rhythm, and decrease serum TG.[7] These factors contribute to improved vascular function, serum lipid levels, and secondary coronary disease prevention. Heart disease risk prediction studies indicate a relative risk of 0.35 with a 1% increase in energy intake from alpha-linolenic acid.[20] The inverse association between omega-3 fatty acid and CVD is more significant for fatal cardiovascular events than nonfatal MI. In fact, the benefits of increasing dietary intake of fish and fish oil are greater for those patients with higher risk of CVD or those with established CHD at levels of two to three servings of oil-rich fish per week.[22] Long-term epidemiological studies examining health characteristics of females have shown a 30% lower risk of CVD with two or more servings of fatty fish per week.[22]

Several clinical trials have investigated the effects of fish and fish oil after cardiovascular events such as MI or diagnosed coronary artery disease. The Gruppo Italiano per lo Studio della Sopravvivenza nell'Infarto Miocardio (GISSI) Prevenzione Trial showed that 1 g/day of omega-3 fatty acids lowered overall risk of death and coronary death from 6.8 to 4.8% following an MI.[9] Also, both the DASH diet study and Lyon Diet Heart Study have shown significant improvements in CVD outcomes by increasing the amount of omega-3 fatty acids in the diet of study subjects.

OMEGA-6 FATTY ACIDS

Contrary to the recent popularity of alpha-linolenic acid in research and the press, omega-6 fatty acids are less widely debated. The most predominant omega-6 fatty acid is linoleic acid, which also is a physiologically essential fatty acid. Linoleic acid is the biologic precursor to arachidonic acid, another physiologically active compound. Sources of this fatty acid are vegetables and vegetable oil such as corn, soybean, safflower, and sunflower oils. Epidemiological studies researching the long-term effects of a diet high in linoleic acid demonstrate a relative risk for fatal CHD of 0.58 with a 5% change in energy intake from saturated fat.[20] In clinical trials, linoleic acid has reduced both LDL-C and HDL-C levels when used in substitution for saturated fat in the diet.[18] Although the cardioprotective effects of linoleic acid are not as pronounced as those of alpha-linolenic acid, both essential fatty acids are important to incorporate in any heart-healthy regimen.

CHOLESTEROL

Another important dietary factor to consider is total dietary cholesterol. Sources of cholesterol in the U.S. diet include egg yolk, high-fat meats, and high-fat dairy products. Dietary cholesterol has been well researched and is known to increase plasma cholesterol[18] as well as the TC to HDL ratio,[7] an important risk factor for CVD.

CARBOHYDRATE

Carbohydrate is an important nutritional factor to consider when managing patients with CVD. The appropriate level of carbohydrate in the diet is of much debate, especially with the emergence of low-carbohydrate, high-protein diets. Clinical trials demonstrate that carbohydrate has the same effects on LDL-C levels as does monounsaturated fatty acids, however, higher intake of carbohydrate can also decrease protective HDL-C levels and increase plasma TG concentration.[7] A potential mediator for this outcome may be the inclusion of high fiber in a high-carbohydrate diet. This will be discussed later.

The glycemic index of foods is one method of determining the most beneficial source of carbohydrate to incorporate in the diet. The glycemic index is essentially a measure of the ability of the carbohydrate source to raise blood glucose levels over a specific period of time following ingestion. Those foods with a high glycemic index raise blood glucose levels to high concentrations in shorter periods of time than do low glycemic index foods. Recommendations from the ATP III advise against the use of glycemic index of foods as the determinate factor in carbohydrate selection due to the lack of research and available information regarding the validity of the measurement.

An important factor to consider when designing diet patterns for patients with CVD is the presence or absence of metabolic syndrome and insulin resistance. As discussed previously, metabolic syndrome is prevalent in the United States today and may be present in several patient populations. For these groups of individuals, with or without diabetes mellitus, alteration of carbohydrate levels to less than 50% of total calories may be the most efficient method for managing blood glucose concentrations.

FIBER

Fiber is a critical element in the development of dietary patterns for individuals throughout the life cycle. Fiber is particularly important for patients with CVD for many reasons. As a bulking agent, fiber may provide a sense of satiety, which may prevent overeating and contribute to weight loss. Dietary fiber also binds bile acids, which causes the body to metabolize cholesterol into bile acid, a method shown to reduce levels of TC. For diabetic patients, fiber facilitates the regulation of blood glucose, important for prevention of long-term consequences of the disease, such as retinal, renal, and cardiovascular complications.

Fiber has two forms, soluble and insoluble; the difference is in the digestibility of the grain. Dietary sources of fiber are whole grains, nuts, legumes, fresh fruits, and fresh vegetables. The refinement process for grains removes the majority of the fiber as well as essential fatty acids, phytochemicals, vitamins, and minerals. Soluble fiber comes from oats, guar, pectin, and psyllium; conversely, cellulose and lignin are insoluble fibers. The AHA recommends three or more servings per day of whole grains.[23] This is because intake of whole grain foods is inversely associated with both coronary artery disease and ischemic stroke.[19] Specifically, an increase in soluble fiber of 5 to 10 g/day can decrease LDL-C by as much as 5%.[7]

ANTIOXIDANTS

With the popularity of dietary supplements, several research efforts have been devoted to the cardioprotective effects of antioxidants. In theory, high levels of antioxidants could prevent the initial oxidative damage to lipoproteins, which progresses into coronary atherosclerosis. Biologically important antioxidants in this research are beta-carotene, alpha-tocopherol (vitamin E), ascorbic acid (vitamin C), and selenium.[7] It is accepted that fruits and vegetables, also high in antioxidants, are associated with a reduced risk of CVD due to the results of several epidemiological studies showing greater life expectancy and lower risk of coronary artery disease with higher intakes of vitamin E, vitamin C, and beta-carotene.[24] However, it is difficult to determine which elements of these foods are at work in the cardioprotective effects of fruits and vegetables.

Several studies have attempted to demonstrate the protective effects of antioxidants as taken in supplemental form and pharmacologic dosing. Vitamin E, alpha-tocopherol, has been widely scrutinized as a new "miracle drug" in the battle against CVD. Vitamin E acts to promote normal formation of red blood cells, and function of the nervous and immune systems.[25] Vitamin E also scavenges the peroxyl radical and impedes lipid peroxidation. Also important in this antioxidant system are vitamin C, beta-carotene, and selenium, all of which act to regenerate vitamin E to a physiologically active form. When studied experimentally in several clinical-controlled trials, supplementation with vitamin E showed no significant protective effect.[25,26] Another study, HDL-Atherosclerosis Treatment Study (HATS), evaluated the effects of drug therapy and antioxidant therapy on HDL-C. Patients were given an antioxidant mix of 800 IU of vitamin E, 1000 mg of vitamin C, 25 mg of beta-carotene, and 100 μg of selenium daily. Despite increased plasma vitamin levels and improved resistance to LDL-C peroxidation, there was no significant arteriographic evidence of improvements in CVD progression.[27] The U.S. Preventive Task Force concluded that the evidence was inadequate to justify recommending vitamins A, E, and C, multivitamins, or antioxidant combinations for the prevention of CVD.[28]

Polyphenols are a different class of antioxidants significant in slowing the progression of CVD. These compounds, present in red wine, grape juice, chocolate, and tea, may protect LDL-C particles from oxidation, much in the same manner as alpha-tocopherol.[24] Studies have demonstrated improvement in vascular function with polyphenolic compounds using flow-mediated vasodilation.[5]

ALCOHOL

The ATP III recommends moderate intake of alcohol — one drink per day for women and two drinks per day for men. One drink is defined as 5 oz of wine, 12 oz of beer, or 1.5 oz of liquor. This recommendation is based on the established *J*-shaped relationship between alcohol consumption and total mortality. Protective effects of alcohol are unknown and may relate more to psychological effects.

As mentioned previously, red wine may have cardioprotective elements. Despite this, results from the Framingham study demonstrated protective effects of alcohol only from stroke and only in those individuals aged 60 to 69 years.[23]

SOY

The overall benefits of incorporating soy into a heart-healthy diet are vast. Of all foods and compounds found in food, soy may have the largest span of influence in nutritional intervention in CVD. Many elements of soy are important to chronic disease, but soy protein may have the most influence when discussing CVD. Dietary intakes of soy protein of 25 g/day, in combination with a diet low in saturated fats and cholesterol, can lower LDL-C levels by as much as 5%.[7] In fact, even modest intakes of soy protein have been proven to decrease serum cholesterol, TG, and the atherogenic small LDL-C molecules. Soy protein is also known to improve vascular reactivity, decrease oxidative damage, act as an anti-inflammatory agent, reduce platelet aggregation, and control serum concentrations of homocysteine and C-reactive protein (CRP).[29] There is a dose–response relationship between soy protein and CVD. Effectively raising daily intake of soy protein above 25 g/day may prove unrealistic when counseling patients in nutrition intervention.

STEROLS AND STANOLS

Secondary prevention studies have demonstrated a significant 6 to 15% reduction in LDL-C without altering HDL or triglyceride concentrations through the addition of 2 to 3 g/day of plant sterols and stanols.[7] This result is equivalent to substituting 8% of saturated fatty acids in the diet with polyunsaturated or monounsaturated fats.[30] Plant sterols and stanols are compounds isolated from soybeans and tall pine-tree oils which are usually incorporated into commercial margarines. They act to reduce blood cholesterol levels by inhibiting the absorption of dietary cholesterol. Sterols and stanols are structurally similar to cholesterol but are not as readily absorbed from the gastrointestinal (GI) tract. Only about 1–15% of plant sterols and stanols are absorbed.[30] Trials have also shown that plant sterols and stanols enhance outcomes of pharmaceutical and nutritional interventions in CVD.[23] It is critical to consider the caloric intake when patients are consuming these products, as some adjustments may need to be made to accommodate for the increases in the fat source to meet recommendations for plant sterols and stanols. Secondary to the mechanism by which sterols and stanols prevent cholesterol absorption from the gut, excessive intake of these nutrients may reduce the absorption of fat-soluble vitamins.

FLAVONOIDS AND PHYTOCHEMICALS

The study of flavonoids and phytochemicals are areas of research gaining popularity in the prevention and treatment of chronic disease. There are more than 5000 phytochemicals identified with more still undiscovered.[31] These complex molecules act as antioxidants and are thought to reduce the risk of chronic disease because of their antioxidant properties. Flavonoids and phytochemicals are found in fruits, vegetables, and soy. As previously established, high intakes of fruits and vegetables are inversely associated with the risk of mortality from CVD and with the incidence of MI.[31] Flavonoids and phytochemicals may contribute to the protective properties of these foods. Major classes of these compounds are quercetin, kaempferol, myricetin, apigenin, luteolin, catechins, and soy isoflavones. These classes are present in apples, tea, broccoli, onions, and tofu.[32] Research has not yet confirmed intakes of flavonoids and reduced risk of CVD.

DIETARY PATTERNS

Despite the evidence that individual nutrients affect disease risk, the most important element to incorporate into any nutrition intervention is an overall healthy diet pattern, counsel patients to include protective nutrients and exclude those nutrients that may put them at unnecessary risk.

Well-designed, long-term epidemiological investigations have examined dietary patterns and their effects on risk of CVD. The Nurses' Health Study and Health Professionals' Follow-Up Study deducted two different dietary patterns from their cohorts, each with vastly different long-term consequences. The "Prudent" dietary pattern consisted of a diet high in fruits and vegetables, legumes, fish, poultry, and whole grains. This is similar to the "Mediterranean" and DASH dietary patterns that have proven benefits in secondary prevention of CVD. The second dietary pattern was termed "Western." Subjects consumed diets higher in red and processed meats, sweets and desserts, fried foods, and refined grains. The Western dietary pattern resulted in higher biochemical markers of inflammation (e.g., CRP), homocysteine, insulin, and decreased plasma folate.[19]

The Lyon Diet Heart Study formulated a Mediterranean dietary pattern that lowered the risk for recurrent heart disease by 50–70% compared to the control group.[23] The Mediterranean diet in this study was characterized by:

- 30% total calories from fat
- 8% total calories from saturated fat
- 13% total calories from monounsaturated fat
- 4.6% total calories from polyunsaturated fat
- 200 mg of cholesterol per day

Analysis of several dietary intervention trials indicates that the amount of fat in the diet is more indicative of CVD risk than the type of fat being consumed. Dietary patterns low in saturated fat and high in dietary fiber show improvement in cardiovascular risk factors, regardless of the amount of fat in the diet.

The inclusion of unsaturated foods in the diet improves CVD risk factors and outcomes without adversely affecting body weight or lipoprotein concentrations when caloric levels are controlled. Foods with established cardioprotective benefits are fruits and vegetables, whole grains, nuts, and fish. Along with this, the Adventist Health Study demonstrated that the frequency of nut consumption was inversely associated with CVD risk independent of other risk factors.[33] Analysis of nut studies shows that individuals who include nuts in their diets more than five times per week lower lifetime risk of CHD by 12%.[33]

PHARMACOLOGICAL INTERVENTIONS IN CARDIOVASCULAR DISEASE

Numerous studies over the past decade have demonstrated the efficacy of the use of pharmacological agents in the treatment of CVD. Table 9.3 reviews some of the major studies that support the use of drug therapy to alter lipid profiles in the treatment of CVD. Five of these studies demonstrated a decrease in coronary events, including CVD-related mortality, by

TABLE 9.3
Major Cardiovascular Trials and Findings

Trial	Description	Major Outcome
Scandinavian Simvastatin Survival Study (4S)	Secondary intervention study using simvastatin	38% ↓ in LDL-C resulting in 30%↓ in major coronary events
Program on the Surgical Control of the Hyperlipidemias (POSCH)	Secondary intervention study using ileal bypass	38% ↓ in LDL-C, 4% ↑ in HDL-C resulting in 28% ↓ in CHD mortality
Cholesterol and Recurrent Events (CARE)	Secondary intervention study using pravastatin	3–35% ↓ in LDL-C, dependent upon baseline levels, resulting in 24% overall ↓ in CHD mortality
Long-term Intervention with Pravastatin in Ischemic Disease (LIPID)	Secondary intervention study using pravastatin	25% ↓ in LDL-C resulting in 29% ↓ in major coronary events
West of Scotland Coronary Prevention Study (WOSCOPS)	Primary intervention study using pravastatin	25% ↓ in LDL-C resulting in a total mortality ↓ of 22%
The Air Force/Texas Coronary Atherosclerosis Prevention Study (AFCAPS/TexCAPS)	Primary intervention study using lovastatin	26% ↓ in LDL-C resulting in 40% ↓ in fatal or nonfatal MI
Veterans Affairs Cooperative Studies Program High-Density Lipoprotein Cholesterol Intervention Trial (VA-HIT)	Secondary intervention study using gemfibrozil	6% ↑ in HDL-C resulting in 22% ↓ of fatal and nonfatal MI
Lipoprotein and Coronary Atherosclerosis Study (LCAS)	Secondary intervention study using diet plus fluvastatin	Progression of atherosclerosis was ↓ as a result of an ↑ in HDL-C
Cholesterol Lowering Atherosclerosis Study (CLAS)	Secondary intervention study using colestipol and niacin	43% ↓ in LDL-C, 37% ↑ in HDL-C resulted in 25% ↓ of CHD events
HDL-Atherosclerosis Treatment Study (HATS)	Secondary intervention study comparing the use of niacin plus simvastatin versus simvastatin alone	Niacin + simvastatin resulted in 70% ↓ of CHD events versus 25–30% ↓ with simvastatin alone

Continued

TABLE 9.3 (Continued)
Major Cardiovascular Trials and Findings

Trial	Description	Major Outcome
Stanford Coronary Risk Intervention Program (SCRIP)	Secondary observational and intervention study using multiple risk factor intervention	Participants with dense LDL-C had 40% greater progression of coronary lesions versus participants with buoyant LDL-C; 79% ↓ in atherosclerosis with intervention
Diet and Reinfarction Trial (DART)	Secondary intervention study using fish and fish oil supplements	33% ↓ in CHD mortality
The Lyon Diet Heart Study	Secondary intervention study using Mediterranean diet	65% ↓ in CHD mortality
The Gruppo Italiano per lo Studio della Sopravvivenza nell'Infarto Miocardio (GISSI) Prevenzione Trial	Secondary intervention study using EPA + DHA and statin therapy	30% ↓ in CHD mortality
Framingham Heart Study	Observational study	Low HDL-C levels correlated to the development of CHD in both males and females
Helsinki Heart Study	Primary intervention study using gemfibrozil	9% ↑ in HDL-C, 35% ↓ in TG, and 8% ↓ in LDL-C with 34% ↓ of coronary events
Heart and Estrogen/Progestin Replacement Study (HERS)	Secondary intervention study using HRT	No notable benefits from HRT on CHD
Lifestyle Heart Trial (LHT)	Secondary intervention study using low fat and nutrient-rich plant-based foods	↓ LDL-C 37%
St. Thomas Atherosclerosis Regression (STAR)	Secondary intervention study using low fat and nutrient-rich plant-based foods	↓ LDL-C 22%

Source: Adapted from Kreisberg, R. and Oberman, A., *J. Clin. Endocrinol. Metab.*, 87, 423, 2002.
Adapted from National Cholesterol Education Program, Third report of the expert panel on detection, evaluation, and treatment of high blood cholesterol in adults (Adult Treatment Panel III), NIH Pub. No.02-5215, National Heart, Lung, and Blood Institute, Bethesda, MD, 2002.
Adapted from Carlson, J.J. and Monti, V., *J. Cardiopulm. Rehabil.*, 23, 322, 2003.

lowering serum LDL-C through the use of statin drugs. Simvastatin, pravastatin, and lovastatin were all successfully used to lower LDL-C by 25–38%, with a resulting 22–40% decrease in major coronary events.[6]

Two studies evaluated the use of fibrates to reduce coronary events through the increase in serum HDL-C. Serum HDL-C was increased 6–9% with the use of gemfibrozil that resulted in 22–34% decrease in CVD events. Combination therapies, drug + drug, drug + diet, drug + dietary supplement, were also studied in four trials. All studies produced a similar decrease in coronary events as with monodrug therapy.[6]

ATP III continues to recommend TLC diet therapy as a primary prevention strategy. Based on the studies discussed above, however, if the TLC diet has failed to produce the desired lipid levels after 12 weeks, ATP III recommends the initiation of drug therapy as an adjunct treatment.[3] Statins are recommended as the primary drug of choice because of their ability to dramatically influence LDL-C levels with few negative side effects. Statins, or 3-hydroxy-3-methylglutaryl (HMG)-CoA reductase inhibitors, have been shown to reduce LDL-C by 18–55%. Statins inhibit the production of endogenous cholesterol in the liver, which increases the expression of the LDL receptors, thereby decreasing serum levels. Statins have also been shown to reduce TG by 7–30%, and increase HDL-C by 5–15%. Statins have been shown to be efficacious as a short-term therapy; however, trials are continuing to examine their long-term safety. Cholestasis and active liver disease are contraindications for statin therapy. Transaminase elevation has been noted, but not reported as statistically significant, and usually returned to normal levels after a reduction in the statin dose. Myopathy has also been noted as a potential side effect, but is primarily seen in individuals with a complex medical history.[7]

Besides statins' lipid-lowering properties, they seem to also possess antioxidant, anti-inflammatory, and vasodilating properties. Since the development of atherosclerosis is largely a function of oxidation, and coronary events are in part a result of inflammation and vasoconstriction, these additional properties only increase the efficacy of statin drugs in the treatment of CVD.[6]

The bile sequestrant cholestyramine is recommended as the second choice for drug therapy. Bile sequestrants bind bile acid in the intestines, which again inhibits the production of endogenous cholesterol and increases the expression of LDL receptors that decreases serum levels. Bile sequestrants have been shown to reduce LDL-C by 15–30% when used as a monotherapy. When used with other LDL-C lowering agents, bile sequestrants enhance their effectiveness and may lower LDL-C up to 70%. As sequestrants are not absorbed by the intestines, GI complaints are their primary side effect, including constipation, bloating, and nausea. Sequestrants should not be taken concurrently with other medications because of their absorption-altering properties. Rather, other medications should be taken 1–2 hours before or 4–6 hours after sequestrants. The only contraindication for the use of this drug because of limited effectiveness is familial dysbetalipoproteinemia.[7]

Although niacin is a highly effective lipid-altering drug, it is problematic concerning patient compliance because of its side effects. While statins and bile sequestrants are notable for reducing LDL-C levels, niacin is equally effective at increasing HDL-C and decreasing TG. Niacin has been shown to reduce TG by 20–50% and increase HDL-C by 15–35%.[6] Niacin inhibits lipoprotein synthesis, reduces the production and release of endogenous VLDL-C, and decreases the catabolism of apolipoprotein A1. Side effects include epidermal flushing, GI distress, hepatotoxicity, and gout. Flushing seem to be lessened with the sustained-release formulations, but these appear to increase the rate of hepatic toxicity.[34] Because it reduces insulin sensitivity, it can exacerbate hyperglycemia in people with type 2 diabetes. Niacin is contraindicated in people with chronic liver disease, severe gout, and peptic ulcer disease.[7]

Fibric acids are another classification of drugs used in the treatment of CVD. Fibrates are most notable for their ability to decrease TG levels. By increasing the catabolism of VLDL-C, fibrates may reduce TG by 20–50%. The most common side effect of fibrates is GI distress. They are contraindicated for patients with hepatic or renal insufficiency.[7]

The newest class of lipid-lowering drugs is cholesterol absorption inhibitors. In October 2002, Food and Drug Administration (FDA) approved ezetimibe for the treatment of hyperlipidemia.[35] By inhibiting the absorption of cholesterol in the intestines, ezetimibe is able to reduce LDL-C levels up to 20% when used as a monotherapy. Due to the synergistic mechanisms of statin drugs and cholesterol absorption inhibitors, additional benefits may be seen when they are used as combination therapy. Minor side effects such as back and joint pain and diarrhea have been noted. Long-term effects are not known, but these drugs are contraindicated for individuals with liver dysfunction.[36]

Combination drug therapy is another option for the treatment of dyslipidemia that has failed to respond to monotherapies. It is quite common for patients to exhibit multiple lipid abnormalities that would benefit from pharmacological agents with differing mechanisms. In the Cholesterol Lowering Atherosclerosis Study (CLAS) both colestipol and niacin were used to achieve a 25% decrease in CVD events. Similarly, HATS utilized a combination of simvastatin and niacin for a 70% decrease in CVD events versus a 25–30% decrease with simvastatin monotherapy.[6]

Statins, bile sequestrants, niacin, and fibrates are the drug therapies available for the treatment of CVD. New pharmacological agents are continuously under development. Regardless of monotherapy or combination drug therapy, the TLC diet continues to be an efficacious primary and secondary treatment for patients with CVD.

NEW INSIGHTS INTO CARDIOVASCULAR DISEASE

All the research in CVD cause and effects notwithstanding, novel concepts continually emerge. The following section highlights new areas of interest in the enduring study of CVD.

FAD DIETS

Discussion of dietary intakes of fat and CVD would not be complete without mentioning the widely exercised high-protein, low-carbohydrate diet. The theory behind a low-carbohydrate diet lies in the physiological role of carbohydrate in insulin secretion. By starving the body of carbohydrate, less insulin is secreted. This prevents lipogenesis and encourages lipolysis for glucose production; thereby reducing adipose tissue and preventing further enlargement of fat cells. The apprehension that some health professionals have regarding recommendation of a high-protein, low-carbohydrate diet is that patients consuming a diet high in protein unavoidably ingest large amounts of fat. Typically, animal fats provide the majority of fats in a high-protein diet, consequently, a diet high in saturated fat. Also, low-carbohydrate diets limit intake of essential nutrients such as fiber, vitamins, and minerals that are found at high concentrations in carbohydrate-containing foods such as fruits, vegetables, and whole grains.

Research on the long-term effects of these specialized diets is limited, despite the existence of these diets for over 30 years. Available randomized, clinically controlled trials last from 6 weeks to 1 year in follow-up with relatively undersized sample sizes. Results from these trials show significant difference in weight loss between low-carbohydrate diets and conventional diets at 3 and 6 months; however, no significant differences in weight loss after 1 year of diet intervention. Traditional dietary approaches resulted in significantly higher TG after 1 year than the low-carbohydrate diet, while the low-carbohydrate diet raised HDL-C levels significantly more than the conventional diet.[37] Further analysis revealed those subjects consuming a low-carbohydrate diet consumed far fewer calories per day than those patients using standard dietary protocol. The essential question is, "Do the effects of short-term significant weight loss from a low-carbohydrate diet outweigh the potential negative outcomes?"

Dieting is not an easy task in which to succeed. Some researchers have approximated that dieters will gain back weight lost within 1 to 5 years about 80–85% of the time.[38] In reality, the ability of individuals to maintain a low-carbohydrate diet for an extended period of time is untested. While in the short term these diets may prove beneficial for weight reduction, sustainable improvements in cardiovascular events and lipid profiles are yet to be documented. Furthermore, studies of short duration have shown a low-carbohydrate, high-protein diet to increase serum levels of homocysteine, lipoprotein(a), and CRP, which potentially place patients at risk for CVD.[39]

Homocysteine

Homocysteine is a sulfur-containing amino acid formed in the metabolism of methionine, another amino acid. Homocysteine propagates atherosclerotic factors, such as increasing platelet aggregation, inducing oxidative stress, promoting smooth muscle cell proliferation, causing damage to vascular walls,[2] and inhibiting the vasodilatory effects of nitric oxide.[40] Homocysteine levels are inversely related to plasma concentrations and dietary intakes of the B-vitamins, folate, pyridoxine (B-6), and cobalamin (B-12) secondary to their roles in homocysteine metabolism.[40,41] Cigarette smoking and caffeine intake have been linked to hyperhomocysteinemia. Hyperhomocysteinemia can also be attributed to inherited metabolic disorders, which predispose individuals to CVD.[42]

Observational studies have linked hyperhomocysteinemia to CVD risk for MI, stroke, and hypertension regardless of other independent risk factors.[40–43] Above-optimal levels of fasting homocysteine (>12 μmol/l) more than double the risk of CVD in men and women independent of traditional risk factors.[41,42] The possibility of lowering homocysteine, thereby reducing CVD risk, is established and meta-analysis reveals significant results.

- Supplementation with folic acid (500–1000 μg/day) resulted in a 25% reduction of homocysteine.
- Supplementation with cobalamin (500 μg/day) resulted in a 7% reduction of homocysteine.
- Supplementation with pyridoxine (250 μg/day) had no significant effect on fasting homocysteine levels,[41] but decreased postmethionine homocysteine levels by 20–30%.[42]

Observational studies have put forth weaker correlations between homocysteine and CVD risk than have case-controlled studies[43]; however, it may be prudent to recommend vitamin supplementation in patients with hyperhomocysteinemia for two reasons — these supplements are considered safe at pharmacologic doses, and relative to the cost of prescription medications, multivitamin supplements are inexpensive.

C-Reactive Protein

CRP is in a class of acute-phase proteins produced by the liver in response to inflammatory cytokines. It is this inflammatory process which, potentially, contributes to plaque instability and cardiovascular events. Contemporary literature suggests CRP, when slightly increased above normal levels, may predict CVD events in otherwise asymptomatic people.[2] In fact, measuring CRP concentrations may prove beneficial in determining risk for all individuals despite Framingham risk assessment scores.[44] Research has been unable to determine if inflammatory proteins such as CRP are solely markers for inflammation, signaling damage or instability in vessel walls or, if CRP and other acute-phase proteins contribute to the progression of atherosclerosis.[45] In prospective studies, CRP is also directly associated with abdominal obesity and type 2 diabetes mellitus, both independent risk factors for CVD and potential risks for developing metabolic syndrome.[2] Use of CRP is of limited specificity in those cases of concurrent inflammatory processes, i.e., rheumatoid arthritis or Crohn's disease.[2,45]

Epidemiological studies following dietary intakes associate intake of omega-3 and omega-6 fatty acids with inflammatory markers such as CRP. Interestingly, with low intakes of omega-3 fatty acids, dietary consumption of omega-6 fatty acids correlated to higher levels of inflammatory markers, while diets high in omega-3 fatty acids resulted in the lowest concentrations of inflammatory markers regardless of dietary intakes of omega-6 fatty acids.[45] Studies have shown significant reductions in CRP concentrations with weight loss, moderate alcohol consumption, exercise, and use of statin drugs.[46]

LIPOPROTEIN(a)

Lipoprotein(a) is emerging as a new risk factor for CVD. Unfortunately, concentrations of lipoprotein(a) are genetically determined and are not altered by changes in diet or activity level.[2] The mechanism of the effects of lipoprotein(a) on CVD is varied; the most critical action may be the inactivation of fibrinolysis in endothelial injury preventing the dissolution of clots and promoting vessel occlusion.[2]

NUTRACEUTICALS AND SUPPLEMENTS

An emerging industry relevant to the prevention and treatment of CVD is nutritional supplement sales. Annual sales have grown consistently and exceeded $20 billion in 1997.[47] When utilized as pharmacological interventions, nutritional supplements are known as "nutraceuticals." In scientific literature, nutraceuticals comprise any food or part thereof used to prevent disease or improve health.[48] Popular supplements today include herbal and botanical supplements as well as nutraceuticals. ATP III does not recommend supplement usage in patients with CVD due to the lack of sound evidence regarding the safety and efficacy of available supplements. Regardless of the ATP III recommendations, patients will continue to purchase and self-medicate with nutritional supplements. Therefore, it is critical that health-care providers interview patients concerning the use of supplements. Patients at serious risk for adverse effects from nutraceutical and other supplement products include those with hypertension and heart disease.[48]

The safety of over-the-counter nutritional supplements is of great concern. Regulation of these medications is different from pharmaceutical products, and there are no imposed composition or concentration standards for herbal, botanical, or nutritional supplements. Scientific studies are precluded by a lack of standardized formulations, consistency, and reproducibility in commercial supplement products. Available literature investigating specific supplements and CVD is limited to small sample sizes.

Any successful individual nutrition assessment requires comprehensive investigation into medical, surgical, and pharmacological history. Patients may either fail to disclose supplement usage or fail to understand the ramifications of supplement usage when contraindicated with prescription medications.

HORMONE REPLACEMENT THERAPY

The Women's Health Initiative is a primary prevention trial of over 15,000 women studying the health benefits of estrogen plus progestin or placebo in postmenopausal women. Initial results from this trial showed that women receiving hormone replacement therapy were at 22% greater risk for all cardiovascular events. Specifically, coronary disease events and stroke rates were 29 and 41% higher, respectively, in the estrogen plus progestin versus placebo.[49] Because CVD risks are higher for older women, postmenopausal patients for whom hormone replacement therapy has been prescribed may be at even higher risk of CVD outcomes and warrant prudent monitoring.

LDL APHERESIS

LDL apheresis appears to be a new, safe, and efficacious treatment for hyperlipidemia. Through extracorporeal removal of LDL-C particles from the bloodstream, studies have shown a significant reduction in both LDL-C levels as well as lipoprotein(a).[50] LDL apheresis is a time-consuming and costly procedure and is therefore limited to individuals with elevated LDL-C levels that have failed to respond to other traditional treatments, as in the case of familial hyperlipidemia.[8]

UPDATES IN HYPERTENSION

One in four adults has hypertension; prevalence is higher among blacks and older persons.[51] High blood pressure is a risk factor for chronic disease such as stroke, MI, renal failure, heart failure, atherosclerosis, and dementia.[51] Systolic blood pressure is evidenced to be a stronger predictor of CVD risk than is diastolic blood pressure.

The goal of treatment in hypertension is to prevent CVD, thus, mortality from cardio-vascular events. Risk reduction for stroke, CVD, and death from cardiovascular causes is lowered 40, 16, and 20%, respectively, with marginal changes in systolic (10–12 mmHg) and diastolic (5–6 mmHg) blood pressures.[51] As with CVD, dietary modifications should be initiated in most patients with hypertension before pharmacological interventions. In fact, lifestyle modifications alone can control hypertension in 59% of patients for at least 4 years.[51] Those exceptions include patients with established CVD, diabetes, or high-risk CVD factors. In these patients, drug therapy should be combined with lifestyle modifications.

Overall changes in lifestyle should include dietary changes as well as increasing aerobic physical activity to 30 min daily, limiting alcohol, quitting smoking, and maintaining ideal body weight. In fact, for every 1 kg weight loss, blood pressure can be reduced by at least 1 mmHg.[51] The DASH trial showed significant changes in systolic and diastolic blood pressures after a diet composed of high intakes of fruits and vegetables, low-fat dairy products, restricted saturated fat, and sodium limited to 2.4 g/day.[9] A diet high in fruits and vegetables also provides high intakes of potassium, calcium, and magnesium, which have been linked to lower CVD risk. After 8 weeks following the DASH diet, study participants had lowered their systolic blood pressure by 11.4 mmHg and diastolic blood pressure by 5.5 mmHg. In fact, the DASH diet proved to be an effective replacement for drug therapy in Stage I hypertension.[23]

Also important to note is the role of antihypertensive medications. Most medications have been known to reduce blood pressure by 10–15% in controlled clinical trials. Selection of medications depends on several factors: age, sex, coexisting conditions, race or ethnicity, and potential adverse reactions. Each class of antihypertensive medications affects CVD risk differently. Diuretics and β-blockers reduce risk of stroke, CHD, and mortality from CVD. Angiotensin-converting enzyme (ACE) inhibitors reduce risk of stroke, CHD, major cardio-vascular events, death from cardiovascular causes, and all-cause mortality. Calcium channel blockers reduce risk of stroke, major cardiovascular events, and death from cardiovascular causes but do not reduce risk of CHD, heart failure, or all-cause mortality.[51]

SUMMARY

The study of CVD is pertinent to multiple disciplines. Understanding the implications of nutritional, medical, pharmacological, and behavioral interventions for patients with CVD greatly improves outcomes. Studies over the past decade have shown considerable insight into the management of this disease, which has led to the development of innovative treatment methodologies. Research continues to support traditional therapies in CVD while generating contemporary modalities (Textbox 9.1 and Textbox 9.2).

Textbox 9.1   Fish Oil and Cardiovascular Disease

Interest in the cardioprotective effects of fish oils first began in the 1980s after a connection between the low occurrence of CVD in Greenland Eskimos and their diet, high in marine sources omega-3 fatty acids.[1] Research was impeded at that time given the unstable nature of the fatty acids in formulated supplements. Advances in research now allow fish oil supplements to remain stable in preparation, improving the validity and reliability of clinical trials. Stable fish oils are those that contain a mixture of natural antioxidants, which prevent rancidity. Unstable oils are those that contain only the natural amounts of vitamin E, these are more likely to break down during purification and processing. Stable fish oil is now known for its more potent effects on cardiovascular outcomes versus unstable oils. In many studies, fish oils have proven to reduce mortality from coronary artery disease, reduce plasma triglycerides, increase HDL-C, and inhibit inflammatory processes by affecting platelet aggregation, vasoconstriction, and neutrophil function.[1]

The proposed mechanism of action for fish oils in CVD is its regulation of inflammation. Omega-3 fatty acids in fish oils replace inflammatory fatty acids (derived from omega-6 fatty acids) in cell membranes and regulate the function of inflammatory mediators.[1] Other cardioprotective effects and mechanisms of action include antiarrhythmic and antithrombotic properties, and improvement in endothelial function.[2]

Appropriate doses of fish oil supplements are still controversial as there are some questions as to potential side effects of prolonged use of fish oils. Studies have demonstrated positive outcomes with 15 ml of natural, stable fish oil (containing 5 g of omega-3 PUFA) daily for 6 months. However, long-term supplementation of 1 g daily of omega-3 fatty acids for over 3 years has proven beneficial as well.[1] The American Heart Association proposed the following recommendations regarding fish oil supplementation in 2002. Notice that fish oil supplementation is utilized in secondary prevention of CVD:

- Patients without CVD: Eat a variety of fatty fish at least twice weekly
- Patients with CVD: Take 1 g of PUFA daily
- Patients with hypertriglyceridemia: Take 2–4 g of PUFA[2]

[1]Saldeen, T.G. and Mehta, J.L., Dietary modulations in the prevention of coronary artery disease: a special emphasis on vitamins and fish oil, *Curr. Opin. Cardiol.*, 17, 559, 2002.

[2]Din, J.N., Newby, D.E., and Flapan, A.D., Omega 3 fatty acids and cardiovascular disease — fishing for a natural treatment, *BMJ*, 328, 30, 2004.

CASE STUDY

A 67-year-old man presents to the Registered Dietitian after being diagnosed with coronary artery disease with the following pertinent anthropometric and laboratory measurements:

BMI (kg/m^2)	34
BP (mmHg)	145/90
Waist-to-hip ratio	1.2
Cholesterol (mg/dl)	215
LDL-C (mg/dl)	150
HDL-C (mg/dl)	35

Diet history revealed that the patient eats two large meals a day, usually at fast-food restaurants because he works 12-h shifts and has to eat on the go. He dislikes vegetables, prefers fruit juices, and likes red meat and fried chicken. He drinks 36 oz of soda per day with about 12 oz of water. The patient does have ice cream or cookies before retiring for the evening.

What would your dietary recommendations be for this gentleman? What changes would you make to his current diet pattern and how would you encourage the patient to make these changes? What other laboratory values are critical to monitoring this patient? What medications, if any, would you expect this patient to be started on?

Five years later the same patient presents in your office s/p CABG × 3 with the following pertinent laboratory measurements and a BMI of 32 kg/m^2 (Textbox 9.3):

Cholesterol (mg/dl)	250
LDL-C (mg/dl)	140
HDL-C (mg/dl)	38
TG (mg/dl)	250
Creatinine (mg/dl)	1.6
BUN (mg/dl)	25

What would you now recommend for this patient given his diet intake is not significantly different from his intake 5 years ago except for the fact that he is now drinking diet soda? The patient was also told by a friend to try a high-protein or low-carbohydrate diet. What do you suggest? What other possible risk factors would you consider in assessing this patient? (Textbox 9.4, Textbox 9.5, and Textbox 9.6).

Textbox 9.2   Garlic

The German Commission E indicates garlic as an important dietary measure to treat CVD, and international research has also shown garlic's benefit in high blood pressure as well.[1] One of the problems in study methods is the multitude of preparations and extracts available and used in various interventional studies. Studies have demonstrated statistically significant hypocholesterolemic effects of garlic supplementation of 600–900 mg/day in adults with hypercholesterolemia. One 12-week study showed a significant reduction in cholesterol and LDL-C with daily supplementation of 220 mg of garlic powder in enteric-coated tablets (the equivalent of 2–3 g of fresh garlic). Tablets were coated to protect the active enzyme in garlic, alliinase, which converts alliin to allicin. Allicin is the active compound in the plant, thought to be responsible for the beneficial health effects.[2]

Selection and dosing of garlic supplements is debatable. Many professionals recommend 600–900 mg/day of standardized garlic extract. The most common side effect in garlic supplementation is halitosis; odorless preparations are available, but these may not be as biologically active as the chemical substances included to limit the odor damage active ingredients in the garlic. Adverse events in limited cases have been reported with individuals consuming more than 1 g of garlic per day (about 2 cloves).[1] Researchers propose that garlic may have an antiplatelet effect which may cause abnormal bleeding in some individuals. Because of the potential negative outcomes, it is prudent to recommend patients include more garlic as part of a balanced diet and those choosing to supplement with garlic should be monitored by a health professional.

[1]Chagan, L. et al., Use of alternative pharmacotherapy in management of cardiovascular diseases, *Am. J. Man Care*, 8, 270, 2002.

[2]Kannar, D. et al., Hypocholesterolemic effect of an enteric-coated garlic supplement, *J. Am. Coll. Nutr.*, 20, 225, 2001.

Textbox 9.3   The Anti-Inflammatory Diet

Recently, many researchers have evaluated the role of inflammation in CVD. Inflammation appears to be a key driver into the development and progression of atherosclerosis. In fact, measuring C-reactive protein, an acute-phase inflammatory marker, along with LDL-C has provided better prognostic information for CVD risk than just LDL-C alone, at all levels of the Framingham risk assessment.[1] Because of the possible connection, research into dietary interventions in modulating inflammatory processes is prevalent.

Of all the possible actions inflammation may play in CVD and atherosclerosis, there are three actions that have potential nutrient interventions. First, inflammation contributes to the instability of plaques in vessel walls. Lipid lowering is the most potent means of reducing plaque inflammation. There are several means of lowering blood lipid levels cited throughout this text. Also inflammation releases free radicals, which cause lipid peroxidation and vasoconstriction. Fish oil supplementation, fiber, vitamins E and C, and niacin could potentially play a role in reducing the release of free radicals. Lastly, damaging inflammation increases with an imbalance of nitric oxide and oxidants. Nutrients that contribute to maintaining this balance are arginine, vitamins C and E, antioxidant nutrients, folic acid, and niacin.[2]

One study[3] evaluated plasma concentrations of vitamin B-6, pyridoxal-5'-phosphate (PLP), and inflammation, specifically, plasma levels of C-reactive protein and fibrinogen. Researchers found an inverse relationship between vitamin B-6 concentrations and the two markers of inflammation. This result was independent of traditional CVD risk factors. The mechanism of action is still unknown, but PLP plays an important role in inflammation and thrombosis.[3] Further research should evaluate the relationship of PLP to homocysteine concentrations as that may also hold significance in the prevention and treatment of CVD.

Research has also looked into dietary patterns in altering inflammatory processes versus supplementation with individual nutrients. Studies in vegetarian dietary patterns have proven to have marked effects on hemostasis and thrombotic factors, lowering platelet aggregation and fibrin formation.[4] These vegetarian patterns are typically higher in anti-inflammatory phytochemicals than are typical, "Western" dietary patterns. For example, catechins and procyanidins from foods containing cocoa prevent platelet aggregation *ex vivo*.[4] Anthocyanins from red wine or purple grape juice may increase HDL-C and also have antithrombotic properties compared to similar amounts of orange or grapefruit juice, or white and red grape juice.[4]

[1]Ridker, P.M., High-sensitivity C-reactive protein, inflammation, and cardiovascular risk: from concept to clinical practice to clinical benefit, *Am. Heart J.*, 148, S19, 2004.

[2]Osiecki, H., The role of chronic inflammation in cardiovascular disease and its regulation by nutrients, *Alt. Med. Rev.*, 9, 42, 2004.

[3]Friso, S. et al., Low plasma vitamin B-6 concentrations and modulation of coronary artery disease risk, *Am. J. Clin. Nutr.*, 79, 992, 2004.

[4]Rajaram, S., The effect of vegetarian diet, plant foods, and phytochemicals on hemostasis and thrombosis, *Am. J. Clin. Nutr.*, 78 (Suppl.), 552S, 2003.

Textbox 9.4   Potential Pitfalls

With approximately 25–50% of Americans utilizing complementary or alternative medicine to treat chronic disease,[1] it is important to understand potential drug–nutrient interactions with frequently prescribed pharmaceutical interventions for CVD. As mentioned throughout, many dietary and herbal interventions for CVD have antiplatelet actions. Patients on warfarin are at particular risk for bleeding when also supplementing with feverfew, garlic, ginger, ginko biloba, dashen, ginseng, or St. John's wort.[1] Patients taking other antiplatelets such as aspirin may be at similar risk for bleeding while supplementing garlic concurrently with warfarin.[2] Many herbs, such as Echinacea and kava-kava, interact with the physiological activity of amiodarone.[1] Kyushin has been shown to interfere with digoxin assays and St. John's wort may decrease serum digoxin levels.[1]

[1]Miller, K.L., Liebowitz, R.S., and Newby, L.K., Complementary and alternative medicine in cardiovascular disease: a review of biologically based approaches, *Am. Heart J.*, 147, 401, 2004.

[2]Chagan, L. et al., Use of alternative pharmacotherapy in management of cardiovascular diseases, *Am. J. Man Care*, 8, 270, 2002.

Textbox 9.5   Glycemic Load and Inflammation

With an established connection between C-reactive protein, inflammation, and CVD risk, many researches are attempting to discover links between diet and C-reactive protein. Of these links, glycemic load may be of particular significance. The mechanism of action for high glycemic load foods to increase plasma C-reactive protein is not completely understood; but the effect of glycemic load on insulin resistance results in a proinflammatory state and increased production of C-reactive protein.[1] Data extrapolated from NHAHES III showed that the amount of dietary fiber was inversely associated with serum levels of C-reactive protein. This relationship existed regardless of any previous history of CVD or diabetes and was only statistically significant for individuals with plasma C-reactive protein levels less than 10 mg/l.[2]

Another study of middle-aged women reported a significant association between quality and quantity of carbohydrate intake and levels of C-reactive protein.[1] In fact, study participants in the highest quintile of dietary glycemic load had a mean C-reactive protein concentration nearly two times higher than those participants with the lowest dietary glycemic load. This dose–response relationship between the glycemic load and plasma C-reactive protein was more pronounced in study participants with a BMI over 25 kg/m^2,[1] indicating that overweight and obese patients are more at risk with a diet high in glycemic load foods than those patients at a healthy body weight.

[1]Liu, S. et al., Relation between a diet with a high glycemic load and plasma concentrations of high-sensitivity C-reactive protein in middle-aged women, *Am. J. Clin. Nutr.*, 75, 492, 2002.

[2]Ajani, U.A., Ford, E.S., and Mokdad, A.H., Dietary fiber and C-reactive protein: findings from National Health and Nutrition Examination Survey data, *J. Nutr.*, 134, 1181, 2004.

Textbox 9.6   Future Directions

New advances in the prevention and treatment of CVD emerge continuously. A few of these advances are worth mentioning for future study. Policosanol is a compound derived in Cuba and used extensively in South America and the Caribbean to lower cholesterol levels. Policosanol may lower cholesterol and LDL-C by inhibiting HMG-CoA reductase. Studies from Cuba looking at supplementation of 5–10 mg/day suggested a lipid-lowering effect of 15–20%. Other benefits of policosanol could be its antiplatelet and antioxidant properties.[1]

Red rice yeast is another area of interest for future research. A product of the yeast, Monacolin K, inhibits HMG-CoA reductase. Monacolin K is one active component of lovastatin. Small studies have evidenced hypocholesterolemic effects of red rice yeast, along with an increase in HDL-C. Because of its similarity to lovastatin, patients taking red rice yeast must consider potential drug interactions when used in combination with niacin, macrolides, or cyclosporine.[1]

Gugulipid has been an important element in Indian medicine (Ayurveda) for thousands of years and continues to be used as a lipid-lowering agent today. A small study showed mild hypocholesterolemic effects of 50 mg of gugulipid supplemented for 24 weeks in comparison to a placebo group. Both groups were encouraged to consume a diet rich in fruits and vegetables. Because of the limited research and available information, gugulipid should be considered for patients with mild hypercholesterolemia and only under the supervision of a professional.[1]

[1]Miller, K.L., Liebowitz, R.S., and Newby, L.K., Complementary and alternative medicine in cardiovascular disease: a review of biologically based approaches, *Am. Heart J.*, 147, 401, 2004.

GLOSSARY

Adult Treatment Panel III: Collaborative group of the National Cholesterol Education Program developed to summarize research into CVD and provide recommendations for health-care professionals.

Atherosclerosis: Development of plaque on small vessel walls.

Body mass index: Ratio of weight in kilograms divided by height in square meters, used as an indicator of weight status.

C-reactive protein: Acute-phase protein, marker for and proponent of inflammatory response in atherosclerosis.

Cholesterol: Obtained from dietary and endogenous sources, necessary for cell membrane structure, abnormal levels associated with CVD risk.

Coronary artery disease: Diminished oxygen supply to the heart muscle due to the presence of atherosclerotic lesions in coronary vessels.

Glycemic index: The effect on blood sugar levels in comparison to an equivalent amount of a standard source of carbohydrate, usually glucose or white bread.

Glycemic load: Product of a food's glycemic index multiplied by the carbohydrate content, a more appropriate indicator of glucose and insulin response than the glycemic index.

High-density lipoprotein cholesterol: Carrier lipoprotein, high levels known to be cardioprotective.

Homocysteine: Sulfur-containing amino acid, byproduct of methionine metabolism, high levels associated with CVD risk.

Hypertension: High blood pressure, more than 130/90 mmHg.

Lipoprotein(a): Particle similar to LDL, largely genetically controlled, may be highly thrombotic in atherosclerotic lesions.

Low-density lipoprotein cholesterol: Lipoprotein associated with cardiovascular risk, susceptible to oxidation.

Myocardial infarction: Occlusion of cardiac arteries causing inadequate blood supply to heart muscle cells with the potential for tissue damage.

National Cholesterol Education Program: Branch of the National Institute of Health developed in 1985 to address the public health concerns of hyperlipidemia.

Omega-3 fatty acids: Fatty acid chains which are precursors for anti-inflammatory leukotrienes and prostaglandins.

Omega-6 fatty acids: Fatty acid chains which are precursors for inflammatory leukotrienes and prostaglandins.

Oxidation: Damage caused by free radicals, which contributes to atherosclerosis.

Plant sterols and stanols: Plant equivalent of animal cholesterol, mostly nondigestible by the gastrointestinal tract.

Stroke: Occlusion of blood vessels in the cerebrovascular system.

Triglycerides: First step in fat metabolism composed of three fatty acid chains attached to a glycerol backbone.

REFERENCES

1. Cardiovascular Disease Statistics, American Heart Association, accessed January 13, 2004 at http://www.americanheart.org/presenter.jhtml?identifier = 4478.
2. Hackam, D.G. and Anand, S.S., Emerging risk factors for atherosclerotic vascular disease, *JAMA*, 290, 932, 2003.
3. Safeer, R. and Ugalat, P., Cholesterol treatment guidelines update, *Am. Fam. Physician*, 65, 871, 2002.
4. Talbert, R., Role of the National Cholesterol Education Program Adult Treatment Panel III Guidelines in Managing Dyslipidemia, *Am. J. Health Syst. Pharm.*, 60 (Suppl. 2), S3, 2003.
5. Carlson, J.J. and Monti, V., The role of inclusive dietary patterns for achieving secondary prevention cardiovascular nutrition guidelines and optimal cardiovascular health, *J. Cardiopulm. Rehabil.*, 23, 322, 2003.
6. Kreisberg, R. and Oberman, A., Lipids and atherosclerosis: lessons learned from randomized control trials of lipid lowering and other relevant studies, *J. Clin. Endocrinol. Metab.*, 87, 423, 2002.
7. National Cholesterol Education Program, Third report of the expert panel on detection, evaluation, and treatment of high blood cholesterol in adults (Adult Treatment Panel III), NIH Pub. No.02-5215, National Heart, Lung, and Blood Institute, Bethesda, MD, 2002.
8. Kurtoglu, E. et al., Effects of lipoprotein apheresis on oxidative stress and antioxidant status in familial hypercholesterolemic patients, *Int. J. Artif. Organs*, 26, 1039, 2003.
9. Sacks, F.M. and Katan, M., Randomized clinical trials on the effects of dietary fat and carbohydrate on plasma lipoproteins and cardiovascular disease, *Am. J. Med.*, 113, 13S, 2002.
10. Fang, J. et al., Exercise, body mass index, caloric intake, and cardiovascular mortality, *Am. J. Prev. Med.*, 25, 283, 2003.
11. Bonow, R. and Eckel, R., Diet, obesity, and cardiovascular risk, *N. Engl. J. Med.*, 21, 2057, 2003.
12. Physical activity and health: a report of the surgeon general, accessed January 12, 2004 at http://www.cdc.gov/nccdphp/sgr/summ.htm.
13. Eckel, R. and Krauss, R., American Heart Association call to action: obesity as a major risk factor for coronary heart disease, *Circulation*, 97, 2099, 1998.
14. Zeman, F.J., *Clinical Nutrition and Dietetics*, 2nd ed., Macmillan, New York, 1993, chap. 10.
15. Step I, step II and TLC diets, accessed January 8, 2004 at http://www.americanheart.org/presenter.jhtml?identifier = 4764.
16. Hunt, S. and Groff, J., *Advanced Nutrition and Human Metabolism*, West Publishing Company, St. Paul, 1990, chap. 16.
17. Health implications of dietary fiber, accessed December 1, 2003 at http://www.eatright.org/Public/Other/index_adar2_0702.cfm.
18. Schaefer, E.J., Lipoproteins, nutrition, and heart disease, *Am. J. Clin. Nutr.*, 75, 191, 2002.
19. Hu, F.B., Plant-based foods and prevention of cardiovascular disease: an overview, *Am. J. Clin. Nutr.*, 78, 544S, 2003.

20. Ascherio, A., Epidemiological studies on dietary fats and coronary heart disease, *Am. J. Med.*, 113, 9S, 2002.

21. Lee, K.W. and Lip, G.Y.H., The role of omega-3 fatty acids in the secondary prevention of cardiovascular disease, *QJM*, 96, 465, 2003.

22. Hu, F.B. and Willet, W.C., Optimal diets for the prevention of coronary heart disease, *JAMA*, 288, 2569, 2002.

23. Kris-Etherton, P.M. et al., Recent discoveries in inclusive food-based approaches and dietary patterns for reduction in risk for cardiovascular disease, *Curr. Opin. Lipidol.*, 13, 397, 2002.

24. Nuttall, S.L., Kendall, M.J., and Martin, U., Antioxidant therapy for the prevention of cardiovascular disease, *QJM*, 92, 239, 1999.

25. Pruthi, S., Allison, T.G., and Hensrud, D.D., Vitamin E supplementation in the prevention of coronary heart disease, *Mayo Clin. Proc.*, 76, 1131, 2001.

26. Hodis, H.N. et al., Alpha-tocopherol supplementation in healthy individuals reduces low-density lipoprotein oxidation but not atherosclerosis: the vitamin E atherosclerosis prevention study (VEAPS), *Circulation*, 106, 1453, 2002.

27. Brown, B.G. et al., Simvastatin and niacin, antioxidant vitamins, or the combination for the prevention of coronary disease, *N. Engl. J. Med.*, 345, 1583, 2001.

28. U.S. Preventative Task Force, Routine vitamin supplementation to prevent cancer and cardiovascular disease: recommendations and rationale, *Ann. Int. Med.*, 139, 51, 2003.

29. Anderson, J.W., Diet first, then medication for hypercholesterolemia, *JAMA*, 290, 531, 2003.

30. Katan, M.B. et al., Efficacy and safety of plant stanols and sterols in the management of blood cholesterol levels, *Mayo Clin. Proc.*, 78, 965, 2003.

31. Liu, R.H., Health benefits of fruit and vegetables are from additive and synergistic combinations of phytochemicals, *Am. J. Clin. Nutr.*, 78, 517S, 2003.

32. Sesso, H.D. et al., Flavonoid intake and the risk of cardiovascular disease in women, *Am. J. Clin. Nutr.*, 77, 1400, 2003.

33. Sabaté, J., Nut consumption, vegetarian diets, ischemic heart disease risk, and all-cause mortality: evidence from epidemiologic studies, *Am. J. Clin. Nutr.*, 70, 500S, 1999.

34. Boden, W., Therapeutic implications of recent ATP III guidelines and the important role of combination therapy in total dyslipidemia management, *Curr. Opin. Cardiol.*, 18, 278, 2003.

35. FDA Orange Book, accessed September 9, 2004 at http://www.accessdata.fda.gov/scripts/cder/ob/docs/obdetail.cfm?Appl_No = 021445&TABLE1 = OB_Rx.

36. Brucket, E. et al., Perspectives in cholesterol-lowering therapy: the role of ezetimibe, a new selective inhibitor of intestinal cholesterol absorption, *Circulation*, 107, 3125, 2003.

37. Foster, G.D. et al., A randomized trial of a low-carbohydrate diet for obesity, *N. Engl. J. Med.*, 348, 2082, 2003.

38. Tapper-Gardzina, Y., Cotugna, N., and Vickery, C.E., Should you recommend a low-carbohydrate, high-protein diet? *Nurs. Pract.*, 27, 52, 2002.

39. Gau, G.T., The search for the perfect heart-healthy diet, *Mayo Clin. Proc.*, 78, 1329, 2003.

40. Rodrigo, R. et al., Implications of oxidative stress and homocysteine in the pathophysiology of essential hypertension, *J. Cardiovasc. Pharmacol.*, 42, 453, 2003.

41. Graham, I.M. and O'Callaghan, P., Symposium: vitamins, homocysteine, and cardiovascular risk, *Cardiovasc. Drug Ther.*, 16, 383, 2002.

42. Haynes, W.G., Hyperhomocysteinemia, vascular function and atherosclerosis: effects of vitamins, *Cardiovasc. Drug Ther.*, 16, 391, 2002.

43. Homocysteine Studies Collaboration, Homocysteine and risk of ischemic heart disease and stroke, *JAMA*, 288, 2015, 2002.

44. Torres, J.L. and Ridker, P.M., Clinical use of high sensitivity C-reactive protein for the prediction of adverse cardiovascular events, *Curr. Opin. Cardiol.*, 18, 471, 2003.

45. Pischon, T. et al., Habitual intake of $n-3$ and $n-6$ fatty acids in relation to inflammatory markers among U.S. men and women, *Circulation*, 108, 155, 2003.

46. Hirschfield, G.M. and Pepys, M.B., C-reactive protein and cardiovascular disease: new insights from an old molecule, *QJM*, 96, 793, 2003.

47. Wood, M.J. et al., Use of complimentary and alternative medical therapies in patients with cardiovascular disease, *Am. Heart J.*, 145, 806, 2003.

48. Hardy, G., Hardy, I., and Ball, P.A., Nutraceuticals — a pharmaceutical viewpoint: part II, *Curr. Opin. Clin. Nutr. Metab. Care*, 6, 661, 2003.

49. Writing Group for Women's Health Initiative Investigators, Risks and benefits of estrogen plus progestin in healthy postmenopausal women, *JAMA*, 288, 321, 2002.

50. Otto, C. et al., Efficacy and safety of a new whole-blood low-density lipoprotein apheresis system (Liposorber D) in severe hypercholesterolemia, *Artif. Organs*, 27, 1116, 2003.

51. August, P., Initial treatment of hypertension, *N. Engl. J. Med.*, 348, 610, 2003.

Nervous System

Ame Golaszewski and Leo McCluskey

CONTENTS

INTRODUCTION

There is a complex relationship between nutrition and the nervous system. Disorders of both the peripheral nervous system (PNS) and central nervous system (CNS) may disrupt normal physiologic processes by which food is desired, acquired, masticated, swallowed, and digested. Optimizing and maintaining adequate nutrition may prove to be quite challenging for individuals faced with some neurological disorders. As a result, secondary malnutrition and dehydration may complicate the neurologic process. Primary nutritional disorders that produce calorie, protein, or vitamin deficiency states may cause transient or permanent PNS or CNS dysfunction. Toxins, purposefully or inadvertently ingested, may also injure the nervous system.

In this chapter, we review some common neurological disorders that may adversely affect nutrition. We also discuss primary nutritional and toxic disorders that may secondarily affect the CNS or PNS.

NEUROLOGICAL APPROACH[1]

The neurological assessment of any clinical problem begins with a determination of the anatomic localization of the disease process. Neurologists use the history of the presenting symptoms and the neurologic examination to localize disease processes to the CNS (brain and spinal cord), PNS (lower motor neurons [LMN], sensory neurons, cranial or peripheral nerves, neuromuscular junction, and muscle). Neurologists then attempt to define the cause of the disorder with diagnostic testing (e.g., body fluid analysis, neuroimaging, and electrophysiology). An understanding of pertinent neurologic anatomy is therefore essential for an understanding of nutritional disorders caused by neurologic disease or nutritional disorders that produce neurologic dysfunction.

NEUROANATOMY

APPETITE AND FOOD-SEEKING BEHAVIOR

During the preabsorptive phase, the sight, smell, or thought of food may trigger a sensation of hunger, reflex production of saliva, gastric secretions, and gastrointestinal hormones. The anterior frontal lobes direct attention and motor planning necessary to fulfill food interest. The lateral hypothalamus contains the so-called "feeding center" that triggers the sense of hunger and initiates food-seeking behavior. Destructive lesions here can lead to involuntary starvation.

Ingestion of food distends the lumen of the stomach and proximal small intestine. Digestion of food releases the nutrient constituents of fats, amino acids, and sugars. Ingestion and digestion trigger systemic release of gastrointestinal hormones including cholecystokinin, bombesin, gastrin, secretin, glucagon, insulin, somatostatin, neurostatin, substance P, and pancreatic polypeptide. These hormones stimulate the ventromedial hypothalamus, the so-called satiety center. They also inhibit the hypothalamic-feeding center. This serves to reduce feeding activity during the absorptive phase of eating. Lesions involving the satiety center portion of the hypothalamus can lead to overeating and obesity. During the post-absorptive phase, hormones such as leptin, produced by adipose tissue, also serve to curb appetite. Leptin may accomplish this by lowering brain levels of natural cannabinoids that act to stimulate appetite.[2-14]

MOTOR SYSTEM[1,15]

Residing in the motor cortex within the posterior aspect of the frontal lobes, upper motor neurons (UMN) that provide voluntary control of skeletal muscles are ordered in a somatotopic (body map) or homuncular pattern. The axons of these first-order neurons descend through the central white matter (centrum semiovale) of the cerebral hemispheres, the posterior limb of the internal capsule, the cerebral peduncle of the midbrain, the pontine base, and the pyramids of the medulla. At the medullary level, the axons cross or decussate to the opposite side and continue to descend as the corticospinal tract in the posterolateral aspect of the spinal cord. Axons emanating from UMN residing in head and neck portions of the homunculus synapse with brain stem LMN grouped within brain stem motor nuclei. LMN axons exit the brain stem via the oculomotor (III), trochlear (IV), trigeminal (V), abducens (VI), facial (VII), glossopharyngeal (IX), vagus (X), spinal accessory (XI), and hypoglossal (XII) cranial nerves (CN) to innervate muscles of the head and neck. Descending axons emanating from UMN residing in the axial and limb portions of the homunculus synapse with LMN residing in the anterior gray matter (anterior horn) of the spinal cord. Axons from these neurons exit the spinal cord via the anterior or motor roots and travel to target muscles via the brachial or lumbar plexi and peripheral limb nerves.

SENSORY SYSTEM[1,15]

Sensory receptors located in soft tissues and bones transmit painful, thermal, mechanical, discriminative touch, and proprioceptive information via first-order peripheral sensory axons that traverse peripheral limb nerves, brachial or lumbar plexi, and sensory or posterior roots to reach the posterolateral aspect of the spinal cord. In the spinal cord, fibers responsible for carrying pain and temperature sensation cross anterior to the central canal and ascend via the spinothalamic tract in the anterolateral aspect of the cord. Head and neck pain and temperature sensory fibers enter the brain stem via CN (V, VII, IX, and X) and join ascending limb fibers in their ascent to the thalamus where they synapse with second-order sensory neurons.

Axons from these second-order neurons traverse the anterior limb of the internal capsule and the corona radiate to synapse with third-order sensory neurons in the sensory strip of the parietal lobe.

Fibers carrying fine touch and proprioception sensation travel rostrally in the posterior column to the level of the cervicomedullary junction where they synapse with neurons in the cuneate (arm) and gracillis (leg) nuclei. Axons from these second-order neurons cross to the opposite side of the brain stem and travel rostrally via the medial lemniscus to synapse with third-order neurons in the thalamus. As with the spinothalamic tract, head and neck fibers enter the brain stem via CN (V, VII, IX, and X) and join the medial lemniscus. Axons from thalamic neurons travel rostrally to synapse with cortical neurons. As with the motor cortex, neurons within the sensory cortex are somatotopically organized.

Afferent information from taste receptors located on the anterior two thirds of the tongue travels with the chorda tympani portion of the facial (VII) nerve to the nucleus of the tractus solitarius. Taste receptors located on the posterior one third of the tongue project to the same region via the glossopharyngeal (IX) nerve. Taste information is then relayed to regions of the thalamus, hypothalamus, and amygdale. From the thalamus, taste information is sent to the sensory cortex.

Olfactory information from smell receptors located in the superior aspect of the nasal cavity travels through the cribriform plate of the skull to synapse with neurons within the olfactory bulbs. Axons from olfactory bulb neurons travel in the olfactory tracts to reach the amygdala, septal nuclei, prepyriform cortex, the entorhinal cortex, hippocampus, and the subiculum. Some of these brain regions are considered to be part of the limbic system, a region of the brain concerned with motivation, emotion, and certain kinds of memory. The septal nuclei and amygdala contain regions known as the "pleasure centers." The hippocampus is concerned with memory and the association of certain stimuli with food. Olfactory axons also project to the thalamus and from there to the frontal cortex for conscious recognition. There are many forward and backward connections between each of these brain centers (Table 10.1).

TABLE 10.1
List of Cranial Nerve Lesions That May Impact Nutrition

Structure	Sympathetic Stimulation	Parasympathetic Stimulation
Iris (eye muscle)	Pupil dilation	Pupil constriction
Salivary glands	Saliva production reduced	Saliva production increased
Oral and nasal mucosa	Mucus production reduced	Mucus production increased
Heart	Heart rate and force increased	Heart rate and force decreased
Lung	Bronchial muscle relaxed	Bronchial muscle contracted
Stomach	Peristalsis reduced	Gastric juice secreted; motility increased
Small intestine	Motility reduced	Digestion increased
Large intestine	Motility reduced	Secretions and motility increased
Liver	Increased conversion of glycogen to glucose	
Kidney	Decreased urine secretion	Increased urine secretion
Adrenal medulla	Norepinephrine and epinephrine secreted	
Bladder	Wall relaxed	Wall contracted
	Sphincter closed	Sphincter relaxed

AUTONOMIC SYSTEM[1,15]

The autonomic nervous system (ANS) is divided into sympathetic and parasympathetic efferent and afferent portions. The central and peripheral components of the ANS regulate salivary and other glandular secretions and control gastrointestinal motility. The efferent ANS is organized into a three-neuron circuit. In both the parasympathetic and sympathetic portions, the first- and second-order neurons are located within the CNS while the third-order neurons are located in the periphery. There are important anatomic and physiologic distinctions between the two portions (Table 10.1).

In the parasympathetic division, the first-order neurons are located within the frontal lobe, temporal lobe, amygdale, and hypothalamus. Second-order neuron cell bodies are located in the brain stem and sacral portion of the spinal cord. The axons of second-order neurons exit these locations and travel to synapse with third-order neurons organized into ganglia located in or near the target organ. Hence the parasympathetic division has a long second order but a short third-order axon. The neurotransmitter of all three neurons of the parasympathetic system is acetylcholine. The parasympathetic system increases salivary, mucus, and gastrointestinal secretion production and accelerates gastrointestinal motility.

In the sympathetic division, first-order neurons are located in the hypothalamus while second-order axons are located in the thoracic and upper lumbar portion of the spinal cord. Second-order axons exit the spinal cord and travel to third-order neurons organized into the paravertebral sympathetic chain, midline accessory ganglia in the retroperitoneum, or to the adrenal medulla. Third-order axons travel to target organs via peripheral nerves or arteries. The neurotransmitter of the first- and second-order sympathetic neurons is acetylcholine. In nearly all circumstances, save for innervation of sweat glands, norepinephrine is the transmitter of the third-order sympathetic neuron. The sympathetic system decreases salivary, mucus, and gastrointestinal secretion and reduces gastrointestinal motility.

Second-order parasympathetic axons from the superior salivatory nucleus exit the brain stem via the VII nerve to supply the sublingual and submandibular salivary glands. Second-order parasympathetic neurons from the inferior salivatory nucleus exit the brain stem via the IX nerve to supply the parotid gland. The axons of the facial (VII) and glossopharyngeal (IX) nerves synapse with the third-order neurons located in local organ related ganglia (pterygo-palatine, otic, submandibular, and celiac). Second-order parasympathetic axons from the dorsal motor nucleus exit the brain stem via the X nerve to supply the gallbladder, bile duct, pancreas, and secretory components of the stomach along with all the other components of the gastrointestinal tract. The vagus (X) also supplies the smooth musculature of the lower two thirds of the esophagus, stomach, small intestine, and colon to the splenic flexure.

Afferent parasympathetic and sympathetic activity originates in sensory receptors located with innervated structures. The sensory autonomic axons of these receptors reach the spinal cord and brain stem by traveling within cranial or spinal nerves. Within the spinal cord, these axons can synapse with regional autonomic neurons or they can ascend to the brain stem or hemispheric level. In this way, afferent autonomic activity can directly influence efferent sympathetic and parasympathetic outflow.

Swallow[16]

The oral phase of swallowing consists of mastication (masseter, temporalis, and pterygoid muscles innervated by CN (V)) and formation of a food or liquid bolus that is voluntarily propelled into the oropharynx by the tongue (tongue muscle innervated by CN (XII)). Maintenance of food or liquid within the oral and proximal pharyngeal cavity depends upon the input from sensory afferents (V, IX). Facial musculature (VII) maintains lip closure while soft palatal closure of the nasopharynx (IX, X) prevents nasal regurgitation of the bolus. Once the bolus enters the pharynx (pharyngeal phase), afferents located in the mucosa and musculature of the pharynx relay sensory information via the glossopharyngeal (IX) and vagus (X) nerves to the solitary nucleus and solitary. After processing, motor output is directed via the vagus (X) to initiate a swallowing sequence, modify an already ongoing swallowing sequence, or even to abort the process. Vagal (X) motor efferents produce a rostral to caudal contraction of the skeletal musculature contained in the proximal one third of the esophagus (esophageal phase). Continuation of peristalsis by the smooth muscle of the distal two thirds of the esophagus is under the control of a local neural plexus located in the esophageal wall.

Cough[16]

Nonvolitional or reflex coughing is a defensive mechanism mediated by sensory afferent activity in the trigeminal (V), glossopharyngeal (IX), and vagus (X) nerves and motor efferent activity in the phrenic nerve (innervating the diaphragm), the vagus (X), and glossopharyngeal nerve (IX). Irritation of the nose and nasopharynx (V), the oropharynx (IX), and the larynx and upper tracheobronchial portion of the respiratory tract (X) can trigger a cough. From a nutritional perspective, the most important trigger for coughing is a solid or liquid bolus that is inappropriately swallowed and allowed to impact sensory receptors in the mucosa of the larynx or upper tracheobronchial tree. When stimulated, these receptors produce sensory action potentials that travel toward the medulla via myelinated vagal sensory afferent fibers ending in or near the nucleus of the tractus solitarius. It is here that the incoming sensory information is processed and a reflex motor output is produced via intrinsic brain stem connections with motor neurons that supply the muscles of the respiratory system (diaphragm, intercostals), larynx, and bronchial tree. The voluntary act of coughing accurately mimics the reflexive variety that can be initiated in the frontal motor region and most likely bypasses the medullary control center.

A cough starts with a deep inspiration that is followed by a forced expiration against a closed glottis. The elastic recoil of the chest aids muscular contraction. Intrathoracic pressure rises precipitously during this compressive phase. Once the glottis opens, air flows at high velocity during the expulsive phase. Airflow mobilizes both tracheobronchial secretions and inappropriately swallowed liquids or solids. While glottic closure is important, patients incapable of this maneuver can produce an effective cough as long as respiratory muscular strength is preserved.

Gag[16]

The gag reflex consists of pharyngeal elevation and constriction with tongue retraction. It is produced in response to sensory stimulation of the pharyngeal wall, posterior tongue, tonsils, or faucial pillars. Stimulation of these regions can trigger vomiting via reflex retrograde contraction of the stomach and esophagus. The sensory afferents reach the medulla via the glossopharyngeal (IX) nerve while the motor efferents travel in the vagus (X) nerve.

NEUROLOGICAL DISORDERS

A variety of CNS and PNS diseases may disrupt motor, sensory and autonomic anatomy, and physiology required for the maintenance of adequate nutrition (Table 10.2). Although disorders of smell and taste are not life threatening, they too may negatively impact nutrition (Table 10.3 and Table 10.4). Anosmia or hyposmia are the terms used to describe the inability

TABLE 10.2
Neurologic Lesions That Impact Nutrition

	Possible Consequences
Cranial nerves[a]	
CN I (olfactory)	Smell and possibly taste deficit
CN V (trigeminal)	Numbness of lips and tongue
	Weakness of masseter/pterygoid/temporalis muscles
CN VII (facial)	Weakness of lips/cheek
	Drooling, biting of cheek
	Reduced salivation (submandibular and sublingual)
	Altered taste anterior two thirds of tongue
CN IX (glossopharyngeal)	Reduced palatal sensation
	Reduced gag reflex
	Reduced salivation (parotid)
CN X (vagus)	Reduced palatal and pharyngeal muscle strength
	Nasal regurgitation of fluids > solids
	Dysphagia
	Reduced laryngeal muscular strength
	Hoarseness, aspiration of liquids > solids
	Reduced autonomic efferent innervation of GI tract
	Gastroparesis, reduced intestinal transit time
	Constipation, ileus
CN XII (hypoglossal)	Tongue weakness
	Reduced ability to manipulate foods
	Reduced ability to imitate swallow
Brain and brain stem	
Posterior frontal lobe	Weakness of contralateral lower > upper face, tongue palate, pharynx, vocal cord, arm, leg
Parietal lobe	Contralateral sensory loss and neglect
Occipital lobe	Contralateral hemifield visual loss
Hypothalamus	Obesity, starvation
Degenerations of brain (Alzheimer's)	Cognitive deficits, altered dietary habits, eventually dysphagia
Frontotemporal dementia	Impulsive or altered dietary habits, eventually dysphagia
Basal ganglia	Movement disorders
Substantia nigra	Parkinson's disease
Putamen/globus pallidus	Parkinsonism
Subthalamus	Chorea, ballism (increased metabolic demand)
Cerebellum	Ipsilateral ataxia, tremor
Brain stem	Combination of cranial nerve deficits with associated ipsilateral or contralateral weakness or sensory loss
Muscle/neuromuscular junction	
Facial weakness	Weakness of lips/cheek, drooling, biting of cheek
Palatal weakness	Nasal regurgitation of fluids > solids
Tongue weakness	Reduced ability to manipulate foods and initiate swallow
Vocal cord weakness	Increased risk of aspiration
Hand/arm weakness	Reduced ability to eat with implements/hand
Peripheral nerve	
Neuropathy involving arms/hands	Reduced ability to eat with implements/hand
Autonomic neuropathy	Gastroparesis, reduced transit time, constipation, ileus

[a]Haerer, A.F., *DeJong's The Neurologic Examination*, 5th ed., J.B. Lippincott Company, Philadelphia, 1992.

TABLE 10.3
Disorders of Smell

Common Causes	Less Common Causes	Uncommon Causes
Nasal and sinus disease (e.g., allergic or vasomotor rhinitis, chronic sinusitis, nasal polyps, adenoid hypertrophy)	Medications	Neoplasm or brain tumor (e.g., osteoma, olfactory groove, or cribriform plate meningioma, frontal lobe tumor, temporal lobe tumor, pituitary tumor, aneurysm, esthesioneuroblastoma, melanoma, squamous cell carcinoma)
Upper respiratory infection	Cocaine abuse (intranasal)	Psychiatric conditions (e.g., malingering, schizophrenia, depression, olfactory reference syndrome)
Head trauma (e.g., frontal skull fracture, occipital injury, nasal fracture)	Toxic chemical exposure (e.g., benzene, benzol, butyl acetate, carbon disulfide, chlorine, ethyl acetate, formaldehyde, hydrogen selenide, paint solvents, sulfuric acid, trichloroethylene)	Endocrine disorders (e.g., adrenocortical insufficiency, Cushing's syndrome, diabetes mellitus, hypothyroidism, primary amenorrhea, pseudohypoparathyroidism, Kallmann's syndrome, Turner's syndrome, pregnancy)
Cigarette smoking	Industrial agent exposure (e.g., ashes, cadmium, chalk, chromium, iron carboxyl, lead, nickel, silicone dioxide)	Epilepsy (olfactory aura)
Neurodegenerative disease (e.g., Alzheimer's disease, Parkinson's disease, multiple sclerosis)	Nutritional factors (e.g., vitamin deficiency, trace metal deficiency, malnutrition, chronic renal failure, liver disease, cancer, acquired immunodeficiency syndrome)	Migraine headache (olfactory aura)
Age	Radiation treatment of head and neck	Cerebrovascular accident
	Congenital conditions (e.g., congenital anosmia, Kallmann's syndrome)	Sjögren's syndrome
		Systemic lupus erythematosus

to smell or a reduction of the ability to smell, respectively. Ageusia is the term used to describe the inability to taste. Dysphagia is the most common cause of nutritional difficulty encountered in neurologic disease. Dysmotility of the stomach, small intestine, or large intestine produced by neurologic disease may also impact nutrition.

DYSPHAGIA[16]

Patients describe the symptom of dysphagia (Greek *phagia* "to eat" and *dys* "difficulty" or "disordered") as a sensation of food hindered in its passage from the mouth to the stomach. Neurologic disorders produce dysphagia by disrupting the intricately coordinated sensory (afferent) and motor (efferent) control of swallowing (Table 10.5). Dysphagia may involve the

TABLE 10.4
Disorders of Taste

Common Causes	Less Common Causes	Uncommon Causes
Oral and perioral infections (e.g., candidiasis, gingivitis, herpes simplex, periodontitis, sialadenitis)	Nutritional factors (e.g., vitamin deficiency, trace metal deficiency,[203] malnutrition, chronic renal failure, liver disease,[204] cancer, acquired immunodeficiency syndrome)	Psychiatric conditions (e.g., depression, anorexia nervosa, bulimia)
Bell's palsy	Tumor or lesions associated with taste pathways (e.g., oral cavity cancer, neoplasm of skull base)	Epilepsy (gustatory aura)
Medications	Head trauma	Migraine headache (gustatory aura)
Oral appliances (e.g., dentures, filling materials, tooth prosthetics)	Toxic chemical exposure (e.g., benzene, benzol, butyl acetate, carbon disulfide, chlorine, ethyl acetate, formaldehyde, hydrogen selenide, paint solvents, sulfuric acid, trichloroethylene)	Sjögren's syndrome
Dental procedures (e.g., tooth extraction, root canal)	Industrial agent exposure (e.g., chromium, lead, copper)	Multiple sclerosis
Age	Radiation treatment of head and neck	Endocrine disorders (e.g., adrenocortical insufficiency, Cushing's syndrome, diabetes mellitus, hypothyroidism, panhypopituitarism, pseudohypoparathyroidism, Kallmann's syndrome, Turner's syndrome)

oral phase (bolus formation followed by propelling the bolus into the pharynx), the pharyngeal phase (propelling the bolus through the pharynx, past the trachea, and into the upper esophagus), or the esophageal phase (propelling the bolus through the esophagus to the stomach). Usually solid or liquid boluses progress from the mouth to the stomach within 10 s. When this rapid and orderly progression of rostral to caudal muscular contraction fails to develop in the esophagus, the bolus can distend the lumen and cause a sense of discomfort and even pain.

Thin liquids are more difficult to swallow than solids. Even mild dysfunction of pharyngeal muscular function may produce liquid dysphagia. Patients may initially describe the need for multiple liquid swallows and when weakness is more significant swallowing of thin liquids may be accompanied by coughing, choking, and other symptoms of aspiration (tearing, strained speech, and strained inspiration with stridor). Patients will often note that they cannot rapidly swallow or "chug" liquids like they have become accustomed to in the past. They may, however, be able to handle smaller amounts of liquids by drinking through a straw or sipping from a cup. They may note that thicker consistency liquids are more easily swallowed. Patients with significant liquid dysphagia may also have coexisting difficulty in handling saliva and other oropharyngeal secretions. Such patients may spontaneously cough or choke upon their own secretions. More severe pharyngeal dysphagia is accompanied by

TABLE 10.5
Neurologic Causes of Dysphagia

Cerebrovascular disorders — arterial
Ischemic stroke
Intracerebral hemorrhage
Subarachnoid hemorrhage
Arteriovenous malformation — hemisphere, brain stem, posterior fossa
Vascular dementia
Cerebrovascular disorders — venous
Venous sinus occlusion
Cortical venous occlusion
Inflammatory/demyelinating disease
Multiple sclerosis
Acute disseminated encephalomyelitis
Neoplastic disorders
Hemispheric tumors — benign, malignant
Brain stem and posterior fossa tumors — benign, malignant
Infectious disorders
Botulism
Diphtheria
Poliomyelitis
Prion disorders (e.g., Creutzfeldt–Jakob)
Motor neuron disorders
Amyotrophic lateral sclerosis
Primary lateral sclerosis
Progressive bulbar palsy
Poliomyelitis and post-polio muscular atrophy syndrome
Kennedy's syndrome (progressive spinobulbar muscular atrophy)
Muscular disorders
Oculopharyngeal muscular dystrophy
Myotonic muscular dystrophy
Polymyositis, dermatomyositis, and inclusion body myositis
Congenital myopathies
Metabolic myopathies
Mitochondrial myopathies
Neuromuscular junction disorders
Myasthenia gravis
Congenital myasthenia
Lambert Eaton myasthenic syndrome
Peripheral nerve disorders
Acute inflammatory demyelinating polyneuropathy (Guillain–Barré)
Chronic inflammatory demyelinating polyneuropathy
Movement disorders
Parkinson's disease
Parkinsonism
Dystonia
Lewy body disease
Huntington's disease
Dementing disorders
Alzheimer's disease
Frontotemporal dementia

solid dysphagia. Patients with significant liquid and particularly solid dysphagia will often note that time necessary to consume their meal is considerably longer.

DIETARY CONSEQUENCES OF NEUROLOGICAL DISEASE

Neurological disease processes affect nutrition by injuring structures that play a role in one or more aspects of eating and digestion. The nervous system is intimately involved in appetite, food acquisition and food preparation, placement of food within the oral cavity, oral manipulation of food, chewing, swallowing, digestion, and transit of food from esophagus to the colon. While dysphagia is the most common neurologic symptom that disturbs nutrition, lesions of the CNS or PNS may negatively impact many other aspects of normal nutrition.

STROKE

Stroke is the third leading cause of death in the United States behind heart disease and cancer. Each year about 700,000 people in the United States have a stroke; nearly 500,000 of these are first events. Approximately, 4 million Americans are living with the effects of stroke. About one third have mild impairments, one third are moderately impaired, and one third are severely impaired. Strokes can be classified as either ischemic or hemorrhagic. Hemorrhagic stroke can be further divided into intracerebral hemorrhage or subarachnoid hemorrhage.[1]

Eighty-eight percent of strokes are ischemic strokes. This occurs when blood flow in one or more brain arteries is interrupted by a blood clot. Most commonly, this is the end result of the accumulation of atherosclerosis that progressively narrows the lumen of the artery culminating in the formation of a local clot or thrombus. Arterial occlusion may also occur if an embolus, a clot from the heart or from the proximal cerebral arteries that dislodges and travels more to distal and smaller arteries, occludes the lumen. If collateral arterial circulation fails to provide blood to the perfused region in time, the tissue will undergo irreversible ischemic necrosis. At times, this is accompanied by the subsequent development of hemorrhage in the injured area. This is termed hemorrhagic stroke or hemorrhagic conversion of an ischemic stroke. The neurologic deficit that follows an ischemic stroke depends upon the size of the lesion, the region or regions affected, and the neurological functions served by each of the involved areas.[1]

Nine percent of strokes result from intracranial hemorrhage. This occurs when one or more arteries within the brain parenchyma rupture forcing arterial blood under pressure into the surrounding brain region. Most often this occurs as a result of weakening of the wall of small arteries or arterioles that is the result of long-standing hypertension. Less commonly, this may result from bleeding from a congenital malformation of blood vessels known as an arteriovenous malformation. Three percent of strokes are the result of subarachnoid hemorrhage. This occurs when one or more arteries outside of the brain parenchyma but within the skull rupture spilling arterial blood into the space outside the brain that is lined with the meningeal membrane known as the pia and arachnoid. This most often occurs as a result of the formation of an aneurysm at areas of congenital weakness within the arterial wall.[1,17]

The initial medical goal for any stroke patient is clinical stabilization. Once a definitive cause of the stroke is determined, medical therapy, which may include anticoagulation and manipulation of blood pressure, is initiated. Patients with subarachnoid hemorrhage may undergo neurosurgical clipping of the offending aneurysm. Once a patient is medically stable, other therapies including nutrition can be addressed. A swallowing evaluation, performed by a speech pathologist, can provide valuable insight into the extent of dysphagia and the dietary or feeding modifications necessary to safely feed patients who have suffered a stroke. The speech pathologist can recommend an appropriate consistency of the liquid and solid components of the diet or any compensatory swallowing strategies that may serve to decrease the risk of aspiration of feeding into the airway.

Diets modified in liquid consistency often involve the use of commercial thickening agents to produce "thickened liquids." This may decrease the risk of aspiration. Nutritional recommendations should reflect information obtained from the swallowing evaluation as well as any appropriate dietary restrictions necessary for related and unrelated medical conditions. This may include the management of hypertension and hyperlipidemia. The provision of small, frequent meals, consisting of nutrient-dense foods, is often needed to meet the nutritional needs of the stroke patient with dysphagia. Although dysphagia that follows stroke may improve within days or possibly weeks after the event, some individuals may have persistent and severe swallowing dysfunction. If oral intake remains suboptimal, or risk of aspiration is high, enteral nutrition via tube feeding, nasogastric or gastric, may be necessary until adequate swallowing function returns.[17] Documentation of the caloric and protein content of oral intake and serial weights may assist in assessing the need for supplemental enteral nutrition.

Efforts of the medical team should be directed toward preventing malnutrition and dehydration, minimizing the risk of aspiration, maintaining the patients' overall health, and managing stroke risk factors (Table 10.6).[18] The combination of a balanced diet, behavioral modifications, and medication compliance often results in reduction of stroke risk. Low-fat, low-cholesterol diets may be indicated for obese individuals or those with evidence of a significant elevation of cholesterol or triglycerides at an increased risk for stroke. Supplementation with vitamin B_{12} and folic acid may be recommended to further reduce stroke risk related to possible elevated levels of serum homocysteine.

AMYOTROPHIC LATERAL SCLEROSIS[19–24]

Amyotrophic lateral sclerosis (ALS) is a lethal, degenerative neurological disorder of unknown cause that is characterized by the progressive loss of UMN or LMN that is responsible for the control of voluntary skeletal muscle. The weakness of ALS begins in the muscles of one body segment (cranial, cervical, thoracic, lumbosacral) and over a variable period of time (months to years) progresses through the original segment of onset and then spreads to the other segments. Limb onset is most common (70%). Bulbar onset, weakness that begins in muscles of the head and neck, is less common (25%). Respiratory muscle onset is the least common (1%). When ALS begins in a limb, it often follows a pattern of progression in the

---

TABLE 10.6
Risk Factors for Stroke

Obesity (BMI > 30 kg/m^2)
Diabetes
Hypertension
Hypercholesterolemia
High dietary fat intake
Age > 65 years
Gender — male
Race — African American
Elevated homocysteine levels; limited intake of vitamin B_{12}, vitamin B_6, and folic acid

Sources: From Victor, M. and Ropper, A.H., *Adams and Victor's Principles of Neurology*, 7th ed., McGraw-Hill, New York, 2000; Selhub, J. et al., *N. Engl. J. Med.*, 1995, 322(5): 286.

---

onset limb (arm or leg), followed by the development of progressive weakness in the contralateral limb of the same segment (arm to arm; leg to leg), then the ipsilateral limb of the other segment (arm to leg; leg to arm), and eventually to bulbar musculature.

ALS is a remarkably variable disorder. There is no "typical" segment of onset, pattern of segment-to-segment spread, pattern of UMN versus LMN involvement, speed of progression, or overall course. As a result, ALS may impact nutrition as one of the first or one of the last symptoms of the disease. Indeed, some individuals with ALS never develop nutritional difficulties. For those with bulbar onset disease, oral or pharyngeal dysphagia may be the initial manifestation of the disease. For those with limb onset, weakness of oropharyngeal musculature occurs later during the clinical course. Nearly all ALS patients die of neuromuscular respiratory failure as a result of the progressive weakness of respiratory muscles. Patients with severe bulbar muscular weakness with or without associated respiratory muscular weakness also face the prospect of dying of malnutrition and dehydration.

ALS-related weakness may compromise nutrition in a number of ways. Frequently, multiple factors are present in the same individual. Each factor must be addressed to provide for maintenance of adequate nutrition and hydration:

1. *Bulbar muscular weakness*: Weakness of bulbar musculature may produce oral or pharyngeal dysphagia, difficulty in managing the increase in oropharyngeal secretions that occur reflexively during feeding, and masticatory muscle (masseter, temporalis, pterygoid) weakness. As a result of one or more of these problems, eating becomes progressively more difficult. Mealtimes become ever longer and accompanied by coughing, choking, and drooling. In order to consume the calories necessary to avoid weight loss, patients may find that they have to eat slowly for hours at a time. Eating is transformed from a pleasurable, social experience to an anxiety-provoking, labor-intensive, and embarrassing chore.

   Serial testing by a speech pathologist will provide an assessment of the ever-increasing degree of bulbar dysfunction. Adaptive mechanical strategies can be suggested and modified when appropriate. A nonchew or soft diet can be recommended for those with masticatory difficulties. Changing the consistency of liquids from thin to thicker can be recommended for those with pharyngeal dysphagia. Changing the consistency of food from solid to puree can be recommended for those with oral dysphagia. Small, more nutrient, and calorically dense meals can also be recommended for these individuals. Excessive oropharyngeal secretions can be reduced with the use of anticholinergic medications or managed more effectively with use of a suction device. While all of these modifications may prove to be effective for a time, nearly all compensatory measures will fail as the disease progresses. A gastrostomy tube (G-tube) should be suggested to individuals with significant dysphagia who continue to lose weight despite their best efforts.

2. *Upper extremity weakness*: ALS patients with significant hand and arm weakness may have considerable difficulty with eating. Patients who live alone or who have minimal help with meal preparation may find it physically difficult to prepare food. Individuals with arm and hand weakness may find that their ability to use utensils and to move food from the plate to the mouth may also be compromised. As in the case of bulbar weakness, mealtimes may be prolonged; patients may be embarrassed by their inability to prevent spilling of food or drink.

   Occupational therapy can offer adaptive equipment to patients with upper extremity dysfunction that negatively impacts nutrition. Built up silverware that is easier to grip and manipulate may help for a time. For those with proximal weakness, supporting and elevating the arm may allow for independent eating. For those without any ability to self-feed, automated feeders are available although costly.

3. *Depression*: Reactive depression is common in ALS. Because of the ever-worsening physical deterioration that characterizes this disease, depression may occur throughout the clinical course from the time that the initial diagnosis is made to the terminal stages. Vegetative signs of depression may include a reduction of appetite.

   Depression is a treatable complication of ALS. There are multiple antidepressants to choose from so that it is often possible to lift depression without any significant adverse side effects.

4. *Loss of appetite and early satiety*: At times ALS patients experience a loss of appetite. Although potentially related to vegetative symptoms of depression or to the side effect of medications, loss of appetite may be difficult to explain. This may be accompanied by a sense of fullness after eating even small amounts of food. Such early satiety may be in part attributed to a reduction in the speed of gastric emptying.

   Loss of appetite may respond to use of medroxyprogesterone (Megace). Early satiety secondary to delayed gastric emptying may respond to prokinetic agents such as metoclopropamide or to the antibiotic erythromycin.

5. *Respiratory muscular weakness*: ALS patients often develop diaphragmatic weakness that may compromise breathing. When severe patients may notice that they become dyspneic following meals. This occurs because the weakened diaphragm must descend against the increased intra-abdominal pressure produced by gastric filling. At times, patients become winded and fatigued after eating even a small amount of food. This may contribute to poor nutrition.

   Small and frequent, calorie-dense meals may assist ALS patients with significant respiratory muscular weakness who experience dyspnea associated with eating. These patients can also use a breathing support device known as noninvasive positive pressure ventilation (NIPPV). NIPPV can be used for those with dyspnea that exacerbates during and following meals. While most of the patients cannot master the ability to eat with NIPPV on, nearly all patients can successfully relieve dyspnea in the post-prandial stage by using NIPPV.

   Despite adaptive equipment, compensatory strategies and altered food or liquid consistencies, malnutrition and dehydration may prevail in ALS. If nutritional status is not closely monitored, malnutrition and dehydration may occur in a relatively short span of time. A feeding tube can provide an alternative and supplemental or complete means of delivering nutrition, hydration, and medication. Although G-tubes are most commonly placed endoscopically, surgical and interventional radiological means of placement are also available. Usually the procedure is performed using conscious sedation or another form of anesthesia. Since ALS patients with significant respiratory muscle weakness are at increased risk for an anesthetic complication, respiratory status must be taken into account when considering this procedure.

OTHER MOTOR NEURON DISORDERS

ALS is the most common adult motor neuron disease. Other less common forms of motor neuron disease may also compromise nutrition. Progressive muscular atrophy (PMA) is a progressive LMN disorder. Primary lateral sclerosis (PLS) is a progressive UMN disorder. Progressive bulbar palsy (PBP) is a progressive UMN and LMN disorder affecting bulbar musculature. PMA, PLS, and PBP are usually considered to be variants of ALS. Kennedy's disease, also known as spinobulbar muscular atrophy, is a slowly progressive, inherited

(X-linked) LMN disorder. Spinomuscular atrophy (SMA) is an inherited LMN disorder. In its most severe forms, it occurs in infancy with severe feeding difficulties and eventually death by progressive neuromuscular respiratory failure. It can present later in childhood and even in adulthood with slowly progressive LMN weakness that may involve bulbar and respiratory musculature. Poliomyelitis is an acute infectious viral infection of the LMNs. It can produce severe and diffuse weakness, including bulbar muscle dysfunction that can improve or even resolve. However, 20 or more years later, patients can develop a slowly progressive LMN weakness known as post-polio muscular atrophy syndrome. This weakness may involve muscles essential for maintaining nutrition.

Multiple Sclerosis[1]

Multiple sclerosis (MS) is a chronic disorder of CNS white matter caused by an autoimmune or inflammatory attack upon myelin, the insulating material surrounding axons of the brain and spinal cord. PNS myelin that surrounds axons of the spinal and peripheral nerves is immunologically distinct from CNS myelin and therefore not involved in MS. The typical lesion of MS, the MS plaque, is an area of demyelination and inflammation that occurs in the white matter of the brain or spinal cord. Demyelination of axons produces axonal conduction failure. The neurological deficit produced by each MS plaque is determined by the function of these affected axons. Remyelination that occurs with healing or resolution of the MS plaque may reestablish lost function. While an MS plaque may occur as a purely demyelinating lesion that spares axons, particularly brisk inflammation may produce secondary axonal loss. As a result, the deficit produced by an MS plaque may persist or resolve incompletely.

MS occurs in three clinical forms. Relapsing–remitting MS is characterized by the sub-acute (days to weeks) development of an initial neurological deficit that persists for a time (weeks to months) and then resolves. This episode may then be followed by another that most commonly occurs in a region of the brain or spinal cord that is anatomically distinct from the first. Commonly the deficit resolves. Over time patients with relapsing–remitting MS have multiple recurrences that are separated in time and in neuroanatomic space. Patients with relapsing–remitting MS may eventually enter a phase of the disease, characterized by gradual worsening rather than acute to subacute relapse followed by improvement. This clinical form of the disease is known as secondary progressive MS. Some patients with MS never manifest a relapsing–remitting form of the disorder but develop gradually progressive deficits. This form is known as primary progressive MS.

MS may produce dysphagia in two ways. Demyelination or secondary axon loss may disrupt UMN control of one or more of the brain stem motor and sensory nuclei or it may disrupt the motor and sensory output of one or more brain stem motor and sensory nuclei involved in the process of chewing and swallowing. A similar, albeit anatomically distinct, process may affect descending UMN pathways such as the corticospinal tract or ascending sensory tracts such as the dorsal columns or spinothalamic tracts. This may produce weakness or sensory disturbance of the arms or legs. The resulting motor weakness or dyscoordination may compromise the acts of procuring, preparing, and eating food. The adaptive and compensatory nutritional strategies reviewed when discussing ALS are applicable to the similar difficulties encountered in MS.

The medical treatment for severe exacerbations of MS is high-dose intravenous steroids, usually solumedrol, followed by a tapering oral dose of steroids, usually prednisone. Steroid therapy may promote hyperglycemia, increased appetite, weight gain, and fluid retention. Chronic immunomodulating therapy for MS includes the use of interferon and at times cytotoxic therapy with medications such as methotrexate. Interferon use may be complicated by diarrhea. Methotrexate may produce anorexia and nausea. Methotrexate is a known folate antagonist. Supplemental folinic acid, a form of folate that does not interfere with methotrexate absorption, is recommended with methotrexate therapy. Depending upon the type of medical treatment used, dietary intake, serum glucose levels, daily weights, and urine output should be assessed and monitored.

Some have considered diet to be a contributing environmental risk factor for the development of MS. Animal fats and dairy foods high in saturated fat have been proposed as possible contributors to the etiology of MS. This is in part based on the report that the incidence of MS fell during World War II ostensibly because of limited resources of dietary fat. This theory has not been universally accepted particularly because of lack of control data. Swank and Dugan[25] have even reported findings, suggesting that a low-fat diet (commonly known as the "Swank diet") improved disease progression. Review of epidemiologic and case–control studies of MS and dietary risk factors suggests that there is no definitive correlation between MS and diet.[26]

Hayes et al.[27] hypothesized that insufficient vitamin D_3 intake may be a risk factor for MS. Further research is needed to investigate the protective role of vitamin D_3 in MS before recommending vitamin D supplementation to all patients with MS. Although there is no substantial evidence linking MS solely to any one particular nutritional factor, the benefit of nutrition intervention is invaluable in the management of dysphagia and medical complications.

ALZHEIMER'S DISEASE AND OTHER DEMENTIAS[1]

Dementia can be broadly defined as a progressive and irreversible loss of intellectual skills in two or more areas such as language, memory, visual and spatial abilities, judgment, or abstract thinking that is significant to affect daily life. Dementia is not a disease but a broad category of symptoms that accompanies certain diseases or conditions. Well-known causes of dementia include Alzheimer's disease (AD), dementia related to multiple strokes (multi-infarct dementia), dementia associated with Parkinson's disease (PD), dementia associated with Huntington's disease, Creutzfeldt–Jakob disease, frontotemporal dementia (FTD), and diffuse Lewy body disease. Other disorders that may mimic or cause dementia include brain tumors, head injury, nutritional deficiency (e.g., vitamin B_{12} deficiency, thiamine deficiency, niacin deficiency), acquired immunodeficiency syndrome (AIDS), encephalitis, syphilis, drug intoxication, and hypothyroidism. Depression may also mimic dementia.

AD is a progressive, degenerative disease that destroys some cortical and subcortical neurons. AD is the commonest form of dementia in individuals of 65 years or older.[28] The risk of developing AD increases with age. It is believed that less than 5% of individuals between 60 and 75 years have AD. Up to one half of individuals >85 years may have AD. The U.S. prevalence of AD is approximately 4 million. Each year approximately 250,000 people in the United States are diagnosed with AD. Other than a postmortem examination, there is no definitive test for AD. However, a premortem diagnosis with an accuracy of 90% can be achieved using a combination of the medical history, physical examination, laboratory evaluation, neuroimaging, and neuropsychological testing.

Persons with AD lose cognitive function, including memory and language, develop mood disturbances, and gradually lose physical abilities, eventually dying of their disease. Although variation exists from one individual to another, AD does follow a progressive course and it can be divided into general stages:

- The early stage of AD features includes recent (versus distant or long-term) memory loss, language difficulty (e.g., difficulty naming, following commands), problems with abstract thinking, diminished ability to perform normal activities of daily living (ADL) and simple tasks, and mood changes.

- The intermediate stage features include worsening of the memory losses, wandering and getting lost, a need for assistance with bathing, eating and dressing, and increasing agitation. Though people in this stage can still walk, they are at risk for falls and injuries.
- In the severe (or terminal) stage of AD, patients are completely dependent on others. They lose all memory, cannot walk, and cannot do anything for themselves at all. They are incontinent.
- End-stage AD is characterized by coma and then death.

Nutritional intervention becomes increasingly important as AD progresses. In the early stage, nutritional goals remain similar to those of healthy individuals of same age and gender. These individuals may require no or minimal assistance. As the disease advances, patients require ever-increasing assistance in food acquisition and preparation as well as in eating. Weight loss is a significant problem as AD progresses. Alzheimer's patients may lose the ability to recognize hunger or thirst, thus forgetting to eat meals or take insufficient fluids potentially promoting malnutrition and dehydration. Caloric needs may increase due to the increase in physical activity, though measured resting energy expenditure is not increased.

The AD Association suggests the following strategies to combat the limited nutritional intake across the spectrum of the disease:

- Serve several small meals rather than three large ones.
- Serve finger foods or the meal in the form of a sandwich.
- Do not serve steaming or extremely hot foods or liquids.
- Limit highly salted foods or sweets if the person has a chronic health problem, such as diabetes or hypertension.
- Fill in gaps between regular meals with healthy snacks.

If individuals have trouble in swallowing, the AD Association recommends the following:

- Blending the food or alternating small bites of food with a drink
- Substituting fruit juice, gelatin, foods cooked with water, sherbet, fruit, or soup
- Serving mashed potatoes rather than fried potatoes
- Offering bite-size pieces of cooked meat, turkey, or chicken salads instead of sliced meat

It is prudent to set aside plenty of time for meals and give the person enough time to swallow before presenting the next bite or drink. It is also suggested that the individual may sit at a 90° angle to avoid backup of food into the throat. Mealtimes should be supervised to assess actual oral intake. If oral intake continues to decline, or the patients are no longer capable of feeding themselves, enteral nutrition support may be indicated.

Controversy still exists regarding the placement of feeding tubes in this population. Feeding tubes may prolong life but it is uncertain if they positively impact quality of life. Adding to the difficulty, at that time a feeding tube may be clinically indicated, the patient is unlikely to have capacity to participate in the decision. This places the burden of decision making upon a surrogate. Thus, it is essential that healthcare providers discuss the pros and cons of feeding tube insertion with patients when they still possess the capacity to decide and that in turn patients discuss their feelings with their family or caregivers. Patients can formalize an advance directive in the form of a living by specifying their desires regarding feeding tube insertion. Patients can also appoint a durable medical power of attorney for healthcare to make this decision.[29–33] Optimally, the patient will inform the surrogate of their feelings in regard to feeding tube insertion. The option of withdrawal of nutrition and hydration support adds to the difficult decision-making process of the families and caregivers of those suffering from AD. It is again essential to discuss this with patients while they have the capacity to make an informed choice. Depending upon the progression of AD, this discussion may occur months to years before the implementation of the patients' choice. Patients who elect to have a feeding tube placed may stipulate that it should be removed or that feeding or hydration be discontinued at some point. Commonly patients and caregivers who opt to discontinue feeding and hydration do so at a time when the ability to communicate ceases.

PARKINSON'S DISEASE[1]

Parkinson's Disease (PD) is a chronic, progressive, irreversible neurodegenerative disease, characterized by the loss of neurons in the part of the brain known as the substansia nigra.[34] Nigral neurons project to large, deep gray matter structures in the cerebral hemispheres known as the corpus striatum. The neurotransmitter of the nigral neurons is dopamine. This dopaminergic nigral to striatal (nigrostriatal) pathway and other circuits within the corpus striatum, some of which use the neurotransmitter acetylcholine, provide background control of motor movements and balance.

The actual cause of neuronal loss in PD remains unknown. Both genetics and environment may play a role in the development of PD. Increasing evidence suggests that PD has a genetic component. A recent study of twins showed that PD before the age of 50 years is strongly genetic.[35] The same study did not find a genetic contribution to PD after the age of 50 years. The exposure to environmental factors such as well water and agricultural pesticides may increase one's risk of developing PD. Other environmental toxins possibly linked to PD include carbon monoxide and carbon disulfide. It is possible that these environmental toxins may contribute to abnormal free-radical formation and lead to PD.[34] For unknown reasons, smoking and coffee reduce the risk of developing PD.[36–41] Some researchers believe that there may be a protective substance in cigarettes and coffee. Others suggest that the substances themselves are irrelevant, and that people with addictive behaviors have a brain chemistry that makes them more resistant to PD.[36] Despite these claims regarding smoking, it is not recommended that individuals begin or continue smoking in order to prevent PD.

The four cardinal symptoms of PD are tremor of the hands, arms, legs, jaw, and face; rigidity or stiffness of the limbs and trunk; bradykinesia or slowness of movement; and postural instability or impaired balance and coordination. PD sometimes is described as early, moderate, or advanced:

- *Early* disease describes the stage when a person has a mild tremor or stiffness but is able to continue work or other normal daily activities. This often refers to a person who has been newly diagnosed with PD.
- *Moderate* disease describes the stage when a person begins to experience limited movement. A person with moderate PD may have a mild to moderate tremor with slow movement.
- *Advanced* disease describes the stage when a person is significantly limited in activity, despite treatment. Daily changes in symptoms, medication side effects that limit treatment, and loss of independence in ADL are common. A person with advanced PD may have significant changes in posture and movement, speech problems, and frequent changes in movement.

PD may also be described by five stages:

- *Stage I* (*mild or early disease*): Symptoms affect only one side of the body.
- *Stage II*: Both sides of the body are affected, but posture remains normal.
- *Stage III* (*moderate disease*): Both sides of the body are affected, and there is mild imbalance during standing or walking. However, the person remains independent.
- *Stage IV* (*advanced disease*): Both sides of the body are affected, and there is disabling instability while standing or walking. The person in this stage requires substantial help.
- *Stage V*: Severe, fully developed disease is present. The person is restricted to a bed or chair.

PD patients in Stages IV and V may experience nutritional difficulties. Slowed movements of the arms and hands as well as gait imbalance compromise food acquisition, preparation, and eating. Slowed movements of the tongue and pharynx compromise swallowing and the handling of oropharyngeal secretions. Patients may have sialorrhea or coughing and choking upon their own secretions. Patients with dysphagia are at risk for aspiration pneumonia. Slowed gastrointestinal transit times may delay gastric emptying, producing early satiety, and slow intestinal motility, producing constipation.[42]

PD does not require a special diet. Adequate fluid and fiber should be incorporated to prevent constipation. Smaller, frequent meals are suggested if gastric motility is impaired. Food and liquid consistencies may need to be altered and other compensatory strategies employed if individuals have dysphagia. A feeding tube can help to provide adequate nutrition and hydration as well as decrease the risk of aspiration in PD cases with severe dysphagia.

The most common medications used in the treatment of PD include levodopa, dopamine agonists, anticholinergics, and catechol-*O*-methyltransferase (COMT) inhibitors.[34] The drug–nutrient interactions between levodopa and dietary protein, and levodopa and pyridoxine and aspartame, are a major nutritional focus when treating with patients with PD. Certain circulating proteins are thought to compete for transport in the gastrointestinal tract varying the rate of absorption of levodopa into the circulation and eventually the brain. Thus, limiting dietary protein intake during the day may enhance the uptake of levodopa. Most often a high load of dietary protein is taken at the evening meal. Following this type of diet may help to prevent circulating levodopa fluctuations, which may in turn, assist in reducing some symptoms of PD. As long as dietary protein intake is adequate to meet estimated requirements, it does not matter nutritionally when this protein is consumed throughout each day. This type of diet manipulation remains controversial.[43,44]

Dopamine agonists are medications that activate the dopamine receptor. Dopamine agonists are associated with many short-term side effects such as nausea, vomiting, dizziness, confusion, and hallucinations.[34] COMT inhibitors block the metabolism of dopamine. They can increase the effectiveness of levodopa, thus possibly reducing PD symptoms. Anticholinergics are used to restore the balance between brain dopamine and acetylcholine in the corpus striatum. The reduction of acetylcholine acts to decrease tremor and muscle stiffness. Anticholinergics can impair memory and thinking, especially in older individuals; therefore, they are used judiciously for the treatment of PD.[34] Anticholinergic medications may reduce the production of oropharyngeal secretions. While this condition may improve sialorrhea and difficulty with pharyngeal secretion clearance, anticholinergic use may increase the thickness or tenacity of these secretions. Maintaining adequate hydration may ameliorate this problem. When severe, this can also be addressed by using guaifenesin.

GUILLAIN–BARRÉ SYNDROME[1]

Guillain–Barré syndrome (GBS), also known as acute inflammatory demyelinating polyradiculoneuropathy (AIDP), is an immune-mediated disorder of the PNS characterized by a subacutely progressive ascending or descending paralysis that may lead to respiratory muscle compromise and, if untreated, possibly death. GBS is the most common cause of acute neuromuscular paralysis in persons living in developed countries. The onset of GBS is preceded about one half of the time by an infectious process. The weakness of GBS may worsen over a period of 1 to 4 weeks after onset. Weakness then plateaus for a variable period of time (days to months) after which strength gradually improves.[45–49]

The level of nutritional intervention that is required depends upon the severity and distribution of weakness. Patients with bulbar muscle weakness and dysphagia may require alterations in liquid or solid diet consistency.[50] Up to 20% of patients with GBS require mechanical ventilation. Ventilated patients require a temporary alternate route for nutrition such as a nasogastric tube to provide nutritional support to maintain lean body mass. Further complicating nutritional management, GBS patients may be hypermetabolic (requiring increased calories) and catabolic due to endocrine, infectious, and inflammatory mechanisms associated with the disease process.[28]

Nutritional intervention for GBS is typically acute and short term. Most of those affected with GBS recover within days to months without significant complications. Fifteen to twenty percent of patients may be left with neurological deficits, some of which may be severe.[28,45,49,51–55] Those requiring mechanical ventilation for more than about 10 days will require conversion from an endotracheal tube to a tracheostomy tube. These individuals and those with persisting bulbar dysfunction may also require placement of an alternate long-term route for administration of nutrition and medications.

MYASTHENIA GRAVIS AND MYOPATHY

Myasthenia Gravis (MG) is an autoimmune disorder, characterized by the production of antibodies that bind to the skeletal muscle membrane acetylcholine receptor (AchR). Acetylcholine that is released from the motor nerve terminal has two potential fates. Some will be destroyed by an enzyme, acetylcholinesterase, located at the nerve–muscle junction. The remainder will bind to the AchR, a transmembrane receptor protein, and initiate muscle contraction. The AchR antibody disrupts neuromuscular transmission by binding to Ach receptor. Some of these antibodies physically block the receptor or reduce its function. Antibody binding to the AchR also causes some receptors to be destroyed reducing the total number of receptors at the nerve–muscle junction.[1,28,56–60]

The cardinal symptom of MG is muscular fatigue and weakness. The ocular, facial, bulbar, neck extensor and flexor, proximal and distal arm and leg, and respiratory muscles are those most commonly involved in MG. Patients with bulbar muscle dysfunction may suffer significant dysphagia and are at risk for malnutrition, dehydration, and aspiration. The location of weakness is used to divide MG patients into two categories. The weakness of ocular MG is confined to the lids and extraocular muscles. The weakness of generalized MG may not only involve the eye but also involve other nonocular musculature.

Myasthenic weakness often fluctuates. Some patients may experience exacerbations of weakness followed by periods of apparent normality. Others may experience chronic persistent weakness that may periodically worsen. Myasthenic crisis is defined as an exacerbation of weakness that includes significant weakness of bulbar or respiratory musculature. Because of its life-threatening potential, MG crisis is a medical emergency.

The current treatment available for MG consists of symptomatic and immunomodulating interventions. Symptomatic drugs are confined to those that block the acetylcholinesterase enzyme. Drugs such as pyridostigmine and neostigmine reduce the enzymatic destruction of Ach at the nerve–muscle junction, make more Ach available for interaction with the AchR, improve muscle contraction, and thereby increase muscle strength. Immunomodulating medications reduce the production of AchR antibody and the immune response to antibody binding to the receptors in the muscle cell membrane. The corticosteroid, prednisone, is commonly used. Because of the potential for steroid medications to produce significant side effects (glucose intolerance, hypertension, weight gain, osteoporosis, cataracts, stomach ulcers), other agents, referred to as steroid-sparing drugs, are often used in conjunction with prednisone. Steroid-sparing drugs include azathioprine, methotrexate, cyclosporine, and mycophenolate mofetil. Intravenous immunoglobulin or plasmapheresis is used to treat MG crisis.[1,28,56–60]

Nutritional interventions in MG focus upon safe feeding and weight control. Patients in MG crisis with significant bulbar or respiratory muscular weakness that requires invasive ventilation may require a temporary, alternative route for enteral nutrition. Small, frequent, calorically dense meals can be administered to patients with less significant dysphagia or to those with fatigable swallowing muscles. A speech therapist should evaluate swallowing function and assess a safe consistency level for oral diet. Since the physical activity of patients with MG may be limited, dietary counseling for weight control is the basis of long-term nutritional intervention. Thus, nutrition counseling along with low-fat, low-carbohydrate diet modifications may be required if a patient is hyperglycemic and overweight due to MG medications.

Myopathy is the generic term used to describe disorders of muscle. Various myopathic disorders involve skeletal muscles used for food acquisition, food preparation, placement of food within the oral cavity, oral manipulation of food, chewing, swallowing, and transit of food in the proximal one third of the esophagus. Muscular dystrophy (MD) is a progressive, destructive disorder of skeletal muscle that is often attributable to a genetic defect in some aspect of muscle cell structure and function. The muscular dystrophies that are most likely to affect nutrition are Duchenne and Becker MD, oculopharyngeal MD, and myotonic MD. The inflammatory myopathies are autoimmune disorders that produce muscle cell destruction. The inflammatory myopathies that are most likely to affect nutrition are polymyositis (PM), dermatomyositis (DM), and inclusion body myositis (IBM). Compensatory nutritional strategies employed in MG and other neurological disorders are similarly employed in myopathy. PM and DM are often treated with the same immunomodulating agents used in MG. IBM does not respond to these medications.[1]

Neurotrauma

Head Trauma

The normal brain consumes 25% of the body's resting energy expenditure, with glucose as the primary source of energy.[61] The resting energy expenditure in patients with severe head trauma, as measured by indirect calorimetry, is generally increased from 135 to 165% of that predicted by the Harris–Benedict equation and remains elevated for at least 3 weeks.[62–66]

An increase in urinary nitrogen loss is also seen initially in post-head trauma. Steroid administration and immobility contribute to elevated urinary nitrogen losses. The increase in nitrogen loss is related to muscle loss and increased protein turnover. This elevation in resting energy expenditure and increased nitrogen loss suggests hypermetabolism and hypercatabolism, which have long been observed in patients following severe head trauma.[67] Positive nitrogen balance is impossible to attain within the first 2 weeks after severe head trauma. Nutritional therapy of severe head trauma patients thus should include a regimen adequate in calories to compensate for hypermetabolism as well as sufficient protein to promote nitrogen balance. An average of 1.6–2.2 g protein/kg body weight may be necessary to achieve nitrogen balance.[68–70] Enteral or parenteral nutrition support is usually required for this patient population as part of the initial nutritional treatment. Enteral nutrition remains the nutritional "route" of choice for trauma patients. Recent research suggests early enteral feeding to head-injured patients promotes improved neurologic recovery, reduces infective and total complications, but does not change the ultimate outcome.[71]

Barbiturate therapy, specifically pentobarbital, may be necessary for individuals with post-head trauma to reduce intracranial pressure (ICP). The use of barbiturate treatment has been shown to decrease energy requirements to nearly 76% of that predicted by the Harris–Benedict equation as well as reduce nitrogen excretion (11.2 $\pm$ 4 g nitrogen versus 19.5 $\pm$ 3.3 g nitrogen).[72] Nutrition regimens should be adjusted to compensate for these effects.

Spinal Cord Trauma

Metabolic rates in spinal cord trauma patients are variable — depending on time frame post-spinal trauma. Metabolic rates are decreased post-spinal injury as compared to controls.[67] It has been noted that the higher the lesion on the spinal cord, the lower the energy requirement. Elevated nitrogen loss is seen post-spinal cord injury.[73–76] This is due in part from muscle wasting and acute high-dose steroid therapy. Research suggests that often positive nitrogen balance may be unattainable for weeks after a spinal injury occurs.[76]

Acutely, spinal cord injury patients become a unique nutritional challenge due to their decreased caloric need in combination with their increased protein requirements. These patients will continue to lose weight during the initial phase of the injury, despite adequate calorie and protein supplementation due to increased muscle loss. Depending upon the location of the injury, enteral or parenteral nutritional therapy, or supplemental nutrition, may be necessary for long-term nutrition support. Serial transport proteins and routine weights may assist the assurance of adequate nutritional therapy.

Spinal cord injury patients, who are bed-bound or wheel chair-bound, are more prone to pressure ulcers. Close monitoring of skin integrity and serial transport proteins may assist with long-term nutritional goals to prevent skin breakdown and possibly assist with wound healing.

BRAIN NEOPLASM

Tumors or neoplasms of the brain may require extensive resection. Depending upon the location and size of the tumor, varying levels of nutritional intervention may be indicated for patients. Unfortunately, there is no general nutritional recommendation for individuals with previous cranial resection. The nutrition assessment should be tailored to each individual case. If dysphagia is evident after tumor removal, altered diet consistencies or supplemental enteral nutrition may be necessary for the provision of adequate nutrition. Nutritional intake should be closely monitored to assess the need for tube-feeding or parenteral nutrition, or simply assistance with meals. Calorie counts may assist in assessing actual oral intake. Various medications used to assist with ICP control may promote electrolyte imbalances, blood glucose, and intakes and outputs. Daily monitoring of these parameters may aid in nutritional recommendations and management.[1]

NEUROLOGIC CONSEQUENCES OF NUTRITIONAL DEFICIENCY

THIAMINE (VITAMIN B_1)

Traditionally known as beriberi (translated as extreme weakness), thiamine deficiency can have both CNS and PNS manifestations. Milder degrees of thiamine deficiency cause isolated peripheral sensory neuropathy. More severe deficiency produces Wernicke's encephalopathy and Korsakoff's syndrome. Wernicke's encephalopathy includes the classic triad of confusion, ataxia, and abnormalities of eye movements. While most patients will respond to parenteral administration of thiamine, residual impairment of recent memory and confabulation, the Korsakoff's syndrome, may persist.[1,77–88]

CYANOCOBALAMIN (VITAMIN B_1)

Vitamin B_{12} deficiency from any cause can produce dysfunction of peripheral sensory nerves, the dorsal and lateral columns of the spinal cord (subacute combined deficiency), and the brain. As a result, distal paresthesias, sensory ataxia, memory loss, and other cognitive change, as well as lower extremity spastic weakness are the commonest manifestations. Both a peripheral neuropathy and myelopathy may exist in the same individual. Neurologic manifestations may occur in the absence of anemia or morphological changes of peripheral white blood cells. Serum methylmalonic acid and homocysteine levels rise as a result of the deficiency and can serve as a way to both confirm the diagnosis and increase the specificity of borderline normal vitamin B_{12} determinations.[1,89–103]

FOLIC ACID

Folic acid is essential for vitamin B_{12}-dependent methyl donor function. It is perhaps not surprising that folic acid deficiency has been associated with polyneuropathy, myelopathy, dementia, and neurocognitive disorders. However, the role of folate deficiency in such disorders is somewhat controversial. For example, asymptomatic elderly patients may demonstrate low folate levels. The most convincing example of a role for folate in neurologic disease is that of patients with subacute combined deficiency with normal vitamin B_{12} levels, extremely low folate levels, poor responses to vitamin B_{12} supplementation, and good response to folate supplementation. Although folate deficiency has been associated with peripheral neuropathy, this is most often seen in the setting of alcoholism or a combined nutritional deficiency syndrome. As a result, a direct role for folate in the production of polyneuropathy remains controversial. Both vitamin B_{12} and folate deficiency may produce elevations of homocysteine. Elevated homocysteine levels have recently been associated with an increased risk of atherosclerosis and as a result an increased vascular risk for stroke and heart disease. Supplementation with vitamin B_{12}, folate, and vitamin B_6 is often offered to patients with vascular risk.[97,104–106]

VITAMIN D

Adult vitamin D deficiency results in the skeletal pathology known as osteomalacia or osteoporosis. As with other causes of osteomalacia, vitamin D-related osteomalacia is accompanied by bone pain, muscular weakness, and muscular atrophy. Muscle pathology and electrophysiologic studies may indicate the presence of a myopathy. Symptoms usually respond promptly to vitamin D replacement.[27,92,107]

Tocopherol (Vitamin E)

Vitamin E deficiency from any cause is most commonly associated with cerebellar ataxia, oculomotor abnormalities, and peripheral neuropathy with loss of proprioceptive and vibration senses. The disorder known as Bassen–Kornzweig syndrome, or abetalipoproteinemia, is associated with low levels of vitamins A and E. Patients develop progressive ataxia, areflexia, and retinitis pigmentosa.[108–118]

Nutrition-Related Neurotoxins[16,119]

Some ingestible neurotoxins may contaminate food or drink and thereby affect the CNS or PNS. Mercury, arsenic, and *Clostridium botulinum* (produced botulism) are three common neurotoxic agents. Some symptoms of neurotoxin ingestion include tremor, nausea, vomiting, diarrhea, polyneuropathy, dysphagia, respiratory weakness, or encephalopathy. Recovery from neurotoxin poisoning depends upon the extent of exposure, amount ingested, and type of toxin.[120–127]

NEUROLOGIC CONSEQUENCES OF SOME SPECIFIC GASTROINTESTINAL DISORDERS

Celiac Disease

Approximately 10% of patients suffering from this disorder may develop either CNS or PNS dysfunction. CNS manifestations may include dementia, cerebellar ataxia, myelopathy, encephalopathy, brain stem encephalitis, progressive multifocal leukoencephalopathy, chronic, progressive leukoencephalopathy, progressive myoclonic ataxia, seizures, isolated CNS vasculitis; and a syndrome that includes celiac disease with encephalopathy and bilateral occipital calcifications. PNS manifestations include peripheral neuropathy and myopathy. While some of the CNS (vitamin B_{12} and vitamin E) and PNS complications (vitamins B_{12}, B_6, and E for neuropathy and vitamin D, potassium for myopathy) may be related to nutritional deficiencies, in most circumstances this is not the case. In some circumstances, the neurologic complications along with the gastrointestinal manifestations of celiac disease may respond to a gluten-free diet.[128–153]

Inflammatory Bowel Disease

Patients with ulcerative colitis and Crohn's disease may uncommonly develop neurologic manifestations. Arterial and venous thrombosis is believed to relate to a hypercoagulable state associated with these disorders. CNS vasculitis may also occur. Other CNS complications include seizures and myelopathy with or without vitamin B_{12} deficiency. There is an increased incidence of MS in patients with these disorders. Peripheral neuropathy including axonal sensory motor polyneuropathy, AIDP (GBS), multiple mononeuropathies related to vasculitis, and plexopathy has also been reported in patients with both ulcerative colitis and Crohn's disease. Myopathy has been reported in association with Crohn's disease.[92,154–156]

Whipple's Disease

This infectious disease is produced by a bacterium (*Tropheryma whippelii*). It is most common in men in their fourth to sixth decade of life. Whipple's disease is a systemic disorder that may have both gastrointestinal (diarrhea, malabsorption, weight loss, cachexia) and extraintestinal (arthritis, chronic cough, pleuritic chest pain, congestive heart failure, pericarditis, lymph-adenopathy, skin hyperpigmentation) manifestations. The nervous system is a common extraintestinal manifestation. Neurologic consequences of Whipple's disease include demen-tia, ocular motility disturbance, involuntary movements, seizures, peripheral neuropathy, myopathy, and ataxia.[115,157–170]

GUILLAIN–BARRÉ SYNDROME ASSOCIATED WITH *CAMPYLOBACTER*

Approximately 30 to 40% of GBS (AIDP) cases follow infection with *Campylobacter jejuni*. Infection occurs by oral ingestion of the bacterium obtained via fecal–oral contact or inappropriate handling of foods (particularly chicken). GBS associated with *C. jejuni* infec-tion is typically more severe. There is more frequent need for respiratory support with mechanical ventilation and a greater chance of residual disability.[171–195]

GASTRIC SURGERY

Gastric surgery is performed for many reasons including gastric and duodenal ulcers, malig-nancies, and the treatment of morbid obesity. Loss of intrinsic factor secretory function after gastric surgery results in malabsorption of vitamin B_{12}. Symptomatic vitamin B_{12} deficiency, manifested as peripheral neuropathy, myelopathy, or encephalopathy, may occur with a delay of months to years determined by the amount of already stored vitamin B_{12}. Wernicke's encephalopathy, myelopathy, and cerebellar ataxia have been reported to occur following gastric surgery for obesity.[196–200]

CLINICAL TIP

WARFARIN (COUMADIN®) TREATMENT

Warfarin is an anticoagulant medication used to increase prothrombin time and decrease platelet aggregation. High levels or varying levels of dietary vitamin K can inhibit the effects of warfarin. Therefore, individuals receiving warfarin therapy need to avoid excessive intake and maintain a consistent intake of dietary vitamin K in order to maximize the drug's effects (Table 10.7).

PHENYTOIN (DILANTIN®) TREATMENT

Phenytoin is an anticonvulsant medication often used to treat or prevent seizures. The effects of phenytoin can be altered or decreased with simultaneous enteral nutrition administration.

TABLE 10.7
Dietary Sources of Vitamin K[a]

Oils: Canola or soybean oil (exposure to fluorescent and sunlight rapidly destroys vitamin K in oils)
Vegetables: Asparagus, broccoli, brussel sprouts, cabbage (green raw), cauliflower, chayote leaf, chickpeas (garbanzo beans), chive (raw), collard greens, coriander leaf, cucumber peel, endive, green tomato, kale, lettuce, scallions (green onions), seaweed (extremely high levels), soybeans, spinach, swiss chard, turnip greens, and watercress
Others: Beef, chicken and pork liver, egg yolk, green tea leaves, algae (purple laver and hijiki), apples with green peel

[a] 50 μg or more vitamin K per 100 g.

Source: From Pronsky, Z.M., *Food Medication Interactions*, 12th ed., Food–Medication Interactions, Birchrunville, 2002, p. 357.

Enteral nutrition decreases the bioavailability of phenytoin. Therefore, if a patient is receiving enteral nutrition along with enteral phenytoin, the feeding should be held 2 h before and 2 h after each phenytoin dose to maximize the bioavailability of the medication. If the intravenous form of phenytoin is used, there is no need to hold enteral feeds.[201]

CLINICAL TIP

Proposed Alternative Therapies Used in MS[202]

- Imagery is a psychological process that unites communication between perception and actual body changes; thought to lessen anxiety and have the individual feel more in control of the illness.
- Massage is thought to assist in muscle relaxation, pain relief, and stress reduction.
- Pulsing magnetic field therapy is thought to alter calcium transport across membranes, improving nerve conduction; spasticity is reduced and muscle energy is improved.
- Vitamin B complex and vitamin C supplementation are thought to decrease fatigue and alleviate stress.
- Herbal therapy include astragalus or milk vetch root and ginseng to treat fatigue, chamomile as an antispasmodic, St. John's wort as an antidepressant, and valerian as an antianxiety and an antispasmodic.
- Aromatherapy is thought to stimulate different areas of the brain promoting relaxation and decreasing anxiety.
- Acupuncture is thought to assist in increasing circulation and energy, decreasing muscle spasm and anxiety.

It should be noted that these MS alternative therapies have not been extensively studied to make strong recommendations for or against their use.

CLINICAL TIP

Feeding Tubes

A feeding tube is a silicone or polyurethane catheter or tube that is inserted into the gastrointestinal tract to provide an alternate route for nutrients, liquids, or medications. The most common type of long-term feeding tube is placed into the stomach. Most tubes needed for a short period of time (<4 weeks) are temporarily inserted into either the nose or the mouth, with the feeding tube tip terminating in the stomach or small bowel.

There are two general types of stomach tubes: a percutaneous endoscopic gastrostomy (PEG) tube and a G-tube. The differences between two types of stomach tubes are how each is inserted and how each is held in place.[50] A PEG tube is usually inserted via an endoscope under conscious sedation and local anesthesia. A rubber-type bumper inside the stomach wall, as well as a rubber-type bumper on the surface of the skin, holds the PEG tube in place where the tube exits the body. A G-tube is a surgically placed tube requiring general anesthesia and intubation for placement. The G-tube is surgically stitched to the skin to hold it in place.

Another type of long-term feeding tube can be placed into the jejunum. This type of tube can be either surgically or endoscopically inserted. A jejunal feeding tube is smaller in diameter than that of the stomach tube, and its tip resides in the small intestine. The main difference between stomach and jejunal feeding tubes, other than their size and location, is their requirement for different feeding schedules.

Enteral feeds can be administered in one of the following three ways: bolus, gravity-drip, or continuous. A bolus feeding is administered via a syringe directly into the feeding tube multiple times each day. A gravity-drip feeding requires a feeding bag with tubing. The enteral formula is poured into the bag and allowed to drip slowly into the feeding tube via gravity. The continuous feeding method also uses a feeding bag and connective tubing, but also requires a pump to regulate the rate of enteral formula administration. All three methods can be used for stomach tubes, however; only continuous administration can be used with jejunal tubes.

Several possible factors must be considered when choosing either a stomach or a jejunal feeding tube. If the aspiration risk is extremely high, severe gastroesophageal reflux is present, if there is some anatomical obstruction in or near to the stomach, or if the patient has had a partial or complete gastrectomy, a jejunal feeding tube may be indicated. However, even if the above is true, a PEG tube may be the only option, if an individual is not safe to undergo general anesthesia.

Although these tubes are termed "feeding tubes," other reasons exist for the placement of feeding tubes. Many times if swallowing function is deteriorating or significantly impaired, it may be difficult to take prescribed oral medication and maintain adequate fluid intake. Therefore, a feeding tube may be indicated to provide an alternate route for oral medications and possibly prevent dehydration.

CLINICAL CASE STUDY

L.K., a 43-year-old female, presents to the hospital emergency room with global (expressive and receptive) aphasia and right facial droop. She was in her usual state of health before this event as per L.K.'s family. No documented weight gain or loss before admission.

Past Medical History

L.K.'s family reports a history of hypertension (HTN), seizure disorder, gastroesophageal reflux disease (GERD), and total abdominal hysterectomy (TAH). L.K. was taking metoprolol, phenytoin, and ranitidine before admission. L.K. has no known drug or food allergies.

Social History

L.K.'s family reports that L.K. usually consumes a "fairly healthy diet." L.K. reportedly drinks "socially." No reported history of tobacco use or drug abuse.

Family History

L.K.'s family history is positive for the presence of stroke and high cholesterol.

Review of Systems

General: L.K. appears lethargic upon examination
GI/abdomen: No vomiting or diarrhea
Neurologic: History of seizures, CT scan shows left-hemispheric stroke

PHYSICAL EXAMINATION

Vital Signs

Temperature: 98.6°F
Heart rate: 80 BPM
Respiratory rate: 16 BPM
Blood pressure: 135/95 mmHg
Height: 5′6″ (168 cm)
Current weight: 134 lb (61 kg)
Usual weight: 134 lb (61 kg)
BMI: 21.6 kg/m^2
General: Well-developed female who appears in no distress; a nasoenteric tube is seen entering the right nares (terminating beyond the pylorus in the duodenum)
Skin: Normal, appears well-hydrated
Eyes: Pupils are equal and reactive
Cardiac: Heart sounds are normal; no murmurs are present
Chest/Pulmonary: Lungs clear to auscultation and percussion bilaterally
Abdomen: Soft, nondistended, nontender
Extremities: No edema noted
Neurologic: Notable global aphasia with a right facial droop; significant oral and pharyngeal dysphagia (as per swallowing evaluation), right arm > leg weakness
Mental status: Awake, slightly lethargic

Laboratory Data	L.K.'s Values	Normal Values
Hemoglobin	15 g/dl	13.5–17.5 g/dl
Hematocrit	46%	41–53%
Albumin	3.9 g/dl	3.5–5.8 g/dl
Prothrombin time	15 s	11.0–13.2 s
International normalized ratio (INR)	1.0	1.0
Sodium	135	133–143 mmol/l
Potassium	3.5	3.5–5.3 mmol/l
Blood urea nitrogen	12	10–20 mg/dl
Creatinine	0.9	0.8–1.3 mg/dl
Glucose	124	70–99 mg/dl
Calcium	8.9	8.5–10.5 mg/dl
Magnesium	2.1	1.3–2.5 mg/dl
Phosphorus	2.5	2.5–5.0 mmol/l

CURRENT MEDICATIONS

Atenolol 50 mg daily
Phenytoin 300 mg daily
Lansoprazole 30 mg daily
IV fluids (normal saline with 40 meq potassium chloride)

Estimated Nutritional Goals

2100 kcal/day (35 kcal/kg)
75 g protein/day (1.2 g protein/kg)
2100 ml water/day (35 ml/day fluid requirements)

Questions

1. Are any of the laboratory values of nutritional concern?
2. Calculate a tube-feeding goal volume for L.K. using the nutritional goals above. Assume the formula has 1.5 kcal/ml and 55 g protein/l.
3. Are there any special considerations or instructions for the goal tube feeding based on the information above?
4. Calculate any additional fluid L.K. will need in addition to the tube feeding, assuming she is no longer receiving IV fluids (use the total fluid requirements as above). Assume that the tube-feeding formula contains 78% free water.
5. What recommendations would you suggest for L.K.'s follow-up?

Answers to Case Study Questions

1. The serum potassium and phosphorus levels are low normal but remain within acceptable limits. These levels along with magnesium, calcium, and albumin should be monitored as L.K. begins nutrition.

   L.K. does have an elevated glucose suggesting hyperglycemia. No history of diabetes mellitus was reported. L.K. should be monitored closely for additional glucose levels, if the glucose remains consistently over 99 mg/dl without sufficient cause (i.e., medications or IV fluids based containing dextrose), a full work-up for hyperglycemia should be initiated.

2. If L.K. requires 2100 kcal/day, she would need 1400 ml (1.4 l) of a 1.5 kcal/ml formula:

   2100 kcal/day/1.5 kcal/ ml = 1400 ml/day or 1.4 l/day of formula

   The protein requirement should also be taken into account when establishing a tube-feeding goal. If L.K. also requires 75 g protein/day, 1400 ml (1.4 l) of the above formula would provide approximately 77 g protein/day:

   55 g protein/l × 1.4 l/day = 77 g protein/day

3. It was stated that L.K.'s nasoenteric tube is beyond the pylorus in the intestine, which requires a continuous administration of tube feeding. Therefore, a 24-h continuous tube-feeding goal would be 58.3 ml/h:

   1400 ml/h/24 h/day = 58.3 ml/h continuous over 24 h

   However, due to L.K. receiving enteral phenytoin daily, the tube feeding needs to be held for a total of 4 h (2 h before and 2 h after) for phenytoin administration. L.K. needs to receive all of her tube-feeding goal over a 20-h period to possibly maximize the absorption of the medication. L.K.'s new tube-feeding goal would be 70 ml/h over 20 h:

   1400 ml/day/20 h/day = 70 ml/h over 20 h

4. If the formula contains 78% free water, and L.K. is going to receive a total of 1400 ml/day, L.K. will receive a total of 1092 ml/day of free water from the tube-feeding formula:

1400 ml $\times$ 0.78 = 1092 ml/day free water from the formula

L.K.'s total fluid requirements are 2100 ml/day. Since L.K. will receive 1092 ml from the tube feeding, she will need an additional 1000 ml/day to attain her required fluids:

2100 ml/day − 1092 ml from tube feeding = 1008 ml needed

Additional water requirements can be administered as flushes via the nasoenteric tube. Flushes may be administered either continuously or via a bolus to provide the required fluid amount. Thus, there are numerous ways to recommend the additional fluid needed for L.K. Examples of two different calculations are listed below:

1000 ml needed/4 = 250 ml every 6 h
or 1000 ml needed/24 h/day = 42(41.7) ml/h

5. L.K. should be evaluated and followed closely by the dietitian and speech pathologist, in addition to the primary team, to assess the need for long-term enteral access. If L.K.'s shows significant improvement, with a relatively short anticipated recovery of swallowing function (<2–4 weeks), no long-term feeding tube may be necessary. If, however, L.K.'s swallowing function does not appear to be improving, or improvement is expected to be a slow process, a long-term feeding tube will need to be addressed. Since, L.K. has global aphasia, she is most likely not capable of making a logical decision regarding long-term enteral access. L.K.'s family will need to be included when deciding upon the placement of a feeding tube.

REFERENCES

1. Victor, M. and Ropper, A.H., *Adams and Victor's Principles of Neurology*, 7th ed., New York: McGraw-Hill, 2000.
2. Altman, J., Weight in the balance, *Neuroendocrinology*, 2002, 76(3): 131.
3. Beglinger, C., Overview. Cholecystokinin and eating, *Curr. Opin. Invest. Drugs*, 2002, 3(4): 587.
4. Wenger, T. and Moldrich, G., The role of endocannabinoids in the hypothalamic regulation of visceral function, *Prostaglandins Leukot. Essent. Fatty Acids*, 2002, 66(2–3): 301.
5. Williams, G., Harrold, J.A., and Cutler, D.J., The hypothalamus and the regulation of energy homeostasis: lifting the lid on a black box, *Proc. Nutr. Soc.*, 2000, 59(3): 385.
6. Williams, G. et al., The hypothalamus and the control of energy homeostasis: different circuits, different purposes, *Physiol. Behav.*, 2001, 74(4–5): 683.
7. Smith, G.P., The controls of eating: a shift from nutritional homeostasis to behavioral neuroscience, *Nutrition*, 2000, 16(10): 814.
8. Stubbs, R.J., Peripheral signals affecting food intake, *Nutrition*, 1999, 15(7–8): 614.
9. Coleman, R.A. and Herrmann, T.S., Nutritional regulation of leptin in humans, *Diabetologia*, 1999, 42(6): 639.
10. Hoebel, B.G., Neuroscience and appetitive behavior research: 25 years, *Appetite*, 1997, 29(2): 119.
11. Hoebel, B.G., Feeding: neural control of intake, *Annu. Rev. Physiol.*, 1971, 33: 533.
12. Rolls, E.T., Taste and olfactory processing in the brain and its relation to the control of eating, *Crit. Rev. Neurobiol.*, 1997, 11(4): 263.
13. Schwartz, M.W., Regulation of appetite and body weight, *Hosp. Pract. (Off. Ed.)*, 1997, 32(7): 109, 117.
14. Schwartz, G.J., The role of gastrointestinal vagal afferents in the control of food intake: current prospects, *Nutrition*, 2000, 16(10): 866.
15. Hendelman, W.J., *Functional Neuroanatomy*, Paperback ed., Boca Raton, FL: CRC Press, 2000, p. 280.
16. Feldman, M., Sleisenger, M.H., and Scharschmidt, B.F., *Gastrointestinal and Liver Disease*, 6th ed., 1998, Philadelphia: W.B. Saunders, 1998.

17. Brunner, C.S., Neurologic impairments, in *Contemporary Nutrition Support Practice*, Matarese, L.E. and Gottschlich, M.M., Eds., St. Louis: W.B. Saunders, 2003.
18. Davaros, A. et al., Effect of malnutrition after acute stroke on clinical outcome, *Stroke*, 1996, 27(6): 1028.
19. Rowland, L.P. and Shneider, N.A., Amyotrophic lateral sclerosis [see comment]. *N. Engl. J. Med.*, 2001, 344(22): 1688.
20. Rowland, L.P., How amyotrophic lateral sclerosis got its name: the clinical-pathologic genius of Jean-Martin Charcot, *Arch. Neurol.*, 2001, 58(3): 512.
21. Rowland, L.P., Primary lateral sclerosis: disease, syndrome, both or neither? [comment], *J. Neurol. Sci.*, 1999, 170(1): 1.
22. Rowland, L.P., What's in a name? Amyotrophic lateral sclerosis, motor neuron disease, and allelic heterogeneity [comment], *Ann. Neurol.*, 1998, 43(6): 691.
23. Rowland, L.P., Diagnosis of amyotrophic lateral sclerosis, *J. Neurol. Sci.*, 1998, 160(Suppl. 1): S6.
24. Mitsumoto, H., Chad, D.A., and Pioro, E., *Amyotrophic Lateral Sclerosis*, 1st ed., Contemporary Neurology Series, Oxford: Oxford University Press, 1997, p. 481.
25. Swank, R.L. and Dugan, B.B., Effect of low saturated fat diet in early and late cases of multiple sclerosis, *Lancet*, 1990, 336: 37.
26. Lauer, K., Diet and multiple sclerosis, *Neurology*, 1997, 49(Suppl. 2): S55.
27. Hayes, C.E., Cantorna, M.T., and Deluca, H.F., Vitamin D and multiple sclerosis, *Soc. Exp. Biol. Med.*, 1997, 216: 21.
28. Matarese, L.E., *Contemporary Nutrition Support Practice*, 2nd ed., St. Louis: W.B. Saunders, 2003, p. 384.
29. Kearnes, P., Nutrition in neurological injury, *Nutr. Clin. Pract.*, 1991, 6(6): 211.
30. Gillick, M.R., Sounding board: rethinking the role of tube feeding in patients with advanced dementia, *N. Engl. J. Med.*, 2000, 342(3): 206.
31. Finucane, T.E., Christmas, C., and Travis, K., Tube feeding in patients with advanced dementia: a review of the evidence, *J. Am. Med. Assoc.*, 1999, 282(14): 1365.
32. Meier, D.E. et al., High short-term mortality in hospitalized patients with advanced dementia: a lack of benefit of tube feeding, *Arch. Intern. Med.*, 2001, 161(4): 2001.
33. Sanders, D.S. et al., Survival analysis in percutaneous endoscopic gastrostomy feeding: a worse outcome in patients with dementia, *Am. J. Gastroenterol.*, 2000, 95(6): 1472.
34. The Cleveland Clinic Movement Disorders Program, D.o.N., *Parkinson's Disease*, 2002, WebMD.com.
35. Tanner, C.M. et al., Parkinson disease in twins, *JAMA*, 1999, 281: 341.
36. Ross, G.W. et al., Association of coffee and caffeine intake with the risk of Parkinson disease, *JAMA*, 2000, 283: 2674.
37. Tan, E.K. et al., Dose-dependent protective effect of coffee, tea, and smoking in Parkinson's disease: a study in ethnic Chinese, *J. Neurol. Sci.*, 2003, 216(1): 163.
38. Marder, K. and Logroscino, G., The ever-stimulating association of smoking and coffee and Parkinson's disease, *Ann. Neurol.*, 2002, 52(3): 261.
39. Louis, E.D. et al., Parkinsonian signs in older people: prevalence and associations with smoking and coffee, *Neurology*, 2003, 61(1): 24.
40. James, W.H., Coffee drinking, cigarette smoking, and Parkinson's disease [comment], *Ann. Neurol.*, 2003, 53(4): 546.
41. Hernan, M.A. et al., A meta-analysis of coffee drinking, cigarette smoking, and the risk of Parkinson's disease, *Ann. Neurol.*, 2002, 52(3): 276.
42. Atienza-Montero, E. et al., Nutritional considerations of Parkinson disease, Proceedings of Meeting, National Parkinson's Foundation, in *What Causes Parkinson's?* Los Angeles, CA, May 1990.
43. Berry, E.M. et al., A balanced carbohydrate: protein diet in the management of Parkinson's disease, *Neurology*, 1991, 41(8): 1295.
44. Karestaedt, P.J. and Pincus, J.H., Protein redistribution diet remains effective in patients with fluctuating parkinsonism, *Arch. Neurol.*, 1992, 49(2): 149.
45. Winer, J.B., Guillain Barre syndrome, *Mol. Pathol.*, 2001, 54(6): 381.

46. Van Koningsveld, R. et al., Mild forms of Guillain–Barre syndrome in an epidemiologic survey in the Netherlands, *Neurology*, 2000, 54(3): 620.

47. van der Meche, F.G. et al., Guillain–Barre syndrome: multifactorial mechanisms versus defined subgroups, *J. Infect. Dis.*, 1997, 176(Suppl. 2): S99.

48. van der Meche, F.G. and van Doorn, P.A., Guillain–Barre syndrome, *Curr. Treat. Options Neurol.*, 2000, 2(6): 507.

49. Ropper, A.H., Severe acute Guillain–Barre syndrome, *Neurology*, 1986, 36: 429.

50. Rombeau, J.L. and Rolandelli, R.H., *Clinical Nutrition Enteral and Tube Feeding*, 3rd ed., Philadelphia: W.B. Saunders, 1997.

51. Asbury, A.K., Arnason, B.G., and Adams, R.D., The inflammatory lesion in idiopathic polyneuritis, *Medicine*, 1969, 48: 173.

52. Asbury, A.K., New concepts of Guillain–Barre syndrome, *J. Child. Neurol.*, 2000, 15(3): 183.

53. Briscoe, D.M. and McMenamin, J.B., Prognosis in Guillain–Barre syndrome, *Arch. Dis. Child.*, 1987, 62: 733.

54. Cole, G.F. and Matthew, D.J., Progress in severe Guillain–Barre syndrome, *Arch. Dis. Child.*, 1987, 62: 288.

55. Group, G.-B.S., Plasmapheresis and acute Guillain–Barre syndrome, *Neurology*, 1985, 35: 1096.

56. Shelton, G.D., Myasthenia gravis and disorders of neuromuscular transmission, *Vet. Clin. North Am. Small Anim. Pract.*, 2002, 32(1): 189, vii.

57. Shelton, G.D., Disorders of neuromuscular transmission, *Semin. Vet. Med. Surg. (Small Anim.)*, 1989, 4(2): 126.

58. Sanders, D.B., Clinical neurophysiology of disorders of the neuromuscular junction, *J. Clin. Neurophysiol.*, 1993, 10(2): 167.

59. Neal, G.D. and Clarke, L.R., Neuromuscular disorders, *Otolaryngol. Clin. North Am.*, 1987, 20(1): 195.

60. Drachman, D.B., Myasthenia gravis, *N. Engl. J. Med.*, 1994, 330(25): 1797.

61. Kaufman, H. et al., General metabolism in head injury, *Neurosurgery*, 1987, 20(2): 254.

62. Clifton, G. et al., The metabolic response to severe head injury, *J. Neurosurg.*, 1984, 60: 687.

63. Moore, R., Najarian, M., and Konvolinka, C., Measured energy expenditure in severe head injury, *J. Trauma*, 1989, 29(12): 1633.

64. Fruin, A., Taylor, C., and Pettis, L., Caloric requirements in patients with severe head injury, *Surg. Neurol.*, 1986, 25: 25.

65. Harris, J. and Benedict, F., *A Biometric Study of Basal Metabolism in Man*, Washington, D.C.: Carnegie Institute, 1919.

66. Young, B. et al., Metabolic and nutrition sequelae in the non-steroid treated head injury patient, *Neurosurgery*, 1985, 17(5): 784.

67. Zaloga, G.P., *Nutrition in Critical Care*, St. Louis: Mosby-Year Book, 1994.

68. Ott, L., Young, B., and McClain, C., The metabolic response to brain injury, *J. Parenteral Enteral Nutr.*, 1987, 11(5): 488.

69. Bivins, B., Twyman, D., and Young, B., Failure of nonprotein calories to mediate protein conservation in brain-injured patients, *J. Trauma*, 1986, 26: 980.

70. Twyman, D., High protein enteral feedings: a means of achieving positive nitrogen balance in head injured patients, *J. Parenteral Enteral Nutr.*, 1985, 9(6): 679.

71. Taylor, S.J. et al., Prospective, randomized, controlled trial to determine the effect of early enhanced enteral nutrition on clinical outcome in mechanically ventilated patients suffering head injury, *Crit. Care Med.*, 1999, 27(11): 2525.

72. Fried, R. et al., Barbiturate therapy reduces nitrogen excretion in acute head injury, *J. Trauma*, 1989, 29(11): 1558.

73. Chin, D.E. and Kearns, P., Nutrition in the spinal-injured patient, *Nutr. Clin. Pract.*, 1991, 6: 213.

74. Kolpek, J. et al., Comparison of urinary urea nitrogen excretion and measured energy expenditure in spinal cord injured and non-steroid treated severe head trauma patients, *J. Parenteral Enteral Nutr.*, 1989, 13: 277.

75. Kaufman, H.H. et al., General metabolism in patients with acute paraplegia and quadriplegia, *Neurosurgery*, 1985, 16: 309.

76. Rodriguez, D.J. et al., Obligatory negative nitrogen balance following spinal cord injury, *J. Parenteral Enteral Nutr.*, 1991, 15: 319.
77. Munir, A. et al., Wernicke's encephalopathy in a non-alcoholic man: case report and brief review, *Mt. Sinai J. Med.*, 2001, 68(3): 216.
78. Homewood, J. and Bond, N.W., Thiamin deficiency and Korsakoff's syndrome: failure to find memory impairments following nonalcoholic Wernicke's encephalopathy, *Alcohol*, 1999, 19(1): 75.
79. Cook, C.C. and Thomson, A.D., B-complex vitamins in the prophylaxis and treatment of Wernicke–Korsakoff syndrome, *Br. J. Hosp. Med.*, 1997, 57(9): 461.
80. Cook, C.C., Hallwood, P.M., and Thomson, A.D., B vitamin deficiency and neuropsychiatric syndromes in alcohol misuse, *Alcohol*, 1998, 33(4): 317.
81. McEntee, W.J., Wernicke's encephalopathy: an excitotoxity hypothesis, *Metab. Brain Dis.*, 1997, 12(3): 183.
82. Zubaran, C., Fernandes, J.G., and Rodnight, R., Wernicke–Korsakoff syndrome, *Postgrad. Med. J.*, 1997, 73(855): 27.
83. Diamond, I. and Messing, R.O., Neurologic effects of alcoholism, *West J. Med.*, 1994, 161(3): 279.
84. Heye, N. et al., Wernicke's encephalopathy — causes to consider, *Intensive Care Med.*, 1994, 20(4): 282.
85. Lindberg, M.C. and Oyler, R.A., Wernicke's encephalopathy, *Am. Fam. Physician*, 1990, 41(4): 1205.
86. Yellowlees, P.M., Thiamin deficiency and prevention of the Wernicke–Korsakoff syndrome. A major public health problem, *Med. J. Aust.*, 1986, 145(5): 216.
87. Harper, C.G., Giles, M., and Finlay-Jones, R., Clinical signs in the Wernicke–Korsakoff complex: a retrospective analysis of 131 cases diagnosed at necropsy, *J. Neurol. Neurosurg. Psychiatry*, 1986, 49(4): 341.
88. Perkin, G.D. and Handler, C.E., Wernicke–Korsakoff syndrome, *Br. J. Hosp. Med.*, 1983, 30(5): 331, 333.
89. Bonjour, J.P., Vitamins and alcoholism. II. Folate and vitamin B12, *Int. J. Vitam. Nutr. Res.*, 1980, 50(1): 96.
90. Davis, R.E., Clinical chemistry of vitamin B12, *Adv. Clin. Chem.*, 1985, 24: 163.
91. Frenkel, E.P. and Yardley, D.A., Clinical and laboratory features and sequelae of deficiency of folic acid (folate) and vitamin B12 (cobalamin) in pregnancy and gynecology, *Hematol. Oncol. Clin. North Am.*, 2000, 14(5): 1079, viii.
92. Ghezzi, A. and Zaffaroni, M., Neurological manifestations of gastrointestinal disorders, with particular reference to the differential diagnosis of multiple sclerosis, *Neurol. Sci.*, 2001, 22(Suppl. 2): S117.
93. Graham, S.M., Arvela, O.M., and Wise, G.A., Long-term neurologic consequences of nutritional vitamin B12 deficiency in infants, *J. Pediatr.*, 1992, 121(5 Pt 1): 710.
94. Hall, C.A., Pathophysiology of vitamin B12, *Pathobiol. Annu.*, 1979, 9: 257.
95. Lindenbaum, J., Drugs and vitamin B12 and folate metabolism, *Curr. Concepts Nutr.*, 1983, 12: 73.
96. Parnetti, L., Bottiglieri, T., and Lowenthal, D., Role of homocysteine in age-related vascular and non-vascular diseases, *Aging (Milano)*, 1997, 9(4): 241.
97. Reynolds, E.H., Neurological aspects of folate and vitamin B12 metabolism, *Clin. Haematol.*, 1976, 5(3): 661.
98. Skeen, M.B., Neurologic manifestations of gastrointestinal disease, *Neurol. Clin.*, 2002, 20(1): 195, vii.
99. Tefferi, A. and Pruthi, R.K., The biochemical basis of cobalamin deficiency, *Mayo Clin. Proc.*, 1994, 69(2): 181.
100. Weir, D.G. and Scott, J.M., Brain function in the elderly: role of vitamin B12 and folate, *Br. Med. Bull.*, 1999, 55(3): 669.
101. Weir, D.G. and Scott, J.M., The biochemical basis of the neuropathy in cobalamin deficiency. *Baillieres Clin. Haematol.*, 1995, 8(3): 479.
102. Wickramasinghe, S.N., The wide spectrum and unresolved issues of megaloblastic anemia, *Semin. Hematol.*, 1999, 36(1): 3.

103. Wynn, M. and Wynn, A., The danger of B12 deficiency in the elderly, *Nutr. Health*, 1998, 12(4): 215.

104. Reynolds, E.H., Rothfeld, P., and Pincus, J.H., Neurological disease associated with folate deficiency, *Br. Med. J.*, 1973, 2(5863): 398.

105. Reynolds, E.H., Benefits and risks of folic acid to the nervous system, *J. Neurol. Neurosurg. Psychiatry*, 2002, 72(5): 567.

106. Reynolds, E.H., Letter: folate-responsive neuropathy, *Br. Med. J.*, 1976, 2(6026): 42.

107. Dreyfuss, P.M., Vitamin deficiencies, *Prog. Clin. Biol. Res.*, 1980, 39: 239.

108. Grant, C.A. and Berson, E.L., Treatable forms of retinitis pigmentosa associated with systemic neurological disorders, *Int. Ophthalmol. Clin.*, 2001, 41(1): 103.

109. Harding, A.E. et al., Spinocerebellar degeneration associated with a selective defect of vitamin E absorption, *N. Engl. J. Med.*, 1985, 313(1): 32.

110. Harding, A.E., Vitamin E and the nervous system, *Crit. Rev. Neurobiol.*, 1987, 3(1): 89.

111. Muller, D.R., Harries, J.T., and Lloyd, J.K., Vitamin E therapy in abetalipoproteinemia, *Arch. Dis. Child.*, 1970, 45(243): 715.

112. Muller, D.P., Lloyd, J.K., and Wolff, O.H., The role of vitamin E in the treatment of the neurological features of abetalipoproteinemia and other disorders of fat absorption, *J. Inherit. Metab. Dis.*, 1985, 8(Suppl. 1): 88.

113. Muller, D.P., Lloyd, J.K., and Wolff, O.H., Vitamin E and neurological function: abetalipoproteinemia and other disorders of fat absorption, *Ciba Found. Symp.*, 1983, 101: 106.

114. Muller, D.P., Lloyd, J.K., and Wolff, O.H., Vitamin E and neurological function, *Lancet*, 1983, 1(8318): 225.

115. Perkin, G.D. and Murray-Lyon, I., Neurology and the gastrointestinal system, *J. Neurol. Neurosurg. Psychiatry*, 1998, 65(3): 291.

116. Sokol, R.J., Vitamin E and neurologic deficits, *Adv. Pediatr.*, 1990, 37: 119.

117. Iannaccone, S.T. and Sokol, R.J., Vitamin E deficiency in neuropathy of abetalipoproteinemia, *Neurology*, 1986, 36(7): 1009.

118. Tanyel, M.C. and Mancano, L.D., Neurologic findings in vitamin E deficiency, *Am. Fam. Physician*, 1997, 55(1): 197.

119. Mount, M.E. and Feldman, B.F., Practical toxicologic diagnosis, *Mod. Vet. Pract.*, 1984, 65(8): 589.

120. Clarkson, T.W., Metal toxicity in the central nervous system, *Environ. Health Perspect.*, 1987, 75: 59.

121. Krigman, M.R., Bouldin, T.W., and Mushak, P., Metal toxicity in the nervous system, *Monogr. Pathol.*, 1985, 26: 58.

122. Winship, K.A., Toxicity of inorganic arsenic salts, *Adverse Drug React. Acute Poisoning Rev.*, 1984, 3(3): 129.

123. Greenhouse, A.H., Heavy metals and the nervous system, *Clin. Neuropharmacol.*, 1982, 5(1): 45.

124. Bahiga, L.M., Kotb, N.A., and El-Dessoukey, E.A., Neurological syndromes produced by some toxic metals encountered industrially or environmentally, *Z. Ernahrungswiss*, 1978, 17(2): 84.

125. Thomas, D.G., Infant botulism: a review in South Australia (1980–89), *J. Paediatr. Child Health*, 1993, 29(1): 24.

126. Watters, M.R., Organic neurotoxins in seafoods, *Clin. Neurol. Neurosurg.*, 1995, 97(2): 119.

127. Watters, G.V. and Barlow, C.F., Acute and subacute neuropathies, *Pediatr. Clin. North Am.*, 1967, 14(4): 997.

128. Wills, A.J. and Unsworth, D.J., The neurology of gluten sensitivity: separating the wheat from the chaff, *Curr. Opin. Neurol.*, 2002, 15(5): 519.

129. Wills, A.J., The neurology and neuropathology of coeliac disease, *Neuropathol. Appl. Neurobiol.*, 2000, 26(6): 493.

130. Pengiran Tengah, D.S., Wills, A.J., and Holmes, G.K., Neurological complications of coeliac disease, *Postgrad. Med. J.*, 2002, 78(921): 393.

131. Hadjivassiliou, M., Grunewald, R.A., and Davies-Jones, G.A., Gluten sensitivity as a neurological illness, *J. Neurol. Neurosurg. Psychiatry*, 2002, 72(5): 560.

132. Hadjivassiliou, M., Grunewald, R.A., and Davies-Jones, G.A., Idiopathic cerebellar ataxia associated with celiac disease: lack of distinctive neurological features, *J. Neurol. Neurosurg. Psychiatry*, 1999, 67(2): 257.

133. Hadjivassiliou, M. et al., Clinical, radiological, neurophysiological, and neuropathological characteristics of gluten ataxia, *Lancet*, 1998, 352(9140): 1582.

134. Hadjivassiliou, M. et al., Does cryptic gluten sensitivity play a part in neurological illness? *Lancet*, 1996, 347(8998): 369.

135. Vaknin-Dembinsky, A., Eliakim, R., and Steiner, I., Neurological deficits in patients with celiac disease, *Arch. Neurol.*, 2002, 59(4): 647.

136. Hanagasi, H.A. et al., A typical neurological involvement associated with celiac disease, *Eur. J. Neurol.*, 2001, 8(1): 67.

137. Ozge, A., Karakelle, A., and Kaleagasi, H., Celiac disease associated with recurrent stroke: a coincidence or cerebral vasculitis? *Eur. J. Neurol.*, 2001, 8(4): 373.

138. Luostarinen, L., Pirttila, T., and Collin, P., Coeliac disease presenting with neurological disorders, *Eur. Neurol.*, 1999, 42(3): 132.

139. Pellecchia, M.T. et al., Cerebellar ataxia associated with subclinical celiac disease responding to gluten-free diet, *Neurology*, 1999, 53(7): 1606.

140. Muller, A.F. et al., Neurological complications of celiac disease: a rare but continuing problem, *Am. J. Gastroenterol.*, 1996, 91(7): 1430.

141. Muller, A.F., The neurological complications of celiac disease, *Am. J. Gastroenterol.*, 1997, 92(3): 540.

142. Tietge, U.J., Schmidt, H.H., and Manns, M.P., Neurological complications in celiac disease, *Am. J. Gastroenterol.*, 1997, 92(3): 540.

143. Auricchio, S., Gluten sensitivity and neurological illness, *J. Pediatr. Gastroenterol. Nutr.*, 1997, 25(Suppl. 1): S7.

144. Collin, P. and Maki, M., Celiac disease — even a neurological disorder, *J. Pediatr. Gastroenterol. Nutr.*, 1997, 24(1): 116.

145. Collin, P. and Maki, M., Associated disorders in coeliac disease: clinical aspects, *Scand. J. Gastroenterol.*, 1994, 29(9): 769.

146. Pfeiffer, R.F., Neurologic dysfunction in gastrointestinal disease, *Semin. Neurol.*, 1996, 16(3): 217.

147. Usai, P. et al., Autonomic neuropathy in adult celiac disease, *Am. J. Gastroenterol.*, 1996, 91(8): 1676.

148. Unsworth, D.J., Gluten sensitivity and neurological dysfunction, *Lancet*, 1996, 347(9005): 903.

149. Kelkar, P., Ross, M.A., and Murray J., Mononeuropathy multiplex associated with celiac sprue, *Muscle Nerve*, 1996, 19(2): 234.

150. Ackerman, Z. et al., Neurological manifestations in celiac disease and vitamin E deficiency, *J. Clin. Gastroenterol.*, 1989, 11(5): 603.

151. Mulder, C.J. and Tytgat, G.N., Coeliac disease and related disorders, *Neth. J. Med.*, 1987, 31(5–6): 286.

152. Kinney, H.C. et al., Degeneration of the central nervous system associated with celiac disease, *J. Neurol. Sci.*, 1982, 53(1): 9.

153. Morris, J.S., Ajdukiewicz, A.B., and Read, A.E., Neurological disorders and adult coeliac disease, *Gut*, 1970, 11(7): 549.

154. Lossos, A. et al., Neurologic aspects of inflammatory bowel disease, *Neurology*, 1995, 45(3 Pt 1): 416.

155. Lossos, A. et al., Peripheral neuropathy and folate deficiency as the first sign of Crohn's disease, *J. Clin. Gastroenterol.*, 1991, 13(4): 442.

156. Topper, R., Gartung, C., and Block, F., Neurologic complications in inflammatory bowel diseases, *Nervenarzt*, 2002, 73(6): 489, quiz 500.

157. Albers, J.W., Nostrant, T.T., and Riggs, J.E., Neurologic manifestations of gastrointestinal disease, *Neurol. Clin.*, 1989, 7(3): 525.

158. Adams, M. et al., Whipple's disease confined to the central nervous system, *Ann. Neurol.*, 1987, 21(1): 104.

159. Chan, R.Y., Yannuzzi, L.A., and Foster, C.S., Ocular Whipple's disease: earlier definitive diagnosis, *Ophthalmology*, 2001, 108(12): 2225.
160. Brown, A.P. et al., Whipple's disease presenting with isolated neurological symptoms. Case report, *J. Neurosurg.*, 1990, 73(4): 623.
161. De Coene, B. et al., Whipple's disease confined to the central nervous system, *Neuroradiology*, 1996, 38(4): 325.
162. Cooper, G.S. et al., Central nervous system Whipple's disease: relapse during therapy with trimethoprim–sulfamethoxazole and remission with cefixime, *Gastroenterology*, 1994, 106(3): 782.
163. De Jonghe, P. et al., Cerebral manifestations of Whipple's disease, *Acta Neurol. Belg.*, 1979, 79(4): 305.
164. Coria, F. et al., Whipple's disease with isolated central nervous system symptomatology diagnosed by molecular identification of *Tropheryma whippelii* in peripheral blood, *Neurologia*, 2000, 15(4): 173.
165. Flemmer, M.C. and Flenner, R.W., Current insights in Whipple's Disease, *Curr. Treat. Options Gastroenterol.*, 2003, 6(1): 13.
166. Fantry, G.T. and James, S.P., Whipple's disease, *Dig. Dis.*, 1995, 13(2): 108.
167. Knox, D.L., Bayless, T.M., and Pittman, F.E., Neurologic disease in patients with treated Whipple's disease, *Medicine (Baltimore)*, 1976, 55(6): 467.
168. Halperin, J.J., Landis, D.M., and Kleinman, G.M., Whipple disease of the nervous system, *Neurology*, 1982, 32(6): 612.
169. Louis, E.D. et al., Diagnostic guidelines in central nervous system Whipple's disease, *Ann. Neurol.*, 1996, 40(4): 561.
170. Manzel, K., Tranel, D., and Cooper, G., Cognitive and behavioral abnormalities in a case of central nervous system Whipple disease, *Arch. Neurol.*, 2000, 57(3): 399.
171. Willison, H.J. and Yuki, N., Peripheral neuropathies and anti-glycolipid antibodies, *Brain*, 2002, 125(Pt 12): 2591.
172. Willison, H.J. and O'Hanlon, G.M., The immunopathogenesis of Miller Fisher syndrome, *J. Neuroimmunol.*, 1999, 100(1–2): 3.
173. Okuda, B. et al., Fulminant Guillain–Barre syndrome after *Campylobacter jejuni* enteritis and monospecific anti-GT1a IgG antibody, *Intern. Med.*, 2002, 41(10): 889.
174. Onodera, M. et al., Acute isolated bulbar palsy with anti-GT1a IgG antibody subsequent to *Campylobacter jejuni* enteritis, *J. Neurol. Sci.*, 2002, 205(1): 83.
175. Nachamkin, I. et al., Ganglioside GM1 mimicry in *Campylobacter* strains from sporadic infections in the United States, *J. Infect. Dis.*, 1999, 179(5): 1183.
176. Nachamkin, I. et al., *Campylobacter jejuni* from patients with Guillain–Barre syndrome preferentially expresses a GD(1a)-like epitope, *Infect. Immun.*, 2002, 70(9): 5299.
177. Nachamkin, I. et al., Molecular population genetic analysis of *Campylobacter jejuni* HS:19 associated with Guillain–Barre syndrome and gastroenteritis, *J. Infect. Dis.*, 2001, 184(2): 221.
178. Nachamkin, I., Allos, B.M., and Ho, T., *Campylobacter* species and Guillain–Barre syndrome, *Clin. Microbiol. Rev.*, 1998, 11(3): 555.
179. Nachamkin, I., Chronic effects of *Campylobacter* infection, *Microbes Infect.*, 2002, 4(4): 399.
180. Nachamkin, I., *Campylobacter* enteritis and the Guillain–Barre syndrome, *Curr. Infect. Dis. Rep.*, 2001, 3(2): 116.
181. Nachamkin, I., Microbiologic approaches for studying *Campylobacter* species in patients with Guillain–Barre syndrome, *J. Infect. Dis.*, 1997, 176(Suppl. 2): S106.
182. Prasad, K.N., Pradhan, S., and Nag, V.L., Guillain–Barre syndrome and *Campylobacter* infection, *Southeast Asian J. Trop. Med. Public Health*, 2001, 32(3): 527.
183. Prasad, K.N., Dixit, A.K., and Ayyagari, A., *Campylobacter* species associated with diarrhea in patients from a tertiary care centre of north India, *Indian J. Med. Res.*, 2001, 114: 12.
184. Yuki, N., Taki, T., and Handa, S., Antibody to GalNAc–GD1a and GalNAc–GM1b in Guillain–Barre syndrome subsequent to *Campylobacter jejuni* enteritis, *J. Neuroimmunol.*, 1996, 71(1–2): 155.
185. Yuki, N. et al., Association of *Campylobacter jejuni* serotype with antiganglioside antibody in Guillain–Barre syndrome and Fisher's syndrome, *Ann. Neurol.*, 1997, 42(1): 28.

186. Yuki, N. et al., Close association of Guillain–Barre syndrome with antibodies to minor mono-sialogangliosides GM1b and GM1 alpha, *J. Neuroimmunol.*, 1997, 74(1–2): 30.

187. Yuki, N., Tagawa, Y., and Handa, S., Autoantibodies to peripheral nerve glycosphingolipids SPG, SLPG, and SGPG in Guillain–Barre syndrome and chronic inflammatory demyelinating poly-neuropathy, *J. Neuroimmunol.*, 1996, 70(1): 1.

188. Yuki, N. et al., Serotype of *Campylobacter jejuni*, HLA, and the Guillain–Barre syndrome, *Muscle Nerve*, 1992, 15(8): 968.

189. Yuki, N., Odaka, M., and Hirata, K., Acute ophthalmoparesis (without ataxia) associated with anti-GQ1b IgG antibody: clinical features, *Ophthalmology*, 2001, 108(1): 196.

190. Yuki, N. and Miyatake, T., Guillain–Barre syndrome and Fisher's syndrome following *Campylobacter jejuni* infection, *Ann. NY Acad. Sci.*, 1998, 845: 330.

191. Yuki, N. et al., Acute motor axonal neuropathy and acute motor-sensory axonal neuropathy share a common immunological profile, *J. Neurol. Sci.*, 1999, 168(2): 121.

192. Yuki, N., Koga, M., and Hirata, K., Is *Campylobacter* lipopolysaccharide bearing a GD3 epitope essential for the pathogenesis of Guillain–Barre syndrome? *Acta Neurol. Scand.*, 2000, 102(2): 132.

193. Hadden, R.D. et al., Preceding infections, immune factors, and outcome in Guillain–Barre syn-drome, *Neurology*, 2001, 56(6): 758.

194. Hadden, R.D. et al., Guillain–Barre syndrome serum and anti-*Campylobacter* antibody do not exacerbate experimental autoimmune neuritis, *J. Neuroimmunol.*, 2001, 119(2): 306.

195. Hadden, R.D. and Gregson, N.A., Guillain–Barre syndrome and *Campylobacter jejuni* infection, *Symp. Ser. Soc. Appl. Microbiol.*, 2001, 30: 145S.

196. Banerji, N.K. and Hurwitz, L.J., Nervous system manifestations after gastric surgery, *Acta Neurol. Scand.*, 1971, 47(4): 485.

197. Abarbanel, J.M. et al., Neurologic complications after gastric restriction surgery for morbid obesity, *Neurology*, 1987, 37(2): 196.

198. Feit, H. and Glasberg, M.R., Neurologic complications of gastric partitioning, *Arch. Neurol.*, 1986, 43(7): 642.

199. Feit, H. et al., Peripheral neuropathy and starvation after gastric partitioning for morbid obesity, *Ann. Intern. Med.*, 1982, 96(4): 453.

200. Brannegan, R.T., Complications in gastric bypass, *Arch. Phys. Med. Rehabil.*, 1987, 68(10): 745.

201. Gilbert, S., Hatton, J., and Magnuson, B., How to minimize the reaction between phenytoin and enteral feeding: two approaches, *Nutr. Clin. Pract.*, 1996, 11(1): 28.

202. Newland, P., The use and effectiveness of alternate therapies in multiple sclerosis, *J. Neurosci. Nursing*, 1999, 31(1): 43.

203. Ahlskog, J.E. et al., Guamanian neurodegenerative disease: investigation of the calcium metabo-lism/heavy metal hypothesis, *Neurology*, 1995, 45(7): 1340.

204. Akesson, B. et al., Effect of experimental folate deficiency on lipid metabolism in liver and brain, *Br. J. Nutr.*, 1982, 47(3): 505.

205. Selhub, J. et al., Association between plasma homocysteine concentration and extracranial carotid-artery stenosis, *N. Engl. J. Med.*, 1995, 322(5): 286.

206. Pronsky, Z.M., *Food Medication Interactions*, 12th ed., Birchrunville: Food–Medication Inter-actions, 2002, p. 357.

11 Upper Gastrointestinal System

Andrea Avery and Pamela Williams

CONTENTS

The upper gastrointestinal (GI) system encompasses the mouth, pharynx, esophagus, stomach, and duodenum.

The mouth is the portal of entry to the digestive tract. Initiation of the digestive process begins as food is chewed by the teeth. The enzymatic activity of salivary amylase simultaneously softens and initiates the chemical breakdown of the food bolus.

Pathologic conditions affecting the mouth, such as tooth and gum disease may affect nutritional status. Poorly fitted dentures and other oral appliances may make eating uncomfortable, even painful to the point of significant weight loss, especially in the elderly. Oral infections primarily include microbially induced, such as gingivitis and thrush, and virally induced, such as those due to herpes simplex viruses.

The esophagus serves as a muscular conduit, which propels the food boluses in an organized fashion to the stomach. This transit takes approximately 6 s for completion. At the end of the esophagus is a muscular area of narrowing called the lower esophageal sphincter, which guards the entryway to the stomach. This sphincter is usually closed until passage to the stomach is imminent.

The esophagus may be plagued with various disorders involving problems with muscular movement; narrowing of the lumen due to strictures, rings, webs, or tumors; esophageal inflammation may occur due to chronic gastroesophageal reflux. Thrush and *Candida* may also infect the esophagus. In addition, extrinsic injury may occur to the esophageal lining from ingested pills, caustic injury from accidental or intentional ingestion of lye, and other substances.

The digestive process in the stomach is both mechanical as well as chemical. The mucosal lining contains glands that produce hydrochloric acid and the proenzymes pepsinogen I and II.

Many bacteria contained in food are destroyed by hydrochloric acid. The stomach produces the protein intrinsic factor, which binds vitamin B_{12} and is critical for its absorption in the ileum.

The top two third of the stomach serves primarily as a reservoir and can hold quite a large volume of food with minimal increase in pressure. The lower one third performs the mixing and grinding function as well as propulsion into the small intestine. Between 2 and 4 h is required for the stomach to perform its various functions.

Numerous stomach maladies may occur due to poor dietary habits, external stressors, as well as functional and anatomic abnormalities. Some of the more common ones include nausea and vomiting, dyspepsia, hiatal hernia, *Helicobacter pylori* infection, and various motility disorders.

The duodenum comprises the first 12 in. or so of the small intestine and is considered part of the upper GI system, given its immediate continuation just after the stomach. Special structures, called Brunner's glands, produce fluid to protect the duodenum from the potential erosiveness of stomach acid. Other glands serve to secrete mucous and the digestive enzyme pepsinogen II. In addition, secretions from the pancreas and biliary system enter here to do their part in the digestive process. The relative acidity of the duodenum allows for easier absorption of iron, folic acid, calcium, copper, thiamin, zinc, vitamins A and B_2. In conditions of low acidity, deficiency of these nutrients may occur in some individuals.

NAUSEA AND VOMITING[1,2]

Nausea refers to a sensation of impending vomiting, the feeling of aversion to food, or generalized feelings of uneasiness of the stomach. Vomiting, in contrast, is an active, sometimes violent process, associated with retching and often heralded by increased salivation and profound nausea. Regurgitation, not to be confused with vomiting, is usually an effortless occurrence, often related to posture and associated with a weak GI sphincter. Patients often relate a bitter or sour taste in the mouth.

Anxiety is a leading cause of nausea and vomiting. This is true in adults, particularly so in young children and adolescents. The earlier vomiting occurs after eating (i.e., within seconds to several minutes), the less likely there is to be a physical cause, and more probable the psychological causes.

Medications are often found to be the cause of nausea and vomiting. Common offenders are nonsteroidal anti-inflammatory drugs (NSAIDs), digoxin, opiates, and L-dopa. Alcohol is another culprit especially in young individuals with early morning vomiting. In females of childbearing age pregnancy, especially during the first trimester, may cause nausea and vomiting.

Motion sickness is another cause of nausea and vomiting and is usually made obvious by the activities during which it occurs. Food poisoning is another cause, usually apparent given recent history of suspect food intake or other individuals who ingested the same food having similar symptoms.

A more ominous cause of vomiting may be a neurologic condition, specifically, brain tumors. This fortunately is rare and is characterized by the absence of nausea or warning signs. Early morning occurrence and associated headache are common.

Some medical conditions such as diabetes with gastroparesis and chronic kidney disease are often associated with nausea and vomiting. Cancer patients may experience nausea and vomiting as a side effect of various chemotherapy medications.

Therapeutic invention for nausea and vomiting involves abstaining from obvious causative dietary or social habits. If alcohol is the problem complete abstinence may be necessary. Any psychological pathology or triggers need to be addressed. If any of the other aforementioned conditions are present, treatment of that condition is warranted and often will result in resolution of the nausea and vomiting.

Medications are sometimes used to afford the individual some relief. Metoclopramide, a promotility agent, is useful in diabetics as well as nondiabetics with chronic symptoms. Specific antiemetics such as phenergan and compazine provide symptomatic relief. Ondansetron is used in patients receiving chemotherapy.[3] Tetrahydrocannabinol, the active agent in marijuana, is sometimes used as well.

DYSPEPSIA, GASTROESOPHAGEAL REFLUX DISEASE, AND ULCERS[4–9]

Dyspepsia is a generic term that refers to nonspecific abdominal discomfort and is usually characterized by gas, heartburn, abdominal distention, and for some, cramping. Peptic ulcers may account for 15 to 25% of dyspepsia and gastroesophageal reflux may account for 5 to 15% of dyspepsia.[10] Other causes of dyspepsia include gastric or esophageal cancer, biliary tract disease, gastroparesis, pancreatitis, carbohydrate malabsorption, medication, infiltrative diseases such as Crohn's disease and metabolic disturbances.[10] Findings on actual visualization of the esophagus and stomach by a procedure called upper endoscopy are typically normal.

Gastroesophageal reflux disease (GERD) occurs due to the weakened pressure of the lower 1 to 2 in. region of the esophagus. Normally there is a brief relaxation with swallowing. Approximately 2 h after eating, the lower esophagus is relatively more relaxed. In persons with GERD, frequent relaxation of the lower esophagus occurs and causes acid-laden stomach contents to enter the esophagus. Individuals have heartburn symptoms related to meals, particularly fatty, spicy, or large meals. Symptoms may occur with bending over or lying down. GERD may also cause nausea, vomiting, which above the region of the esophagus, results in chronic cough, hoarseness, asthma, and dental erosions.

Hiatal hernia is an anatomical abnormality in which the upper portion of the stomach protrudes into the chest through the diaphragm. It does not necessarily cause reflux, although the two may coexist.

Lifestyle changes are first recommended and may result in significant improvement (Table 11.1). Some medications cause relaxation of the lower esophagus and these may need to be discontinued. Medications used to treat reflux are H2 histamine blockers and proton pump inhibitors (PPIs). These medications work to decrease acid output, and aid with healing. Surgery is an option for severe, resistant cases.[11–13]

TABLE 11.1
Lifestyle Modifications to Improve GI Disorders

Consume small to moderate meals

Certain foods may cause symptoms in some individuals. Foods to watch: alcohol, caffeinated beverages, chocolate, citrus, garlic, onions, peppermint, and tomato-based products

Limit fat intake — butter, margarine, oil, mayonnaise, fried foods, animal fat, nuts, etc.

After eating a meal, wait 3 to 4 h before lying down

Certain medications may potentiate symptoms: calcium channel blockers, beta agonists, tranquilizers, anticholinergic agents, alpha-adrenergic agonists, theophylline, nitrates, and sedatives

Losing weight may help reduce the stress around the GI tract and can minimize symptoms

Stop smoking and monitor weight to avoid weight gain associated with smoking cessation

Relaxation techniques

Elevate the head of the bed by 6 in.

Source: From Heidelbaugh, J.J., *Am. Fam. Physician*, 68, 1311, 2003.

Peptic ulcers occur in the duodenum or the stomach and affect one in ten people in the United States. They are usually caused by *H. pylori* infections, but can also develop with long-term use of NSAIDs such as aspirin or ibuprofen, or excessive gastric acid secretion in disorders such as Zollinger–Ellison syndrome.[14–16] Stress or spicy foods do not cause ulcers but can aggravate them.

Patients with ulcer disease tend to have pain that is relieved with food or antacids. The pain generally occurs 1 to 3 h after eating and at night. If abdominal symptoms are associated with loss of weight, difficulty in swallowing, loss of appetite, bleeding, early satiety during a meal, or anemia, cancer may be present.

H. pylori is a spirochete microorganism that is commonly associated with duodenal and gastric ulcers. It is found in the stomach lining of many individuals with ulcer disease. *H. pylori* causes ulcers by weakening the effect of the mucosal lining that protects the stomach. This allows the stomach acid to irritate the stomach or duodenum. *H. pylori* protects itself from the acid by excreting enzymes that neutralize the acid until it burrows itself into the lining. This as well as stomach acid can lead to ulcer development.[17] The body defense mechanisms help to control infection, but unless treated specifically, *H. pylori* remains in the stomach for life.

H. pylori is also associated with nonulcer dyspepsia. However, eradication of *H. pylori* to alleviate symptoms is less well established.[18] Approximately 20% of people less than 40 years old and 50% of those over 60 years have *H. pylori* but most are not affected by ulcers.[17]

Ulcers due to NSAIDs occur because of a decrease in stomach mucous production and decreased blood flow to the lining of the stomach. The stomach is the most common location of the ulcers. The first month of treatment with NSAIDs is the time during which the risk of developing an ulcer is greatest. Elderly persons are particularly at risk as well as anyone who has had prior history of an ulcer.

Prevention and treatment minimizing the dose and use of NSAIDs especially in those with increased risk is recommended. The PPI medications are useful in preventing as well as treating NSAID-induced ulcers.[19,20]

Management of the above conditions begins with dietary and other habitual changes where indicated (Table 11.1). Over-the-counter antacids may be used for occasional symptoms but chronic symptoms require prescriptive medication (Table 11.2). H2 blocker medications such as ranitidine or cimetidine are often the first line of medical treatment prescribed to suppress acid secretion. Another class of medications, the PPIs such as omeprazole, lansoprazole, and others, are often more effective than the H2 blockers in clinical practice.[11,21] If *H. pylori* is found, it should be treated with some combination of antibiotic therapy. Amoxicillin, metronidazole, bismuth, and PPI preparation are few regimens advised for eradication, if *H. pylori* is found in association with ulcer disease.[22] Treatment for *H. pylori*-associated dyspepsia as opposed to ulcer disease remains controversial.[23] There is no consensus that *H. pylori* should be eradicated in these cases.

ESOPHAGEAL INFECTION

Esophageal infection may cause pain on swallowing. Persons at risk for developing these infections are those with immune system deficiencies such as AIDS. Also, persons with diabetes or cancer are more susceptible. Fungal infection due to *Candida* and viral infection due to herpes and cytomegalovirus are the usual ones. Antifungal medicines used include clotrimazole, nystatin, fluconazole, or ketoconazole. Antiviral treatments include acyclovir or ganciclovir.[27]

TABLE 11.2
Common Medication for Dyspepsia, GERD, and Ulcers

Category	Drugs	Purpose
Antacids	Alka-Seltzer, Maalox, Mylanta, Pepto-Bismol, Riopan, Rolaids, Tums	Antacids contain magnesium, calcium, or aluminum to neutralize stomach acid. Magnesium salts may cause diarrhea and aluminum salts may cause constipation. These two minerals are usually combined to balance their actions. Over-the-counter
Histamine receptor antagonists or H2 blockers	Cimetidine (Tagamet) Famotidine (Pepcid) Nizatidine (Axid) Ranitidine (Zantac)	H2 blockers help reduce stomach acid Over-the-counter and prescription
Proton pump inhibitors	Esomeprazole (Nexium) Lansoprazole (Prevacid) Omeprazole (Prilosec) Pantoprazole (Protonix) Raberprazole (Aciphex)	Proton pump inhibitors help reduce stomach acid. Prescription only
Foaming agents	Gaviscon	Foaming agents cover stomach contents with foam thereby reducing acid reflux. Over-the-counter
Prokinetics	Bethanechol (Urecholine) Metoclopramide (Reglan) Metoclopramide (Reglan)	Prokinetics helps increase esophageal sphincter pressure; also helps to increase stomach emptying to minimize acid reflux

Sources: From Ruth, M, et al., *Aliment. Pharmacol. Ther.*, 12, 35, 1997; Liebman, B., *Nutrition Action Newsletter*, April, 2003; Heidelbaugh, J.J., *Am. Fam. Physician*, 68, 1311, 2003.

SWALLOWING PROBLEMS[28]

Swallowing difficulties generally include problems with the transfer of food into the esophagus, pain upon swallowing, and the sensation of food getting stuck, which may be described as chest pain by the individual.

Difficulty in moving food from the mouth to the esophagus usually is due to problems with muscle function or a neurologic disorder. The individual may complain of aspirating food into the lungs or nose when attempting to swallow. Myasthenia gravis, multiple sclerosis, polymyositis, and changes after a stroke may cause such symptoms.

As mentioned earlier, gastroesophageal reflux is quite common and in some, acid irritation of the esophagus may be perceived as a chest discomfort during swallowing. Odynophagia is the term used to describe actual pain upon swallowing. Reflux may be associated with odyrophagia in many cases when drinking hot liquids or alcohol, which further serve to irritate an already acid damaged esophagus.

Herpes and cytomegalovirus infection can cause painful swallowing and a biopsy may be needed to diagnose these conditions. Some pills are notorious for causing potential chemical irritation, especially in those persons whose habit is to take pills with a sip or two of water rather than 6 to 8 oz. Tetracycline, potassium, NSAIDs, quinidine, and alendronate are common medications that cause irritation of the esophagus. The pill-induced damage usually resolves upon taking more liquids with subsequent doses. Some individuals may develop strictures.

Dysphagia is the sensation of food getting stuck during eating or shortly after swallowing. Dysphagia is due to a mechanical obstruction such as a tumor or some abnormal anatomical variation in the esophagus such as a web or ring. Also prolonged history of acid reflux can cause scarring and narrowing known as strictures usually in the lower esophagus.

Postgastrectomy: persons who have had stomach resection can have reflux of alkaline fluids from the intestines into the esophagus. Alkali is actually more injurious to the esophagus than acid from the stomach. Spasm of the esophagus may also occur. The individual usually experiences chest pain and trouble with food sticking in the esophagus. Hot or cold liquids may cause spasms. Treatment consists of several different options: nitrates — to increase blood flow, anticholinergic medicine, Nifedipine — a calcium channel blocker medication that helps relax muscles.[27,29] Surgery is also done in severe cases — the affected section of muscle is removed.

Esophageal pouches or diverticula are anatomical variations that occur in some individuals. When the pouch is full, it compresses the nearby normal area of the esophagus.

Other anatomical variations include esophageal rings and webs — usually thin fibrous tissue that partially obstructs the esophageal lumen at times, especially when eating large pieces of meat — "steakhouse syndrome." The individual notes improvement by drinking fluids or by inducing vomiting.

Strictures or scarred narrowed areas of the esophagus may result from prolonged gastroesophageal reflux. Chronic NSAID use is a contributing factor. Injury to esophageal lining may occur from ingestions of caustic substances or lye; sometimes individuals may deny this in case of intentional ingestion. These persons usually have underlying psychiatric conditions.

Cancerous growth is surely the most ominous cause of dysphagia. Clues are associated with weight loss, poor appetite, bleeding, and anemia.

Management of swallowing difficulty involves treating the underlying cause, especially in the case of a primary muscular or neurologic cause. For infectious causes, antiviral, antifungal medicines are indicated. Evaluation for HIV may also be indicated. Further benefit with dilation is indicated for the various mechanical causes. Treating reflux with H2 blockers or PPIs as well as discontinuing NSAIDs is advised as indicated.

MOTILITY DISORDERS

Achalasia is a general motility disorder of the esophagus due to denervation of the esophageal smooth muscle. The resulting abnormal movement of food contributes to difficulty in swallowing, chest pain, and aspiration. Eventually the esophagus stretches, resulting in retention of food, fluid, and passive regurgitation. Surgical treatment with removal of damaged muscle appears to be an increasingly successful treatment as are dilation procedures. Medications include injection of botulinum toxin (repeated injections are required).[30] Calcium channel blockers and nitrates also provide some relief.[31]

Diffuse esophageal spasm is a condition in which frequent simultaneous contractions occur but with no coordinated movement. Nutcracker esophagus is diagnosed when contractions are accompanied by extremely high esophageal pressure. Chest pain is the most common complaint with these conditions.

In persons with diabetes, the autonomic nervous system responsible for stomach emptying may be affected, causing delayed emptying. Some medications can alter motility, such as anticholinergics, tranquilizers, tricyclic antidepressants, calcium channel blockers, and nicotine.[32] No particularly good treatment presently exists. Metoclopramide and domperidone are sometimes useful, as is erythromycin.

POSTGASTRECTOMY

One out of ten individuals develops severe GI symptoms after stomach resection. Nutritional problems are most common with anemia, weight loss, and bone demineralization problems due to calcium loss. Anemia occurs due to absence of the duodenum where much of the body's iron is absorbed and due to decreased intrinsic factor production with subsequent vitamin B_{12} malabsorption. Bacterial growth in the postsurgical loop also causes vitamin B_{12} absorption to decrease.

Vomiting and reflux often occur due to lower esophageal sphincter and muscle disturbance, which results from the surgery. Heartburn, manifesting as abdominal pain after eating, may occur. Injury to the vagus nerve during surgery may result in problems with stomach emptying.

Dumping syndrome refers to symptoms that occur as a result of rapid emptying of the stomach contents into the intestinal tract. This large volume, highly concentrated load causes symptoms of sweating, tiredness, headache, and feeling of faintness. Meals with high carbohydrate content tend to be associated with more severe symptoms, which occur within 30 min after eating. Later, individuals may also experience nausea and vomiting, feeling of bloating, stomach rumbling, and diarrhea. Dumping symptoms are worse shortly after surgery and tend to improve somewhat over time. Reactive hypoglycemia may also be a component of the dumping syndrome. It usually occurs 2 to 4 h after eating with sweating, dizziness, and extreme feeling of hunger. Increased insulin levels are often present, usually in association with high carbohydrate-containing meals.

Management of postgastrectomy disorders includes iron supplementation, vitamin B_{12} supplementation as well as calcium, vitamin D, and other fat-soluble vitamins to replace the losses that occur due to altered gastric and duodenal absorption. Vomiting and reflux symptoms usually respond poorly to antacids. Prokinetic agents such as metoclopramide or domperidone may be helpful as are oral bile salt-binding agents (i.e., cholestyramine). The latter helps to bind the refluxed bile and pancreatic juices that occur after surgery. Having the individual eat small high-protein low-carbohydrate meals can often control dumping symptoms. A diabetes medication acarbose can be used to help delay carbohydrate absorption. In severe cases surgical treatment with intestinal rerouting may be necessary.

ALTERNATIVE NUTRITION THERAPIES

Traditionally, alternative therapies for GI disorders have been nonspecific, meaning that herbs and other substances are often recommended or prescribed to treat symptoms in general rather than a specific disorder. Lay literature offers a plethora of remedies for stomach ailments. Carminative herbs such as peppermint may be recommended for gas and bloating because they help to relax the smooth muscles. Demulcent herbs such as slippery elm are sometimes recommended for heartburn because they are rich in mucilage, which soothes the stomach. While some people report relief from these recommendations, the scientific literature offers benefits or anecdotal evidence. Some studies examining alternative therapies for the upper GI tract are poorly designed but offer insight to the possible uses of these therapies.

Alpha-linolenic acid has inhibited the growth of *H. pylori in vitro* and among 15 patients with *H. pylori* and mild symptoms of dyspepsia. Two grams of fish oil and black currant seed oil were given to patients for 8 weeks. Patients were evaluated for *H. pylori* infection at the end of 8 weeks and at 6 months. *H. pylori* eradication was obtained in 20% of these subjects.[33] *In vitro* studies have shown that in the presence of alpha-linolenic acid, linoleic acid, gamma-linolenic acid, and eicosapentaenoic acid, *H. pylori* growth was inhibited or eradicated.[34]

Cinnamon (*Cinnamomum zeylanicum*) is dried tree bark from the laurel family. It is often used as seasoning or for its aroma as incense and pot-pourris. It has been studied for its effects on *H. pylori*. In one *in vitro* study, researchers found that ethanol and methylene chloride extracts of cinnamon inhibited the growth of *H. pylori*.[35] In another study involving 15 subjects, 80 mg cinnamon in an alcoholic extract was ineffective against *H. pylori*.[36] There is not enough research to support cinnamon as an effective alternative treatment for *H. pylori*.

Chamomile (*Matricaria chamomilla*) has been used for various ailments such as skin disorders and diarrhea, and has been used as a mouthwash to treat inflammation of the membranes within the mouth and throat. Traditionally, it is used as a carminative for nonspecific distress of the GI system.

The benefits of chamomile in the upper GI system are limited in scientific literature. One double-blind, randomized study with 79 children reported that a chamomile extract and apple pectin preparation relieved symptoms of diarrhea in 3 days.[37] In a government clinical trial, chamomile is studied for its ability to alleviate chronic pain associated with bowel disorders in children.[38]

Garlic cloves in the form of an aqueous extract, inhibited the growth of *H. pylori in vitro*. However, the use of garlic was not effective in 15 human subjects who tested positive for *H. pylori*. Each subject ingested 300 mg of dried garlic powder three times daily for 8 weeks but only one subject had a negative breath test but was not tested at a later date to see if the organism had been eradicated. Based on this study and others, garlic has not been recommended for *H. pylori* treatment.[34]

Ginger (*Zingiber officinale Roscoe*), a traditional alternative medicine, has been used to treat nausea and vomiting during pregnancy, to prevent and treat motion sickness and postoperative surgery. Although the symptoms associated with its use are minimal, its use for nausea and vomiting has been controversial.

Several experimental studies inducing motion sickness have evaluated the efficacy of ginger. An early study examined the effect of ginger on motion sickness among subjects who were placed in a rotating chair and found no significant benefits.[39] But a more recent study determined that pretreatment of motion sickness with ginger among 13 subjects reduced the severity of nausea caused by circular vection, thereby lengthening latency before the onset of nausea and shortening recovery time.[40]

In a review article, researchers reported that three double-blind, placebo-controlled randomized controlled trials (RCTs) evaluated ginger for its effectiveness on nausea and vomiting among postoperative subjects and two of these trials reported that ginger was superior to placebo. One study evaluated ginger during both morning sickness and chemotherapy-induced nausea and reported the effectiveness of ginger over the placebo.[41]

In another review article, researchers identified six double-blind RCTs with a total of 675 subjects and a cohort study of 187 subjects. These studies examined ginger's effect during pregnancy. Four of the six RCTs reported benefits with use of ginger as compared to the placebo and two RCTs suggested that ginger is effective in relieving symptoms of nausea and vomiting. These studies also indicated that there were no significant side effects or adverse effects during pregnancy with the use of ginger.[42]

Overall, ginger may be an effective alternative treatment for nausea and vomiting during pregnancy, postoperative surgery, and for motion sickness but further research is needed to confirm its mechanism and effectiveness.

Ginseng (*Panax ginseng, Panax quinquefolius*, and *Eleutherococcus senticosus* or Siberian ginseng) has been recommended for stomach ailments in lay literature but scientific data is limited in supporting ginseng for this use. There is data suggesting that *Panax ginseng* may help reduce the risk of gastric cancer[43] and inhibit HCl–ethanol-induced gastric lesion, aspirin-induced gastric ulcer, acetic acid-induced ulcer, and Shay ulcer.[44]

Peppermint (*Mentha piperita*) has been reported to be one of the most widely used complementary and alternative medicine therapies used for irritable bowel syndrome.[47] It has been used alone or in combination with other therapies. Peppermint has supportive evidence for its use in dyspepsia, irritable bowel syndrome, and as an intraluminal spasmolytic agent during enemas or endoscopy.[46] In 2003, researchers Thompson and Ernest reviewed 17 randomized clinical trials involving the use of peppermint in nonulcer dyspepsia patients. Nine of these studies involved the combination of peppermint and caraway, and symptoms were reduced by these treatments.[47] Whether or not this herb is truly efficacious for GI ailments remains to be seen.

Prebiotics such as fructooligosaccharides (FOS), galactooligosaccharides, and inulin are essentially carbohydrates of relatively short chain length. These carbohydrates are considered to be a nondigestible food that benefits the body by stimulating growth of certain beneficial probiotic-like bacteria in the colon. These low molecular weight carbohydrates are found in artichokes, onions, chicory, garlic, leeks, and in smaller amounts in cereals. Galactooligosaccharides are found in human and cow's milk, and can be produced from lactose. Prebiotics are thought to be beneficial to the GI system if they resist digestive activity and reach the cecum. Prebiotics may also stimulate fermentation, and function as a mild laxative. Flatulence has been reported with the use of prebiotics.[48,49]

Probiotics are live microbial organisms, which improve the intestinal microbial profile. These live microbial organisms are found in foods such as miso, yogurt, and other dairy products, and can be supplied through supplementation. Some of the more popular organisms include lactobacilli and bifidobacteria. They enter the GI system, bypass the digestive activities, and temporarily bring benefits of normal gut flora. Their influence in the gut is temporary and they need to be ingested regularly to maintain any health benefit achieved.[49,50]

Lactobacilli have been used to treat diarrheal diseases and to help reduce GI effects of antibiotic use, especially during treatment of *H. pylori*.[51,52] The mechanism by which these microbial organisms work is not clearly understood since human studies have been observational rather than mechanistic. It has been theorized that these microbial organisms bind to the intestinal wall or bind to certain mutagens on the wall and block adhesion. They are also thought to be effective against intestinal pathogens by blocking invasive microbes.[49]

Researchers report that probiotic study results have been inconsistent, which may be due to different microbial strains, methods of administration, or the investigational procedure. Further studies are needed to confirm the mechanism and effects of probiotics.

Other therapies have been recommended for the health of the upper GI tract but there is minimal research or not enough data to support their use. Some of the recommended herbs include: berberine, black horehound (*Ballota nigra*), chen pi (*Citrus reticulata*), flavonoids, gentain (*Gentaina lutea*), mastic gum (*Pistacia lentiscus*), and vitamin C.[53] (See Textbox 11.1.)

SUMMARY

Although research is beginning to unravel the role of alternative therapies in upper GI disorders, much has yet to be uncovered. Presently, the understanding of conventional treatment for disorders related to *H. pylori* are advanced and effective in many cases, but treatment for other disorders such as nonulcer dyspepsia is not as defined. In these cases, the role of alternative therapies may be beneficial to those who experience symptoms but find no relief with conventional treatment. In addition, patients who suffer from disorders such as nausea and vomiting may benefit from the effective alternative therapies such as ginger, and probiotics or peppermint may be used in the treatment of symptoms related to nonulcer dyspepsia. These treatments are worth following in scientific literature in order to determine their roles alongside conventional treatments.

Textbox 11.1 Drug–Herb Interactions[54,55]	
Chamomile	May increase sedative effect of alcohol, antidepressants, antihistamines, barbiturates, benzodiazepines, narcotics, and sedatives
Garlic	Increases effect of warfarin, antidiabetic drugs, blood pressure-lowering medications, and antiplatelet medications
Ginger	Increases the effect of anticoagulants, antidiabetic drugs (increases hypoglycemic effect), antiplatelet medications, barbiturates, cardiac drugs
	May increase or decrease the effect of antihypertensive medications
	May decrease the effect of antacids, protein pump inhibitors, and H2 antagonists
Panax ginseng	Decreases the effect of warfarin, antipsychotics, and monoamine oxidase inhibitors
	Increases the effect of diabetic medication and the effect of caffeine (increases blood pressure)
	May increase or decrease the effects of blood pressure medications
Peppermint	Increases the effect of calcium channel blockers
	May increase the effect of heartburn associated with calcium channel blockers
Siberian ginseng	Increases the effect of anticoagulants, antiplatelet medication, barbiturates, sedatives, diabetic medications
	May increase blood pressure — avoid taking with blood pressure medications
	Increases or interferes with the effects of antipsychotics and hormones (avoid using Siberian ginseng with these substances)

CASE STUDY

A 51-year-old African American male complained of GI pain in his abdomen. The episodes of pain occurred sporadically for over 2 years and each episode grew progressively worse.

At the time of his first office visit, the patient described pain occurring at the back of his throat and in his chest, as a burning sensation after a high-fat, spicy, or large meal. Sometimes he experienced bloating in his stomach or a dull gnawing pain in his intestines. He also experienced loose bowels or no bowel movement for as long as 5 days. Prior to his first office visit he used over-the-counter treatments such as Gaviscon and Pepcid AC to reduce or relieve his symptoms but now the medicine was ineffective in relieving the pain.

Blood samples were drawn and *H. pylori* antibody serology was done. He was diagnosed with *H. pylori* and GERD. He was treated for *H. pylori* with 500 mg Amoxicillin, 20 mg Omeprazole, and 500 mg Biaxin taken twice a day for 10 days. The patient was instructed to reduce meal size, spicy foods, and fat intake, remain upright at least 3 h after eating a meal, and elevate his head 6 in. whenever he sleeps. He was also instructed that after taking the antibiotics for 10 days, to regularly consume one cup of a yogurt that contained *Lactobacillus bulgaricus, L. reuteri, L. acidophilus*, and *L. casei*. This was to help replace the helpful bacteria in his gut after antibiotic treatment.

After the antibiotic treatment, the patient initially experienced no GI pain or discomfort for 3 weeks but the pain returned. He then started to reduce meal size, fat intake, and spices. He experienced some relief but then he added yogurt to his breakfasts and the pain ceased. On the days he skips yogurt or consumes a high fat or a large volume meal the pain returns. When he returned to the doctor's office, he explained that he did not have symptoms as long as he consumed the yogurt and followed the lifestyle changes recommended by the doctor.

It was recommended that if the symptoms return, he should schedule for an esophagogastroduodenoscopy (EDG) or an upper GI series to determine if *H. pylori* had been eradicated and to see if there was an ulcer present.

REFERENCES

1. Hasler, W.L. and Chey, W.D., Nausea and vomiting, *Gastroenterology*, 125, 1860, 2003.
2. Prakash, C. and Staioro, A., Similarities in cyclic vomiting across age groups, *Am. J. Gastroenterol.*, 96, 604, 2001.
3. Flake, Z.A., Scalley, R.D., and Bailey, A.G., Practical selection of antiemetics, *Am. Fam. Physician*, 69, 1169, 2004.
4. Kurata, J.H., Nogawa, A.N., and Everhart, J.E., A prospective study of dyspepsia in primary care, *Dig. Dis. Sci.*, 47, 747, 2002.
5. Manes, G., et al., Empirical prescribing for dyspepsia: randomised controlled trial of test and treat versus omeprazole treatment, *BMJ*, 326, 118, 2003.
6. McQuaid, K.R. and Isenbag, J.I., Medical therapy of peptic ulcer disease, *Surg. Clin. North Am.*, 72, 285, 1992.
7. NIH Consensus Conference. *Helicobacter pylori* in peptic ulcer disease. NIH consensus development panel on the *Helicobacter pylori* in peptic ulcer disease, *JAMA*, 272, 65, 1994.
8. Jones, M.P., Evaluation and treatment of dyspepsia, *Postgrad. Med. J.*, 79, 25, 2003.
9. Yeomons, N.D., Management of peptic ulcer disease not related to *Helicobacter*, *J. Gastroenterol. Hepatol.*, 17, 488, 2002.
10. Dickerson, L.M. and King, D.E., Evaluation and management of nonulcer dyspepsia, *Am. Fam. Physician*, 70, 107, 2004.
11. Rabeneck, L., et al., A double blind, randomized, placebo-controlled trial of proton pump inhibitor therapy in patients with uninvestigated dyspepsia, *Am. J. Gastroenterol.*, 97, 304S, 2002.
12. Brzana, R.J. and Koch, K.L., Gastroesophageal reflux disease presenting with intractable nausea, *Ann. Intern. Med.*, 126, 704, 1997.
13. El-Serog, H.B. and Sonnenberg, A., Association of esophagitis and esophageal strictures with diseases treated with nonsteroidal anti-inflammatory drugs, *Am. J. Gastroenterol.*, 92, 52, 1997.
14. Whitney, E.N., et al., *Understanding Normal and Clinical Nutrition*, 6th ed., Wadsworth/Thompson Learning, California, 2002.
15. Howden, C.W. and Hunt, R.H., Guidelines for the management of *Helicobacter pylori* infection, *Am. J. Gastroenterol.*, 93, 2330, 1998.
16. Spechler, S.J., American Gastroenterological Association medical position statement on the treatment of patients with dysphagia caused by benign disorders of the distal esophagus, *Gastroenterology*, 117, 229, 1999.
17. National Digestive Disease Information Clearinghouse, *H. pylori* and peptic ulcers, http://digestive.niddk.nih.gov/diseases/pubs/hpylori/, accessed July 29, 2005.
18. Walling, A.D., *Helicobacter pylori* treatment for nonulcer dyspepsia, *Am. Fam. Physician*, 63, 947, 2001.
19. Chan, F.K. and Leung, W.K., Peptic-ulcer disease, *Lancet*, 360, 933, 2002.
20. La, K.C., et al., Lansoprazole for the prevention of recurrences of ulcer complications from long term low-dose aspirin use, *N. Engl. J. Med.*, 345, 2033, 2002.
21. La, K.C., et al., Lansoprazole for the prevention of recurrences of ulcer complications from long term low-dose aspirin use, *N. Engl. J. Med.*, 346, 2033, 2002.

22. Hopkins, R.J., Girardi, L.S., and Turney, E.A., Relationship between *H. pylori* eradication and reduced duodenal and gastric ulcer recurrence: a review, *Gastroenterology*, 117, 229, 1999.

23. Laine, L., Schoenfeld, P., and Fennergy, M.B., Therapy for *Helicobacter pylori* in patients with nonulcer dyspepsia. A meta-analysis of randomized controlled trials, *Ann. Intern. Med.*, 134, 361, 2001.

24. Heidelbaugh, J.J., Management of gastroesophageal reflux disease, *Am. Fam. Physician*, 68, 1311, 2003.

25. Ruth, M, et al., The effect of mosapride, a novel prokinetic, on acid reflux variables in patients with gastro-oesophageal reflux disease, *Aliment. Pharmacol. Ther.*, 12, 35, 1997.

26. Liebman, B., Health issues of the gastrointestinal system, *Nutrition Action Newsletter*, April, 2003.

27. Richter, J.E. and Bradley, L.A., Esophageal chest pain: current controversies in pathogenesis, diagnosis and therapy, *Ann. Intern. Med.*, 110, 66, 1989.

28. Kikendall, J.W., et al., Pill-induced esophageal injury: case reports and review of the medical literature, *Dig. Dis. Sci.*, 28, 174, 1983.

29. Clouse, R.E., Spastic disorders of the esophagus, *Gastroenterologist*, 5, 112, 1997.

30. Storr, M. and Allescher, H.D., Treatment of symptomatic diffuse esophageal spasm by endoscopic injection of botulinum toxin: a prospective study with long term follow up, *Gastrointest. Endosc.*, 54, 754, 2001.

31. Cattau, E.L. and Castell, D.O., Diltrazam therapy for symptoms associated with nutcracker esophagus, *Am. J. Gastroenterol.*, 86, 272, 1991.

32. Clouse, R.E. and Lustman, P.J., Low dose trazodone for symptomatic patients with esophageal contraction abnormalities. A double-blind, placebo controlled trial, *Gastroenterology*, 92, 102, 1987.

33. Frieri, G., et al., Polyunsaturated fatty acid dietary supplementation: an adjuvant approach to treatment of *Helicobacter pylori* infection, *Nutr. Res.*, 20, 907, 2000.

34. Gaby, A.R., *Helicobacter pylori* eradication: are there alternatives to antibiotics? *Altern. Med. Rev.*, 6, 355, 2001.

35. Nir, Y., et al., Controlled trial of the effect of cinnamon extract on *Helicobacter pylori*, *Helicobacter*, 5, 94, 2000.

36. Tabak, M., Armon, R., and Neeman, I., Cinnamon extracts' inhibitory effect on *Helicobacter pylori*, *J. Ethnopharmacol.*, 67, 269, 1999.

37. de la Motte, S., et al. [Double-blind comparison of an apple pectin–chamomile extract preparation with placebo in children with diarrhea], *Arzneimittelforschung*, 47, 1247, 1997. German [abstract only].

38. Treatment of functional abdominal pain in children: evaluation of relaxation/guided imagery and chamomile tea as therapeutic modalities, http://clinicaltrials.gov/ct/gui/c/w2b/screen/ResultScreen/action/GetStudy? order = 2&xml_f . . . Accessed July 20, 2005.

39. Scott, J.R., et al., The effect on motion sickness and oculomotor function of GR 38032F, a 5-HT3-receptor and antagonist with anti-emetic properties, *Br. J. Clin. Pharmacol.*, 27, 147, 1989.

40. Lien, H., et al., Effects of ginger on motion sickness and gastric slow-wave dysrhythmias induced by circular vection, *Am. J. Physiol. Gastrointest. Liver Physiol.*, 284, G481, 2003.

41. Ernst, E. and Pittler, M.H., Efficacy of ginger for nausea and vomiting: a systematic review of randomized clinical trials, *Br. J. Anaesth.*, 84, 367, 2000.

42. Borrelli, F., et al., Effectiveness and safety of ginger in the treatment of pregnancy-induced nausea and vomiting, *Obstet. Gynecol.*, 105, 849, 2005.

43. Yo, A., Diet and stomach cancer in Korea, *Int. J. Cancer*, Suppl 10, 7, 1997.

44. Jeong, C.S., Effect of butanol fraction of *Panax ginseng* head on gastric lesion and ulcer, *Arch. Pharm. Res.*, 25, 61, 2002.

45. Krueger, K.J., et al., Nutritional supplements and alternative medicine, *Curr. Opin. Gastroenterol.*, 20, 130, 2004.

46. Koretz, R.L. and Rotblatt, M., Complementary and alternative medicine in gastroenterology: the good, the bad, and the ugly, *Clin. Gastroenterol. Hepatol.*, 2, 957, 2004.

47. Thompson, C.J. and Ernst, E., Systematic review: herbal medicinal products for non-ulcer dyspepsia, *Aliment. Pharmacol. Ther.*, 16, 1689, 2002.

48. Cummings, J.H., Macfarlane, G.T., and Englyst, H.N., Supplement. Prebiotic digestion and fermentation, *Am. J. Clin. Nutr.*, 73, 415S, 2001.

49. Macfarlane, G.T. and Cummings, J.H., Probiotics and prebiotics: can regulating the activities of intestinal bacteria benefit health? *BMJ*, 318, 999, 1999.
50. Duggan, C., Gannon, J., and Walker, W.A., Protective nutrients and functional foods for the gastrointestinal tract, *Am. J. Clin. Nutr.*, 75, 789, 2002.
51. Sakamoto, I., et al., Suppressive effect of *Lactobacillus gasseri* OLL 2716 (LG21) on *Helicobacter pylori* infections in humans, *J. Antimicrob. Chemother.*, 47, 709, 2001.
52. Wang, K., et al., Effects of ingesting *Lactobacillus-* and *Bifidobacterium*-containing yogurt in subjects with colonized *Helicobacter pylori*, *Am. J. Clin. Nutr.*, 80, 737, 2004.
53. Phytotherapies Monographs. Accessed July 23, 2005, http://www.phytotherapies.org/indications_detail.cfm?id=1121.
54. Jellin, J.M., Batz, F., and Hitchens, K., *Natural Medicines Comprehensive Database*, 2nd ed., Therapeutic Research Faculty, Stockton, CA, 1999.
55. DeBusk, R.M. and Treadwell, P.R., *Herbs as Medicine: What You Should Know*, DeBusk Communications, Tallahassee, Florida, 2000.

12 Promoting Small and Large Bowel Health

Susan Roberts and Mary Krystofiak Russell

CONTENTS

INTRODUCTION

Individuals with gastrointestinal (GI) disease frequently battle nausea, fatigue, and chronic pain.[1] Many of these people turn to alternative healthcare to seek relief.[2] Alternative practices have been shown to provide benefit in management of stress, stimulation of the immune system, and pain reduction[3]; others, such as misuse of herbs, may cause liver damage,[4] or may delay initiation of appropriate conventional care.[5]

This chapter will review five GI concerns: colon cancer, diverticulosis/diverticultitis, irritable bowel syndrome (IBS), inflammatory bowel disease (IBD) (Crohn's disease and ulcerative colitis [UC]), and celiac disease. Etiology and symptoms of each disorder will be included, but discussion will focus primarily on nutritional strategies (traditional and complementary and alternative) used to manage the disorders.

COLON CANCER

INCIDENCE

Colon cancer is a prevalent cancer in the developed countries, including the United States where it is the third most common cancer in males and females.[6] The American Cancer Society estimates over 100,000 new cases of colon cancer will be detected and over 56,000 deaths will be attributed to colon cancer in 2004.[6] When detected early, the five-year relative survival rate is 90%. If regional and lymph node metastasis has occurred, the five-year survival rate drops to 65%, if distant metastases have developed, the rate is 9%.[7] Surgery is the most common treatment for colon cancer, and can be curative in localized early stage disease. Chemotherapy and radiation are needed for individuals with metastases.[7]

SIGNS AND SYMPTOMS

There are typically no symptoms in the early stages. With more advanced disease, rectal bleeding, melana, a change in bowel habits, and lower abdominal cramping may be present. Because of the lack of symptoms in the early stages of colon cancer and the poorer prognosis with more advanced colon cancer, screening for colon cancer is recommended for both men and women at average risk for development of colon cancer, beginning at 50 years of age. Individuals with a family history of colon cancer or a personal history of adenomatous polyps or IBD should undergo earlier and more frequent screening. Common screening tests include fecal occult blood test, flexible sigmoidoscopy, double contrast barium enema, and colonoscopy.[8]

RISK FACTORS

Modifications in diet, body weight, exercise, tobacco, alcohol, and nonsteroidal anti-inflammatory drugs may change the risk for colon cancer.[9,10] The presence of a first-degree relative with a history of colon cancer increases the risk.[11] A recent research focus is the role of insulin resistance and insulin-like growth factors (IGF) in the etiology of colon cancer.[12] While some influences, such as family history, genetic predisposition, and history of IBD, are not controllable, many can be modified to lower colon cancer risk.

PREVENTIVE NUTRITION THERAPY

Diet, body weight, and physical activity are modifiable risk factors for colon cancer development. Researchers have estimated that reducing red meat intake, maintaining a desirable body weight, modest alcohol consumption, and folic acid supplementation, in conjunction with regular exercise and avoidance of tobacco products, could reduce the risk of colon cancer by 70%.[13] A recent multicenter study of more than 3000 asymptomatic people discovered several dietary components that influence colon cancer development. Intake of four or more servings of red meat per week increased risk nearly three times, high-fiber ingestion (at least 8 g/day from cereal) decreased risk by almost half, and adequate calcium intake (at least 900 to 1200 mg/day) reduced risk by almost half.[11]

Meat

Researchers have found increased risk of colon cancer with high red meat intake;[14,15] processed meat also appears to raise risk. Red and processed meat may increase colon cancer incidence by increased excretion of bile acids and damage to DNA. One serving of red or processed meat per week does not substantially increase the risk of colon cancer above no red meat intake. Red meat should be replaced at some meals with fish or chicken, which are not associated with an elevated risk of colon cancer.

Dietary Fat

Studies have found saturated or animal fat intake as an independent risk factor for colon cancer.[14,16] However, a pooled analysis of over 5000 cancer cases did not find dietary fat to influence colon cancer risk.[17] Conversely, polyunsaturated and monounsaturated fats do not increase colon cancer risk, and it has been suggested that olive oil, high in monounsaturated fat, may lower colon cancer incidence.[18] Intake of omega-3 fatty acids, such as those found in fish, has been associated with a decreased occurrence of colon cancer.[19] A diet with less than 30% of calories from total fat and less than 10% of calories from saturated fat is recommended. Additionally, use of omega-3 and monounsaturated fats may be protective,[20,21] but additional research is needed.

Obesity

Excessive energy intake and a sedentary lifestyle, which contribute to obesity, are associated with an increased risk of colon cancer.[22–25] A body mass index (BMI) greater than 30 increases colon cancer risk by two to three times compared to a BMI less than 22.[23] One hypothesis for how obesity influences colon cancer risk is through elevated insulin and IGF-1.[26] An epidemiological study, which found IGF-1 levels predicted colon cancer even after adjustment for BMI, lends support to this theory.[27]

Folic Acid

Significant epidemiological evidence exists supporting folic acid's function in prevention of colon cancer.[28] In two large prospective cohort studies, the Nurses' Health Study and the Health Professionals Follow-up Study, folate intake was inversely associated with colon cancer risk.[28] Additionally, the NHANES I Epidemiologic Follow-up Study, which included over 14,000 patients followed for 20 years, also found that a high folate intake reduced colon cancer risk.[29] Folate's ability to decrease colon cancer risk is likely due to its importance in the methylation, synthesis, and repair of DNA.[30] Based on current evidence, use of a daily multiple vitamin supplement containing 400 μg of folate is recommended.[31] Because alcohol interferes with folate availability, folate supplementation in those with moderate to high alcohol intake is associated with a reduction in colon cancer.[30,31]

Fiber

Fiber has been promoted as protective against colon cancer for over 30 years. Mechanisms by which fiber reduces colon cancer may include dilution of carcinogens in feces, decreased secondary bile acid concentration in the stool, modification in colonic microflora, increased short-chain fatty acid (SCFA) production, and decreased GI transit time.[30] However, current research has cast doubt on fiber's protective role. In several large prospective cohort studies, fiber was not associated with a decrease in adenoma or colon cancer risk.[32–34] Another study was positive and found intake of eight or more grams of cereal fiber was associated with a significant reduction in colon cancer risk.[11] The development of adenomas, which can progress to cancer, is often used as a surrogate end point in colon cancer intervention trials. A number of large prospective, randomized, intervention trials have also had negative results.[35–38] These studies have been criticized for their short duration and dose of fiber. One intervention trial, with a $2 \times 2 \times 2$ factorial design and a four-year follow-up period, examined the effect of wheat bran fiber, a low-fat diet, and β-carotene supplementation on adenoma recurrence in 424 patients.[39] Only those patients who received both the wheat bran fiber and a low-fat diet had a significant decrease in adenoma recurrence. While research has shown that certain fibers do not decrease adenoma recurrence, it is still not clear whether fiber *per se*, or a certain type of fiber, is important in colon cancer prevention. Possibly, only a high-fiber intake in combination with a low-fat diet lowers risk. Abandoning the recommendation to consume a diet with 20–35 g of fiber per day does not appear wise until more research provides a convincing answer.

Fruits and Vegetables

The role of fruits and vegetables in the prevention of colon cancer is not well defined. The long-held belief that a larger intake of fruits and vegetables is protective has been questioned by the results of a number of large prospective cohort studies, which have not found an association between high fruit and vegetable intake and lower colon cancer risk.[40–42] Another prospective cohort study conducted in a population with a habitually low fruit and vegetable consumption and vitamin supplement use did find an inverse relationship between colon cancer development and fruit and vegetable intake.[33] However, the effect was only seen in the lowest quartile, the group consuming less than 2.5 servings per day, and no effect was seen in the upper three quartiles that consumed more fruits and vegetables.[33] These results suggest risk-reduction from a certain level of fruit and vegetable intake. More research is needed before an authoritative recommendation can be made regarding fruit and vegetable consumption and colon cancer risk, although the current guideline of five or more fruits and vegetables daily seem prudent.

Calcium

Calcium, which may act to reduce the damage to colonocytes triggered by bile and fatty acids, has emerged as a chemopreventive agent against colon cancer.[30] Additional mechanisms by which calcium may exert an effect on colon cancer risk have been described.[43] Both cohort and intervention studies have had positive results. A prospective cohort study found that 900 to 1,200 mg of calcium per day reduced colon cancer risk by 50%.[11] Two prospective cohort studies, which included more than 134,000 subjects, revealed an inverse relationship between calcium intake of at least 1,250 mg and distal colon cancer.[44] The Polyp Prevention Study Group showed through a double-blind, randomized prospective trial that supplementation with 1,200 mg of calcium carbonate results in a significant reduction in recurrence of adenomas.[45] The evidence suggests the value of supplement with 1,200 mg of calcium per day as a preventive measure against colon cancer.

Selenium

The efficacy of selenium supplementation in reducing colon cancer risk has not been extensively studied in humans. One prospective, randomized, placebo-controlled trial supplemented diets with 200 μg of selenium and decreased colorectal cancer risk by 60% in the treatment group.[46] A case–control study examining selenium concentrations in toenails found an inverse relationship between toenail selenium levels and the risk of colon cancer.[47] Selenium may lower colon cancer incidence through apoptosis, enhanced immune function, and reduced DNA damage.[30] More extensive research is needed before recommendations can be made for use of selenium in chemoprevention of colon cancer.

COMPLEMENTARY THERAPIES

Many dietary supplements and herbal remedies are promoted for prevention and treatment of all forms of cancer. Unfortunately, high-quality research supporting the efficacy of many of these products is often not available. Adverse effects and drug-herb–supplement interactions can occur. Supplementation with the antioxidant vitamins C and E and β-carotene is common. A large prospective cohort study, the American Cancer Society's Cancer Prevention Study II, investigated the association between risk of colorectal cancer mortality and use of individual supplements of vitamins C and E.[48] The study included over 700,000 men and women with no history of cancer. After 14 years of follow-up, there was no significant association between supplementation and colorectal cancer mortality.[48] Another prospective cohort study also found no consistent support for lower risk of colon cancer with supplemental vitamin E.[49] Dietary β-carotene, α-carotene, lycopene, lutein, zeaxanthin, and β-cryptoxanthin were studied in a case–control trial to evaluate associations between intake of carotenoids and risk of colon cancer.[50] Only dietary lutein was inversely related to colon cancer risk.[50] It is not known if a dietary lutein supplement versus dietary intake of lutein would have the same effect. Research does not support the use of antioxidant supplements for the prevention of colon cancer. However, dietary intake of antioxidants from food sources, such as fruits and vegetables, is recommended due to possible benefits from antioxidants, fiber, and other phytochemicals in these foods.

Both case–control and large prospective cohort studies have shown that a high intake of raw or cooked garlic (ranging from approximately 1 to 9 cloves per week) to lower colon cancer risk.[51–54] However, garlic supplements have not been shown to lower colon cancer risk.[55] The pharmacological activity of garlic is related to several of its components, including allicin and ajoene.[56] Garlic may offer protection against colon cancer through immune stimulation.[57]

Pre- and probiotics may have a potential role in cancer prevention (see Textbox 12.1). These substances are thought to detoxify genotoxins in the intestinal tract.[58] Ingestion of lactic acid bacteria in animal studies has been found to prevent carcinogen-induced colon cancer.[59,60] In humans, epidemiologic studies do not show a consistent relationship between consumption of probiotics via fermented diary products and the risk of colon cancer.[61–64] From evidence available, pre- and probiotics do have a potential preventive role in colon cancer and further research is needed to substantiate this role.

Many other phytochemicals and plant components, including ginseng, quercetin, curcumin, phenols, plant sterols, lignans, inulin, and soy protein, are investigated as preventive. While dietary supplements of chemopreventive agents may appear to be the simplest way to obtain many phytochemicals, their efficacy requires investigation since in many cases, supplements do not always provide the same benefit as the food source.

NUTRITION INTERVENTION

Once colon cancer is present, the nutritional focus is altered. Surgery, chemotherapy, and radiation negatively impact nutrient intake and nutritional status. Cancer patients may

---

Textbox 12.1   Probiotics

Probiotics are helpful bacteria utilized in the treatment of a number of conditions, but most commonly for travelers and antibiotic-associated diarrhea. The intestinal tract is populated with different types of harmless bacteria. The balance of microflora can be upset by illness and antibiotic therapy. Probiotics repopulate the intestinal tract with "friendly" bacteria to restore the balance, and may generate substances, which hinder pathogenic bacterial growth and stimulate the immune system. Examples of probiotics are *Lactobacillus GG*, *L. plantarum*, *L. reuteri*, and *S. boulardii*. Pro- and prebiotics are not one and the same. Prebiotics are complex sugars, such as inulin and fructooligosaccharides, which provide nutrients for the bacteria already in the intestinal tract. Probiotics are found in yogurt, other fermented dairy products, capsules, powders, tablets, and beverages. Because probiotics are classified as a dietary supplement, they are not routinely tested for quality or content. Quality of probiotics products should be evaluated based on the viability of the bacteria, types of bacteria, and enteric protection of the product if it includes bacteria that cannot survive passage through stomach acid.

exhibit alterations in nutrient metabolism and increased production of inflammatory cytokines, which can contribute to the anorexia and malnutrition.[65] The goal of nutrition intervention is to minimize significant loss of lean body mass through management of GI symptoms and optimal nutrient intake.

Medical Nutrition Therapy

Traditionally, resumption of oral intake following GI surgery was dependent on resolution of postoperative ileus. However, research supports the safety of early resumption of an oral diet after colorectal surgery.[66,67] Despite the evidence, nutrient intake following surgery is still commonly low, especially in the first few days after surgery. Henriksen et al. investigated whether randomization to a different postoperative analgesic and enforced mobilization beginning on postoperative day 1 versus standard care would affect postoperative nutrient intake.[68] All study patients were given a clear liquid diet as soon as they were alert, a full liquid diet on day 1, and a general protein-rich diet on day 2. The intervention group consumed approximately 25% more calories and 50% more protein than the control group.[68] This study suggests that a combination of factors, including diet, pain therapy, and activity level, impacts the oral nutrient intake after colorectal surgery. It is unnecessary to wait for bowel sounds and flatus to begin oral intake, which makes it feasible to initiate early oral nutrition for prevention of postsurgical complications. The immune, inflammatory, and gut function effects of preoperative consumption of an oral nutritional supplement, containing arginine, RNA, and omega-3 fatty acids compared to a standard nutritional supplement were studied in a prospective, double-blind trial.[69] Forty colorectal or stomach cancer patients drank either the enriched or control supplement for 7 days before surgery. Compared to the standard supplement, the enriched formula significantly improved gut function parameters and positively altered the inflammatory and immune responses seen after surgery.[69] These results suggest that feeding certain nutrients to GI cancer patients before surgery is another method of improving outcomes. Enteral tube feeding (EN) and parenteral nutrition (PN), may be necessary for some colon cancer patients with significant malnutrition and prolonged inability to take in oral nutrition. Many factors, including prognosis, risk–benefit ratio, and patient desires, must be considered when determining whether to provide EN or PN to a colon cancer patient. In general, a malnourished patient receiving treatment who is unable to consume adequate nutrition via oral intake is a candidate for these modalities. EN is preferred over PN. If the GI tract cannot be used, PN should be considered. However, routine use of PN in cancer patients is not recommended and has not universally been proven beneficial.[70–72]

COMPLEMENTARY INTERVENTIONS

Many individuals with cancer use complementary and alternative medicine (CAM).[73] CAM includes the use of dietary supplements, such as herbs and vitamins. The interest in CAM has led to the establishment of the National Center for Complementary and Alternative Medicine (NCCAM) at the National Institutes of Health (NIH). One of the aims of the NCCAM is to support high-quality research in order to determine the efficacy of CAM, including its role in cancer therapy.

European mistletoe (EM), also known as *Viscum album*, has been used for many years in Europe as a sole and adjuvant therapy in cancer patients and has been shown, in preclinical studies, to have immunoenhancing and cytotoxic effects. EM in combination with gemcitabine, will be studied in an NCCAM-sponsored trial.[74] This study will examine pharmacokinetics of gemcitabine upon exposure to EM as well as safety and toxicity data in solid tumors, including colon cancer. While there is evidence to suggest EM may improve survival in colon cancer, many of the studies have not been consistent or have had methodological shortcomings.[75,76] Before EM can be recommended as a treatment for colon cancer, more rigorous research is needed. Oral EM in higher doses can cause vomiting, diarrhea, abdominal cramping, hepatitis, hypotension, seizures, coma, and death. Patients should not self-medicate with EM due to the potential for serious adverse reactions.[77]

Shark cartilage is another popular dietary supplement among cancer patients studied in advanced colorectal cancer in an NCCAM-sponsored trial. The trial's objectives include evaluating if shark cartilage, along with standard therapy, improves overall survival, impacts toxicity, or improves quality of life (QOL).[78] Shark cartilage inhibits angiogenesis, which is the prevention of new blood vessel growth necessary for tumor growth.[79] Adverse reactions include taste alterations, nausea, vomiting, constipation, hypotension, hyper- and hypoglycemia, hypercalcemia, peripheral edema, and fatigue.[77] Additional research is needed to establish the efficacy of shark cartilage before it can be recommended for colon cancer.

The use of high doses of antioxidant supplements, vitamins E and C, β-carotene, and selenium, during cancer therapy is a controversial issue. One hypothesis proposes multiple antioxidants in high doses along with radiation and chemotherapy will enhance the response to treatment and improve QOL.[80] Others argue against this practice since many chemotherapy agents and radiation destroy cancer cells through oxidation.[81–83] The American Institute for Cancer Research recommends that cancer patients take a standard multivitamin supplement during treatment, until more data are available regarding the safety and benefits of taking higher doses of antioxidants.[84]

DIVERTICULOSIS AND DIVERTICULITIS

Diverticulosis is a common, generally benign condition in Western industrialized countries.[85] Diverticulitis is less prevalent than diverticulosis and can result in a number of serious complications.

DEFINITIONS

Diverticulosis consists of a pocket or pockets of the colonic mucosa membrane herniating outward through the colonic wall's muscle layer.[85] Diverticulitis occurs when these pockets become inflamed or infected.

INCIDENCE

Diverticulosis is rarely seen in individuals less than 30 years of age; the incidence rises with age. Approximately half of all Americans aged 60 to 80 years have diverticulosis; it is present in almost all individuals older than 80 years of age. Diverticulosis develops into diverticulitis in 10 to 25% of the individuals.[86] The etiology of diverticulitis is unclear; it may begin when feces or bacteria are trapped in the diverticula.

ETIOLOGY

Over a lifetime, inadequate intake of dietary fiber is thought to result in morphologic changes in the colon, due to increased colonic pressure and prolonged GI transit time. These changes weaken the wall of the colon, allowing the pockets of diverticula to develop. Another possible cause is weakening of the colonic wall as a natural consequence of aging. It is likely a combination of diet, advancing age, colonic structure and motility, and genetic influences play a role in the development of this condition.[87] Diverticulosis is common in Westernized countries where a low-fiber diet is prevalent, such as the United States, the United Kingdom, and Australia.[86] The average American diet contains only 10–20 g of fiber per day. In the rural areas of Asia and Africa, where a high-fiber diet is consumed, diverticulosis is rare. However, as the rural population moves into urban areas and begins to consume a more Westernized diet, the incidence of diverticulosis increases.[87]

SIGNS AND SYMPTOMS

Diverticulosis usually does not cause any discomfort or symptoms. However, some individuals may experience mild cramps, abdominal distention, and constipation. Diverticulitis, most often in the sigmoid colon, presents with left-sided abdominal tenderness or pain. Individuals may also have fever, nausea and vomiting, chills, and left lower quadrant abdominal cramping. The severity of diverticulitis is dependent on the degree of the infection and presence of complications.

COMPLICATIONS OF DIVERTICULITIS

Complications of diverticulitis may include infections, abscess, perforation, peritonitis, fistula, obstruction, and hemorrhaging. Antibiotic therapy is common and surgical intervention is sometimes necessary.[86]

NUTRITIONAL PREVENTION OF DIVERTICULOSIS

Because a low-fiber diet is implicated in diverticulosis, it follows that a high-fiber (20–35 g/day) diet, especially if high in insoluble fiber, would be preventive. Both soluble and insoluble fibers are important, since their action in the colon differ. However, higher intake of insoluble fiber, particularly cellulose (the predominant insoluble fiber in fruits and vegetables), appears to reduce the risk of development of diverticulosis. Dietary fiber should be added gradually, with careful attention to adequate fluid intake, since fiber draws fluid into the intestine. Table 12.1 provides a list of good food sources of soluble or insoluble fiber.[88] Note that most foods contain some of both types of fiber. One prospective cohort study found that, besides high intake of insoluble dietary fiber, lower fat and red meat intake also lowered the risk of diverticular disease.[89] These researchers also discovered an association between increasing levels of physical activity and reduced risk of diverticulosis.[89]

TABLE 12.1
Good Food Sources of Dietary Fiber

	Grams of Fiber per Serving
Predominantly soluble fiber	
Oats	0.6–6.0
Barley	4.0
Legumes	6–13.5
Some fruits and vegetables	0.5–8.5
Predominantly insoluble fiber	
Whole grain breads, cereals, rice, pasta	1.5–13
Nuts and seeds	1.3–3
Some vegetables	0.5–8.5

Source: From Pennington, J., *Bowes and Church's Food Values of Portions Commonly Used*, 16th ed., J.B. Lippincott, Philadelphia, 1994.

Nutritional Intervention

The nutritional intervention will vary with disease severity. A study by Wunderlich and Tobias[90] suggests the hospitalized patient with diverticulosis or diverticulitis deserves careful nutritional screening. The researchers retrospectively studied which common laboratory parameters could predict the length of hospital stay in 163 patients. They found the presence of low serum albumin and hemoglobin at admission led to a more lengthy hospitalization, even in patients without GI bleeding.[90] Individuals with active diverticulitis with significant nausea and vomiting and abdominal distention, may need to remain *nil per os* initially with provision of adequate intravenous fluids. Usually, the diet can be advanced as tolerated within 3 to 4 days, although more severe cases may require 8 to 10 days to completely resolve. Those individuals who develop more serious complications such as abscess, perforation, peritonitis, obstruction, or fistulas may require EN or PN. Once the diverticulitis has resolved and a normal diet is tolerated, the individual should be counseled to follow dietary recommendations that mirror those for diverticulosis. The dietary treatment for diverticulosis is a high-fiber diet, often utilizing a fiber supplement to ensure adequate fiber intake. In the past, a restriction of foods containing small seeds was enforced due to anecdotal reports, but this is a controversial issue currently due to lack of evidence to support this practice.[86]

Complementary Therapies

Cat's claw, flaxseed, and slippery elm have been utilized as treatments for diverticulitis, but are unproven. Chlorella, methysulfonylmethane, oat bran, and wild yam are suggested as therapies for diverticulosis, but are also not proven therapies.[77] Oat bran and flaxseed are good sources of fiber and could play a role in prevention and treatment of diverticulosis.

IRRITABLE BOWEL SYNDROME

IBS is a functional disorder of the GI tract, which results in abnormal motility.[91] IBS not only can decrease an affected individual's QOL, but also carry other costs such as a significant number of lost workdays and health-care expenses.[91]

Incidence

One in five Americans, or approximately 35 million individuals, has IBS, making it one of the most common GI disorders. IBS occurs more commonly in women than men, and usually begins around the age of 20.[92] IBS is difficult to treat and a combination of therapies, utilizing diet, psychotherapy, and medications, is commonly employed.

Signs, Symptoms, and Diagnosis

IBS symptoms vary from one individual to another and can include abdominal pain, bloating, constipation, diarrhea, and mucus in the stool. The predominant symptoms of IBS are usually abdominal pain or discomfort with a change in stool frequency or consistency. Often, an individual will have one predominant symptom and minimizing the occurrence of this symptom is the focus of treatment. The diagnosis of IBS is a clinical one made by ruling out the presence of organic GI disease, such as IBD or colorectal cancer and by utilizing symptom-based criteria.[93] Several symptom-based criteria have been developed, including the Manning, Rome I, and Rome II criteria. Table 12.2 provides a description of Rome II criteria, the most recently developed of the three.[94]

TABLE 12.2
Diagnostic Criteria for Irritable Bowel Syndrome

Rome II Criteria

Twelve weeks or more, which do not need to be consecutive, in the past 12 months,
  of abdominal pain or discomfort that has two of the following three features:
- Relieved with bowel movement
- Onset associated with a change in frequency of stool
- Onset coupled with a change in appearance of stool

The following symptoms are not essential for the diagnosis, but their presence increases
  confidence in the diagnosis and may be used to identify subgroups of IBS:
- Abnormal stool frequency (>3 per day or <3 per week)
- Abnormal stool consistency (hard or loose) in 25% of bowel movements
- Abnormal stool passage (straining, urgency, or sensation of incomplete evacuation)
  in 25% of bowel movements
- Passage of mucus in 25% of bowel movements
- Bloating or abdominal distention (>25% of days)

Source: From Drossman, D.A., Rome II: a multinational consensus document on
functional gastrointestinal disorders, *Gut*, 45 (Suppl. 11), 1, 1999.

ETIOLOGY

The etiology of IBS is unknown. Individuals with IBS seem to have a more sensitive and reactive colon than usual, which can respond to different triggers such as stress and certain foods. Some areas of research on the etiology of IBS are focusing on the psychology of IBS, visceral hypersensitivity, motility abnormalities, bacterial overgrowth, and the "brain-gut axis."

TRADITIONAL MEDICAL TREATMENT

Pharmacologic therapies commonly prescribed for patients with IBS include antispasmodics, antidiarrheals, laxatives, and antidepressants. One meta-analysis evaluating the effectiveness of antispasmodic medications demonstrated a decrease in abdominal pain and overall global symptoms as compared to placebo.[95] The antispasmodics act primarily to reduce the spasms of smooth muscles in the colon or small intestine. Loperamide, an antidiarrheal agent, has been shown to be more effective than placebo in controlling diarrhea (both frequency and consistency) in IBS.[96,97] In constipation-predominant IBS, use of laxatives may be necessary. Osmotic laxatives are recommended over stimulant laxatives due to less risk of side effects such as abdominal cramping.[93] Tricyclic antidepressants seem to be efficacious in treatment of abdominal pain associated with IBS,[98] and selective serotonin reuptake inhibitors also may be beneficial.[99]

NUTRITIONAL INTERVENTION

A thorough patient interview is the foundation of nutritional intervention in IBS. It is essential to collect information about the predominant symptom (which should guide the treatment plan), food and fluid intake, eating behaviors, stool habits, exercise program, stress, and use of over-the-counter medications and herbal remedies. A food and bowel habit diary will help to reveal whether or not food is playing a role in triggering IBS. It is important to evaluate the sufficiency of dietary intake also. Gee et al. examined the adequacy of the diets of individuals with functional GI disorders, including IBS.[100] They found that affected individuals often consumed diets low in calories, iron, folate, and vitamin A, highlighting the need for careful attention to the adequacy of the diet in IBS sufferers and the possible need for vitamin or mineral supplements.

TRADITIONAL NUTRITION THERAPY

After obtaining a thorough history from the IBS patient, the clinician can develop a medical nutrition therapy (MNT) plan. The American Dietetic Association (ADA) has published an MNT protocol for IBS, which can help to guide the nutritional intervention, monitoring, and expected outcomes.[101] Table 12.3 provides a summary of diet modifications commonly recommended for IBS.[101,102] It is important to ascertain what is pertinent and potentially effective for each individual. For example, it may be unnecessary to provide counseling on lowering intake of caffeine if the individual does not consume caffeine. Also, if a food and GI symptom diary reveals caffeine intake but no relation to IBS symptoms, it may be nonproductive to provide counseling on this particular diet modification. Fiber, which is commonly recommended by physicians for treatment of IBS, has not universally been found to be beneficial in IBS. In those with constipation-predominant IBS, the use of fiber supplements appears efficacious.[93] However, in those with abdominal pain or bloating, increased intake of fiber is likely to worsen the symptoms.

COMPLEMENTARY THERAPIES

Individuals with IBS often turn to alternative therapies, such as herbal or dietary supplements and psychological treatment, due to dissatisfaction with conventional management.[103,104] Physicians recommend these therapies as well, despite the paucity of high-quality research, when the medical therapies offered fail to control symptoms. A number of dietary supplements have been employed to manage IBS. Arrowroot, an edible starch available in powder form, was studied in 11 patients with diarrhea-predominant IBS. Ten milliliters of arrowroot powder, taken three times a day for 1 month, resulted in less diarrhea, constipation, and abdominal pain when compared to a month without arrowroot.[105] A larger randomized study is needed to confirm the findings of this pilot study. Artichoke leaf extract, which possesses antiemetic, antispasmolytic, and carminative properties was found to alleviate IBS symptoms in one study and should be studied in a randomized fashion.[106] Peppermint oil has been successful, likely due to its antispasmodic effects. Two prospective, randomized placebo-controlled trials found enteric-coated peppermint oil capsules to be superior to placebo in the treatment of IBS symptoms.[107,108] Several probiotics, including *Lactobacillus plantarum*, Lacteol fort, and VSL#3, have been studied and found to lessen IBS symptoms.[109–111] Probiotics may be beneficial if an imbalance in GI microflora is part of the etiology of IBS.

Traditional Chinese medicine (TCM), with numerous Chinese herbs, was employed in a double-blind randomized trial including 116 patients. After 16 weeks, TCM, compared to placebo, resulted in global improvement, as assessed by the patient and gastroenterologist, and reduced interference with life by IBS symptoms.[112] Psychological therapies, such as hypnosis, psychotherapy, behavior therapy, and relaxation therapy have also been used to manage IBS. A meta-analysis reported a modest improvement in IBS with psychological therapies versus standard interventions.[113] A number of alternative therapies for the treatment of IBS appear promising and are reasonable options, especially in the patient whose symptoms are not relieved by conventional therapies.

TABLE 12.3
Common Diet Changes Recommended in IBS

Diet Component	Dietary Change	Further Recommendations/Comments
Fiber	Increase fiber intake to 20–35 g/day with more emphasis on increasing intake of fruits and vegetables	• Modify type of fiber (insoluble versus soluble) based on predominant symptoms and tolerance of fiber • Diarrhea — soluble fiber • Constipation — insoluble fiber • Abdominal pain/bloating — increased fiber may not be effective; and elimination of foods and behaviors reported to increase gas may be beneficial
Alcohol	Decrease intake of alcohol	• May not be necessary if alcohol does not trigger symptoms of IBS
Caffeine	Decrease intake of caffeine	• Not necessary unless elicits IBS symptoms • Educate on sources of caffeine
Fat	Decrease intake of fat	Fat may contribute to IBS by: • Stimulation of release of CCK • Malabsorption of fats • Presence of bile salts in colon • Nonabsorbable fats, such as olestra, also may contribute if consumed in large amounts
Meal size and consumption time	Decrease meal size and slow down at meals to chew foods thoroughly	• Overeating at meals can lead to abdominal distention and GI distress • Poorly chewed foods are more difficult to digest and undigested food may lead to malabsorption and GI complaints
Lactose	Minimize intake of lactose (dose of lactose may be important)	• Needed if lactose triggers IBS symptoms • Consider use of lactase supplement • Educate on identifying sources of lactose
Fructose	Decrease intake of large amounts of fructose	• May not lead to IBS symptoms when consumed in small amounts • Present in many processed foods, diet foods, soft drinks, fruits, and fruit juices
Fluid	Take in more than eight cups of fluid per day and avoid large amounts of beverages with high osmolality or sugar content	• Adequate fluid needed to replace fluids lost through diarrhea or to help combat constipation • Decreasing sugar content and osmolarity of liquids can decrease the influx of water into the colon, and reduce the incidence of liquid stools
Sorbitol	Decrease intake of sorbitol	• Sorbitol is a poorly absorbed carbohydrate, commonly added to sugar-free products, chewing gum, and liquid medications • If consumed in large enough quantities, the osmotic load of sorbitol will result in diarrhea
Other foods	Consider elimination of other potential food allergens such as eggs, chocolate, wheat, bran fiber	• Elimination of these foods should be based on recognized intolerance

Sources: From *Medical Nutrition Therapy Across the Continuum of Care*, 2nd ed., The American Dietetic Association, Chicago, 1998, section IV; Suneson, J., *Support Line*, 21, 11, 1999.

INFLAMMATORY BOWEL DISEASE

IBD is chronic and incurable, and affects people of all ages. Onset of the disease often occurs between the second and third decades of life, although first onset may occur later. The symptoms (weight loss, diarrhea, rectal bleeding, abdominal pain, and chronic fatigue) affect the QOL of sufferers, and may impact their ability to hold a job.[114] Traditional medical therapy, including corticosteroids, and surgery may be rejected by some patients, due to the serious side effects of steroids or the perception that conventional therapies do not alleviate symptoms.[114] In one study, current complementary therapy was used among 33% of IBD patients, with one-half of these using the therapy for their IBD.[115] Type of disease (i.e., Crohn's or UC), disease duration, previous hospitalizations and surgeries, and a previous course of intravenous steroids were significantly related to complementary therapy use; vitamins and herbal therapies were most commonly reported.[116] However, little controlled evidence exists for the efficacy of any herbal therapy used for IBD.[115,117–119]

CROHN'S DISEASE

Incidence

Crohn's disease often begins in the second decade of life, and may affect any part of the GI tract. Most commonly the distal ileum and colon are involved, although in approximately 15 to 25% of cases only the small intestine or the colon is affected. The disease affects men and women equally.

Risk Factors

The causes of IBD are not fully identified. Genetic predisposition, altered microflora of the gut, environmental factors, and an altered immune or autoimmune response in the intestinal wall may interact in a complex way. Genetic mutations may be involved. Emotional distress does not cause Crohn's disease. Approximately 20% of those with the disease have a blood relative with some form of irritable bowel disease.

Signs and Symptoms

Most common symptoms are abdominal pain (often in the right lower quadrant), diarrhea, and rectal bleeding, which may be severe enough to cause anemia. Weight loss and fever may also be present. Children may suffer from stunted growth and delayed development. Complications include bowel scarring and strictures, with occasional fistula formation.[120]

INTERVENTION

Medical Treatment

Treatment depends on location and severity of disease and response to any previous treatment; it is long term. The goals of therapy are to manage inflammation, correct nutritional deficits, and manage or relieve symptoms, including diarrhea, pain, and rectal bleeding. Medications such as sulfasalazine, Asacol, Pentasa, and corticosterol can aid in management of inflammation. Immune suppressants such as 6-mercaptopurine are also used, as is infliximab (Remicade), an antitumor necrosis factor substance. Medications can control but not cure the disease. Surgical intervention is very often a component of therapy for Crohn's disease, with 50 to 70% of affected people undergoing at least one operation.[121] Many patients require re-operation, sometimes within the first 1 to 3 years but often at least once more during their lifetime.

Medical Nutrition Therapy

Restoration of nutritional status, and maintenance of that status long term, are key goals. Regular foods, dietary supplements, EN, and PN may be used to achieve nutrition goals; use of the GI tract is always preferable if possible. Possible reasons for the value of enteral nutrition as an effective primary treatment for Crohn's disease include its ability to reverse malnutrition, modify gut flora, reduce gut permeability, and provide trophic nutrients.[122] Because of the effect of corticosteroids on growth rates in children, use of enteral nutrition may be preferable to the pharmacologic therapy in some cases. Chemically defined enteral products have been shown to result in remission rates of 80%.[123] However, these products are unpalatable and expensive, and patient compliance with consumption is often poor. Protein intake of at least 1–1.5 g/kg/day is recommended. A daily multivitamin should be part of the nutrition regimen; additional B and fat-soluble vitamins may be necessary in some cases. Avoiding foods, which exacerbate symptoms, has been the cornerstone of nutrition management. Spices, milk, fiber, and ethanol have been implicated in flares. However, fiber may serve to normalize the intestinal flora; wholesale elimination of fiber from the diet may not be beneficial and periodic attempts to increase fiber intake may be useful. No specific dietary management has been proven successful in all cases of Crohn's disease.

Education is an important part of therapy for Crohn's disease. Information about nutrition management is available from a wide variety of sources, including the Internet (Crohn's and Colitis Foundation at www.ccfa.org) and the media.

Complementary Therapies

The Functional Medicine Research Center advocates investigating the diet of persons with IBD for food irritants, and approaching therapy with the "4 Rs" approach: remove (pathogen microflora, allergens, and potential toxins), replace (nutritional factors lacking or in insufficient quantities), reinoculate (via prebiotic supplements or cultured or fermented foods), and repair (nutrition support of the GI mucosa with material necessary for structure and function).[124] The Natural Medicines Comprehensive Database reports only one compound, *Saccharomyces boulardi*, to be possibly effective in the management of Crohn's disease.[125] Taken orally, this preparation is said to reduce the frequency of stools. Insufficient reliable evidence was available to rate fluoride added to the diet, which appears to increase bone mass in patients with the disease who have lost mass, and chitosan taken orally in combination with ascorbic acid, which may increase excretion of fecal fat and relieve symptoms.[125] Several herbs have anti-inflammatory properties and are labeled "herbal COX-II inhibitors" due to their ability to inhibit the inflammatory cascade of eicosanoids.[124] The following herbs may be used in managing Crohn's disease: 1–2 g/day powdered ginger extract in divided doses (inhibits prostaglandin synthesis; 1200 mg/day of turmeric, in three divided doses manages inflammation, stimulates the immune system, and has antimicrobial and antiviral actions); commonly recommended in Ayurvedic medicine; 30–50 g linseeds, crushed and soaked for 30 min, then mixed in a ratio of 10 parts seeds and 1 part water, soothe the inflamed mucosa due to the seed's mucilaginous qualities and may promote healing.[124] Of note, very little controlled evidence exists for the efficacy of herbal remedies in treatment of IBD.[126–128]

ULCERATIVE COLITIS

Incidence

UC occurs most commonly in people between the ages of 15 and 30, or 50 to 60 years, but a person of any age may develop the disease. Between 15,000 and 30,000 new cases of IBD annually have been reported in the United States.

Risk Factors

The risk factors for UC are similar to Crohn's disease, described earlier.

Signs and Symptoms

Anorexia, nausea, abdominal pain, vomiting, and bloody diarrhea with mucous and purulence commonly occur.[129] The large intestinal mucosa is inflamed, but the inflammation is superficial, rather than transmural as in Crohn's disease. Weight loss is less common in UC than in Crohn's. Complications include colonic perforation, severe bleeding, and toxic megacolon.

INTERVENTION

Medical Treatment

Pharmacologic management of UC, as with Crohn's, involves direct suppression or modification of the host immune or immunoinflammatory response.[130] Corticosteroids are most effective in managing the disease in its acute stages. Other commonly used medications include aminosalicylates such as sulfasalazine and mesalazine, immunosuppressants such as mercaptopurine and cyclosporine A, antibiotics such as metronidazole, bile acid sequestrants such as cholestyramine, and antidiarrheals such as loperamide.[130] Persons with UC of long duration are at increased risk for cancer. In this case, or when disease is severe, complete surgical colectomy may be indicated.

Medical Nutrition Therapy

Unlike Crohn's disease, nutrition therapy does not play a primary role in the management of UC. Neither PN nor EN have been shown to be effective in treating UC.[131] Since UC has been postulated to be a manifestation of enterocyte fuel deficiency,[132] feeding the colon would appear to be the optimal therapy during treatment of the disease. The SCFA acetate, propionate, and butyrate, produced by fermentation of dietary fiber and resistant starch unabsorbed by the GI tract, are the preferred fuel for the human colonyte.[130] SCFA enhance sodium and water absorption and thus counteract diarrhea. Human and animal studies of SCFA have shown a trophic effect on the colonic mucosa, increased bursting pressure of colonic anastomoses, and prevention or improvement of inflammatory changes in the large bowel.[130] Preliminary trials with butyrate enemas have demonstrated effectiveness comparable with corticosteroids and mesalamine enemas in reducing flares of UC.[124] Pectin, which is fermented to SCFA, has been added to enteral tube feeding, but the resultant product has a high viscosity, which complicates infusion. No commercially available feeding formulations, enteral or parenteral, currently contain SCFA.[130]

Complementary Therapies

The Natural Medicines Comprehensive Database reports that Bifidobacteria combined with *Lactobacillus* and *Streptococcus thermophilus* may possibly be effective in preventing an increase in the pathogenic bacteria that may contribute to relapse in some patients.[125] Blond psyllium seeds, 10 g taken orally twice daily, has been shown to be as effective as mesalamine three times daily in preventing relapse, and may also relieve GI symptoms in adult patients.[125] For other compounds, insufficient reliable evidence exists to rate, but there is a suggestion of benefit: folic acid may protect against development of cancer in some patients with UC, bromelain may relieve symptoms in some patients whose symptoms do not respond to conventional pharmacotherapy, Indian Frankincense taken orally may reduce symptoms and wheatgrass taken orally may help manage symptoms of active distal UC.[125] Studies in the Chinese literature reference a variety of herbal therapies for management of UC, but only the abstracts are available in English.[119] The herbal therapies, which included Jiam Pi Ling tablets and RSF-FS concoction enemas, Kui jie qing enemas, and Yuki tang orally with herbal decoction enemas, resulted in marked improvement, compared with controls.[11] However, some of these studies suffered from lack of blinding and randomization. In an Indian study, the effect of the gum resin from *Boswellia serrata* was compared to sulfasalazine; remission rates were 82 and 75%, respectively.[133] Herbal remedies used to manage UC symptoms include those classified as anti-inflammatory (ginger, turmeric, as well as Boswellia), demulcents (linseed, marshmallow root), calmatives (peppermint, chamomile), and "others."[124] Aloe vera is one of the most common herbs used by patients with UC as well as Crohn's, to clear constipation and soothe the inflamed gut.[124] Modified Robert's Formula, a blend of herbs including Echinacea, golden seal, and slippery elm, has no research to document its efficacy or actions, but is frequently recommended by naturopathic physicians for UC.[124] Wagner recommends a "natural supplementation protocol" for many intestinal problems.[134] His individually referenced recommendations include:

- More fiber (preferably psyllium husk)
- Identification of food allergies or sensitivities through elimination diets
- Acidophilus and fructooligosaccharides to aid in integrity of microflora
- Digestive pancreatic enzymes such as bromelain or papain before meals
- Carminative herbs (chamomile, peppermint, fennel, ginger) for antispasmodic effects
- Sedative or nervine tonic herbs such as valerian and St. John's wort for stress relief
- Betaine HCL, a plant-based source of hydrochloric acid, which may improve protein digestion and reduce food sensitivities
- Aloe vera juice, to coat mucous membranes and help manage constipation
- Peppermint oil as an antispasmodic
- Curcuma longa, gingko bilboa, and Cat's claw as anti-inflammatory agents

CELIAC DISEASE

INCIDENCE

Celiac disease, also known as gluten-sensitive enteropathy or celiac sprue, is an autoimmune disease. Individuals with celiac disease have an inappropriate T-cell-mediated immune response to gluten, which results in mucosal damage to the small intestine. Prevalence is variably estimated at 1 of 133, 1 of 250, and 1 of 4700 persons in the United States, with a higher incidence in those with relatives who have the disease.[135,136] Celiac disease may be under-diagnosed in the United States, for several reasons[136]:

- Celiac symptoms can be attributed to other disorders
- Many physicians are not knowledgeable about the disease
- Few U.S. laboratories are experienced and skilled in testing for celiac disease

Twenty percent of cases occur in adults over 60 years of age, but the majority of cases are diagnosed during the period from infancy to young adulthood.[137]

ETIOLOGY

Ingestion of gluten by sensitive individuals initiates the disease.[138] Gluten, the protein in flour and grains such as wheat, barley, rye, and possibly oats, contains four peptides: gliadins, glutenins, albumins, and globulins.[139] The prolamin fraction of wheat gluten, gliadin, contains the amino acid peptide sequence that results in an immune response. The offending prolamin fraction in rye is secalin, and in barley, hordein.[140] Intestinal villi become flattened and inflamed, and malabsorption results.[138]

Signs and Symptoms

Noncompliance with dietary restrictions results in diarrhea, abdominal cramps, malabsorption, failure to thrive, and an increased risk of lymphoma.[141] Even with attentive dietary therapy, the precipitating condition continues to exist, and any dietary gluten will cause mucosal changes, which may flare immediately or remain latent for 8 weeks or longer.[135] Continued "yo yo" compliance and noncompliance with the diet may eventually cause chronic ulcerative jejunoileitis and extraintestinal manifestations, with increased risk of malignant disease.[135] Early diagnosis and strict dietary compliance may decrease the risk of intestinal malignancies as well as markedly improve symptoms.[142] Secondary nutrition concerns include anemia, osteopenia, osteoporosis, and vitamin K-related coagulopathy. Dermatitis herpeteformis (a form of celiac disease that also involves the skin), muscle and joint pain, thyroiditis, type 1 diabetes, hepatic steatosis, infertility, systemic lupus erythematus, rheumatoid arthritis, and psychiatric syndromes may be seen in patients with celiac disease.[135]

Intervention

Medical Treatment

Elimination of gluten from the diet is the cornerstone of therapy. Electrolyte and fluid replacement may be needed, and vitamin and mineral supplementation (including calcium and vitamin D) are required.[135] Truly refractory cases of celiac disease may require therapy with immunosuppressive or anti-inflammatory agents such as azathioprine, cyclosporine, and corticosteroids.[139] Shan et al.,[143] in 2002, identified a 33-amino acid peptide fraction from gliadin that triggers the inflammatory response. This fragment appears to be the same in other grains that contain gluten. Preliminary studies have shown that the destruction of the peptide fragment by bacterial endopeptidase prevented the typical immunological response seen in celiac disease. There is hope that oral endopeptidase enzymes could be used by sensitive individuals, allowing consumption of gluten-containing foods without symptoms.[135]

Medical Nutrition Therapy

The complete details of the dietary treatment of celiac disease are published elsewhere.[135,144] Traditionally, wheat (including spelt, triticale, and kamut), rye, barley, and oats are eliminated. Lifelong adherence to a gluten-free diet, meaning total elimination of gluten from all foods and medications, is essential for treatment. Foods, which contain these peptide sequences are ubiquitous, so dietary compliance impacts QOL as well as food consumption habits of affected individuals.[138] Hidden sources of gluten include additives, preservatives, and stabilizers that are found in processed food, medications, and even mouthwash. Some researchers counsel avoidance of grains such as quinoa, amaranth, wild rice, oats, and millet[145–147] while Kasarda[148] considers these acceptable. The need to eliminate oats from the diet has been challenged.[149] While wheat starch in other countries may be sufficiently low in gluten to be acceptable, celiac organizations in North America do not recommend consumption of wheat starch products, or of oats.[135] Care must be taken to assure that acceptable grains (corn, potato, rice, soybean, tapioca, buckwheat, and according to some, quinoa, amaranth, wild rice, and millet) and products made from them are not contaminated with gluten during processing.

At diagnosis, many individuals are malnourished and will require vitamins, minerals, additional protein, and fluid and electrolytes if diarrhea has been severe. Appropriate treatment of anemia with folic acid, vitamin B_{12}, or iron; administration of calcium and vitamin D to manage bone disorders; and supplementation with vitamins A, E, and K depleted by steatorrhea may be needed.[135] Once dietary management is initiated, individuals should continue to take a daily multivitamin, which contains at least 100% of the daily reference intakes (DRI). Medium Chain triglycerides (MCT) oil adds easily absorbed energy to the diet, although its palatability may be a problem. A low-lactose or low-fructose diet may help in controlling initial symptoms, although consistent use of such a diet may not be needed.[135] Additional information is available at www.niddk.nih.gov/health/digest/pubs/celiac, www.gluten.net, and www.glutenfree.com.

Complementary Therapies

Rakel[150] does not refer to celiac disease in his textbook *Integrative Medicine*. The Natural Medicines Comprehensive Database reports no compounds with an effectiveness rating.[125] Carob, lipase, pantothenic acid, and spleen extract are reportedly used by some patients with the disease; no information on results is available.[125]

CASE STUDY

SW is a 38-year-old female nurse who presents to her family practitioner once again with long-term complaints of bloating, diarrhea, inability to maintain weight, and foul-smelling stools. She is 5'5" tall and weighs 115 lb; her highest weight has been 125 lb. Family history is remarkable for one sister and her mother with similar symptoms; her father and two other siblings did not exhibit these symptoms. Social history is remarkable for the recent death of her father, after a long illness including a prolonged intensive care unit stay. She recently completed a dual master's degree in health-care administration and business administration and changed her job. She admits that her diet could use some improvement but states that she tries to eat in a healthful way. The physician has referred her to the registered dietitian for evaluation.

1. What additional information about this patient's diet and eating patterns would be useful?
2. What complementary therapies may prove helpful in management of her condition?

GLOSSARY

Apoptosis: Programmed cell death as signaled by the cell nuclei in normally functioning human and animal cells when the age or condition of the cell dictates. This normal process is absent in cancer cells.

Chemoprevention: The use of natural or laboratory-made substances to prevent cancer.

Cytokines: Nonantibody proteins secreted by inflammatory leukocytes and some nonleukocyte cells that act as intercellular mediators.

Gluten: A protein found in flour and grains such as wheat and barley, which contains a prolamin fraction that provokes an immune response in individuals with celiac disease.

Inflammatory bowel disease: A chronic disease involving the interaction of host microflora, genetic predisposition, environmental factors, and an abnormal immune or autoimmune reaction in the intestinal wall, manifested as Crohn's disease or UC.

Phytochemicals: Plant chemicals that are thought to provide health benefits such as prevention of cancer and heart disease.

Short-chain fatty acids: Fatty acids with 4 to 6 carbons. Butyrate, acetate, and propionate are readily absorbed by the human colon and comprise 85% of the short-chain fatty acids produced in the human colon.

REFERENCES

1. Giese, L., A study of alternative health care for gastrointestinal disorders, *Gastroenterol. Nurs.*, 23, 19, 2000.
2. Sutherlan, L., Alternative medicine: what are our patients telling us? *Am. J. Gastroenterol.*, 83, 1154, 1988.
3. Passant, H., A holistic approach to the ward, *Nursing Times*, 86, 26, 1990.
4. McGinnis, L., Alternative therapies, *Cancer*, 67, 1788, 1991.
5. Eisenburg, D., Advising patients who seek alternative medical therapies, *Ann. Intern. Med.*, 127, 61, 1997.
6. Jemal, A. et al., Cancer Statistics 2004, *CA Cancer J. Clin.*, 54, 8, 2004.
7. www.cancer.gov, Cancer Facts and Figures 2003, accessed 1/23/04.
8. Smith, R.A., Cokkinides, V., and Eyre, H.J., American Cancer Society Guidelines for the Early Detection of Cancer, 2004, *CA Cancer J. Clin.*, 54, 41, 2004.
9. Giovannucci, E., Modifiable risk factors for colon cancer, *Gastroenterol. Clin. North Am.*, 31, 925, 2002.
10. Chan, A.T. et al., A prospective study of aspirin use and the risk of colorectal adenoma, *Ann. Intern. Med.*, 140, 157, 2004.
11. Lieberman, D.A. et al., Risk factors for advanced colonic neoplasia and hyperplastic polyps in asymptomatic individuals, *JAMA*, 290, 2959, 2003.
12. Giovannucci, E., Nutrition, insulin, insulin-like growth factors and cancer, *Horm. Meta. Res.*, 35, 694, 2003.
13. Platz, E.A. et al., Proportion of colon cancer risk that might be preventable in a cohort of middle-aged US men, *Cancer Causes Control*, 11, 579, 2000.
14. Willet, W. et al., Relation of meat, fat, and fiber intake to the risk of colon cancer in a prospective study among women, *N. Engl. J. Med.*, 323, 1664, 1990.
15. Giovannuci, E. et al., Intake of fat, meat, and fiber in relation to the risk of colon cancer in men, *Cancer Res.*, 54, 2390, 1994.
16. Goldbohm, R., van den Brandt, P., and van't Veer, P., A prospective cohort study on the relation between meat consumption and the risk of colon cancer, *Cancer Res.*, 54, 718, 1004.
17. Howe, G. et al., The relationship between dietary fat intake and the risk of colorectal cancer: evidence from the combined analysis of 13 case–control studies, *Cancer Causes Control*, 8, 215, 1997.
18. Stoneham, M. et al., Olive oil, diet, and colorectal cancer: an ecological study and a hypothesis, *J. Epidemiol. Community Health*, 54, 756, 2000.
19. Caygill, C. and Hill, M., Fish, $n-3$ fatty acids and human colorectal health and breast cancer mortality, *Eur. J. Cancer Prevent.*, 4, 329, 1995.
20. Yang, C. et al., Fish consumption and colorectal cancer: a case-reference study in Japan, *Eur. J. Cancer Prevent.*, 12, 109, 2003.
21. Levi, F. et al., Macronutrients and colorectal cancer: a Swiss case–control study, *Ann. Oncol.*, 13, 369, 2002.
22. Boutron-Ruault, M. et al., Energy intake, body mass index, physical activity, and colorectal adenoma–carcinoma sequence, *Nutr. Cancer*, 39, 50, 2001.
23. Ford, E., Body mass index and colon cancer in a national sample of adult US men and women, *Am. J. Epidemiol.*, 150, 309, 1999.
24. Martinez, M. et al., Physical activity, obesity, and risk for colon cancer in women, *Am. J. Epidemiol.*, 143, S73a, 1996.

25. Giovannucci, E. et al., Physical activity, obesity, and risk for colon cancer and adenoma in men, *Ann. Intern. Med.*, 122, 327, 1995.
26. Giovannucci, E., Insulin, insulin-like growth factors and colon cancer: a review of the evidence, *J. Nutr.*, 131, 3109S, 2001.
27. Ma, J. et al., Prospective study of colorectal cancer risk in men and plasma levels of insulin-like growth factor-1 and IGF-binding protein 3, *J. Natl. Cancer Inst.*, 91, 620, 1999.
28. Wei, E. et al., Comparison of risk factors for colon and rectal cancer, *Int. J. Cancer*, 108, 433, 2004.
29. Su, J. and Arab, L., Nutritional status of folate and colon cancer risk: evidence from NHANES I Epidemiologic Follow-up Study, *Ann. Epidemiol.*, 11, 65, 2001.
30. Mason, J., Nutritional chemoprevention of colon cancer, *Sem. Gastroenterol.*, 13, 143, 2002.
31. Willet, W., Diet and cancer, *Oncologist*, 5, 393, 2002.
32. Gaard, M., Tretli, S., and Loken, E., Dietary factors and risk of colon cancer: a prospective study of 50,535 Norwegian men and women, *Eur. J. Cancer Prevent.*, 5, 445, 1996.
33. Terry, P. et al., Fruits, vegetables, dietary fiber, and risk of colorectal cancer, *J. Natl. Cancer Inst.*, 93, 525, 2001.
34. Fuchs, S. et al., Dietary fiber and the risk of colorectal cancer and adenoma in women, *N. Engl. J. Med.*, 340, 169, 1999.
35. McKeown-Eyssen, G. et al., A randomized trial of a low fat, high fiber diet in the recurrence of colorectal polyps, *J. Clin. Epidemiol.*, 47, 525, 1994.
36. Schatzkin, A. et al., Lack of effect of a low-fat, high-fiber diet on the recurrence of colorectal polyps, *N. Engl. J. Med.*, 342, 1149, 2000.
37. Alberts, D. et al., Lack of effect of a high-fiber cereal supplement on the recurrence of colorectal adenoma, *N. Engl. J. Med.*, 342, 1156, 2000.
38. Bonithon-Kopp, C. et al., Calcium and fibre supplementation in prevention of colorectal adenoma recurrence: a randomized intervention trial, *Lancet*, 356, 1300, 2000.
39. MacLenna, R. et al., Randomized trial of intake of fat, fiber, and β-carotene to prevent colorectal adenomas, *J. Natl. Cancer Inst.*, 87, 1760, 1995.
40. Voorips, L. et al., Vegetable and fruit consumption and risks of colon and rectal cancer in a prospective, cohort study, *Am. J. Epidemiol.*, 152, 1081, 2000.
41. Michels, K. et al., Prospective study of fruit and vegetable consumption and incidence of colon and rectal cancers, *J. Natl. Cancer Inst.*, 92, 1740, 2000.
42. Steinmetz, K. et al., Vegetables, fruit, and colon cancer in the Iowa Women's Health Study, *Am. J. Epidemiol.*, 139, 1, 1999.
43. Lamprecht, S. and Lipkin, M., Chemoprevention of colon cancer by calcium, vitamin D and folate: molecular mechanisms, *Nat. Rev.*, 3, 601, 2003.
44. Wu, K. et al., Calcium intake and risk of colon cancer in women and men, *J. Natl. Cancer Inst.*, 94, 437, 2002.
45. Baron, J. et al., Calcium supplements for the prevention of colorectal adenomas, *N. Engl. J. Med.*, 340, 101, 1999.
46. Clark, L. et al., Effects of selenium supplementation for cancer prevention in patients with carcinoma of the skin, *J. Am. Med. Assoc.*, 276, 1957, 1996.
47. Ghadirian, P. et al., A case–control study of toenail selenium and cancer of the breast, colon, and prostate, *Cancer Detect. Prevent.*, 24, 305, 2000.
48. Jacobs, E. et al., Vitamin C and vitamin E supplement use and colorectal cancer mortality in a large American Cancer Society cohort, *Cancer Epidemiol. Biol. Prevent.*, 10, 17, 2001.
49. Wu, K. et al., A prospective study on supplemental vitamin E intake and risk of colon cancer in women and men, *Cancer Epidemiol. Biol. Prevent.*, 11, 1298, 2002.
50. Slattery, M. et al., Carotenoids and cancer, *Am. J. Clin. Nutr.*, 71, 575, 2000.
51. Steinemtz, K. et al., Vegetables, fruit, and colon cancer in the Iowa Women's Health Study, *Am. J. Epidemiol.*, 139, 1, 1994.
52. Witte, J. et al., Relation of vegetable, fruit, and grain consumption to colorectal adenomatous polyps, *Am. J. Epidemiol.*, 144, 1015, 1996.

53. LeMarchand, L. et al., Dietary fiber and colorectal cancer risk, *Epidemiology*, 8, 658, 1997.
54. Fleischauer, A., Poole, C., and Arab, L., Garlic consumption and cancer prevention: meta-analyses of colorectal and stomach cancers, *Am. J. Clin. Nutr.*, 72, 1047, 2000.
55. Dortant, E., van den Brandt, P., and Goldbohm, R., A prospective cohort study on the relationship between onion and leek consumption, garlic supplement use and risk of colorectal carcinoma in the Netherlands, *Carcinogenesis*, 17, 477, 1996.
56. Lamm, D. and Riggs, D., The potential application of *Allium sativum* (garlic) for the treatment of bladder cancer, *Urol. Clin. North Am.*, 27, 157, 2000.
57. Ali, M., Thomson, M., and Afzal, M., Garlic and onions: their effect on eicosanoid metabolism and its clinical relevance, *Prostaglandins Leukot. Essent. Fatty Acids*, 62, 55, 2000.
58. Wollowski, I., Rechkemmer, G., and Pool-Zobel, B., Protective roles of probiotics and prebiotics in colon cancer, *Am. J. Clin. Nutr.*, 73 (Suppl.), 451S, 2001.
59. Rowland, I. et al., Effect of *Bifidobacterium longum* and inulin on gut bacterial metabolism and carcinogen-induced aberrant crypt foci in rats, *Carcinogenesis*, 19, 281, 1998.
60. Challa, A. et al., *Bifidobacterium longum* and lactulose suppress azoxymethane-induced colonic aberrant crypt foci in rats, *Carcinogenesis*, 18, 517, 1997.
61. Kampman, E. et al., Fermented dairy products, calcium and colorectal cancer in the Netherlands cohort study, *Cancer Res.*, 54, 3186, 1994.
62. Kearney, J. et al., Calcium vitamin D, and dairy foods and the occurrence of colon cancer in men, *Am. J. Epidemiol.*, 143, 907, 1996.
63. Young, T. and Wolf, D., Case–control study of proximal and distal colon cancer and diet in Wisconsin, *Int. J. Cancer*, 42, 167, 1988.
64. Peters, R. et al., Diet and colon cancer in Los Angeles County, California, *Cancer Causes Control*, 3, 457, 1992.
65. McNamara, M., Alexander, H., and Norton, J., Cytokines and their role in the pathophysiology of cancer cachexia, *J. Parenter. Enteral. Nutr.*, 16 (Suppl. 6), 50S, 1992.
66. Bufo, A. et al., Early postoperative feeding, *Dis. Colon. Rectum*, 37, 1260, 1994.
67. Reissman, P. et al., Is early oral feeding safe after colorectal surgery? A prospective randomized trial, *Ann. Surg.*, 222, 73, 1995.
68. Henriksen, M., Hansen, H., and Hessov, I., Early oral nutrition after elective colorectal surgery: influence of balanced analgesia and enforced mobilization, *Nutrition*, 18, 263, 2002.
69. Braga, M. et al., Gut function and immune and inflammatory responses in patients perioperatively fed with supplemented enteral formulas, *Arch. Surg.*, 131, 1257, 1996.
70. Fasth, S. et al., Postoperative complications in colorectal surgery in relation to preoperative clinical and nutritional state and postoperative nutritional treatment, *Int. J. Colorec. Dis.*, 2, 87, 1987.
71. Vitello, J., Nutritional assessment and the role of preoperative parenteral nutrition in the colon cancer patient, *Sem. Surg. Oncol.*, 10, 183, 1994.
72. Dixon, D. et al., Total parenteral nutrition as an adjunct to chemotherapy of metastatic colorectal cancer, *Cancer Treat. Rep.*, 65 (Suppl. 5), 121, 1981.
73. Richardon, M., Biopharmacologic and herbal therapies for cancer: research update from NCCAM, *J. Nutr.*, 131, 3037S, 2001.
74. Mansky, P. et al., Mistletoe and gemcitabine in patients with advanced cancer: a model for the phase I study of botanicals and botanical–drug interactions in cancer therapy, *Integ. Cancer Ther.*, 2, 345, 2003.
75. Kienle, G., Mistletoe in cancer — a systematic review of controlled clinical trials, *Eur. J. Med. Res.*, 8, 109, 2003.
76. Ernst, E., Schmidt, K., and Steuer-Vogt, M., Mistletoe for cancer? A systematic review of randomised clinical trials, *Int. J. Cancer*, 107, 262, 2003.
77. www.naturaldatabase.com, Natural Medicines Comprehensive Database, accessed 3/5/04.
78. http://nccam.nih.gov, National Center for Complementary and Alternative Medicine, accessed 3/5/04.
79. Gingras, D., Neovastat — a novel antiangiogenic drug for cancer therapy, *Anticancer Drugs*, 14, 91, 2003.

80. Prasad, K. et al., High doses of multiple antioxidant vitamins: essential ingredients in improving the efficacy of standard cancer therapy, *J. Am. Coll. Nutr.*, 18, 13, 1999.

81. Labriola, D. and Livingston, R., Possible interactions between dietary antioxidants and chemotherapy, *Oncology*, 13, 1003, 1999.

82. Salganik, R.I. et al., Dietary antioxidant depletion: enhancement of tumor apoptosis and inhibition of brain tumor growth in transgenic mice, *Carcinogenesis*, 21, 909, 2000.

83. Kong, Q. and Lillehei, K.O., Antioxidant inhibitors for cancer therapy, *Med. Hypotheses*, 51, 405, 1998.

84. Norman, H.A. et al., The role of dietary supplements during cancer therapy, *J. Nutr.*, 133, 3794S, 2003.

85. Eastwood, M., Colonic diverticula, *Proc. Nutr. Soc.*, 62, 31, 2003.

86. http://www.niddk.nih.gov, The National Digestive Diseases Information Clearinghouse of The National Institutes of Health, accessed 2/3/04.

87. Simpson, J., Scholefield, J.H., and Spiller R.C., Pathogenesis of colonic diverticula, *Br. J. Surg.*, 89, 546, 2002.

88. Pennington, J., *Bowes and Church's Food Values of Portions Commonly Used*, 16th ed., J.B. Lippincott, Philadelphia, 1994.

89. Aldoori, W.H., The protective role of dietary fiber in diverticular disease, in *Dietary Fiber in Health and Disease*, Kritchevsky, D. and Bonfield, C., Eds., Plenum Press, New York, 1997, chap. 29.

90. Wunderlich, S.M. and Tobias, A., Relationship between nutritional status indicators and length of hospital stay for patients with diverticular disease, *J. Am. Diet. Assoc.*, 92, 429, 1992.

91. Villanueva, A., Dominguez-Muñoz, J.E., and Mearin, F., Update in the therapeutic management of irritable bowel syndrome, *Dig. Dis.*, 19, 244, 2001.

92. http://www.webmd.com, WebMD Health website, accessed 1/23/04.

93. Somers, S.C. and Lembo, A., Irritable bowel syndrome: evaluation and treatment, *Gastroenterol. Clin. North Am.*, 32, 507, 2003.

94. Drossman, D.A., Rome II: a multinational consensus document on functional gastrointestinal disorders, *Gut*, 45 (Suppl. 11), 1, 1999.

95. Poynard, T., Naveau, S., Mory, B., and Chaput, J.C., Meta-analysis of smooth muscle relaxant in the treatment of irritable bowel syndrome, *Aliment. Pharmacol. Ther.*, 8, 499, 1994.

96. Cann, P. et al., Role of loperamide and placebo in management of irritable bowel syndrome, *Dig. Dis. Sci.*, 29, 239, 1984.

97. Efskind, P., Bernkley, T., and Vatn, M., A double-blind, placebo-controlled trial with loperamide in irritable bowel syndrome, *Scan. J. Gastroenterol.*, 31, 463, 1996.

98. Jackson, J. et al., Treatment of functional gastrointestinal disorders with antidepressant medications: a meta-analysis, *Am. J. Med.*, 108, 65, 2000.

99. Clouse, R. et al., Antidepressant therapy in 138 patients with irritable bowel syndrome: a five-year clinical experience, *Aliment. Pharmacol. Ther.*, 8, 409, 1994.

100. Gee, M. et al., Nutritional status of gastroenterology outpatients: comparison of inflammatory bowel disease with functional disorders, *J. Am. Diet. Assoc.*, 85, 1591, 1985.

101. *Medical Nutrition Therapy Across the Continuum of Care*, 2nd ed., The American Dietetic Association, Chicago, 1998, section IV.

102. Suneson, J., Irritable bowel syndrome: a practical approach to medical nutrition therapy, *Support Line*, 21, 11, 1999.

103. Smart, H., Mayberry, J., and Atkinson, M., Alternative medicine consultations and remedies in patients with irritable bowel syndrome, *Gut*, 27, 286, 1986.

104. Koloski, N. et al., Predictors of conventional and alternative health care seeking for irritable bowel syndrome and functional dyspepsia. *Aliment. Pharmacol. Ther.*, 17, 841, 2003.

105. Cooke, C. et al., Arrowroot as a treatment for diarrhoea in irritable bowel syndrome patients: a pilot study, *Arq. Gastroenterol.*, 37, 20, 2000.

106. Walker, A., Middleton, R., and Petrowicz, O., Artichoke leaf extract reduces symptoms of irritable bowel syndrome in a post-marketing surveillance study, *Phytother. Res.*, 15, 58, 2001.

107. Liu, J. et al., Enteric-coated peppermint oil capsules in the treatment of irritable bowel syndrome: a prospective, randomized, trial, *J. Gastroenterol.*, 32, 765, 1997.

108. Kline, R. et al., Enteric-coated, pH-dependent peppermint oil capsules for the treatment of irritable bowel syndrome in children, *J. Pediatr.*, 138, 125, 2001.

109. Nobaek, S. et al., Alteration of intestinal microflora is associated with reduction in abdominal bloating and pain in patients with irritable bowel syndrome, *Aliment. Pharmacol. Ther.*, 17, 895, 2003.

110. Kim, H. et al., A randomized controlled trial of a prebiotic, VSL#3, on gut transit and symptoms in diarrhea-predominant irritable bowel syndrome, *Aliment. Pharmacol. Ther.*, 17, 895, 2003.

111. Halpern, G. et al., Treatment of irritable bowel syndrome with Lacteol fort: a randomized, double-blind, cross-over trial, *Am. J. Gastroenterol.*, 91, 1579, 1996.

112. Bensoussan, A., Treatment of irritable bowel syndrome with Chinese herbal medicine, *JAMA*, 280, 1585, 1998.

113. Spaneir, J., Howden, C., and Jones, M., A systematic review of alternative therapies in the irritable bowel syndrome, *Arch. Intern. Med.*, 163, 265, 2003.

114. Scott, C., Verhoef, M., and Hilsden, R., Inflammatory bowel disease patients' decision to use complementary therapies: links to existing models of care, *Comp. Ther. Med.*, 11, 22, 2003.

115. Hilsden, R., Scott, C., and Verhoef, M., Complementary medicine use by patients with inflammatory bowel disease, *Am. J. Gastroenterol.*, 93, 697, 1998.

116. Verhoef, M., Scott, C., and Hilsden, R., A multimethod research study on the complementary therapies among patients with inflammatory bowel disease, *Altern. Ther.*, 4, 68, 1998.

117. Rawsthorne, P. et al., An international survey on the use and attitudes regarding alternative medicine by patients with inflammatory bowel disease, *Am. J. Gastroenterol.*, 94, 1298, 1999.

118. Moody, G., et al., The role of complementary medicine in European and Asian patients with inflammatory bowel disease, *Public Health*, 112, 269, 1998.

119. Langmead, L., Chitnis, M., and Rampton, D., Complementary therapies in GI patients: who uses them and why? *Gut*, 46 (Suppl. II), A22, 2000.

120. Sitrin, M., Nutrition support in inflammatory bowel disease, *Nutr. Clin. Pract.*, 7, 53, 1992.

121. Patel, H. et al., Surgery for Crohn's disease in infants and children, *J. Pediatr. Surg.*, 32, 1063, 1997.

122. Griffiths, A. et al., Meta-analysis of enteral nutrition as the primary treatment of active Crohn's disease, *Gastroenterology*, 108, 1056, 1995.

123. Teahon, K. et al., Practical aspects of enteral nutrition in the management of Crohn's disease, *J. Parenter. Enteral. Nutr.*, 19, 365, 1995.

124. Lutz, R., Inflammatory bowel disease, in *Integrative Medicine*, Rakel, D., Ed., W.B. Saunders, Philadelphia, 2002, chap. 39.

125. www.naturaldatabase.com, accessed 3/7/04.

126. Langmead, J. and Rampton, D., Review article: herbal treatment in gastrointestinal and liver disease-benefits and dangers, *Aliment. Pharmacol. Ther.*, 15, 1239, 2001.

127. Rawsthorne, P. et al., An international survey of the use and attitudes regarding alternative medicine by patients with inflammatory bowel disease, *Am. J. Gastroenterol.*, 94, 1298, 1999.

128. Moody, G. et al., The role of complementary medicine in European and Asian patients with inflammatory bowel disease, *Public Health*, 112, 269, 1998.

129. Dudrick, S., Latifi, R., and Schrager, R., Nutritional management of inflammatory bowel disease, *Surg. Clin. North Am.*, 71, 609, 1991.

130. Wall-Alanso, E., Sullivan, M., and Byrne, T., Gastrointestinal and pancreatic disease, in *Contemporary Nutrition Support Practice, A Clinical Guide*, Matererese, L. and Gottscjlich, M., Eds., W.B. Saunders, Philadelphia, 2003, chap. 31.

131. Hanauer, S., Medical therapy of ulcerative colitis, *Lancet*, 342, 412, 1993.

132. Sagar, P. and Macfie, J., Pouchitis, colitis, and deficiencies of fuel, *Clin. Nutr.*, 14, 13, 1995.

133. Gupta, I. et al., Effects of Boswellia serrate gum resin in patients with ulcerative colitis, *Eur. J. Med.*, 2, 37, 1997.

134. Wagner, D., Complementary healthcare practices: thoughts on complementary approaches to intestinal disease, *Gastroenterol. Nurs.*, 26, 41, 2003.

135. Beyer, P., Medical nutrition therapy for lower gastrointestinal tract disorders, in *Krauses' Food, Nutrition, and Diet Therapy*, 11th ed., Mahan, K. and Escott-Stump, S., Eds., W.B. Saunders, Philadelphia, 2004, chap. 30.

136. Celiac disease, National Digestive Diseases Information Clearinghouse, http://digestive.niddk.nih.gov/ddiseases/pubs/celaic/index.htm, accessed 1/28/2004.

137. Farrell, R. and Kelly, C., Celiac sprue, *N. Engl. J. Med.*, 346, 180, 2002.

138. Lee, A. and Newman, J., Celiac diet: its impact on quality of life, *J. Am. Diet. Assoc.*, 103, 1533, 2003.

139. Trier, J., Diagnosis of celiac sprue, *Gastroenterology*, 115, 211, 1998.

140. Thompson, T., Wheat starch, gliadin, and the gluten-free diet, *J. Am. Diet. Assoc.*, 101, 1456, 2001.

141. Janatuinen, E. et al., A comparison of diets with and without oats in adults with celiac disease, *N. Engl. J. Med.*, 333, 1033, 1995.

142. Green, P. et al., Characteristics of adult celiac disease in the USA: results of a national study, *Am. J. Gastroenterol.*, 96, 126, 2001.

143. Shan, L. et al., Structural basis for gluten intolerance in celiac sprue, *Science*, 297, 2275, 2002.

144. Hornick, B. et al. Eds., Celiac disease, in *Manual of Clinical Dietetics*, 6th ed., The American Dietetic Association, Chicago, 2002.

145. Thompson, T., Do oats belong in a gluten-free diet, *J. Am. Diet. Assoc.*, 97, 1413, 1997.

146. Maki, M. and Collin, P., Coeliac disease, *Lancet*, 349, 1755, 1997.

147. Recommendations made to individuals on gluten-free diets, *Natl. Res. Newslett.*, 19, 18, 2000.

148. Kasarda, D., Defining cereals toxicity in coeliac disease, in *Gastrointestinal Immunology and Gluten-Sensitive Disease*, Feighery, C. and O'Farrelly, F., Eds., Oak Tree Press, Dublin, 1994, pp. 203–220.

149. Janatuinen, E. et al., No harm from five year ingestion of oats in coeliac disease, *Gut*, 50, 332, 2002.

150. Rakel, D., *Integrative Medicine*, W.B. Saunders, Philadelphia, 2003.

13 Liver Disease

Roschelle Heuberger

CONTENTS

PHYSIOLOGY AND FUNCTION OF THE NORMAL LIVER

The liver is the most complex organ in the body, performing a myriad of metabolic functions. It is also one of the largest organs, weighing approximately 3 lb. The normal liver is smooth, glistening, and deeply pigmented. The tissue itself is highly perfused and divided into two main lobular components, right and left. Approximately 1.5 l of blood circulates through the tissue per minute from both the portal and hepatic vasculature. Capillary beds form sinusoids within the liver, and these irregular spaces are lined with a variety of highly specialized cells. Accompanying the vasculature are the interlobular bile ducts, which converge to form the common bile duct.[1]

The normal liver is primarily comprised of hepatocytes (>80%), followed by Kupffer, stellate, ductal epithelial, sinusoidal endothelial, and other phagocytic cells. Each has multiple functions within the organ. The liver has a remarkable capacity for increasing the production of these specialized cells in response to injury, stress, or sepsis, thus regenerating itself and recovering relatively rapidly after acute adverse conditions.[2]

Hepatocytes are essential to the deamination, transamination, and overall metabolism of amino acids. They are responsible for the catabolism of ammonia, urea, and other nitrogenous by-products. These cells are also the sites of redox reactions for the metabolism of a variety of compounds, including the micronutrients. Enzyme systems present within the hepatocytes are responsible for the detoxification of numerous drugs, hormones, environmental contaminants, and synthetic compounds obtained through the food and water supplies. Hepatocytes house alcohol dehydrogenase (ADH) and acetaldehyde dehydrogenase systems, the microsomal ethanol-oxidizing and cytochrome P-450 enzyme systems, for the detoxification of ethanol. The liver is the primary site for the detoxification of drinking alcohol.[3]

Kupffer's cells are the largest single warehouse for fixed macrophages, which remove particulate matter and foreign particles. They are also responsible for cytokine production, toxin removal, and detoxification as well as chemokine feedback to nearby specialty cells. Hepatic stellate cells, probably best known for retinoid storage, are also central to the production of collagen and the development of cicatrix formation in liver tissue in response to severe injury. Bile duct epithelial cells facilitate the transport of bile by regulating flow, sinusoidal endothelial cells participate in the production of sticky coatings and the engulfing of dead or foreign cells through endocytosis, and the free-motion phagocytes tag and eliminate organisms.[4]

The liver is also the chief regulatory and homoeostatic organ for a variety of processes. The liver functions in the regulation of blood glucose and glycogenesis, glycogenolysis, gluconeogenesis, and pentose metabolism. The liver synthesizes plasma proteins and is responsible for the bulk of protein metabolism, the urea cycle, and the disposition of amino acids, thus participating in overall feedback of total body protein anabolism and catabolism.[5] The liver regulates, produces, and disposes insulin-like growth factor, prothrombin, fibrinogen, micronutrient transport proteins as well as many other signaling components, which are central to normal function. Micronutrient storage, activation, conversion, and cleavage also occur in the hepatocytes. In addition to retinoids, the liver stores tocopherols, 1,25-dihydroxycholecalciferol, and small quantities of phyloquinone and menaquinone. The minerals iron, zinc, copper, and magnesium are stored in the liver as are the carotenoids and holocyanocobalamin.[6] Hepatocytes are also responsible for the conversion of carotenoids to retinoids, the activation of 1,25-dihydroxycholecalciferol, and the transformation of folate to 5-methyl tetrahydrofolate (5-THF). The liver is also responsible for the bulk of conversions among ketones, aldehydes, alcohols, and esters and the disposition of their metabolic intermediates.

Bile, cholesterol, fatty acid synthesis, and metabolism are also critical functions of liver cells. Mitochondrial beta-oxidation of fatty acids, the mevalonate and cholesterol synthesis cycles, and chenodeoxycholate and cholate production are under genetic, environmental, and homeostatic controls in the normal liver.[7] Bile aids in the digestion and absorption of essential fatty acids, fat-soluble vitamins, and other fat-soluble components. It is a route for the excretion of a variety of by-products of metabolism and aids in the resorption of nutrients from the lower gut. Bile also serves as a route for the excretion of bilirubin. After disposition of fatty acids, the conjugates of trihydroxy bile acid and cholic acid are resorbed from the distal small bowel by an active sodium-dependent transport process and the dihydroxy acids are resorbed passively with no additional energy expenditure. Some acids are excreted in the feces and may carry additional nonabsorbed fat-soluble components with them.[8]

Hepatocytes are sensitive to insulin, glucagon, and steroid hormones. Insulin and steroid hormones increase the production of hepatic proteins and glucagon and various cytokines provide negative feedback, decreasing production, and increasing catabolism. The liver is responsible for the catabolism of the steroid hormones, such as testosterone, estrogen, progesterone, and aldosterone.[9]

Alcohol is predominantly metabolized in the liver. This is especially true in women, who have little to no gastric ADH. Ethanol and its metabolite acetaldehyde are converted to acetate, which can then enter circulation or be converted to acetyl CoA. The acetyl CoA can then enter the tricarboxylic acid cycles (TCA) for adenosine triphosphate (ATP) production or fatty acid synthesis.[10]

Drugs and environmental agents are also handled by the liver and a variety of enzyme systems exist for detoxification. These systems are generally rate limited. There are genetic and environmental influences on the capacity for drug detoxification. Upregulation of enzyme production usually occurs with repeated exposure over time. The phenomenon of tolerance is a consequence often seen with these enzyme families. The kinetics of pharmacological agents and environmental contaminants are variable among individuals due to the genetic and environmental differences on upregulation.[11]

Certain plant compounds fall into the category of agents that require liver detoxification. Some herbal products, select fungi, and certain berries have large quantities of potential toxins that are handled by the liver and are often hepatotoxic. Cellular response to alkaloids and other such compounds varies by individual and effective dose. Environmental contaminants such as lead and mercury can also permanently affect hepatocytic function.[12]

Due to the integral role the liver plays in homeostasis and its centrality to the function of multiple organ systems, injury or functional decline results in a ripple effect that further complicates the clinical picture. Consequences of liver disease include pancreatitis, gallbladder disease, portal hypertension, nephropathy, encephalopathy, and multiple organ failure.[13]

EPIDEMIOLOGY

The term "liver disease" encompasses a wide variety of conditions, with varied etiologies and classifications. The National Center for Health Statistics (NCHS) reported that the number of discharges for patients with chronic liver disease or cirrhosis was 360,000 in the year 2000, which represents a considerable burden on the healthcare system. The classification of "chronic liver disease" by the Centers for Disease Control (CDC) encompasses hereditary, infectious as well as environmentally induced conditions. Prevalence estimates for chronic liver disease are highest for males across all races and ages, with the exception of women in the 75- to 84-year age groups, where estimates are higher due to increasing numbers of women living longer than men.[14,15]

Overall prevalence estimates for chronic liver disease have risen from 1997–1998 to 2000–2001. This increase is seen consistently across genders, all races, and all age groups. Non-Hispanic Black males aged 45 to 64 years have the highest estimates for liver disease according to NCHS 2000–2001 data at 3.0% in comparison to Caucasian males (2.1%), non-Hispanic Black females (1.3%), and Hispanic males (2.2%). Overall age-adjusted data for adults in the United States peak at 50 to 64 years at a 1.6% prevalence estimate and then decline with advancing age.[16]

Viral hepatitis is differentiated from alcoholic hepatitis by the CDC. In the United States, viral hepatitis infections have increased for all strains and subtypes. Non-Hispanic Black males, aged 45 to 54 years, represent the group most affected, with crude rates of 12 per 100,000 persons in 2000–2001. This represents an increase of 77% in the last decade in this subgroup alone. The crude rate for all adults in the United States in 2001–2202 is 2 per 100,000. Overall mortality from viral hepatitis has increased by 84% since 1985. These statistics do not represent institutionalized populations, such as incarcerated individuals or long-term treatment facility patients where rates are higher. Adjustment for age did not significantly alter the rates for hepatitis infection or mortality.[17]

CDC data show the diagnosis of malignant neoplasms of the liver and intrahepatic bile ducts increase with age in all races and in both males and females. Mortality increases with increasing age. Diagnosis and mortality for neoplastic liver disease have increased over the last few decades. Age-adjusted mortality rates for both sexes, all races, aged 65 to 74 years, were 24 per 100,000 in 2000–2001 in comparison to 16 per 100,000 in 1985. Death from neoplastic liver disease was significantly higher in males and in non-Hispanic Blacks.[18]

Chronic liver disease is associated with nutritional deficiencies. The CDC reports a slight decrease in overall rates of nutritional deficiency since 1985, from 11 per 100,000 to 10 per 100,000. Older White females and non-Hispanic Black males are the groups most affected. Rates were highest in the oldest old (85 years and older). Age-adjusted rates (65–74 years) in 2000–2001 for White females were 24 per 100,000 and non-Hispanic Black males were 42 per 100,000. General malnutrition makes up the majority of the categorization of nutritional deficiency in NCHS data. According to 2002, the overall age-adjusted mortality rate for malnutrition in the United States is 1.2 per 100,000 standardized population.[19]

Chronic liver disease or cirrhosis was listed as the seventh leading cause of death nationally in persons with 25–64 years of age in 2000. The rates for younger persons (under age of 45 years) are less due to the length of time required to manifest the condition. American Indians and Alaskan Natives were at greatest risk for mortality across gender and age; males had greater mortality for liver disease than females across age and race. Age-adjusted rates for chronic liver disease or cirrhosis are presented in Table 13.1. The primary cause of mortality is broken down into alcoholic liver disease and other chronic liver disease or cirrhosis. The age-adjusted rates for alcoholic liver disease can be found in Table 13.2. There is a secondary categorization that includes alcohol-induced deaths and accidental poisoning or exposure to noxious substances. The age-adjusted rates for alcohol-induced deaths and poisoning are detailed in Table 13.3. These latter categorizations are for the most part mechanistically mediated via hepatotoxicity and therefore are included in this section.[20,21]

Data from the National Health Interview Survey conducted by the United States Department of Health and Human Services (USDHHS) along with the CDC with noninstitutionalized persons interviewed in 2001 found that 1.3% of interviewees reported were having liver disease. Of those reporting chronic disease a greater number were poor, 45–64 years of age, males, and lived in the western United States. Percentages were increased among Alaskan Natives, American Indians, and persons reporting of two or more races.[22]

Heavy lifetime alcohol intake is a major factor in the prevalence of liver disease. It is notable that early onset of heavy and binge drinking is associated with peak mortality rates

TABLE 13.1
NCHS Age-Adjusted Death Rates per 100,000 U.S. Standard Population for Chronic Liver Disease or Cirrhosis by Race and Gender, 1970–2000[a]

	1970	1980	1990	1995	2000
All persons	17.8	15.1	11.1	9.9	9.5
Males	24.8	21.3	15.9	14.2	13.4
Females	11.9	9.9	7.1	6.2	6.2
White	16.6	13.9	10.5	9.7	9.6
Non-Hispanic Black	28.1	25.0	16.5	12.0	9.4
American Indian or Alaskan Native	—	45.3	24.1	27.4	24.3
All cause mortality — all persons	1222.6	1039.1	938.7	909.8	869.0

[a]All ages are included in the above estimates. Note that mortality estimates for groups of age 45 years and older are higher.

Source: From Fried, V.M., Prager, K., MacKay, A.P., and Xia, H., in *Health, United States, 2003*, National Center for Health Statistics, Hyattsville, MD, 2003, pp. 136–137.

TABLE 13.2
NCHS Death Rates per 100,000 U.S. Standard Population for Alcoholic Liver Disease by Race and Gender, 1981–2001[a]

	1981	1990	1995	2000	2001
All persons	12.2	10.7	10.1	9.3	9.3
Males	19.0	17.2	16.5	15.2	14.9
Females	6.6	5.6	4.8	4.2	4.6
White	11.8	10.4	10.0	9.3	9.4
Non-Hispanic Black	19.4	17.7	13.9	10.0	10.0
American Indian or Alaskan Native	41.5	31.1	32.2	26.1	26.9

[a]All ages are included in the above estimates. Note that mortality estimates for groups of age 45 years and older are higher.

Source: From Fried, V.M., Prager, K., MacKay, A.P., and Xia, H., in *Health, United States, 2003*, National Center for Health Statistics, Hyattsville, MD, 2003.

from liver disease in persons older than 45 years. The age-adjusted lifetime drinking status percentages for current drinkers over the age of 18 years are shown in Table 13.4. Heavy drinking is greatest in persons of 18–44 years, with highest rates seen in American Indians, Alaskan Natives and in persons of two or more races. Rates were higher with less years of formal education, among the poor, and in divorced individuals. Males are more likely than females to be heavy alcohol consumers, binge drinkers, and lifetime current drinkers. Persons living in the western United States were more likely to report increased intake of alcoholic beverages over their lifetime; however, binge drinking was highest in the Midwest. Urban dwelling is also associated with higher drinking rates, but binge drinking was higher among rural dwellers. American Indians, Alaskan Natives, and non-Hispanic White women were more likely to be binge drinkers than women from other race groups.[23] Trends in heavy alcohol consumption and binge drinking are shown in Table 13.4. Alcoholic liver disease rates parallel these trends in consumption.[24,25]

Older age and normally occurring changes in the hepatocytes adversely affect prognosis with alcoholic liver disease, chronic liver disease, and cirrhosis. Due to the long period required for the progression of the disease to symptomatic stages, information regarding risk factors for the development of the disease must be routinely assessed for all patients early

TABLE 13.3
NCHS Age-Adjusted Death Rates per 100,000 U.S. Standard Population for Alcohol-Induced Deaths and Accidental Poisoning or Exposure to Noxious Substances for 2001–2002[a]

	2001	2002
Alcohol-induced deaths	6.9	6.2
Accidental poisoning and exposure to noxious substances	4.9	5.1

[a]All ages are included in the above estimates.

Source: From National Center for Health Statistics, *National Vital Statistics Reports*, Vol. 52, No. 13, NCHS, Hyattsville, MD, 2004.

TABLE 13.4
NCHS Percent Distributions: U.S. Alcohol Consumption for Current Drinkers, 1997, 2001

Characteristic	Both Sexes		Male		Female	
	1997	2001	1997	2001	1997	2001
Age adjusted — 18 years and older						
Light	69.6	68.8	59.5	59.1	81.0	79.6
Moderate	22.5	23.4	31.8	32.6	12.0	13.0
Heavy	7.9	7.9	8.7	8.3	7.0	7.3
Binge drinking among current drinkers						
1–12 days/year	18.5	17.1	22.0	19.9	14.6	14.0
>12 days/year	15.6	15.3	23.4	22.8	6.8	7.0
Binge drinking on more than one occasion per year among current drinkers						
18–44 years	42.4	41.4	54.6	52.3	28.7	29.2
45–64 years	25.3	23.8	36.1	34.7	12.9	11.9
65 years and older	11.2	8.2	17.8	13.1	4.4	3.1
Caucasian	33.3	31.8	44.4	42.0	20.9	20.7
Non-Hispanic Black	23.6	20.6	31.7	27.5	14.9	12.5
American Indian, Alaskan Native	54.5	34.6	70.5	35.9	38.4	27.9
Asian	25.5	23.2	30.7	28.9	16.6	12.9
Hispanic	36.8	32.2	46.3	41.9	22.3	17.9
Two or more races	44.0	41.6	53.1	59.9	31.5	24.3
Urban	31.6	30.1	42.4	39.9	19.8	19.1
Rural	34.8	32.8	45.7	42.2	21.2	22.5
Northeast	31.3	30.0	43.1	41.4	18.9	18.8
Midwest	33.8	33.6	44.7	44.4	21.6	22.4
South	30.9	27.9	40.5	36.1	19.2	18.0
West	33.4	31.7	44.6	41.4	20.8	20.1

Source: From Fried, V.M., Prager, K., MacKay, A.P., and Xia, H., in *Health, United States, 2003*, National Center for Health Statistics, Hyattsville, MD, 2003.

on. Male gender, Alaskan Native or American Indian, impoverished socioeconomic status, drinking history, and other indicators may be useful to the clinician in the determination and prevention of chronic liver disease.[26]

MANIFESTATIONS (PATHOPHYSIOLOGY)

Liver disease may be caused by a variety of factors. Regardless of etiology, the symptomatology of acute and chronic liver disease presents as malaise, weakness, anorexia, nausea, vomiting, and alterations in glycemic control. It may be accompanied by frank malnutrition.[27] In acute, self-limiting conditions that result in hepatocytic injury, decreased oral intake, malabsorption, and gastrointestinal disturbances usually resolve before the onset of frank malnutrition and there are minimal long-term consequences. Chronic liver disease is most often associated with long-term nutritional consequences, frank malnutrition, and permanent metabolic alterations.[28,29]

Alcoholic liver disease presents with more complications, as a result of underlying inflammatory response, cellular death, and the alcohol intake itself. Chronic alcohol ingestion has its own set of metabolic sequelae. Alcohol metabolism causes a rise in reduced nicotinamide adenine dinucleotide (NADH), which effectively shuts down the TCA cycle and interrupts the normal cellular redox state.[30] This change in redox state decreases beta-oxidation of fatty acids and promotes synthesis and retention of fatty acids, glycerol, triglycerides, and apolipoproteins. Hypoglycemia is also compounded by decreases in hepatic glycogen reserves and gluconeogenesis, the latter occurring via suppression by ethanol and the secondary depression of the TCA cycle.[31]

Fatty component buildup leads to steatosis or fatty liver, which progresses to inflammation or hepatitis over time. The inflammatory response is worsened by the continued ingestion of ethanol. Alcoholic hepatitis in the early stages is still reversible, but with continued insults, the cytokine production as a result of the inflammatory response increases and results in a cascade of reactions that lead to a rapid progression of liver cell death. Once the number of dead hepatocytes reaches a critical mass, a diagnosis of cirrhosis may be inevitable. There is no reversal of cirrhosis from any etiology, and the progression to cirrhosis is fastest with continued alcohol ingestion. Diabetics, morbidly obese persons and persons incurring rapid weight loss, often exhibit nonalcoholic steatosis, which results in the same progression of the disease.[32,33] The incidence of nonalcoholic steatohepatitis (NASH) is increasing due to the rise in obesity and diabetes. Bariatric surgery and rapid weight loss can also induce steatosis.[34]

Severe liver disease is often accompanied by portal hypertension, alterations in colloid pressure, and the subsequent involvement of pancreatic, gastrointestinal, renal, and pulmonary systems.[35] If unchecked, encephalopathy may ensue, with frank psychosis, confabulation, and ataxia, loss of neuromuscular function, flapping tremor, coma, and eventually death. Third spacing, cushinoid appearance, and chronic febrile states may accompany the disease.[28]

Manifestations of liver disease may be classified into the following categories: abnormal histological findings on a liver biopsy, overt signs and symptoms of severe liver disease (including anthropometry), abnormal laboratory and other biochemical indicators of liver function.[36] Visual inspection of the diseased liver may show fatty infiltrates, enlargement, edematous structures, scarring, darkening, and shriveling of the tissue. Overt signs and symptoms (not including the manifestations of concomitant malnutrition) may include jaundice, darkening of the urine, melena, steatorrhea, loss of lean body mass, ascites, spider nevii, esophageal varices, discoloration of the sclera, gynecomastia, itching, dysguesia, and epigastric pain.[37] Encephalopathic patients exhibit overt symptomatology according to four stages:

- Stage 1 — confusion, sleep, disturbances
- Stage 2 — confabulation, disorientation
- Stage 3 — somnolence, aggression when awake
- Stage 4 — comatose[38]

Biochemical indicators vary with the etiology of the disease.[39] Primary indicators include elevations in the liver enzymes alanine aminotransferase (ALT), aspartate aminotransferase (AST), serum lactic dehydrogenase (LDH); elevations in hepatic function tests for excretion, such as total serum bilirubin, direct serum bilirubin, serum bile acid levels, ammonia, and urea; elevations in urinary bilirubin and urobilinogen; and elevations in hepatocytic plasma membrane function tests such as gamma-glutamyl transpeptidase and 5′ nucleotidase.[40]

Fecal fat determinations may be useful for liver disease-induced steatorrhea. Blood glucose monitoring is indicated for hypoglycemia associated with hepatocytic dysfunction and indicators of dyslipidemia, such as triglycerides, very low-density lipoprotein (VLDL) levels, and apolipoprotein profiles should be checked.[41] In addition, measures of the plasma proteins synthesized by the liver are useful in determining the extent of hepatocytic damage. These include prothrombin, albumin, globulin, ferritin, transferrin, transcobalamin, ceruloplasmin,

TABLE 13.5
Biochemical Indicators in Liver Disease: Normal Ranges for Select Indices

Biochemical Indicators	Normal Range
Compound indicators	
Creatinine-height index (CHI) for LBM[a] catabolism	0–5% Deficit
Serum indicators	
Albumin	3.0–5.0 g/dl
Triglycerides	<200 mg/dl
Total cholesterol	<200 mg/dl
Ferritin	12–200 ng/ml
Transferrin	200–400 mg/dl
Retinol-binding protein	2.1–6.4 mg/dl
Glucose — fasting	70–110 mg/dl
Blood urea nitrogen	5–20 mg/dl
Bilirubin, total	0.1–1.0 mg/dl
Alkaline phosphatase (AlkP)	25–140 units/l
Aspartate aminotransferase (AST)	1–40 units/l
Alanine aminotransferase (ALT)	0–45 units/l
Excretion indicators	
Urinalysis bilirubin	0 units/dl
Urinalysis urobilinogen	0.1–1.0 units/dl
Quantitative fecal fat	<5 g fat/24 h

[a]LBM: lean body mass.

Source: From Pagana, K.D. and Pagana, T.J., *Manual of Diagnostic and Laboratory Tests*, Mosby Publishing, St. Louis, MO, 2002.

retinol-binding protein, alpha-antitrypsin, and select apolipoproteins. Table 13.5 depicts normal levels of biochemical indices for select liver-associated proteins. Newer and more sensitive tests of liver function are also developed, but are not yet readily available in most clinical settings. These include liver holotranscobalamin levels, metallothionine subtypes, aminotransferase profiles, and hepatic arginase assays.[42–45] Additional considerations when evaluating the above biochemical indices include time of the day the sample was obtained, variation in methodology between laboratories, and individual variation in normal ranges.[46]

For the assessment of viral, autoimmune, and inherited liver disease, titers for the following antigenic complexes may be determined through biochemical assay.[47,48] IgM and IgG anti-HAV for hepatitis virus A, IgM and IgG anti-HBV for hepatitis virus B, anti-HBC and HCV-RNA for hepatitis C, IgM and IgG anti-HDV for hepatitis virus D, and IgM and IgG anti-HEV for viral hepatitis E.

Low ceruloplasmin levels, alterations in transferrin saturation, and ferritin may be used for the diagnosis of Wilson's disease.[14] Abnormal ferritin and transferrin levels may be used to determine hereditary hemochromatosis and low alpha-antitrypsin levels may be diagnostic for alpha-antitrypsin deficiency disease, another inherited disorder leading to liver disease.[49,50]

Primary biliary cirrhosis (PBC) and primary sclerosing cholangitis (PSC), both immune-mediated disease states, will evidence elevated or abnormal circulating autoantibodies, immunoglobulins, cell-mediated immune proteins, and human leukocyte antigen subtypes.[51] Other diseases that have clinical manifestations that include liver damage will impact biochemical indicators but must be confirmed using alternate methods of diagnosis. These include rheumatoid arthritis, systemic lupus erythymatosis, scleroderma, morbid obesity, sequelae to rapid weight loss or bypass surgery, long-term parenteral nutrition, primary or metastatic cancers, and HIV or AIDS.[52,53] Finally, there are a small number of parasitic, bacterial, fungal, and cryptogenic liver diseases along with the liver diseases of pregnancy.[54-58] Their incidence is low as they are considered rarities and their overt signs and symptoms are extremely variable.

End-stage liver disease (ESLD) with acute renal failure will evidence biochemical alterations consistent with both hepatic disease states and renal insufficiency. Fluid, electrolyte, and osmotic status indicators will be abnormal.[59,60] Oliguria, hemolysis, metabolic acidosis, and marked third spacing may progress rapidly.[61] Portal hypertension and systemic hypertension also cause rapid lung involvement and changes in pulmonary function indicators. If hemorrhage and varices occur as a result of the hypertensive crises, visualization may require endoscopic or imaging procedures for diagnostic determination.[62] Chronic bleeds will be associated with biochemical indices of iron deficiency anemia. Pancreatitis is also seen frequently in this population.[63]

Hepatic osteodystrophy, a form of osteopenia, occurs in liver disease and is worsened by renal complications as well as by the treatments offered for both disease states.[64] Corticosteroid administration may quickly further the progression of osteopenia in these patients. Bone density scans, fecal fat determinations for steatorrhea-related vitamin and mineral losses, hepatic enzyme assays, and specific protein analysis of osteoblastic function may be useful in the assessment of the osteopenic manifestations of ESLD and hepatorenal syndrome.[65]

COMPLICATIONS

Malnutrition and specific nutritional deficiencies are complications of liver disease. The phenomenon is multifactorial in nature. Mechanisms include poor intake due to anorexia, nausea, vomiting; inappropriate dietary intake due to socioeconomics or other factors such as alcohol ingestion. Malabsorption and steatorrhea occur due to dysregulation of bile acid production, micronutrient transporter synthesis, macronutrient disposition, and increased excretion of both macro- and micronutrients.[66] In addition, decreased storage capacity for glycogen, vitamin A, vitamin K, zinc, iron, and copper, decreased transporter protein synthesis, and decreased activation capacity for vitamin D and folate result in systemic dysregulation.[67] Often the treatment of liver disease furthers malnutrition. Pharmacological agents used in treatment often have side effects, which include anorexia, nausea, gastrointestinal distress, fatigue, and electrolytic disturbances. Surgical procedures also have a marked impact on nutritional status and nutrition support is often instituted. If comorbid conditions such as renal disease or pancreatitis exist, the clinical picture worsens.[68]

Malnutrition seen in hepatic disease is mediated through cytokines and the inflammatory cascade, among other factors.[69] Fatty streaking results in phagocytic infiltration and the subsequent release of cytokines such as tumor necrosis factor (TNF) and the interleukin (IL-1, 6, 8) series.[70] These in turn mediate muscle catabolism via the liver and its production of cell signals, plasma proteins, and feedback on glucocorticoids and other steroid hormones. Hypercatabolism and an increase in resting metabolic rate are most often seen with acute febrile state, although hypercatabolism may persist in chronic disease, especially with alcoholic hepatitis leading to cirrhosis.[71]

Malnutrition mediated through cytokines has specific micronutrient features. Zinc homeostasis is adversely affected, with hepatic zinc sequestered and unavailable. Depletion of total body zinc (minus hepatic zinc) results in low serum zinc levels with a concomitant increase in ceruloplasmin and circulating copper. The prooxidant nature of copper furthers cellular damage in the hepatocyte. Hepatocytic injury also decreases the availability of iron, as the production of transferrin is impaired.[72] This may result in iron overload in the hepatocyte and iron is also a potent prooxidant. Additional consequences include toxicity from fat-soluble vitamins, especially vitamin A with a decreased production of retinol-binding protein and decreased ability for conversion between retinals, retinols, and retinaldehydes.[73]

In the presence of continual ingested alcohol, hepatocytes have decreased ability to mount negative phase responses to inflammation, activate folate, conserve thiamine, and modulate conversion to vitamin D_3.[74–76] Because of ADH and acetaldehyde dehydrogenase dependence on zinc as a cofactor, increased zinc needs cannot be met. Through independent mechanisms on folate status, alcohol and liver disease impact homocysteine levels, which is a potent prooxidant, a risk factor for cardiovascular and cerebrovascular disease and a contributor to further hepatic injury.[77–79]

Gender studies on continual ingestion of large amounts of alcohol have found increased risk of cirrhosis, hormonal changes, certain cancers, and gallbladder disease in women.[80] Women are at greater risk due to differential effects of ethanol on detoxification enzymes.[81] Women do not have appreciable amount of gastric ADH, have higher circulating blood levels of ethanol postingestion, and have decreased induction of hepatic detoxification enzymes.[82] Women have higher morbidity and mortality related to alcohol-induced pathogenesis.[83,84] Women have increased aromatization of androgens to estrogens with ethanol consumption, which is thought to act as a promoter to carcinogenesis in sex hormone sensitive cancers such as breast and endometrial cancers.[85–89]

In either gender, diminution of total oxidative stress may also provide some protection against liver injury regardless of the etiological basis. Because inflammation results in systemic response, fewer resources are available to counteract the damage from oxidation overall. Antioxidant species such as glutathione, metallothionine, ethyl pyruvate, gamma-tocopherols, and vitamin C may prove to be protective due to their free-radical scavenging potential.[90–92]

Folate and cyanocobalamine may also provide protection from elevated homocysteine levels, which also increase systemic stress. Carotenoids are also influential in systemic oxidative stress and in addition to acting as general antioxidants do not pose the toxicity potential of preformed vitamin A in the injured hepatocyte.[93]

Hypercatabolism mediated through cytokine involvement impacts macronutrient metabolism. Diminished gluconeogenesis, glycogenesis, glycogenolysis, and glycogen storage capacity coupled with increased needs results in glycemic dysregulation.[94] Utilization of muscle for the provision of substrates results in muscle wasting and an increase in deamination and urea cycle activities. Nitrogenous waste is increased but hepatorenal capabilities are diminished.[95] This results in elevations in levels of serum ammonia, blood urea nitrogen, and hepatic enzymes.

Because of the liberation of aromatic amino acids (AAA) from muscle breakdown and the utilization of the branched-chain amino acids (BCAA) for energy by tissues during depressed gluconeogenesis in liver disease, an imbalance in the ratio of AAA:BCAA results.[96] The amino acid transporters that cross the blood–brain barrier (BBB) are competitive and an increase in AAA results in decreased transport of BCAA across the BBB. This deficiency of BCAA in the brain coupled with increasing levels of ammonia, a potent cerebral toxin, alters neurotransmission.[97] This is thought to be a contributing factor to the development of hepatic encephalopathy. Other contributors may include fluid and electrolyte shifts, sepsis, hypo- or hyperglycemia, and constipation.

Hepatic encephalopathy may be further worsened by zinc sequestering, poor intake leading to malnutrition and general alterations in metabolism. Bleeding increases the load of nitrogenous waste, renal complications decrease nitrogenous waste removal, and by-products of bacterial degradation in the gut all serve to increase ammonia levels.[98] Encephalopathy may also present with electrolytic abnormalities, metabolic alkalosis, and multiple organ-system failure.[99] Negative nitrogen balance is usually present and worsens with restrictions on dietary intake of protein that occurs as the disease progresses.[100]

Wernicke–Korsakoff syndrome is differentiated from hepatic encephalopathy, as it is a nutrient deficiency (thiamine) in the alcoholic patient with liver disease. The clinical features include abnormal mental status, ocular abnormalities such as nystagmus, and altered gait. Thiamine deficiency with some of the clinical manifestations of beri beri can be seen in a small percentage of malnourished alcoholics with liver disease and Wernicke–Korsakoff syndrome. Not all malnourished alcoholic patients will develop the syndrome.[101] The changes are mediated by a diminution of thiamine pyrophosphate (TPP), the active cofactor for metabolic pathways including the hexose monophosphate shunt. In patients exhibiting the syndrome, there is an existing aberration in TPP activation, which gets expressed under conditions of poor thiamine intake and increased alcohol consumption. Because the central nervous system (CNS) is dependent on TPP as cofactor for hexose metabolism, Wernicke–Korsakoff patients exhibit far reaching neurological abnormalities.[102]

The injured liver is unable to handle lipolysis, lipogenesis or cyclization, elongation, desaturation, interesterification, and intermediate metabolism of triglycerides, fatty acids, and sterols. In addition, the synthesis, recycling, and metabolism of bile acids are negatively impacted.[103] Cholesterol, lipoprotein, and steroid hormone metabolism are also adversely affected. As a result of bile salt dysregulation fats, fat-soluble vitamins and certain drugs are malabsorbed. Steatorrhea with fatty foul-smelling stool occurs along with fat-soluble vitamin loss. With an already impoverished diet, energy loss, vitamin and other nutrient losses, the patient rapidly progresses to malnutrition.[104] If comorbid pancreatitis exists, the clinical picture worsens with the absence of pancreatic enzymes, altered gastric motility, cholestasis, and electrolytic disturbances.

Apolipoprotein synthesis is impaired which alters the trafficking of lipids and sterols.[105] Declines in fatty acid oxidation and the increase in NADH from alcohol ingestion result in fatty streaking and fibrosis. Decreased availability of two-carbon fragments and acetyl CoA leads to deficits in ATP. These deficits coupled with other metabolic aberrations result in lethargy and weakness, hallmarks of alcoholic, viral, and other forms of hepatitis.[106]

In NASH, high-fat diet, obesity, diabetes, visceral adiposity, and rapid weight loss have all been shown to contribute to fibrosis.[107] Alterations in fat metabolism, insulin sensitivity, changes in glucose transporter activity, changes in transcription of lipoprotein lipase, and hormone sensitive lipase all contribute to the advent of fatty streaking and fibrosis, but the inflammatory response and production of cytokines such as TNF initiate the latter changes. Levels of systemic oxidative stress and lipid peroxidation are the deciding factors, which develop NASH.[108,109]

Portal hypertension, the increase in pressure due to limited blood flow through and around the liver, is also a concomitant event in liver disease.[110] It is partially mediated via alterations in hepatic production and metabolism of plasma proteins, release of feedback hormones such as ADH, catecholamines, etc. and the retention of sodium. Ascites and peripheral edema are common. Fluid and electrolytic disturbances are frequent. Esophageal varices occur, further depressing intake.[111]

In primary hepatic carcinogenesis as well as in cancer that has metastasized to the liver, the clinical picture is further complicated by the increased metabolic stress of the mutated, rapidly dividing cells. Because rapid cell division increases protein demand, folate and zinc needs, the already diminished hepatic capacity is further taxed. Surgical resection and chemotherapeutic agents also increase nutritional demands.[112,113] Side effects of both the carcinogenesis and the treatment for the disease result in poor postoperative (p.o.) intake, increases in the number of days spent without any oral intake (n.p.o.), and worsening profile of serum indicators of nutritional status and liver function. Many chemotherapeutic agents

TABLE 13.6
Common Therapeutic Agents and Their Select Nutritional Consequences

Therapeutic Agent or Class	Nutritional Consequences
Methotrexate	Dysregulation of folate metabolism and excretion, mucositis, anorexia, nausea, vomiting, dysguesia
Cisplatin	Anorexia, nausea, vomiting, dysguesia, diarrhea
Gemcitabine	Anorexia, nausea, vomiting, dysguesia, diarrhea or constipation
Ironotican	Anorexia, nausea, vomiting, dysguesia, diarrhea or constipation
5-Fluorouracil	Mucositis, anorexia, nausea, vomiting, dysguesia
Cyclosporine	Nausea, vomiting, diarrhea
Glucocorticoids	Hyperglycemia, decreased calcium absorption with increased excretion, vitamin D dysregulation, appetite dysregulation, fluid shifts, electrolytic abnormalities
Interferon	Dry mouth, dysguesia, stomatitis, dysphagia, nausea, vomiting, dyspepsia, abdominal pain, diarrhea or constipation, flatulence
Spiranolactone	Hyperkalemia, thirst, anorexia, dehydration, weight loss
Lactulose	Increased gut motility, increased gastric emptying, fluid loss, electrolytic disturbances, nausea, vomiting, cramps, diarrhea

Source: From Pronsky, Z.M., et al., *Food–Medication Interactions*, 13th ed., Food–Medication Interactions, Birchrunville, PA, 2003.

have specific interactions with vitamins and minerals, such as methotrexate and folate. All indices for nutriture, liver function, inflammation, and oxidative stress should be carefully monitored. Table 13.6 depicts common therapeutic agents and their potential side effects in terms of nutritional status.[114]

An idiopathic feature of severe, chronic liver disease is pruritus. Because the liver is also responsible for immunocompetence, breaking the skin increases the risk for infection, with systemic sepsis occurring in a large percentage of those patients. Again, sepsis and wound healing increase hypercatabolic states and protein, zinc, folate, and many other macro- and micronutrients are adversely affected. Pruritus affects the majority of patients with PBC, and may be severe and unresponsive to treatment.[115] Cholestasis in liver disease in general is associated with unremitting pruritus and an estimated 10% of patients experience severe depression, sleep disturbance, and fatigue, which may lead to suicide. The itching follows a circadian rhythm starting at the feet and hands then spreading over the entire body. Excoriation, hyperpigmentation, and cicatrix formation result from repeated scratching.[116] Wound healing is depressed in these patients and the level of malnutrition correlates strongly with delays.

PBC is of unknown etiology, but destroys the intrahepatic bile ducts and culminates in the portal inflammation that results in liver disease.[117] It seems to affect women between 35 and 60 years of age, and has familial predisposition.[118] Recent evidence suggests that it may in fact be mediated by dysregulation of endogenous retinoids and the conversion of retinyl esters to retinoic acid, the most biologically active form of vitamin A. Retinoic acid is a potent cell mediator, binding to the nuclear receptor superfamily and regulating transcription and subsequent gene expression for morphology, growth, enzyme production, cell differentiation, and more.[119] The inherited abnormal immunoregulation seen in PCB and the similarities to hypervitaminosis A in terms of clinical signs and symptoms lead to the hypothesis that PCB is related to abnormal accumulations of retinoids and subsequent hepatotoxicity.[120,121]

PSC is another disease of unclear etiology, which affects more men and has strong familial predisposition. Many of these patients also have inflammatory processes occurring elsewhere, such as comorbid inflammatory bowel disease or osteodystrophic disease.[122] The bile ducts are affected both intra- and extrahepatically, with inflammation progressing to liver disease. PSC is associated with the same clinical manifestations as other liver disease states and similar patterns of malabsorption leading to malnutrition. In addition, several other inherited diseases, which are systemic in nature, will follow the same progression of inflammation leading to fibrosis and chronic liver disease with the same nutritional issues.[123] Sarcoidosis, systemic lupus, and rheumatoid arthritis are examples.

Wilson's disease, an inherited disorder of copper excretion, presents with inflammation, fibrosis, hepatic disease, and chronicity due to the accumulation of copper in the hepatocytes. Low levels of ceruloplasmin and impaired excretion result in increasing cellular destruction and cytokine activation. In addition, copper is a prooxidant and causes further damage upon accumulation.[124]

Oxidative stress increases from copper and is further aggravated by poor nutritional status. Antioxidant levels, degree of malnutrition, degree of hepatic decompensation, and levels of glutathione peroxidase, metallothionein, and other enzyme systems that mitigate peroxidation impact the progression and mortality from the disease.[125] Because of the impact zinc and metallothionine levels have on copper, aggressive zinc administration is warranted upon diagnosis.[126] Zinc binding of copper, its competition with copper for carriers across the enterocyte, and its competition for transport in the hepatocyte can mitigate the accretion of copper and prevent the severe and fatal progression of the disease if transplantation fails.[127]

Hereditary hemochromatosis, a disease of iron accumulation and hepatotoxicity, is seen more frequently in males than females. Parenchymal cells become overloaded with iron, a potent prooxidant.[128] The homozygous form of the disease is mediated via an increase in the expression of the divalent metal ion transporter in the enterocytes of the upper small intestine, and a mutation in the gene responsible for regulation of iron homeostasis, a negative feedback process with hepatic involvement.[129] Excessive iron absorption and hepatic storage coupled with increasing hepatic decompensation result in a decrease in the ability of the hepatocyte to mobilize iron for transport out to other tissues.[130] Excessive iron blocks the absorption, storage, transport, and metabolism of other divalent cations such as zinc and copper, and the increases in the levels of free iron due to decreased hepatic production of transporter proteins speeds pathogenesis. The prooxidant nature of free iron further enhances the process.[131]

HIV and AIDS also present with comorbid hepatic disease, from both the infection and from the treatment.[132] This clinical picture is further complicated by the number of hepatitis variant coinfected individuals.[133] Dyslipidemia and steatosis from highly active antiretroviral therapy (HAART) present with visceral and trunkal adiposity and syndrome X (metabolic syndrome). Infection and viral replication also impact hepatic function. Malnutrition and ketosis are comorbid to the infection as well as to the complications.[134] Hepatic decompensation, viral load, coinfection status, and poor intake are all associated with depressed immunological response. Many of the drugs used to treat the primary infection and comorbid conditions associated with HIV and AIDS have hepatotoxic effects.[135] Indices of nutritional status, immunocompetence, and hormonal homeostasis must be carefully monitored.

Total parenteral nutrition (TPN) has also been associated with the induction of liver disease, although the etiology is unclear. Overfeeding, refeeding, and other factors have been attributed to the inflammatory response and lipid infiltration seen in TPN induction.[136] Photooxidation of multivitamin solutions in the admixture may contribute to the steatosis seen in a small percentage of individuals receiving TPN.[137] Alternatively, deficiencies in conjugated bile acids or the amino acid composition of the formulation may mediate the progression.[138,139]

Poor oral intake due to anorexia, nausea, vomiting, dysguesia, poor socioeconomic status, depression, medication side effects, comorbid conditions, etc. furthers hepatic decompensation.[140] High fat, antioxidant poor, dietary patterns may be both causal as well as promotional to hepatic steatosis.[141,142] Diabetes, obesity, and gastrointestinal surgery also may result in or increase the progression of hepatic decompensation.[143]

Transplantation is often indicated in ESLD. Transplantation has its own set of nutritional concerns. Before transplant, aggressive nutrition support is usually required for the malnutrition and associated complications of liver disease. Posttransplantation, risk for malnutrition increases, with days NPO with surgery, poor p.o. intake, hypercatabolic state from surgery, comorbidities, and increased needs for wound healing and immunocompetence.[144] Iatrogenic infection and food safety are two additional risks. Drug–nutrient interactions are frequent in this population. Immunosuppressive, antibiotic, and glucocorticoid regimens are difficult to adhere to, are poorly tolerated, and have a wide array of nutritional effects.[145]

Acute hepatic failure due to viral or traumatic causes and fulminant hepatitis present differently than chronic liver disease in terms of the nutritional manifestations.[146] Fulminant hepatitis is sudden onset, occurs in the absence of underlying hepatic or systemic conditions and is accompanied by hepatic encephalopathy. The etiology is variable; it can be traumatic, viral, or toxic. Liver "dialysis" or plasmapheresis, which is currently tested may aid in decreasing the effects of acute hepatic failure in the near future.[147] Preexisting malnutrition is not usually present, but the disease itself as well as the absence of specific nutrients such as choline, carnitine, and glutamine from nutritional formulations may cause deterioration in nutritional status. This results in the need for acute nutritional management of hypercatabolism, encephalopathy (if present), and the inflammatory response until the recovery phase.

NUTRITIONAL MANAGEMENT

Nutritional management in liver disease must be tailored to the individual needs due to the high rates of comorbidities and malnutrition in this population. Etiological considerations must also be addressed before constructing the treatment plan. Acute or chronic illness will impact the decision-making process. A detailed history, matrices of drug–nutrient interactions, biochemical, anthropometric, and clinical indicators must be thoroughly evaluated. If possible, patient input into the nutritional care plan should be obtained to enhance compliance. Follow-up care must be monitored with frequent assessment of all indices as the patient progresses.[148] It is also useful to note that end of life issues must be considered with this patient population, and a frank discussion of hydration and feeding at the end of life must be undertaken with the patient and caregivers. A check of legal documentation and patient wishes should be performed.[149]

Sensitivity and specificity of laboratory testing must be addressed.[150] It is usually cost prohibitive to obtain biochemical indicators that are either sensitive or specific enough to determine appropriate treatment, therefore the clinician must carefully evaluate the data obtained from a variety of sources, and make the best determination of an appropriate nutrition care plan.[151] Because of the complexities of the disease, it is critical to obtain repeated measurements of all potentially important indicators over time. Initial screening should include anthropometric data, with attention paid to muscle mass, measures of visceral adiposity, assessment of edema, or ascites. Bedside bioimpedance (BIA) may be useful in this regard.[152] Several studies using height-standardized resistance and reactance for BIA have shown excellent precision in evaluating body composition in patients with ascites, edema, and fluid shifts with cirrhosis.[153–155] Over time, fluid intake and output should be routinely assessed along with changes in girth, scale weight, muscle mass loss, and peripheral skin turgidity.[156] Because osteopenia is a risk with liver disease, bone density and vitamin K measurements over time are useful.[157]

The evaluation of level of malnutrition should be done with dietary recall, food frequency, and intake history including alcohol intake, supplement use, herbal use, drug use, and environmental contaminant exposure.[158] The use of assessment tools such as the subjective global assessment (SGA) or setting specific procedures may be appropriate for a preliminary screening, but will require additional information once risk has been determined.[159] For critically ill patients, enteral and parenteral recommendations will require more specific indicators. Oral feeding is always preferable, but if oral feeding is contraindicated, or if it is inadequate for increased needs, nutrition support should be initiated as soon as possible.[78]

Nitrogen balance, measures of muscle catabolism, serum proteins, liver enzymes, hematopoetic function tests, and immunological competence assays and electrolyte panels are all potentially useful data that should be considered in concert, due to the impact of liver disease on systemic function.[160,161] Because hypoglycemic events are common in liver disease, blood glucose should be continually monitored. Renal function must be monitored periodically through both biochemical indicators and urinary output.[162] Fecal fat should be assessed in steatorrhea, and if possible, levels of fat-soluble vitamins should be determined.[163] In alcoholic patients, the water-soluble vitamins should be assayed, along with measures of serum zinc, iron, copper, and oxidative stress, when possible.[164] Because of the dangers of supplementation in this population, it is not advisable to routinely recommend vitamin A, copper, and iron. Individual nutrients should be supplemented on an as-needed basis to correct deficiency or to improve antioxidant status.[165]

Fluid and electrolyte monitoring is especially important with ascites. Sodium restrictions are indicated in ascites and peripheral edema.[166] The restriction should be graded to the level of fluid retention, diuretic administration, and urinary output. Generally, mild to moderate restrictions of <2 g of sodium per day are initiated, then amended over time. Fluids may be restricted if hemodilution is evidenced by rapid, precipitous drops in plasma proteins over short-term sequential laboratory measurements. Alternately, sudden shifts in electrolyte panel values may indicate the need for fluid restrictions (electrolyte). Otherwise, fluids should initially be liberal (>1.5 l) and amended as needed. If a potassium-sparing diuretic is used for edema, potassium levels must be monitored and salt substitutes are avoided.[167]

Metabolic state should be assessed, and in the event of hypercatabolism the calculation of energy requirements for dry weight should be multiplied by mild stress factors.[168] Comorbid conditions or surgery compound this effect and therefore the stress factor is increased to 1.5–1.75 times the basal energy expenditure calculations. Metabolic carts provide useful data in this regard, but are not often available for use in the clinical setting. Overfeeding in this population can worsen steatosis, so the provision of excess energy should be avoided.[95]

Protein recommendations for this population are still controversial. The consensus is that total protein should not be restricted, but supplementation or restriction of specific amino acids in ESLD and hepatic encephalopathy remains contentious. Guidelines provided by the American Society for Parenteral and Enteral Nutrition Evidence suggest that BCAA-enriched formula should only be used if the patient is unresponsive to pharmacotherapy.[169] The Canadian Society for Parenteral and Enteral Nutrition guidelines state that there is insufficient evidence to make recommendations for BCAA use.[170] However, recent evidence points to the contrary. Several studies have reevaluated the evidence that support the use of BCAA in hepatic failure and encephalopathy.[171,172] Reexamination of data collected regarding restriction of AAA and supplementation with BCAA has shown value in decreasing the progression of hepatic failure and improvements in function in patients. In the case of ESLD and encephalopathy, BCAA should be increased and AAA decreased in the admixture or in the modular formulations. Use of enteral products that have been specifically formulated for hepatic disease is another option for both tube feeding and p.o. supplementation.[173] Specialized enteral formulas are enriched with BCAA and have a high caloric density, which is utilized for the hypercatabolic, fluid-restricted patient. BCAA may provide enough calories to prevent catabolism of body proteins, will alter the ratio of BCAA:AAA, and increase competitive carriage across the BBB, decreasing abnormalities in neurotransmission and thus improving hepatic encephalopathy.[174] It must be noted however that the results of clinical trials of both intravenous (IV) and enteral BCAA administration in acute and chronic encephalopathy are mixed and more research into cost efficacy is required. For hypercatabolic patients without encephalopathy, total protein should be given at ranges of 1.2–1.5 g/kg dry body weight (DBW)/day. Encephalopathic patients may benefit from the provision of 1.2 g/kg DBW/day protein, with the bulk as BCAA.[175] The protein requirements increase with transplant, surgery, sepsis, and number of comorbid conditions.[176]

Fat should represent 30% of calories with medium-chain triglycerides used in steatorrhea and malabsorption. The exceptions are retroviral therapy-induced hepatosteatosis, and alcoholic hepatitis, as there has been evidence to suggest that long-chain saturated fatty acids may actually be beneficial to the reduction of hepatotoxicity by their ability to alter fatty acid metabolism.[177] Carbohydrate should make up the difference. Dysregulation of glycemic control and the inability for the damaged hepatocyte to metabolize carbohydrate and glycogen make monitoring of glycemic response critical. If carbohydrate is poorly tolerated, fat can be increased slightly, but levels over 40% of calories should be avoided in this population.[178]

In Wilson's disease, management involves chelation of copper and the administration of zinc. Foods containing significant levels of copper should be avoided; a listing of high copper foods can be found in Table 13.7. Zinc acetate is administered at 150 mg/day.[127] There has also been evidence from animal models that administration of excess histidine may lower copper levels and normalize hepatic enzymes, and soy protein may do the opposite.[179,180] In hemochromatosis, chelation and low iron diets are recommended. Patients may require education regarding the use of cast iron skillets, acid-enhancing iron absorption, and the iron content of common foods.[181]

In NASH, especially if the patient is ambulatory, diabetic, obese, and has dyslipidemic profiles, energy-controlled, low fat, moderate carbohydrate diet is advised. A high-fiber diet

---

TABLE 13.7
Foods Containing High Levels of Copper[a]

Food Groups	High Copper Content per Serving	Food Groups	High Copper Content per Serving
Meats	Organ meats	Starches	Dried peas, beans, lentils
	Lamb, pork		Sweet potato
Poultry	Game birds		Millet, barley
Fish	Shellfish		Wheat germ and bran
Meat substitutes	Soy, gelatin	Fruits, vegetables	Mushrooms
	Nuts, seeds		Dried fruits
Miscellaneous	Yeast extracts, Marmite		Avocado
	Instant breakfast beverages	Desserts, sugars	Cocoa, chocolate, licorice

[a]Copper content of foods varies greatly depending on soil conditions, geographical origin, contaminants, processing techniques, and water table conditions. Copper estimates are highly variable.

Source: From Leiber, C.S., in *Modern Nutrition in Health and Disease*, 9th ed., Shils, M.E. and Olson, J.A., Eds., Lippincott, Williams & Wilkins, Baltimore, MD, 1999, pp. 1177–1179 (Appendix A-23a).

plan is recommended. Administration of antioxidants, such as vitamins E and C, has been shown to be helpful in decreasing the progression of fibrotic disease.[165]

Acute liver disease is not usually accompanied by malnutrition, and upon resolution is unremarkable in terms of nutritional consequences. Patients should be managed as hypercatabolic with the provision of increased calories, protein, and water-soluble vitamins during the preicteric and icteric phases. Cryptogenic chronic liver disease should be managed as ESLD and hepatic carcinoma must be attended to as both ESLD and cancer, with the specific chemotherapeutic agents used as the determinant of nutritional therapy.[182] In surgical resection, immunocompetence and wound healing require careful consideration of zinc levels in addition to increased caloric needs and prolonged periods of poor intake and days NPO. Nutrition support in these patients must be monitored for signs of refeeding syndrome, overfeeding, and further steatosis. Early initiation of permissive underfeeding may be appropriate for these patients.[183]

Osteopenia is critical to the discussion of liver disease. Prolonged bed rest, loss of lean body mass, malnutrition, alcohol intake, increased calcium excretion, hormonal imbalance affecting calcium homeostasis worsen the already existing deficits incurred by hepatic failure to activate vitamin D and regulate the cell signals involved in calcium absorption, transport, and assimilation. Calcium, vitamin D, and vitamin K must be monitored closely. Supplementation must be carefully undertaken in this population as the risk for toxicity is high.[184]

Comorbid renal failure in the hepatic patient takes precedence in terms of nutritional management. Renal restrictions should be implemented and additional changes made to accommodate the consequences of liver failure. Chronic liver disease with or without comorbid conditions may result in multiple organ-system failure. Nutritional management in these cases is both critical and difficult.[185]

Transplant and chemotherapy patients must be carefully followed to ensure adherence to nutritional management and food safety guidelines. Calorically dense, nutrient-dense, cold, palatable foods are indicated in nausea, vomiting, and anorexia. Small frequent meals, liquids between meals, and snacks throughout the day are indicated in early satiety. Oral supplementation is preferable if possible. Risk of infection often contraindicates other routes of nutrient administration. Well-washed bottled water and thoroughly cooked foods are some considerations for food safety. Consistent monitoring and educational reinforcement is important for this population.[186]

Hepatic disease and its management also involve a discussion of supplementation, herbal use, and toxicity from ingested naturally occurring or chemically formulated compounds. Hepatotoxicity can result from supplement poisoning, either accidental or through megadosing. Certain herbal preparations have been associated with hepatic consequences. Certain poisonous mushrooms, seaweed, plants, and berries incur severe acute hepatic failure or hepatorenal syndrome. Alternatively, specific herbal and supplement use has been shown to be effective in the treatment of hepatic disease. Patients should be monitored for supplement and herbal use.

ALTERNATIVE TREATMENTS

S-adenosyl methionine (SAM-e), milk thistle (silymarin, silibinin, silybin), turmeric, green tea, betaine, and glycyrrhizin (licorice root derivative) have been used for the treatment of hepatic diseases. There has been considerable interest in these compounds from the pharmacological standpoint, as their mechanisms of action remain unclear, despite their seeming efficacy and a concomitant rise in use. Thirty percent of hepatic outpatients reported herbal use and among transplant recipients, use was estimated as 20%.[187,188]

SAM-e is an intermediary in methionine metabolism. It is a methyl donor, which partici-pates in a host of reactions involving numerous enzymes, metabolic pathways, and is the precursor for glutathione, a potent antioxidant. The liver is the primary site of the intermediate metabolism involving methyl donation, and a by-product of the use of SAM-e is homocysteine and its precursors and metabolites. Homocysteine is a potent oxidant and has implications in a variety of disease states, most notably vascular disease. Homocysteine metabolites include betaine, cystathionine, methylglycine, and polyamines through cyanocobalamine and tetra-hydrofolate mediation.[189] SAM-e also controls activation and utilization of folate through allosteric feedback. SAM-e utilization is increased in recovery from tissue injury.[190]

In chronic liver disease, methionine metabolism is impaired and failure is due to low methionine adenosyltransferase (MAT) levels. Increasing oxidative stress in the form of nitrous oxide levels and reactive oxygen species inactivate MAT types I and III. This inactivation is reversible, but requires glutathione, the end product of methionine:homocys-teine metabolism, whose intermediary metabolism requires SAM-e.[191] This condition has implications in hepatocarcinogenesis, hepatitis, cirrhosis, secondary cholestasis (such as in cholestasis of pregnancy), fibrosis, nonalcoholic steatosis, alcoholic liver injury, and acute hepatic injury.[192] Hepatocellular recovery and regeneration are dependent on the appropriate expression and activation of MAT subtypes, which require SAM-e. SAM-e may decrease risk from further morbidity and mortality in hepatic patients.[193,194]

Methionine cannot be directly administered to patients as a result of dysregulation of the intermediary metabolism. SAM-e administration does not have the same potential for tox-icity and therefore has been shown to conditionally replace the need for methionine, and decrease the wasting of pyridoxine, cyanocobalamin, and tetrahydrofolate. SAM-e's influ-ence on glutathione and its allosteric control also make it suitable for combating the effects of ethanol in terms of oxidative stress and the toxicity of the intermediate acetaldehyde on hepatocytes. Ethanol depresses glutathione, acetaldehyde increases the level of reactive oxygen species, and fatty acid peroxidation increases with continued ingestion of alcohol. Administration of SAM-e despite claims of poor intrahepatic uptake was associated with attenuation of ethanol-induced oxidative stress and pathogenic cell membrane alter-ations.[195,196] Dosages for adults are 400–800 mg/day, and SAM-e has also been purported to be useful in promoting joint health and emotional well-being.

Milk thistle (silymarin, sililibin, silybin) has been used in the treatment of liver disorders. A member of the daisy family, the seeds are high in flavones, including silybin, betaine, and linolenic and linoleic acids. The compounds are not water soluble and their absorption is purportedly low. The constituents are excreted via biliary routes. These flavinols decrease liver enzymes, alter histology of hepatocytes, decrease fibrosis, and improve functional capacity of many specific liver cells (including Kupffer's cells). Milk thistle's active constitu-ents may improve intercellular regulation mechanisms, which are protective for acute injury. The effects are thought to be mediated via decreased lipid peroxidation, decreased overall oxidative stress, protection against glutathione depletion, inhibition of lipoxygenase, and the concomitant decrease in the formation of leukotrienes from hepatocytic membrane polyun-saturated fatty acids as well as other anti-inflammatory processes.[197,198]

Milk thistle displays hepatoprotective properties in both acute and chronic liver disease states. Cellular, animal, and clinical data point to utility in administration of milk thistle for accidental or intentional poisoning by known hepatotoxins. Animal studies appear to suggest protection against fetal alcohol syndrome damage. Cellular studies have evidenced protection against environmental contaminant hepatotoxicity and clinical studies have shown benefit for patients with chronic liver disease with few side effects. Preliminary clinical studies have found that silymarin improves liver function tests and symptomatology in chronic viral hepatitis, but not acute viral infection.[199] The results for silymarin seem to be dependent on etiological considerations as well as acuity.

In a randomized controlled trial of silymarin in cirrhotic patients, results suggested that mortality rates were reduced regardless of the etiological basis, but the effects were more pronounced in alcoholic cirrhosis.[200] In clinical trials with nonhuman primates (baboons), alcoholic induction of hepatic fibrosis was decreased with the administration of silymarin. Measures of specific markers of hepatic fibrosis (collagen type I factors) were used in the evaluation of the effects of supplementation under controlled conditions. Morphological and biochemical parameters evidence hepatoprotective effects over time.[201]

Decreased gastrointestinal absorption and poor bioavailability of silymarin confound many studies. Silybin as a lipophilic phosphatidylcholine complex was absorbed well and retained in circulation at higher concentrations. While without known major side effects, milk thistle may have laxative properties in high doses. The standard dose for an adult is 250–900 mg/day in two to three divided doses.[197,202] Because of absorption issues, the active ingredients should be evaluated on product labels and the supplement should be taken with a mixed meal. Patients should be asked about supplement usage as it has been reported that approximately 30% of patients use "alternative agents," most commonly milk thistle preparations of unknown composition.[203] Patients must also be advised of the potential for herb–medication interactions. There has been concern regarding silymarin and its interference with interferon and ribavarin therapies for hepatitis.[204]

Turmeric (*Curcuma longa*), a member of the ginger family, is thought to have hepatoprotective effects and anti-inflammatory properties. Curcumin (diferuloylmethane) and the volatile oils in turmeric are thought to be the active constituents. They are poorly absorbed and their bioavailability is questionable. Toxicity is low, they have antioxidant effects *in vitro*, and animal studies have shown moderate antihepatotoxigenic effects. The polyphenolics present in green tea (*Camellia sinensis*) are thought to be the active constituents. Absorption of these compounds is dose-dependent. Hepatoprotective effects are thought to be mediated via antioxidant potential afforded by the catechins in green tea. Catechins have been used in the treatment of acute and chronic hepatitis and hepatocarcinogenesis in animal models with some success, although further research is needed in this area. Toxicity risks are low, but patients must be advised to consume decaffeinated green tea solids. Pepper may enhance the activity of green tea polyphenols. Licorice root (glycyrrhizin, glycyrrhin, *Glycyrrhiza glabra*) has been known to have antitussive, expectorant, laxative, and anti-inflammatory effects. The active constituents include flavinoids, isoflavones, coumarins, phytosterols, and triterpenoids. The constituents are metabolized hepatically and excretion is biliary. They act as free-radical scavengers in a wide array of cellular subtypes, increase the activity of cytochrome P-450 in phase I detoxification and have antiviral activity *in vivo*. Oral dosing may be beneficial in patients with viral hepatitis (acute and chronic). Dosages of the tincture for adults are 750 mg/day, or 7.5 g of the crude root. Toxicity effects include pseudoaldosteronism. Licorice is contraindicated with many other medications and in persons with histories of hypertension, renal disease, portal or pulmonary hypertension. Patients should be educated regarding the use of licorice root.[205,206]

Betaine is a naturally occurring by-product of methionine and choline metabolism in cycles mediated by SAM-e. NASH and misclassified cryptogenic cirrhosis, where a central role for lipoperoxidation has been postulated, may benefit from betaine administration, due to its ability to increase levels of SAM-e, and thus protect from the progression of steatohepatitis in these patients. Pilot studies have shown promise in terms of betaine administration for NASH patients with limited adverse events.[207] A good deal of research must be done in this area, before any recommendations regarding betaine can be made. Other experimental approaches have been used in the treatment of liver diseases and its complications, and will be briefly addressed in the following section.

EXPERIMENTAL THERAPIES

In the areas of surgical procedures for liver disease, drug treatment of specific aspects of liver disease, transplantation, treatment for the symptomatology and complications of the disease as well as in the arena of hepatorenal syndrome and multiple organ-system failure, the advents have been too far reaching to be covered with any great depth in this section. Specific technical information regarding surgical procedures, pharmaceutical trials, advances in transplantation, and critical illness management are best acquired through their respective peer-reviewed journals. However, a brief overview of select novel approaches includes the use of photoablation (also known as radio frequency and radio-frequency thermal ablation) of cancerous tissue, where surgical procedures rely on focused near infrared light to penetrate tumor sites. This procedure is directed specifically at abnormal tissue and does not harm surrounding viable cells.[208–210]

Drugs under investigation for the treatment of hepatocellular carcinoma include irinotecan, gemcitabine, oxaliplatin, and related chemotherapeutic agents.[211,212] Colchicines are tested for the treatment of PBC when ursodiol and methotrexate prove ineffective.[213,214] Regimens for both viral hepatitis treatment, and HIV or AIDS treatment have been experimentally combined and administered jointly, as the two coinfections have dissimilar manifestations and consequences.[215] It is important to advise patients on HAART about the dyslipidemic effects of the therapy and the impact it has on liver function.

Acupuncture may be useful in hepatic disease if not for the etiological conditions then for pain, symptoms, and complications of the disease.[216] Light banks and ocular phototherapy is tested for the pruritus of liver disease, which due to the mediation by melanin may offer significant relief to a population at risk for suicide from this symptom.[217] Photo banks may also offer emotional benefits to patients. Cocoa extract has been tested in animal models as antioxidants for alcohol-induced hepatic injury. The authors suggest that dietary flavinols such as in cocoa may be of benefit in preventing early fatty infiltration of hepatocytes induced by ethanol intake.[218] Holistic approaches to treatment should always be discussed with the patient and the family.

INDUCTION BY HEPATOTOXIC COMPOUNDS

Hepatic injury includes the induction of the process by hepatotoxic agents, such as naturally occurring poisons, ethanol, certain medications, herbal preparations, environmental contaminants, and incidental contaminants in the food or water supply.

Evaluation of herbal products faces problems in terms of standardization, the use of mixed extracts, differences in harvesting, preparing, and extracting components as well as a dearth in information regarding the activity of the individual compounds in the mixture. Safety and dosage are issues as well. Numerous reports of the toxic effects of herbal remedies have been filed, and hepatotoxicity is the most frequently cited adverse effect.[219] Proven hepatotoxic herbal preparations include chaparral, kava kava, comfrey, and germander.[220–222] In addition, some cases of hepatotoxicity from herbal preparations have resulted from heavy metal contamination of the product or incorrect storage, leading to poisonous fungal growth and microbial toxin production on the material before processing.[219] Poisonous mushrooms, such as the *Amanita phalloides* (death cap mushroom), and other fungi evidence acute severe hepatotoxic effects upon ingestion in minute amounts.[223]

Herbal preparations can also interact with medications or alcohol and result in hepatotoxic effects. Licorice root, for example, may potentate corticosteroid actions. Ethanol and drug metabolites and their influence on the etiology or progression of hepatic disease are of concern in clinical practice. Patients may not be forthcoming with information regarding ethanol or herbal remedy use.[224] A workshop hosted by the National Center for Natural Product Research, the Food and Drug Administration (FDA), and the National Center for Food Safety and Nutrition (NCFSAN) resulted in a protocol for the determination of hepatotoxicity with dietary supplements. The research recommendations described will require intensive effort and cross validation through multiple laboratories. This process has been projected to be costly and not likely to be undertaken by the botanical supplement industry.[225]

1. Describe the indicators of pathophysiology in this patient and their relative significance to the diagnostic and treatment considerations.

Liver function tests show abnormalities consistent with a flare up of hepatitis, which may be due to increasing titers of HCV or the impact of regular alcohol consumption in an already compromised HCV carrier. Fluid shifts are apparent from the physical examination and laboratory values, with epigastric distention, edema, and low-protein levels. Nausea, vomiting, diarrhea, epigastric pain, and hepatomegaly are all consistent with hepatitis. Steatorrhea is evident from the medical history. All symptomatology is consistent with hepatitis and the inability of the liver to function with increasing inflammation.

2. Develop a nutritional treatment plan, educational strategies, and a follow-up protocol for this patient.

Current intake is low in kilocalories, protein, and micronutrients. Poor oral intake may further compromise the patient and extend the duration of the flare-up. Since hepatitis resolution is thought to occur in the vast majority of patients in a relatively short period of time, acute treatment recommendations are appropriate.

Cold palatable foods should be introduced. Highly caloric supplements, moderate in protein and lower in micronutrients such as iron should be given with low-fat ice cream, yogurt, or sorbet. If nausea is present, dry bland foods should be encouraged. Alcohol intake should be eliminated. Patient should be instructed regarding easily digested energy and nutrient-dense food consumption, small frequent meals, liquids taken between meals, and lower fat food substitutions.

Until inflammation and consequent symptoms subside, oral supplementation with a palatable, well-tolerated product should be implemented two to three times per day, between meals. Patient should be closely monitored for improvements in liver function tests, increases in protein status indicators, increases in body weight, and amelioration of overt symptoms such as anorexia, nausea, vomiting, and steatorrhea.[226]

Upon resolution of hepatitis, patient education should include low-fat diet planning, nutrient-dense food choices, and information regarding alcohol use and liver function. Patient should be followed long term for adherence.

3. List alternative treatments or prophylaxes which may be contraindicated in this individual and list those which may be beneficial for this patient. Explain why.

Pepto-Bismol should not be used due to its potential for interacting with medications containing salicylates and decreasing the absorption of micronutrients such as the divalent ions through depression of gastric acid changes in oxidation state.

Milk thistle should be avoided until resolution of hepatitis as it has not been shown to impact acute viral hepatitis outcome and has been shown to cause diarrhea in some patients.

Generic high-potency multivitamins should be avoided until resolution of hepatitis to decrease stress on hepatocytes. Iron, copper, zinc, and the fat-soluble vitamins in high doses may adversely affect hepatocytes during recovery.

SAM-e may offer some protective effects without confounding side effects such as diarrhea seen with milk thistle and has shown promise in acute hepatitis.

Green tea may be an appropriate recommendation for increasing antioxidant capacity, thus reducing damage to hepatocytes without substantial side effects.

CASE STUDY

Client name: Paul K.
Age: 40
Gender: Male
Current body weight: 220 lb
Height: 6′2
Waist to hip ratio: 1.7
Blood pressure: 130/70
Pulse: 122
Temperature: 100.1
Respiration: 82

Current medications and supplements: Pepto-Bismol as needed; Milk thistle 2 tsp once a day
Smoking status: Current: one pack per week when drinking; Lifetime: ten packs per year
Ethanol intake: Six 12 oz dark beers × 3 days per week × 12 months per year × 22 years
No known family history of gastrointestinal or other disease states. No known food or drug allergies.

CC: Lower epigastric pain, nausea, vomiting, diarrhea, anorexia

History: 40-year-old male with intermittent epigastric pain, unintentional weight loss of 15 lb within past 6 months, poor appetite, frequent nausea, and diarrhea, with foul smelling, loose and oily stools on a daily basis. Vomiting is intermittent and not attributable to ingestion of specific foods, time of day is variable, does not resolve with administration of Pepto-Bismol.

Past medical history: Patient is positive for hepatitis C virus (HCV). Patient has had chronic carrier status for HCV since 1980. Titers of immunoglobulin have been low and three rounds of interferon were administered in 1994 after a liver biopsy showed minor steatosis. No further treatment was deemed necessary at that time.

PHYSICAL EXAMINATION

Skin: Smooth, warm, dry, mild pitting edema
Peripheral vascular: Pulse +2 bilaterally, warm, mild pitting edema
Abdomen: Distended, epigastric tenderness, mild hepatomegaly, spleen not enlarged, borborygmus

NUTRITIONAL HISTORY

Usual dietary intake (prior to onset of symptomatology):
Breakfast: 16 oz of espresso and foamed milk (1% fat)
    Two cups total raisin bran
    One cup 1% milk
    One banana

Lunch: 16 oz apple juice
   One apple
   One pear
   Ham, turkey or roast beef and cheese sandwich:
      Two slices 12 grain bread
      Mustard
      Two slices low-fat Swiss cheese
      Four slices lean meat
      Sliced tomato ($\times$3)
      Arugula — quantity unknown
      Alfalfa sprouts — quantity unknown
Dinner: 16 oz water
   One skinless grilled chicken breast or grilled salmon steak or sirloin steak
   Two cups steamed broccoli or green beans or asparagus
   Dinner salad:
      One cup spring mix lettuces
      Six to eight cherry tomatoes
      One red bell pepper
      Half cucumber
      Three scallions
      One eighth cup croutons
      3 tsp low fat, reduced calorie blue cheese dressing
      Two cups fresh mixed berries or other fruits

CURRENT 24-H RECALL

Breakfast: 8 oz of espresso and foamed milk (1% fat)
   One slice dry toast — whole wheat
   Multivitamin 1 tsp once a day (Centrum high potency)
   Milk thistle 2 tsp once a day; unknown dosage
Lunch: 6 oz ginger ale
   Half banana
   Pepto-Bismol
Dinner: 6 oz ginger ale
   One slice dry toast
   Half a cup farina cooked cereal

BIOCHEMICAL INDICES UPON ADMISSION

Albumin: 2.2 g/dl (L)	Total protein: 5.0 g/dl (L)
Prealbumin: 15 mg/dl (L)	Transferrin: 175 mg/dl (L)
BUN: 26 mg/dl (H)	Ammonia: 33 μmol/l (H)
ALT: 77 U/L (H)	AST: 140 U/L (H)
AlkP: 266 U/L (H)	LDH: 720 U/L (H)

REVIEW QUESTIONS

1. Describe the functions of the normal liver in terms of homeostatic control, macro- and micronutrient metabolism, detoxification capacity, and cellular regulatory capabilities.

2. Describe the epidemiological considerations in alcoholic, chronic, and acute liver diseases.
3. List the anthropometric, biochemical, morphological, clinical, and nutritional indicators of liver diseases. Explain their relative significance in terms of diagnostic criteria and treatment modalities.
4. Illustrate how disruption of normal hepatocytic function results in systemic complications, which in turn result in comorbid conditions over time. Detail the nature of these comorbid conditions.
5. Explain the premises behind nutritional management of the following: acute nonviral hepatitis, alcoholic hepatitis, viral hepatitis, cirrhosis, ESLD, encephalopathy, cholestatic liver disease, Wilson's disease, and hemochromatosis.
6. Describe the major alternative and experimental therapies available for the treatment of liver diseases.
7. Describe the induction of hepatotoxicity by exposure to toxins, drugs, herbs, alcohol, and environmental contaminants.

REFERENCES

1. Sheir, D., Butler, J., and Lewis, R., *Hole's Essentials of Human Anatomy and Physiology*, McGraw-Hill, New York, NY, 2003, pp. 137–199.
2. Porth, C., *Pathophysiology*, 6th ed., Lippincott, Williams & Wilkins, Baltimore, MD, 2002, pp. 859–861.
3. Leiber, C., *Medical and Nutritional Complications of Alcoholism*, Plenum Press, New York, 1992, pp. 1–24.
4. Porth, C., *Pathophysiology*, 6th ed., Lippincott, Williams & Wilkins, Baltimore, MD, 2002, pp. 869–879.
5. Stryer, L., *Biochemistry*, 4th ed., Freeman Publishing, New York, 1995, pp. 464–500.
6. Leiber, C.S., Nutrition in liver disorders, in *Modern Nutrition in Health and Disease*, Shils, M.E. and Olson, J.A., Eds., Lippincott, Williams & Wilkins, Baltimore, MD, 1999, pp. 1177–1179.
7. Brody, T., *Nutritional Biochemistry*, 3rd ed., Elsevier, Philadelphia, PA, 1998, pp. 312–344.
8. Leiber, C.S., Nutrition in liver disorders, in *Modern Nutrition in Health and Disease*, Shils, M.E. and Olson, J.A., Eds., Lippincott, Williams & Wilkins, Baltimore, MD, 1999, pp. 1180–1189.
9. Porth, C., *Pathophysiology*, 6th ed., Lippincott, Williams & Wilkins, Baltimore, MD, 2002, pp. 879–884.
10. Leiber, C., *Medical and Nutritional Complications of Alcoholism*, Plenum Press, New York, 1992, pp. 37–44.
11. Katzung, B., *Basic and Clinical Pharmacology*, McGraw-Hill, New York, NY, 2003, pp. 36–57.
12. Braunwald, E., Ed., *Harrison's Principles of Internal Medicine*, 15th ed., McGraw-Hill, New York, NY, 2001, pp. 2579–2587.
13. Braunwald, E., Ed., *Harrison's Principles of Internal Medicine*, 15th ed., McGraw-Hill, New York, NY, 2001, pp. 2562–2566, 2707–2785.
14. Accessed June 1994. www.cdc.gov
15. Fried, V.M., Prager, K., MacKay, A.P., and Xia, H., Chartbook on trends in the health of Americans in *Health, United States, 2003*, National Center for Health Statistics, Hyattsville, MD, 2003, pp. 137–139.
16. Fried, V.M., Prager, K., MacKay, A.P., and Xia, H., Chartbook on trends in the health of Americans in *Health, United States, 2003*, National Center for Health Statistics, Hyattsville, MD, 2003, pp. 136–137.
17. www.cdc.gov/nchs (accessed June 1994).
18. www.cdc.gov/nchs/nvss (accessed June 1994).
19. www.cdc.gov/nchs (accessed June 1994).
20. National Center for Health Statistics, *National Vital Statistics Reports*, Vol. 52, No. 13, NCHS, Hyattsville, MD, 2004.
21. www.cdc.gov/nchs (accessed June 1994).
22. Lucas, J.W., Schiller, J.S., and Benson, V.E., Summary health statistics for United States adults in *National Health Interview Survey, 2001*, National Center for Health Statistics, Hyattsville, MD, *Vital Health Stat.*, 10(218), 28, 2004.

23. Schoenborn, C.A., Adams, P.F., Barnes, P.M., Vickery, J.L., and Schiller, J.S., *Health Behaviors of Adults: United States, 1999–2001*, National Center for Health Statistics, Hyattsville, MD, *Vital Health Stat.*, 10(219), 11, 2004.
24. www.niaaa.nih.gov (accessed June 1994).
25. http://etoh.niaaa.nih.gov/(accessed June 1994).
26. http://aspe.hhs.gov/datacncl/DataDir (accessed June 1994).
27. Flores, D.A. and Aranda-Michel, J., Nutritional management of acute and chronic liver disease, *Semin. Gastrointest. Dis.*, 13, 169, 2002.
28. Hoyumpa, A.M. et al., Hepatic encephalopathy, *Gastroenterology*, 76, 184, 1979.
29. Bergheim, I. et al., Nutritional deficiencies in German middle-class male alcohol consumers: relation to dietary intake and severity of liver disease, *Eur. J. Clin. Nutr.*, 57, 437, 2003.
30. Mira, L. et al., Evidence for free radical generation due to NADH oxidation by aldehyde oxidase during ethanol metabolism, *Arch. Biochem. Biophys.*, 318, 53, 1995.
31. You, M. and Crabb, D.W., Recent advances in alcoholic liver disease. Minireview: molecular mechanism of alcoholic fatty liver, *Am. J. Physiol.*, 287, 1, 2004.
32. Cabre, E. and Gasull, M.A., Nutritional aspects of liver disease and transplantation, *Curr. Opin. Clin. Nutr. Metab. Care*, 4, 581, 2001.
33. Allard, J.P., Other disease associations with non-alcoholic fatty liver disease, *Res. Clin. Gastroenterol.*, 16, 783, 2002.
34. Andersen, T., Gluud, C., Franzmann, M.B., and Christoffersen, P., Hepatic effects of dietary weight loss in morbidly obese subjects, *J. Hepatol.*, 12, 224, 1991.
35. Ishak, K.G., Zimmerman, H.J., and Ray, M.B., Alcoholic liver disease: pathologic, pathogenic and clinical aspects, *Alcohol Clin. Exp. Res.*, 15, 45, 1991.
36. Roongpisuthipong, C. et al., Nutritional assessment in various stages of liver cirrhosis, *Nutrition*, 17, 761, 2001.
37. McGuire, B.M. and Bloomer, J.R., Complications of cirrhosis. Why they occur and what to do about them, *Postgrad. Med.*, 103, 209, 1998.
38. Abou-Assi, S. and Vlahcevic, Z.R., Hepatic encephalopathy: metabolic consequence of cirrhosis often is reversible, *Postgrad. Med.*, 109, 52, 2001.
39. Pagana, K.D. and Pagana, T.J., *Manual of Diagnostic and Laboratory Tests*, Mosby Publishing, St. Louis, MO, 2002.
40. Uchida, T. et al., Alcoholic foamy degeneration — a pattern of acute alcoholic injury of the liver, *Gastroenterology*, 84, 683, 1983.
41. Figuicredo, F.A. et al., Utility of standard nutritional parameters in detecting body cell mass depletion in patients with end stage liver disease, *Liver Transpl.*, 6, 575, 2000.
42. Baker, H. et al., Cobalamin (vitamin B12) and holotranscobalamin changes in plasma and liver tissues in the alcoholic with liver disease, *J. Am. Coll. Nutr.*, 17, 235, 1998.
43. Carrera, G. et al., Hepatic metallothionine in patients with chronic hepatitis C: relationship with severity of liver disease and response to treatment, *Am. J. Gastroenterol.*, 98, 1142, 2003.
44. Clark, J.M., Brarncati, F.L., and Diehl, A.M., The prevalence and etiology of elevated aminotransferase levels in the United States, *Am. J. Gastroenterol.*, 98, 960, 2003.
45. Ikemoto, M. et al., A useful ELISA system for human liver-type arginase, and its utility in diagnosis of liver diseases, *Clin. Biochem.*, 34, 455, 2001.
46. Johnson, D.E., Special considerations in interpreting liver function tests, *Am. Fam. Phys.*, 15, 2223, 1999.
47. Bell, S.A., Faust, H., and Schmidt, A., Auto antibodies to C-reactive protein and other acute phase proteins in systemic autoimmune disease, *Clin. Exp. Immunol.*, 113, 327, 1998.
48. Wendland, B.E., Nutritional guidelines for persons infected with the hepatitis virus: a review of the literature, *Can. J. Diet. Pract. Res.*, 62, 7, 2001.
49. Shione, Y. et al., Iron accumulation in the liver of male patients with Wilson's disease, *Am. J. Gastroenterol.*, 96, 3147, 2001.
50. Kang, J.O., Chronic iron overload and toxicity: clinical chemistry perspective, *J. Am. Soc. Med. Tech.*, 14, 209, 2001.

51. Selmi, C. and Gershwin, M.E., Bacteria and human autoimmunity: the case of primary biliary cirrhosis, *Curr. Opin. Rheumatol.*, 16, 406, 2004.
52. Arnett, F.C. and Reichlin, M., Lupus hepatitis: an under-recognized disease feature associated with autoantibodies to ribosomal-P, *Am. J. Med.*, 99, 465, 1995.
53. Youssef, W.I. and Tavill, A.S., Connective tissue diseases and the liver, *J. Clin. Gastroenterol.*, 35, 345, 2002.
54. Butt, A.A., Aldridge, K.E., and Sanders, C.V., Infections related to the ingestion of seafood. Part II: parasitic infections and food safety, *Lancet Infect. Dis.*, 4, 294, 2004.
55. Singh, S. and Sivakumar, R., Recent advances in the diagnosis of leishmaniasis, *J. Postgrad. Med.*, 49, 55, 2003.
56. Stanley, S.L., Amoebiasis, *Lancet*, 361, 1025, 2003.
57. Butt, A.A., Aldridge, K.E., and Sanders, C.V., Infections related to the ingestion of seafood. Part I: viral and bacterial infections, *Lancet Infect. Dis.*, 4, 202, 2004.
58. Steingrub, J.S., Pregnancy associated severe liver dysfunction, *Crit. Care Clin.*, 20, 763, 2004.
59. Neuschwander-Tetri, B.A., Common blood tests for liver disease. Which ones are most useful? *Postgrad. Med.*, 98, 49, 1995.
60. Addolorato, G. et al., Nutritional status and body fluid distribution in chronic alcoholics compared with controls, *Alcohol Clin. Exp. Res.*, 23, 1232, 1999.
61. Boon, L. et al., Response of hepatic amino acid consumption to chronic metabolic acidosis, *Am. J. Physiol.*, 271, F198, 1996.
62. Rector, W.G., Jr., Portal hypertension: a permissive factor only in the development of ascites and variceal bleeding, *Liver*, 6, 221, 1986.
63. Buchner, A.M. and Sonnenberg, A., Co-morbid occurrence of liver and pancreatic disease in United States military veterans, *Am. J. Gastroenterol.*, 96, 2231, 2004.
64. Shiomi, S. et al., Calcitriol for bone disease in patients with cirrhosis of the liver, *J. Gastroenterol. Hepatol.*, 14, 547, 1999.
65. Lane, N.E., An update on glucocorticoid-induced osteoporosis, *Rheum. Dis. Clin. North Am.*, 27, 235, 2001.
66. Hoffman, A.F., The continuing importance of bile acids in liver and intestinal disease, *Arch. Int. Med.*, 159, 2647, 1999.
67. Preedy, V.R. et al., Protein metabolism in alcoholism. Effects on specific tissues and the whole body, *Nutrition*, 15, 604, 1999.
68. Hampel, H. et al., Risk factors for the development of renal dysfunction in hospitalized patients with cirrhosis, *Am. J. Gastroenterol.*, 96, 2006, 2001.
69. Dammacco, F., Gatti, P., and Sansonno, D., Hepatitis C virus infection mixed cryoglobulinemia and non-Hodgkin's lymphoma: an emerging picture, *Leuk. Lymphoma*, 31, 463, 1998.
70. Trean, J.C., Nutrition and liver diseases, *Curr. Gastroenterol. Rep.*, 1(4), 335, 1999.
71. Tilg, H. et al., Serum levels of cytokines in chronic liver disease, *Gastroenterology*, 103, 264, 1992.
72. Limdi, J.K. and Hyde, G.M., Evaluation of abnormal liver function tests, *Postgrad. Med. J.*, 79, 307, 2003.
73. Harrison, E.H., Lipases and carboxylesterases: possible roles in the hepatic utilization of vitamin A, *J. Nutr.*, 130, 340S, 2000.
74. Salvatore, F. et al., Multivariate discriminant analysis of biochemical parameters for the differentiation of clinically confounding liver diseases, *Clin. Chem. Acta*, 257, 41, 1997.
75. Tsuneoka, K. et al., Osteodystrophy in patients with chronic hepatitis and liver cirrhosis, *J. Gastroenterol.*, 31, 669, 1996.
76. Vitala, K. et al., Serum IgA, IgG and IgM antibodies directed against acetylaldehyde isotopes: relationship to liver disease severity and alcohol consumption, *Hepatology*, 25, 1418, 1997.
77. Halsted, C.H. et al., Metabolic interactions of alcohol and folate, *J. Nutr.*, 132, 236S, 2002.
78. Patton, K.M. and Aranda-Michel, J., Nutritional aspects in liver disease and liver transplantation, *Nutr. Clin. Pract.*, 17, 332, 2002.
79. Mehta, K. et al., Nonalcoholic fatty liver disease: pathogenesis and the role of antioxidants, *Nutr. Rev.*, 60, 289, 2002.

80. Bradley, K.A., Badrinath, S., and Bush, K., Medical risks for women who drink alcohol, *J. Gen. Intern. Med.*, 13, 627, 1998.

81. Kwo, P.Y. et al., Gender differences in alcohol metabolism: relationship to liver volume and effect for adjustment of body mass, *Gastroenterology*, 115, 1552, 1998.

82. Stranges, S. et al., Differential effects of alcohol drinking pattern on liver enzymes in men and women, *Alcohol Clin. Exp. Res.*, 28, 949, 2004.

83. Thun, M.J. et al., Alcohol consumption and mortality among middle aged and elderly US adults, *N. Engl. J. Med.*, 337, 1705, 1997.

84. White, I.R., Altman, D.R., and Nanchahal, K., Alcohol consumption and mortality: modeling risks for men and women of different ages, *BMJ*, 325, 191, 2002.

85. Smith-Warner, S.A. et al., Alcohol and breast cancer in women: a pooled analysis of cohort studies, *JAMA*, 279, 535, 1998.

86. Sarkola, T. et al., The role of the liver in the acute effects of alcohol on androgens in women, *J. Clin. Endocrinol. Metab.*, 86, 1981, 2001.

87. Purohit, V., Can alcohol promote aromatization of androgens to estrogens? A review, *Alcohol*, 22, 123, 2000.

88. Aronson, K., Alcohol: a recently identified risk factor for breast cancer, *CMJA*, 168, 1147, 2003.

89. Emmanuelle, M.A., Wezeman, F., and Emanuelle, N.V., Alcohol's effects on female reproductive function, *Alcohol Res. Health*, 26, 247, 2002.

90. Yadav, D. et al., Serum and liver micronutrient antioxidants and serum oxidative stress in patients with chronic hepatitis C, *Am. J. Gastroenterol.*, 97, 2634, 2002.

91. Yang, R. et al., Ethyl pyruvate ameliorates acute alcohol-induced liver injury and inflammation in mice, *J. Lab. Clin. Med.*, 142, 322, 2003.

92. Zhou, Z. et al., Metallothionine protection against alcoholic liver injury through inhibition of oxidative stress, *Exp. Biol. Med.*, 227, 214, 2002.

93. Leo, M.A. and Leiber, C.S., Alcohol, vitamin A and beta-carotene: adverse interactions including hepatotoxicity and carcinogenicity, *Am. J. Clin. Nutr.*, 69, 1071, 1999.

94. Klover, P.J. and Mooney, R.A., Hepatocytes: critical for glucose homeostasis, *Int. J. Biochem. Cell Biol.*, 36, 753, 2004.

95. Richardson, R.A. and Davidson, H.I., Nutritional demands in acute and chronic illness, *Proc. Nutr. Soc.*, 62, 777, 2003.

96. Leiber, C., *Medical and Nutritional Complications of Alcoholism*, Plenum Press, New York, NY, 1992, pp. 130–134.

97. Btaiche, I.F., Branched-chain amino acids in patients with hepatic encephalopathy, *Nutr. Clin. Pract.*, 18, 97, 2003.

98. Mizock, B.A., Nutritional support in hepatic encephalopathy, *Nutrition*, 15, 220, 1999.

99. Nijveldt, R.J. et al., Elimination of asymmetric dimethylarginine by the kidney and liver: a link to the development of multiple organ failure, *J. Nutr.*, 134, 2848S, 2004.

100. Mascarenhas, R. and Mobarhan, S., New support for branched-chain amino acid supplementation in advanced hepatic failure, *Nutr. Rev.*, 62, 33, 2004.

101. Trusswell, A., Australian experience with the Wernicke–Korsakoff syndrome, *Addiction*, 95, 829, 2000.

102. Butterworth, R., Effects of thiamin deficiency on brain metabolism: implications for the pathogenesis of Wernicke–Korsakoff's syndrome, *Alcohol Alcoholism*, 24, 271, 1989.

103. Ma, X. et al., Gender differences in medium chain dicarboxylic aciduria in alcoholic men and women, *Am. J. Med.*, 106, 70, 1999.

104. Shronts, E.P., Nutritional assessment of adults with end-stage hepatic failure, *Nutr. Clin. Pract.*, 3, 113, 1988.

105. Polaverapu, R. et al., Increased lipid peroxidation and impaired antioxidant enzyme function is associated with pathological liver injury in experimental alcoholic liver disease in rats fed diets high in corn oil and fish oil, *Hepatology*, 27, 1317, 1998.

106. Lieber, C.S., Alcohol and hepatitis C, *Alcohol Res. Health*, 25, 245, 2001.

107. Nair, S. et al., Obesity and female gender increases in breath ethanol concentration: potential implications for the pathogenesis of nonalcoholic steatohepatitis, *Am. J. Gastroenterol.*, 96, 1200, 2001.

108. Lieber, C.S. et al., Model of non-alcoholic steatohepatitis, *Am. J. Clin. Nutr.*, 79, 502, 2004.

109. Harrison, S.A. et al., Nonalcoholic steatohepatitis: what we know in the new millennium, *Am. J. Gastroenterol.*, 97, 2714, 2002.

110. Patch, D., Armonis, A., and Sabin, C., Single portal pressure measurement predicts survival in cirrhotic patients with recent bleeding, *Gut*, 44, 264, 1999.

111. Torres, E., Barros, P., and Calmet, F., Correlation between serum ascites albumin concentration gradient and endoscopic parameters of portal hypertension, *Am. J. Gastroenterol.*, 93, 2172, 1998.

112. Choti, M.A. et al., Trends in long-term survival following liver resection for hepatic colorectal metastases, *Ann. Surg.*, 235, 759, 2002.

113. Bach, N. et al., Methotrexate therapy for primary biliary cirrhosis, *Am. J. Gastroenterol.*, 98, 187, 2002.

114. Pronsky, Z.M. et al., *Food–Medication Interactions*, 13th ed., Food–Medication Interactions, Birchrunville, PA, 2003.

115. Brettler, S., Defenses gone awry: primary biliary cirrhosis, *RN*, 66, 38, 2003.

116. Moses, S., Pruritus, *Am. Fam. Phys.*, 68, 1135, 2003.

117. Parik-Patel, A. et al., Functional status of patients with primary biliary cirrhosis, *Am. J. Gastroenterol.*, 97, 2871, 2002.

118. Fahey, S., The experience of women with primary biliary cirrhosis: a literature review, *J. Adv. Nurs.*, 30, 506, 1999.

119. Carey, E.J., Blan, V., and Kremers, W.K., Osteopenia and osteoporosis in patients with end stage liver disease caused by hepatitis C and alcoholic liver disease: not just a cholestatic problem, *Liver Transpl.*, 9, 1166, 2003.

120. Erickson, J.M. and Mawson, A.R., Possible role of endogenous retinoid toxicity in the pathophysiology of primary biliary cirrhosis, *J. Theor. Biol.*, 206, 47, 2000.

121. Kowalski, T.E. et al., Vitamin A hepatotoxicity: a cautionary note regarding 25,000 IU supplements, *Am. J. Med.*, 97, 523, 1994.

122. Parkes, M. et al., Do steroids help jaundice caused by primary sclerosing cholangitis? *J. Clin. Gastroenterol.*, 33, 319, 2001.

123. Valla, D.C. and Benhamou, J.P., Hepatic granulomas and hepatic sarcoidosis, *Clin. Liver Dis.*, 4, 269, 2000.

124. Filipe, P. et al., Anti- and pro-oxidant effects of urate in copper induced low density lipoprotein oxidation, *Eur. J. Biochem.*, 269, 5474, 2002.

125. Farianti, F. et al., Zinc treatment prevents lipid peroxidation and increases glutathione availability in Wilson's disease, *J. Lab. Clin. Med.*, 141, 372, 2003.

126. Brewer, G.J. et al., Treatment of Wilson's disease with zinc XVI: treatment during the pediatric years, *J. Lab. Clin. Med.*, 137, 191, 2001.

127. Askari, F.K. et al., Treatment of Wilson's disease with zinc. XVII. Initial treatment of the hepatic decompensation presentation with trientine and zinc, *J. Lab. Clin. Med.*, 142, 385, 2003.

128. Motulsky, A.G. and Beutler, E., Population screening in hereditary hemochromatosis, *Ann. Rev. Pub. Health*, 21, 65, 2000.

129. Stone, A. and Schumann, L., Update on hereditary hemochromatosis, *Clin. Adv.*, 72, 74, 1999.

130. Cogswell, M.E. et al., Iron overload, public health and genetics: evaluating the evidence for hemochromatosis screening, *Ann. Int. Med.*, 129, 971, 1998.

131. Ramrakhiani, S. and Bacon, B.R., Hepatology in the new millennium: advances in viral hepatitis, hepatic disorders, and liver transplantation, *Med. Clin. North Am.*, 84, 1085, 2000.

132. Nunez, M. et al., Risk factors for severe liver toxicity following the introduction of HAART, *J. AIDS*, 27, 426, 2001.

133. Cotler, S. and Jensen, D., Treatment of hepatitis C virus and HIV co-infections, *Clin. Liver Dis.*, 5, 1046, 2001.

134. Vanltallie, T.B. and Nufert, T.H., Ketones: metabolism's ugly duckling, *Nutr. Rev.*, 61, 327, 2003.

135. Lewis, J.H., Drug-induced liver disease, *Med. Clin. North Am.*, 840, 1275, 2000.

136. Klein, C.J., Stanek, G.S., and Wiles, C.E., Overfeeding macronutrients to critically ill adults: metabolic complications, *J. Am. Diet. Assoc.*, 98, 795, 1998.
137. Chessex, P. et al., Photo-oxidation of parenteral multivitamins induces hepatic steatosis in a neonatal guinea pig model of intravenous nutrition, *Pediatr. Res.*, 52, 958, 2002.
138. Heubi, J.E. et al., Tauroursodeoxycholic acid (TUDCA) in the prevention of total parenteral nutrition-associated liver disease, *J. Pediatr.*, 141, 237, 2002.
139. Kearns, L.R. et al., Update on parenteral amino acids, *Nutr. Clin. Pract.*, 16, 219, 2001.
140. Wessely, S. and Parinate, C., Fatigue, depression and chronic hepatitis C infection, *Psychol. Med.*, 32, 1, 2002.
141. Daubioul, C. et al., Dietary fructans, but not cellulose, decreases triglyceride accumulation in the liver of obese Zucker fa/fa rats, *J. Nutr.*, 132, 967, 2002.
142. Angulo, P., Medical progress: non-alcoholic fatty liver disease, *N. Engl. J. Med.*, 346, 1221, 2002.
143. Younossi, Z.M. et al., Diabetes and non-alcoholic fatty liver disease: a worrisome combination, *Gastroenterology*, 116, 1292, 1999.
144. Perseghin, G. et al., Resting energy expenditure in diabetic and nondiabetic patients with liver cirrhosis: relation with insulin sensitivity and effect of liver transplantation and immunosuppressive therapy, *Am. J. Clin. Nutr.*, 76, 541, 2002.
145. Newton, S.E., Promoting adherence to transplant medication regimens: a review of behavioral analyses, *J. Transplant. Coord.*, 9, 13, 1999.
146. Lauer, G. and Walker, B., Hepatitis C virus infection, *N. Engl. J. Med.*, 345, 42, 2001.
147. Singer, A. et al., Role of plasmapheresis in the management of acute hepatic failure in children, *Ann. Surg.*, 234, 418, 2001.
148. Villeneuve, J.P. et al., Drug disposition in patients with HBsAg positive chronic liver disease, *Dig. Dis. Sci.*, 32, 710, 1987.
149. Roth, K. et al., Dying with end stage liver disease with cirrhosis: insights from SUPPORT. Study to Understand Prognoses and Preferences for Outcomes and Risks of Treatment, *J. Am. Geriatr. Soc.*, 48, S122, 2000.
150. Whitehead, M.W. et al., A prospective study of the causes of notably raised aspartate aminotransferase of liver origin, *Gut*, 45, 129, 1999.
151. Neuberger, J. and Bryan, S., Clinical economics review: cost effectiveness in the therapy of liver disease, *Aliment. Pharmacol. Ther.*, 11, 61, 1997.
152. Pirlich, M. et al., Bioelectrical impedance analysis is a useful bedside technique to assess malnutrition in cirrhotic patients with and without ascites, *Hepatology*, 32, 1208, 2000.
153. Gugelielmi, F.W., Mastronuzzi, T., and Pietrini, L., The RXc graph in evaluating and monitoring fluid balance in patients with liver cirrhosis, *Ann. NY Acad. Sci.*, 873, 105, 1999.
154. Plauth, M. et al., Weight gain after intrahepatic porto-systemic shunt is associated with improvement in prognostics, *J. Hepatol.*, 40, 228, 2004.
155. Kyle, U.G. et al., Reliable bioelectrical impedance analysis estimates of fat free mass in liver heart and lung transplant patients, *J. Parenter. Enteral Nutr.*, 25, 45, 2001.
156. Sokhi, R.P. et al., Bone mineral density among cirrhotic patients awaiting liver transplantation, *Liver Transpl.*, 10, 648, 2004.
157. Shiomi, S. et al., Vitamin K2 (menatetrenone) for bone loss in patients with cirrhosis of the liver, *Am. J. Gatroenterol.*, 97, 978, 2002.
158. Thorne, D. and Kaplan, K.J., Laboratory indicators of ethanol consumption, *Clin. Lab. Sci.*, 12, 343, 1999.
159. Stephenson, G.R. et al., Malnutrition in liver transplant patients: preoperative subjective global assessment is predictive of outcome after liver transplantation, *Transplantation*, 72, 666, 2001.
160. Intragumtornchai, T. et al., The role of serum ferritin in the diagnosis of iron deficiency anemia in patients with liver cirrhosis, *J. Intern. Med.*, 243, 233, 1998.
161. Veseley, D.L. et al., Hepatitis A induced diabetes mellitus, acute renal failure and liver failure, *Am. J. Med. Sci.*, 317, 419, 1999.
162. Gentilini, P., La Villa, G., and Casini-Raggi, V., Hepatorenal syndrome and its treatment today, *Eur. J. Gastroenterol. Hepatol.*, 11, 1061, 1999.

163. Phillips, J.R. et al., Fat soluble vitamin levels in patients with primary biliary cirrhosis, *Am. J. Gastroenterol.*, 96, 2745, 2001.
164. Loguercio, C. et al., Relationship of blood trace elements to liver damage, nutritional status and oxidative stress in chronic nonalcoholic liver disease, *Biol. Trace Elem. Res.*, 81, 245, 2003.
165. Harrison, S.A. et al., Vitamin E and vitamin C treatment improves fibrosis in patients with nonalcoholic steatohepatitis, *Am. J. Gastroenterol.*, 98, 2485, 2003.
166. Habib, A., Bond, W.M., and Heuman, D.M., Long-term management of cirrhosis. Appropriate supportive care is both critical and difficult, *Postgrad. Med.*, 109, 101, 2001.
167. Morrison, R.T., Edema and principles of diuretic use, *Med. Clin. North Am.*, 81, 689, 1997.
168. Matos, C. et al., Nutrition in chronic liver disease, *J. Clin. Gastroenterol.*, 35, 391, 2002.
169. Aspen Board of Directors and Clinical Guidelines Task Force, Guidelines for the use of parenteral and enteral nutrition in adult and pediatric patients, *J. Parenter. Enteral Nutr.*, 26S, 1SA, 2002.
170. Heyland, D.K., Dhaliwal, R., and Drover, J.W., Canadian Clinical Practice Guidelines for nutritional support in mechanically ventilated critically ill patients, *J. Parenter. Enteral Nutr.*, 27, 355, 2003.
171. Mascarenhas, R. and Mobarhan, S., New support for branched chain amino acid supplementation in advanced hepatic failure, *Nutr. Rev.*, 62, 33, 2004.
172. Moriwaki, H., Branched chain amino acids as a protein energy source in liver cirrhosis, *Biochem. Biophys. Res. Commun.*, 313, 405, 2004.
173. Platell, C. et al., Branched chain amino acids, *J. Gastroenterol. Hepatol.*, 15, 706, 2000.
174. Plauth, M. et al., Long term treatment of latent porto-systemic encephalopathy with branched chain amino acids. A double blind, placebo controlled crossover study, *J. Hepatol.*, 17, 308, 1993.
175. Marchesini, G. et al., Nutritional supplementation with branched chain amino acids in advanced cirrhosis: a double blind, randomized trial, *Gastroenterology*, 124, 1792, 2003.
176. Marchesini, G. et al., Nutritional treatment with branched-chain amino acids in advanced liver cirrhosis, *J. Gastroenterol.*, 35, 7, 2000.
177. Ronis, M.J. et al., Dietary saturated fat reduces alcoholic hepatotoxicity in rats by altering fatty acid metabolism and membrane composition, *J. Nutr.*, 134, 904, 2004.
178. Han, Y. et al., A balanced 5:1 carbohydrate:protein diet; a new method for supplementing protein to patients with chronic liver disease, *J. Gastroenterol. Hepatol.*, 15, 1463, 2000.
179. Xu, H. et al., Excess dietary histidine decreases the liver copper level and serum alanine aminotransferase activity in Long-Evans cinnamon rats, *Br. J. Nutr.*, 90, 573, 2003.
180. Yonezawa, K. et al., Soy protein isolate enhances hepatic copper accumulation and cell damage in LEC rats, *J. Nutr.*, 133, 1250, 2003.
181. Tandon, N. et al., Beneficial influence of an indigenous low-iron diet on serum indicators of iron status in patients with chronic liver disease, *Br. J. Nutr.*, 83, 235, 2000.
182. Riley, T.R. and Bhatti, A.M., Preventive strategies in chronic liver disease: part II, *Am. Fam. Phys.*, 64, 1735, 2001.
183. Sax, H.C. and Bower, R.H., Hepatic complications of total parenteral nutrition, *J. Parenter. Enteral Nutr.*, 12, 615, 1988.
184. Gallego-Rojo, F.J. et al., Bone mineral density and serum insulin like growth factor I and bone turnover markers in viral cirrhosis, *Hepatology*, 28, 695, 1998.
185. Palmer, B.F., Pathogenesis of ascites and renal salt retention in cirrhosis, *J. Investig. Med.*, 47, 183, 1999.
186. Cabelof, D.C., Preventing infection from food borne pathogens in liver transplant patients, *J. Am. Diet. Assoc.*, 94, 1140, 1994.
187. Schuppan, D. et al., Herbal products for liver disease: therapeutic challenge for the new millennium, *Hepatology*, 30, 1099, 1999.
188. Crone, C.C. and Wise, T.N., Survey of alternative medicine use among organ transplant patients, *J. Transplant. Coord.*, 7, 123, 1997.
189. Barak, A.J., Beckenhauer, H.C., and Tuma, D.J., Betaine, ethanol, and the liver: a review, *Alcohol*, 13, 395, 1996.
190. Leiber, C.S. and Packer, L., S-adenosyl methionine: molecular, biological and clinical aspects — an introduction, *Am. J. Clin. Nutr.*, 76, 1148S, 2002.

191. Arias-Diaz, J. et al., *S*-adenosyl methionine protects hepatocytes against the effects of cytokines, *J. Surg. Res.*, 62, 79, 1996.

192. Poli, G., Pathogenesis of liver fibrosis: role of oxidative stress, *Mol. Aspects Med.*, 21, 49, 2000.

193. Bottiglieri, T., *S*-adenosyl-L-methionine (SAM-e): from the bench to the bedside — molecular basis of a pleiotropic molecule, *Am. J. Clin. Nutr.*, 76, 1151S, 2002.

194. Martinez-Chantar, M.L. et al., Importance of deficiency in SAM-e synthesis in the pathogenesis of liver injury, *Am. J. Clin. Nutr.*, 76, 1177S, 2002.

195. Lieber, C.S., *S*-adenosyl-L-methionine: its role in the treatment of liver disorders, *Am. J. Clin. Nutr.*, 76, 1183S, 2002.

196. Carretero, M.V. et al., Inhibition of liver methionine adenosyltransferase gene expression by 3-methylcolanthrene: protective effect of *S*-adenosyl-methionine, *Biochem. Pharm.*, 61, 1119, 2001.

197. Luper, S., A review of plants used in the treatment of liver disease: part one, *Alt. Med. Rev.*, 3, 410, 1998.

198. Dehmlow, C., Erhard, J., and De Groot, H., Inhibition of Kupffer cells functions as an explanation for the hepatoprotective properties of sililibin, *Hepatology*, 23, 749, 1996.

199. Chavez, M.L., Treatment of hepatitis C with milk thistle, *J. Herbal Pharmacother.*, 1, 79, 2001.

200. Ferenci, P. et al., Randomized controlled trail of silymarin treatment in patients with cirrhosis of the liver, *J. Hepatol.*, 9, 105, 1989.

201. Lieber, C.S. et al., Silymarin retards the progression of alcohol-induced hepatic fibrosis in baboons, *J. Clin. Gastroenterol.*, 37, 336, 2003.

202. Gatti, G. and Perucca, E., Plasma concentrations of free and conjugated silybin after oral intake of siliybin–phosphatidylcholine complex (silipide) in healthy volunteers, *Int. J. Clin. Pharm. Ther.*, 32, 614, 1994.

203. Flora, K.D. et al., Milk thistle (*Silybum marianum*) for the therapy of liver disease, *Am. J. Gastroenterol.*, 93, 139, 1998.

204. Giese, L.A., Complementary healthcare practices. Milk thistle and the treatment of hepatitis, *Gastroenterol. Nurs.*, 24, 95, 2001.

205. Luper, S., A review of plants used in the treatment of liver disease: part two, *Alt. Med. Rev.*, 4, 178, 1999.

206. Giese, L.A., Complementary healthcare practices. Herbs and hepatobiliary disease, *Gastroenterol. Nurs.*, 24, 38, 2001.

207. Abdelmalek, M.F. et al., Betaine, a promising new agent for patients with non-alcoholic steatohepatitis: results of a pilot study, *Am. J. Gastroenterol.*, 9, 2711, 2001.

208. Bowles, B.J. et al., Efficacy of radiofrequency thermal ablation in advanced liver tumors, *Arch. Surg.*, 136, 864, 2001.

209. Curley, S.A. et al., Radiofrequency ablation of hepatocellular cancer in 110 patients with cirrhosis, *Ann. Surg.*, 232, 381, 2000.

210. Papadimitriou, J.D. et al., The impact of new technology on hepatic resection for malignancy, *Arch. Surg.*, 136, 1307, 2001.

211. O'Reilly, E.M. et al., A phase II study of irinotecan in patients with advanced hepatocellular carcinoma, *Cancer*, 91, 101, 2001.

212. Taieb, J. et al., Gemcitabine plus oxaliplatin for patients with advanced hepatocellular carcinoma using two different schedules, *Cancer*, 98, 2664, 2003.

213. Lee, Y.M. and Kaplan, M.M., Efficacy of colchicines in patients with primary biliary cirrhosis poorly responsive to ursodiol and methotrexate, *Am. J. Gastroenterol.*, 98, 205, 2003.

214. Jorgensen, R. et al., Results of long-term ursodiol treatment for patients with primary biliary cirrhosis, *Am. J. Gastroenterol.*, 97, 2647, 2002.

215. Nasti, G. et al., Chronic hepatitis C in HIV infection: feasibility and efficacy of interferon alfa-2b and ribavarin combination therapy, *J. AIDS*, 26, 299, 2001.

216. Li, Y. et al., The effect of acupuncture on gastrointestinal function and disorder, *Am. J. Gastroenterol.*, 87, 1372, 1992.

217. Bergasa, N.V. et al., Pilot study of bright-light therapy reflected toward the eyes for the pruritus of chronic liver disease, *Am. J. Gastroenterol.*, 96, 1563, 2001.

218. McKim, S.E. et al., Cocoa extract protects against early alcohol-induced liver injury in the rat, *Arch. Biochem. Biophys.*, 406, 40, 2002.

219. Stedman, C., Herbal hepatotoxicity, *Semin. Liver Dis.*, 22, 195, 2002.

220. Gordon, D.W. et al., Chaparral ingestion: the broadening spectrum of liver injury caused by herbal medications, *JAMA*, 273, 489, 1995.

221. Katz, M. and Sailbil, F., Herbal hepatitis: subacute hepatic necrosis secondary to chaparral leaf, *J. Clin. Gastroenterol.*, 12, 203, 1990.

222. Ridker, P.M. et al., Hepatic veno-occlusive disease associated with the consumption of pyrrolizidine-containing dietary supplements, *Gastroenterology*, 88, 1050, 1985.

223. Perron, A.D., Patterson, J.A., and Yanofsky, N.N., Kumbucha "mushroom" hepatotoxicity, *Ann. Emerg. Med.*, 26, 660, 1995.

224. Fugh-Berman, A., Herb–drug interactions, *Lancet*, 355, 134, 2000.

225. Willett, K.L., Roth, R.A., and Walker, L., Workshop overview: hepatotoxicity assessment for botanical dietary supplements, *Toxicol. Sci.*, 79, 4, 2004.

226. Bunout, D., Nutritional and metabolic effects of alcoholism: their relationship with alcoholic liver disease, *Nutrition*, 15, 583, 1999.

Nutrition and the Pancreas

M. Patricia Fuhrman, Cynthia Payne, Kelly Eiden, Nanette Steinle, and Nick Gonzalez

CONTENTS

INTRODUCTION

The pancreas is a gland located in the abdominal cavity that is essential for digestion and metabolism of macronutrients. It has both endocrine (manufacture of insulin, glucagon, and somatostatin) and exocrine (secretion of enzymes, bicarbonate, electrolytes, and protein) functions. Dysfunction of the pancreas results in malabsorption of nutrients, glucose intolerance, and aberrations of gastrointestinal (GI) secretions. Conventional treatments of pancreatic disorders include pancreatic enzyme replacement therapy, insulin therapy, diet modification (low fat for pancreatitis, carbohydrate and fat modification for diabetes), and feeding modality manipulation (specialized nutrition support including enteral nutrition (EN) and parenteral nutrition (PN)). Complementary and alternative treatments of pancreatic disorders include herbs, prebiotics and probiotics, and omega-3 fatty acids and other anti-inflammatory nutrients. When the pancreas becomes inflamed or diseased as in pancreatitis, there is an increased secretion of enzymes with altered feedback mechanisms leading to adverse sequelae (such as diarrhea and abdominal pain). This chapter will address normal pancreatic anatomy and physiology as well as diseases of the pancreas and their treatment.

ANATOMY AND PHYSIOLOGY OF THE PANCREAS

Anatomically, the pancreas is located in the upper epigastrium in the retroperitoneal area, adjacent to the duodenum, behind the stomach (Figure 14.1).[1] In the adult, the pancreas is about 10–15 cm in length (5–7 in.) with a wide head, narrow body, and tapering tail. The head of the pancreas fits tightly into the c-shaped duodenum. The superior mesenteric and hepatic arteries supply blood; the portal, splenic, and superior mesenteric veins drain the pancreas.

There are several ducts associated with the pancreas that facilitate the transport of pancreatic enzymes and enzymatic precursors into the GI tract. The dorsal duct (duct of Santorini) is located in the body and the tail of the pancreas, and the ventral duct (duct of Wirsung) is located in the head of the pancreas. The duct of Wirsung empties into the duodenum along with the common bile duct at the ampulla of Vater.

The vagus nerve innervates the pancreas.[1,2] The vagus receives stimuli from the GI tract and sends information to the brain (afferents) as well as sends stimuli back to the organs of the GI tract (efferents).[1,2] Pancreatic secretions are increased via vagal efferents when the

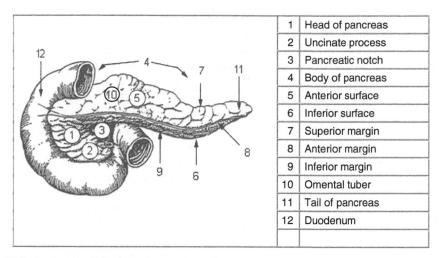

1	Head of pancreas
2	Uncinate process
3	Pancreatic notch
4	Body of pancreas
5	Anterior surface
6	Inferior surface
7	Superior margin
8	Anterior margin
9	Inferior margin
10	Omental tuber
11	Tail of pancreas
12	Duodenum

FIGURE 14.1 Anatomy of the pancreas mesenteric.
The pancreas has three main sections:

- Head: area of pancreas to right of left border of superior vein
- Body: area of pancreas between left border of superior mesenteric vein and left border of aorta
- Tail: area of pancreas between left border of aorta and hilum of spleen

The most common site of primaries is the head of the pancreas. The pancreas has two functional components: endocrine, to produce insulin and other hormones, and exocrine, to produce pancreatic juices for digestion. The pancreas is in direct contact with the stomach, duodenum, spleen, and major vessels of the abdomen.

vagal afferents are stimulated by gastric distention. The pancreas also receives sympathetic innervation from T_5 through T_{10} of the spinal column. Sympathetic stimulation contributes to decreased blood flow and can inhibit pancreatic secretion, impacting both the exocrine and endocrine pancreatic function. Pancreatic secretions can vary in volume and concentration of bicarbonate and enzymes. Volume can be minimal when the bowel is at rest, in contrast to the dramatic increase in pancreatic secretions during digestion.

EXOCRINE PANCREAS AND PANCREATITIS

EXOCRINE FUNCTION OF THE PANCREAS

The term exocrine refers specifically to the production of the various enzymes of the pancreas and their release locally into the duodenum during digestion. The pancreas serves as an important source of the enzymes needed for digestion. The pancreas secretes up to 2.5 l/day of exocrine fluid, such as bicarbonate, electrolytes, protein, and various enzymes.

The cells of the exocrine pancreas are arranged in a very distinctive histologic pattern, clustering in a single epithelial layer of up to 12 cells around a common microscopic space, or lumen, into which the individual cells release their enzyme content upon receiving the appropriate neurological or hormonal signals. These cell arrangements, known as acini, are scattered throughout the pancreas, and in fact make up to 95% of the organ tissue.

The acinar cells secrete the three main categories of digestive enzymes: the proteolytic enzymes, which digest proteins; lipases, which break down various ingested fats and protein; and amylases, which cleave ingested carbohydrates into simpler sugar molecules. The pancreas produces a number of enzymes in each of these three classes, with the greatest diversity found in the proteolytic component. More than a dozen of these protein-digesting enzymes have now been identified, including trypsin, chymotrypsin, carboxypeptidase A, carboxypeptidase B, elastase, aminopeptidase, a series of dipeptidases, tripeptidases, and another form of pepsin, the enzyme also produced by stomach cells. Of all the enzymes, trypsin is secreted in the largest amount. Each of these enzymes breaks down protein at very specific points. Trypsin and chymotrypsin digest complete proteins or large protein fragments into peptide fragments. Dipeptidases and tripeptidases further reduce peptide fragments. Finally, the carboxypeptidases break down any remaining protein remnants into individual amino acids that can be easily absorbed through the intestinal mucosa.

The acinar cells also secrete multiple lipases and esterases, both fat-digesting enzymes that each target specific molecules. Pancreatic lipase reduces triglycerides into free fatty acids and monoglycerides for absorption. Phospholipase separates fatty acids from phospholipids, and cholesterol esterase starts the breakdown of cholesterol esters (CE).

All proteolytic enzymes, particularly trypsin and chymotrypsin, as well as the family of lipases are very powerful enzymes, with the potential to break down or digest proteins and fats within the pancreas tissue itself. Conversely, autodigestion is less of a problem with the amylases. The acinar cells produce these enzymes in inactive precursor forms to protect the pancreas from its proteolytic and lipolytic secretions. For example, the acinar cells manufacture trypsin initially as trypsinogen, chymotrypsin as chymotrysinogen, and the carboxypeptidases in the procarboxypeptidase form, all of which are completely inactive with no proteolytic ability at all. Additionally, lipases appear initially as the inactive colipase.

The acinar cells store these precursors in vacuoles known as zymogen granules, within the cytoplasm until needed for digestion. While the preenzymes remain in their inactive form, the pancreas is protected form various medical problems (for example, pancreatitis) that can arise when these enzymes are released into the surrounding pancreatic tissues, resulting in tissue damage and inflammation. The subsequent sequlae is associated with increased morbidity and mortality. As an added protection, the acinar cells secrete into their own cytoplasm a trypsin inhibitor protein that, as the name implies, helps prevent the activation of trypsin within the cells. Activation of the digestive enzymes occurs in the duodenum. When chyme (a mixture of semifluid food and hydrochloric acid) comes into direct contact with the duodenal mucosa, the epithelial cells secrete enteropeptidase, which activates trypsinogen and forms trypsin. The trypsin then activates chymotrypsinogen. Trypsin and chymotrypsin digest proteins into peptides but cannot digest proteins into single amino acids. Other proteases from the pancreas, for example carboxypeptidase, can break down peptides into amino acids though cleaving of peptides to amino acids is primarily done by peptidases and proteases.

PHASES OF PANCREATIC SECRETION

There are three phases of pancreatic secretion. The first phase, the *cephalic phase*, occurs when the vagus nerve provides direct cholinergic stimulation to the pancreas. Indirect stimulation occurs through release of gastrin from the gastric antrum and vasoactive inhibitory proteins (VIP) from the small intestine. The release of gastrin during the cephalic phase stimulates pancreatic enzyme secretion.

The cephalic phase is followed by the *gastric phase*. The presence of food within the stomach causes gastric dilatation further stimulating the pancreas and release of gastrin. Gastric distention is mediated by the vagus nerve. Gastrin also stimulates pancreatic acini to produce other enzymes needed for digestion.

The third phase, the *intestinal phase*, is similar to the gastric phase. The gastric antrum releases gastrin that, in turn, stimulates hydrochloric acid release into stomach, acidifying the gastric contents. Chyme, arriving into the small intestine, is extremely acidic due to the hydrochloric acid load secreted by the stomach to start the digestive process. The pancreatic enzymes work efficiently only in an alkaline environment, in the pH range above 7. However, when the pH of the duodenum drops below 4.5–5, S cells in the intestinal mucosa release the peptide secretin into the bloodstream. When secretin reaches the pancreas, the hormone signals the cells lining the numerous ducts to secrete copious amounts of the alkaline sodium bicarbonate. In the duodenum, bicarbonate quickly neutralizes the acid effect of chyme, and as the pH quickly rises, the pancreatic enzymes become optimally active.[3]

Partially digested foods, primarily fat and protein, enter the duodenum and cause the release of the enzyme, pancreozymin, which further stimulates pancreatic secretion. VIP is a homologue that further stimulates pancreatic bicarbonate secretion. Undigested protein has minimal, if any, stimulatory effect on pancreatic secretion, but polypeptides, oligopeptides, and amino acids have a marked stimulatory effect on the gland. Ingestion of a combination of amino acids has a greater stimulatory effect on the pancreas than any single amino acid alone. The presence of calcium in the duodenum also stimulates pancreatic enzyme release, and bile salts stimulate both pancreatic enzyme and bicarbonate secretion. GI hormones that stimulate or inhibit the pancreas are interrelated in their function and are often synergistic.

Pancreatic secretory function can be markedly reduced by altering the amount and content of dietary intake. Pancreatic rest, as necessitated by some medical conditions, can be achieved by eliminating oral intake or by administrating inhibitors of pancreatic secretion. The sympathetic nervous system inhibits pancreatic secretion through the splanchnic nerves and circulating catecholamines. GI hormones, which inhibit pancreatic secretion, include glucagon, somatostatin, and pancreatic polypeptide. Pancreatic secretion is inhibited by the presence of trypsin or chymotrypsin in the duodenum.[4]

PANCREATITIS

"Pancreatitis" is a general term that encompasses a wide variation in etiology, clinical course, and treatment. It can be classified as acute (mild, moderate, or severe) or chronic. Common causes of acute pancreatitis include alcohol abuse and biliary tract disease.[5] The incidence of acute pancreatitis varies from 5.4 to 79.8 per 100,000.[6] Acute pancreatitis is generally a mild, self-limiting illness that resolves with 5 to 7 days of supportive therapy.[7] Mild pancreatitis is associated with mild pancreatic edema, minimal enzyme elevation, and relatively low mortality and morbidity. Amylase and lipase levels in mild pancreatitis may be minimally elevated, though levels do not always correlate with the severity of the disease. Patients experience mild episodes of abdominal pain, nausea, vomiting, and anorexia. The majority of patients present with a mild form of pancreatitis that resolves in several days with limited periods of restricted food intake, pain control, and intravenous (IV) fluids.[5] Patients are typically not malnourished and are able to resume their oral diet following symptom resolution. Calorie-free liquids are usually introduced first, and if tolerated, followed by low-fat diet.

Severe cases of pancreatitis can result in organ necrosis resulting from intra- and extra-pancreatic extravasation of pancreatic enzymes. Severe pancreatitis can be life-threatening and is a medical emergency. Severe pancreatitis can lead to loss of fluid and protein due to the escape of enzymes into the abdominal cavities. Specialized nutrition support is often required for patients with moderate to severe pancreatitis. If complications develop, including pseudocyst, abscess, or fistula, a protracted period of increased metabolic and nutritional needs should be anticipated. The overall mortality rate for acute pancreatitis is 10 to 15%, however, mortality can increase as high as 40% in severe acute pancreatitis.[6]

Chronic pancreatitis is a progressive inflammatory disease associated with permanent anatomical and functional damage.[8] The two histomorphological forms of chronic pancreatitis are obstructive and calcifying.[9] Pancreatic pseudocysts have an occurrence rate of 60%

and are complications of pancreatic inflammation and pancreatic calculi. The inflammation can also contribute to stenosis of the common bile duct and duodenum and portal hypertension.[10]

ETIOLOGY OF PANCREATITIS

Acute Pancreatitis

Cholelithiasis is the most common cause of acute pancreatitis in the United States, accounting for approximately 45% of cases.[7] Alcohol and idiopathic or miscellaneous are the causative factors in 35 and 20% of cases, respectively. Pancreatitis secondary to cholelithiasis is usually mild and self-limiting. Acute pancreatitis may also be side effects to a number of pharmacologic agents or medications, including steroids, antibiotics (tetracycline), furosemide, and thiazide diuretics, as well as some antiretrovirals and chemotherapeutic agents. Patients, who are on chronic medications associated with pancreatitis, may suffer repeated bouts and develop a chronic form of the disease. Other causes of acute pancreatitis include hyperlipidemia, direct trauma to the pancreas gland, viral infections, peptic ulcer disease with posterior penetration, and iatrogenic pancreatitis.

Chronic Pancreatitis

It has been hypothesized that recurrent episodes of acute pancreatitis result in development of chronic pancreatitis.[9] A severe relapsing course of acute pancreatitis creates a necrosis–fibrosis sequence that results in permanent pancreatic damage.[11] This progressive sequence contributes to the development of psuedocysts and pancreatic duct stenosis. It has been hypothesized that when severe acute alcoholic-induced pancreatitis results in chronic pancreatitis, it is actually different stages of the same disease.[12] A study revealed that 78% of 140 patients with recurrent alcoholic acute pancreatitis developed chronic pancreatitis.[13]

Chronic pancreatitis is most often associated with chronic ethanol abuse and biliary tract disease. Eighty percent of all cases of chronic pancreatitis in the Western world are related to ethanol abuse.[8] This is often exacerbated by high-fat and high-protein diets, smoking, and inadequate vitamin and mineral intake.[9] The relationship of alcohol and pancreatitis seems well documented in men, but is less clear in women.[14] There does appear to be a "dose–response curve" demonstrating a direct relationship between the mean daily ethanol intake and the risk of chronic pancreatitis. Alcohol stimulates pancreatic secretion and this response is directly proportional to the amount and type of alcohol consumed.

Excessive alcohol intake, >80 g/day for >35 years, is associated with alcohol-induced chronic pancreatitis.[9] Alcohol damages hepatocytes and acinar cells and changes microcirculatory perfusion, all of which predispose to alterations in acinar protein secretion with subsequent protein plug and dutal stone formation.[8] Other nonalcohol etiologies of pancreatitis include tropical chronic pancreatitis, hereditary pancreatitis, and in approximately 10% of cases, the etiology is idiopathic.

Hyperlipidemia is frequently noted in acute and chronic pancreatitis, and may precipitate pancreatitis (levels >1000 mg/dl), or be a sequelae of the disease. Patients with type I, IV, and V hyperlipoproteinemia are more likely to develop recurrent bouts of pancreatitis.[15] Ethanol abuse leading to acute pancreatitis is frequently associated with hypertriglyceridemia. Decreased clearance of lipids has been observed in this group of patients. A triglyceride level should be obtained on admission and monitored throughout nutrition therapy.

Chronic pancreatitis may be an independent risk factor for the development of pancreatic cancer. A study with 2015 chronic pancreatitis patients reported an eightfold increased risk of developing pancreatic cancer.[16] The mortality for patients with chronic pancreatitis is approximately 30 to 40%.[17] Twenty percent of mortality is directly related to the disease itself. Patients with advanced chronic pancreatitis have a shorter life expectancy by 10 to 20 years.[18]

DIAGNOSIS OF PANCREATITIS

A number of laboratory imaging tests have been used to diagnose and monitor patients with pancreatitis. Pancreatitis is determined to be mild, moderate, or severe on the basis of clinical findings, biochemical or laboratory evaluations, and actual pathologic changes. The laboratory data most commonly used are serum amylase and lipase values. A tolerable upper limit (UL) of serum amylase >250 U/L is associated with pancreatitis. However, amylase levels are not always elevated and serum levels return to normal within 3 to 5 days, making it a nonspecific diagnostic tool. Serum lipase >110 U/L is a more sensitive indicator of pancreatitis, since it remains elevated longer and there are few nonpancreatic causes of hyperlipasemia. Generally patients with pancreatitis have amylase levels greater than 1000 units and commonly levels are increased to several thousand units. Hypocalcemia, hyperglycemia, and hypertriglyceridemia are often noted in acute pancreatitis, therefore serum levels of calcium, glucose, and triglycerides become important parameters in assessing and following these patients. As inflammation of the pancreas continues, pancreatic parenchyma damage and atrophy of the pancreatic gland result in decreased endocrine and exocrine function.[9] Patients with chronic recurring pancreatitis often do not present with elevated enzyme levels.

Ranson and coworkers[19,20] defined the severity of the disease by a set of criteria that would predict outcome within 48 h of admission. The presence of three or more of Ranson's criteria is diagnostic for pancreatitis.[21] Mortality is higher in patients who demonstrate three or more of Ranson's criteria. The patient groups who demonstrate five or more of Ranson's criteria have a mortality of 40%. The Acute Physiology and Chronic Health Evaluation (APACHE II) assessment has been used in other critically ill patients (trauma, sepsis, etc.) and has also been applied to assess outcome in pancreatitis.[22,23] Pancreatitis is characterized by an APACHE II score of 8 or more.[21] Within the first 48 h, patients with APACHE II scores <9 were more likely to survive. Patients with scores ≥13 had a significantly higher mortality. Mortality is obviously worse in patients, who develop additional organ failure, such as respiratory, acute renal, hepatic, and cardiovascular failure.

Radiological imaging tests are helpful in the diagnosis and monitoring disease progression. Computerized tomography (CT) scan, in contrast, is the gold standard for diagnosing pancreatic necrosis and peripancreatic collections. Sequential CT scanning is used to monitor the course of pancreatitis and the CT findings have been closely associated with the expected prognosis and mortality. CT scanning is generally recommended to establish the diagnosis, when patients show no improvement in the first 72 h, or in any patient, who demonstrates more than three of Ranson's criteria or an APACHE score ≥9.[24] Patients generally improve clinically before improvement of the CT scan.[25]

Endoscopic retrograde cholangiopancreatography (ERCP) is a valuable means of diagnosing and treating ductal stenosis and stones.[6] The test is invasive, involving the use of x-rays and an endoscope. ERCP can cause pancreatitis, infection, bleeding, and perforation of the duodenum. Magnetic resonance cholangiopancreatography (MRCP), introduced in the early 1990s, is a noninvasive method of diagnosis that images the pancreaticobiliary tree.[6] MRCP is safe and as accurate as CT for diagnosis and grading of acute severe pancreatitis.

SYMPTOMOLOGY OF PANCREATITIS

The process of pancreatic disease begins before symptoms appear and functional abnormalities occur. Subclinical pancreatitis generally begins 10 years before the onset of clinical

TABLE 14.1
Progressive Stages of Chronic Pancreatitis

Stage 1: Subclinical period: Inflammatory infiltration of pancreatic tissue, fibrosis, atrophy of acinar cells,
        calcifications, pancreatic duct strictures
Stage 2: Clinical period: Various degrees of pain, exocrine, and then later, endocrine dysfunction
Stage 3: Burnout period: Global insufficiency of the pancreas, pain subsides

Source: From Strate, T. et al., *Eur. J. Gastroenterol. Hepatol.*, 14, 929, 2002.

symptoms, often in the fourth or fifth decade of life. Chronic pancreatitis is characterized by three stages, subclinical, clinical, and burnout, outlined in Table 14.1.

Pain is the most common and noticeable symptom of pancreatitis. The goal is to identify the etiology of pain, nociceptive versus neuropathic, and provide effective treatment regimens. Potential treatable etiologies of pain include pseudocysts, biliary and duodenal obstruction, and peptic ulceration.[26] The etiology of pain is multifactorial and appears to persist following withdrawal of alcohol and with exocrine and endocrine deficiency.[9] Suspected etiologies of pain include parenchymal and ductal hypertension, and parenchymal inflammation with neural alterations. Pain can be either recurrent or constant. Very few patients do not experience pain during the course of their disease.

Chronic inflammation and the resulting release of various growth factors contribute to irreversible, pathological alterations in the neuroanatomy of the pancreas and its central nervous system connection.[26] This results in an exaggerated and irreversible pattern of neuropathic pain. Resection of the altered parenchyma, primarily the pancreatic head, reduces pain and prevents further inflammation. A correlation has been seen with preoperative pain and increased pancreatic duct pressure as well as increased pressure in the body and tail of the pancreas.[27] Although non-narcotic analgesics are the first line of pain therapy, narcotic anlgesics are often necessary to control the pain.[26] Antisecretory therapy with either H_2-receptor antagonists or proton pump inhibitors reduces acid-induced secretin release from the duodenum, which in turn decreases pancreatic stimulation. The role for octreotide in pancreatitis pain management is controversial.[26] Pancreatic enzyme replacement therapy has also been used for pain control. Despite controversy over the effectiveness of enzymes in ameliorating pain, most clinicians attempt a trial of pancreatic enzyme replacement therapy, especially for patients with idiopathic and early disease. There are inconsistent data concerning the effect of antioxidant therapy for pain reduction.[26]

Pancreatic exocrine secretion normally exceeds the body's enzymatic requirement for nutrient digestion and absorption. Malabsorption does not occur until pancreatic digestive enzyme output is <10% of normal.[28] Exocrine pancreatic function is the initial abnormality to appear. Interference with production and release of pancreatic enzymes results in malabsorption and steatorrhea with subsequent weight loss.[9] Adequate digestion of protein, carbohydrate, and fat requires that the patients receive at least 5 to 10% of the normal maximal digestive enzyme output.[26] Steatorrhea occurs before malabsorption of protein. Pancreatic enzyme replacement therapy may be necessary as the disease progresses. Adequate fat digestion requires that approximately 25,000–40,000 units of lipase per meal be delivered to the duodenum.[29] Each tablet or capsule of commercially available enzymes contains 4,000–20,000 IU lipase. Pancreatic enzymes can be enteric coated and be in the form of minitablets or microspheres. Gastric acid production, resulting in a gastric pH less than 4, can inactivate and reduce the effectiveness of exogenous enzymes. Patients may require 60,000–75,000 units of lipase per meal to avoid malabsorption. Caution must be exercised when

TABLE 14.2
Pancreatic Enzyme Preparations

Enzyme Preparation	Form	Lipase (USP Units) per Pill
Creon[®a]	Enteric-coated minimicrospheres	Available in 5,000, 10,000, or 20,000 units
Viokase[®b] (pancrelipase)	Tablet	Available in 8,000 or 16,000 units
Viokase[b] (pancrelipase)	Powder	16,800 per quarter teaspoon
Ultrase[b]	Enteric-coated microspheres or minitablets	4,500
Ultrase[b] MT	Enteric-coated microspheres or minitablets	Available in 12,000, 18,000, or 20,000 units
Pancrease[®c]	Enteric-coated microspheres	4,500

[a]Registered trademark of Solvay Pharmaceuticals, Inc., Marietta, GA.
[b]Registered trademark of Axcan Pharma, Inc., Birmingham, AL.
[c]Registered trademark of Ortho-McNeil Pharmaceutical, Inc., Spring House, PA.

prescribing higher doses of pancreatic enzymes. Research in cystic fibrosis patients has shown increased risk of fibrotic alterations in the colon with high-dose pancreatic enzyme therapy (greater than 6,000–10,000 units per kg per meal), especially in children.[30,31] Antacids, proton pump inhibitors, H_2-blockers, and enteric-coated enzyme preparations can help decrease the enzyme dose required and increase the effectiveness of enzyme replacement therapy by decreasing destruction of enzymes by gastric acid and increasing the availability of bicarbonate for enzyme release.[26] Pancreatic enzymes that contain particles of >1–2 mm in diameter are retained in the stomach and may not empty in the fed state, thus delaying delivery. Microspheres are acid-resistant enteric-coated pancreatic enzymes that are not released in the stomach. They are small enough to empty from the stomach in conjunction with the food, though different preparations may differ in the amount of time it takes to liberate the lipase within the intestinal lumen, thereby reducing the time for nutrient digestion. Table 14.2 provides some examples of commercially available enzyme preparations.

Endocrine dysfunction resulting in diabetes mellitus (DM) is often a late development (20 years after onset) of pancreatic disease. Approximately 30 to 50% of patients with chronic pancreatitis develop DM. Most of the patients who develop diabetes require insulin therapy. Factors that contribute to the development of diabetes include loss of islet cell function, decreased hormone secretion, and impaired release of glucagon. Irregular energy intake due to malabsorption and alcohol abuse can increase the risk of hypoglycemia and contribute to undertreatment or avoidance of insulin.

Treatment of Pancreatitis

The goals of conservative management of pancreatitis are to limit progression and development of complications; correct endocrine and exocrine dysfunction; and provide pain control.[26] Management of the complications is often the primary focus of therapy. Potential major complications of chronic pancreatitis are listed in Table 14.3.

Management of acute pancreatitis centers on resuscitation, evaluating the severity of the disease, diagnosing and treating the etiology as well as subsequent complications of the disease process.[6] Acute severe pancreatitis is treated with aggressive fluid resuscitation, oxygen supplementation, and support for any failing organ or system.[6] Interstitial fluid accumulation can result in one third of the plasma shifting to the interstitial space. This is

TABLE 14.3
Major Complications Associated with Chronic Pancreatitis

Abdominal pain
Bile duct obstruction
Diabetes mellitus
Duodenal obstruction
Maldigestion
Pancreatic cancer
Pseudocyst
Splenic vein thrombosis with gastric varicies

Sources: From Strate, T. et al., *Eur. J. Gastroenterol. Hepatol.*, 14, 929, 2002; Khalid, A. and Whitcomb, D.C., *Eur. J. Gastroenterol. Hepatol.*, 14, 943, 2002.

responsible for a 23% incidence of renal failure and an 80% mortality rate in acute pancreatitis.[6] Aggressive restoration of vascular volume contributes to electrolyte abnormalities.

Indirect treatment for pain involves endoscopic draining of the main pancreatic duct and cystic cavities, stenting, and removing stones, obstructing the duct.[32] Drainage of symptomatic psuedocysts relieves pain, delays progression of exocrine malfunction, but does not affect endocrine dysfunction.[9] The most straightforward way to directly suppress pain is total or partial pancreatectomy.[32] Approximately half of chronic pancreatitis patients will be treated surgically during the course of their disease.[33] Duodenum-preserving pancreatic head resection and a pylorus-preserving Whipple procedure are preferred to the previously used Whipple procedure for pancreatic resection.[34] Preserving the duodenum contributes to pain relief, while delaying the loss of pancreatic function with an improvement in the patient's quality of life.[9]

NUTRITION AND PANCREATITIS

Nutrition Assessment

The principles of nutrition management with pancreatitis are to provide adequate nutrients to correct altered metabolism and nutritional deficits, avoid overfeeding, reduce pancreatic stimulation, and attenuate the inflammatory process.[35] It has been estimated that 30% of acute pancreatitis patients are malnourished.[36] Patients with severe acute or chronic pancreatitis may be undernourished secondary to the inflammatory process itself or the poor oral intake or malabsorption that accompanies diseases of the pancreas. Approximately 10% of patients with acute hemorrhagic pancreatitis will have significant morbidity and need operative intervention. Most of these patients experience iatrogenic deterioration of their nutritional status, mandating the need for nutrition support.[19,37] Chronic pancreatitis patients are at nutritional risk due to malabsorption, alcohol abuse, and weight loss. Pancreatitis is an inflammatory state, therefore, negative acute phase proteins, albumin, prealbumin, and transferrin, are indicators of severity of illness and not nutritional status.[38]

PANCREATITIS AND NUTRIENT METABOLISM

Physiologic changes that occur with pancreatitis induce a state of hypermetabolism and hypercatabolism, similar to the hormonal alterations seen in critical illness (increased catecholamines, insulin, glucagon). Carbohydrate, protein, and fat metabolism are affected by elevated resting metabolism and energy expenditure. The primary site of digestion and absorption shifts from the proximal bowel to the more distal bowel with chronic pancreatitis.[26]

The delivery of more nutrients to the distal ileum alters normal transit and secretory function of the proximal small bowel. Pancreatic enzyme therapy improves digestion and GI transit, suggesting that malabsorption is both a cause and a consequence of abnormal motor function.

Carbohydrate

Hyperglycemia is a common finding in patients with pancreatitis, even in the absence of underlying DM. The etiology of hyperglycemia is multifactorial and includes increased levels of cortisol and adrenocorticotrophic hormone (ACTH), increased ratio of glucagon to insulin and peripheral insulin resistance, and decreased rate of glucose oxidation.[25] The administration of PN with hypertonic dextrose can further complicate glycemic management. Significant hyperglycemia requiring substantial insulin replacement has been observed in over 80% of patients with pancreatitis.[37] Outcome has been related to the severity of hyperglycemia and the insulin requirements in these patients, with a significant increase in mortality noted in patients requiring greater than 3 units of insulin per hour.[39]

Protein

Hypercatabolism with loss of lean muscle mass, negative nitrogen balance, and increased ureagenesis are all observed in acute pancreatitis.[40] Circulating levels of the major gluconeogenic amino acid, alanine, are decreased, and plasma levels of glutamine are markedly depressed even though other amino acids are rapidly released by skeletal muscle. Decreased plasma alanine and glutamine levels are similar to that seen in other critically ill patients.[41,42] Protein needs in this patient group approach 1.2 to 1.5 g/kg/day.[35] When appropriate energy and protein are provided, the calorie to nitrogen ratio is 100:1. Provision of protein may be affected by renal and hepatic function, presence of sepsis, and the severity of pancreatitis.

Lipid

The concentration of lipase in pancreatic secretions responds to oral fat, though not intravenous fat emulsions. Fat malabsorption is generally seen before carbohydrate or protein malabsorption in alcohol-induced pancreatitis.[26] Fat malabsorption is defined as 7 to 15 g of fat (mild steatorrhea) in the stool and >15 g of fat (severe steatorrhea) with a diet of 100 g of fat per 24 h. In chronic pancreatitis, 30 to 40 g of fat per day in the stool is pathognomonic.[26] Steatorrhea is characterized by loose, greasy, and foul-smelling stools, cramping, bloating, and flatus.[26] Approximately 30% of patients with chronic pancreatitis present with steatorrhea. Although the "gold standard" for identifying steatorrhea is a 72-h fecal-fat collection, while the patient consumes a 100 g fat diet per day, many clinicians agree that a simple qualitative microscopic examination of the stool for fat globules (Sudan stain) is sufficient.[26] Other clinicians simply ask patients if their stools "float."

Micronutrients

Chronic pancreatitis is associated with poor nutrient intake and malabsorption, both of which contribute to increased risk of micronutrient inadequacy and deficiency. Vitamin A and E deficiencies have been reported in patients with chronic pancreatitis.[43] Alcohol-related pancreatitis has the additional risk of vitamin C, riboflavin, thiamin, folic acid, and nicotinic acid deficiencies because of the adverse effect of alcohol on micronutrient intake and absorption.[39] The presence of steatorrhea contributes to losses of divalent cations (calcium, magnesium, zinc) as these cations saponify fatty acids. Although B_{12} malabsorption is common, deficiency is rare.[7]

PANCREATITIS AND ENERGY METABOLISM

Septic patients with pancreatitis are usually hypermetabolic.[44] The hormonal alterations associated with acute pancreatitis and sepsis (increased cortisol and catecholamines) have the overall effect of increasing the resting energy expenditure (REE). However, in the absence of severe infection or sepsis, there is little evidence that chronic pancreatitis increases energy expenditure.[45,46] The need for caloric support varies with the patient's age, height, weight, severity of disease, and associated fever or sepsis.[44,46]

Dickerson et al.[46] evaluated 48 patients with either acute or chronic pancreatitis with or without sepsis. The REE, measured by indirect calorimetry, was compared with predicted energy expenditure, using the Harris–Benedict equation. The REE was significantly greater in septic patients (120 ± 11%) compared to those without sepsis (105 ± 14%). However, REE varied widely in patients with pancreatitis (77 to 139% of predicted energy expenditure). The authors concluded that the Harris–Benedict equation was an unreliable means of determining energy requirements in pancreatitis patients. Sepsis was the critical denominator in determining REE in patients with pancreatitis.

Data indicate that energy requirements are overestimated by the Harris–Benedict equation. REE is most accurately determined by indirect calorimetry. REE elevations of as much.[44–47] as 30 to 50% may be observed in patients with severe, progressive pancreatitis, and in patients with a Ranson's score of ≥6.[44,45] The European Society for Clinical Nutrition and Metabolism (ESPEN) guidelines recommend 25 to 35 kcal/kg/day with severe pancreatitis.[35]

SELECTING THE ROUTE OF NUTRITION DURING PANCREATITIS

Oral Diet and Pancreatitis

An oral diet can be initiated when pain is controlled and pancreatic enzyme levels have normalized.[35] The oral diet should focus on minimizing pancreatic stimulation and limiting disease progression. A low-fat diet with frequent small meals is the cornerstone of therapy. However, the role of fat in exacerbating pancreatitis has not been fully elucidated.[26] A moderate fat diet in conjunction with pancreatic enzyme replacement therapy is recommended when patients have steatorrhea.[7] If steatorrhea does not improve on this regimen, the pancreatic enzymes should be continued with a low-fat diet. Patients should abstain from alcohol. Eighty percent of acute pancreatitis cases are classified as mild. These patients recover within 7 days and require no specialized nutrition support intervention.[48]

Enteral Nutrition

EN is used to support patients with pancreatitis despite previous tendencies to encourage "bowel rest." Initial enteral studies examined the efficacy of elemental diets in the treatment of acute pancreatitis.[49,50] It was postulated that elemental formulas produced less pancreatic stimulation and secretion than polymeric formulas. Early studies in animals with pancreatitis fed an elemental diet showed conflicting data. Some investigators found a significant decrease in the volume and enzyme concentration of pancreatic secretions with elemental feeding,[49,50] while others found an increase in pancreatic secretion.[51–53] Most early studies fed patients via the duodenum instead of the current practice of jejunal feeding. Jejunal administration of formulas is not associated with an increase in pancreatic stimulation.[54] Guan et al.[55] studied animals with pancreatitis and concluded that elemental diets did not stimulate pancreatic secretion and polymeric diets did increase pancreatic exocrine output. The differences between the formulas were attributed to the intact protein in the polymeric diet versus the free amino acids in elemental diets.

Early studies in humans documented the efficacy of elemental diets in pancreatitis.[56,57] Feller et al.[57] retrospectively reviewed 200 patients treated initially with PN, and then converted to EN. Nitrogen balance was achieved and mortality decreased from 21.6 to 14%. Bodoky et al.[58] compared PN with EN in patients with pancreatitis and found no significant differences between pancreatic secretion in the two groups.

Kudsk et al.[59] studied EN in 11 patients with acute pancreatitis. The patients were given jejunostomy feeding with an elemental formula. Over the course of the 31-day follow-up, there was no worsening of pancreatitis. Parekh et al.[60] reported similar results with 17 patients receiving an elemental diet for 16 days. Grant et al.[61] used defined formula diets in patients with severe pancreatitis and reported no diarrhea or worsening of the disease process. However, almost half of the patients in this study required exogenous insulin to maintain blood glucose levels within acceptable range. Other studies have documented the success of repleting patients using enteral feeding without exacerbating symptoms in acute pancreatitis.[62–65] The need for supplemental pancreatic enzymes to facilitate absorption of both elemental and polymeric formulae in severe pancreatic insufficiency has been questioned.[66]

EN is postulated to reduce intestinal permeability and downregulate the inflammatory process.[35] Current evidence suggests that enteral feeding, preferably into the jejunum, is the optimal method of specialized nutrition support in patients with pancreatitis, who are unable to meet nutritional need orally.[35] EN should be discontinued if it increases pain, ascites, or fistula output.[7]

Parenteral Nutrition

"Bowel rest" for treating pancreatitis is directed toward reducing pancreatic secretory volume (primarily bicarbonate) and minimizing enzyme release.[67,68] PN maintains nutritional status during prolonged periods of bowel rest. Several studies have shown improvement in patients with pancreatitis who received PN.[37] Despite the decrease in pancreatic secretions and pain with bowel rest, the efficacy as measured by clinical outcomes has yet to be determined. No clinical trials have demonstrated a reduction of mortality and morbidity with bowel rest.[7] Sax et al.[48] conducted a prospective, randomized trial to evaluate the effect of early PN in acute pancreatitis compared with intravenous fluids alone and analgesia. The PN group had significantly longer hospitalization (16 versus 10 days) and a significantly higher rate of catheter sepsis (10.5 versus 1.5%).[48] Other studies similarly do not confirm clinical benefit of bowel rest and PN in pancreatitis.[69]

Effective management of PN is critical to reduce the risk of metabolic and septic complications. Administration of parenteral glucose should be between 3 and 6 mg/kg/min in severe pancreatitis.[35] Glucose infusion should not exceed 4 to 6 mg/kg/min in euglycemic patients and 3 to 4 mg/kg/min in hyperglycemic or diabetic patients. Excess glucose contributes hyperglycemia, infection risk, cholestasis, fatty liver, and increased risk of mortality and morbidity.[39,70,71] Studies in critically ill patient populations have shown a reduction in mortality and morbidity with blood sugars <110 mg/dl[70] and <140 mg/dl.[71] In general, total energy per day should be provided as 50 to 60% glucose, 15 to 20% protein with the balance supplied by fat. A mixed fuel substrate for energy is recommended in patients with pancreatitis.[41,44,46]

Parenteral lipid emulsions are provided as an energy substrate in patients with pancreatitis. Patients with pancreatitis are at risk of developing hypertriglyceridemia, therefore, serum triglyceride levels should be checked initially and then sequentially throughout therapy. Triglyceride levels should be maintained at less than 400 mg/dl during continuous lipid infusion.[7] Studies have suggested that lipid infusion stimulated pancreatic secretions.[72,73] However, these studies involved patients with inflammatory bowel disease, who were also receiving corticosteroids that may have altered lipid kinetics. Most studies in both animals[51,74,75] and humans[37,74,76-79] have reported that fat emulsions are safe and do not stimulate pancreatic secretion. Most patients with acute pancreatitis without hyperlipoproteinemia or hypertriglyceridemia, tolerate lipid emulsions. The recommended dose of lipid in critically ill patients without hypertriglyceridemia is <1 g/kg/day.[76] The ESPEN guidelines recommend providing lipids up to 2 g/kg/day as long as serum triglycerides are within acceptable limits.[35] Exceeding 1 g of fat/kg/day or 30% of the total energy as lipid should be avoided in septic patients because of associated risk of immunosuppression with long-chain omega-6 fatty acids.[80] Controlled trials have demonstrated no hypertriglyceridemia and no adverse outcome associated with use of lipid emulsions in patients with pancreatitis.[76,81]

Despite trends toward early enteral feeding, PN may be the preferred method of specialized nutrition support in patients who develop complications from pancreatitis (i.e., worsening severe inflammation, abscess formation, pseudocysts, ascites, or fistulas).[82-86] Latifi and coworkers[83,86] postulated that PN reduced pancreatic stimulation and secretions and recommended that PN be given until acute symptoms resolve. This evidence has not been widely supported by other investigators. Jackson et al.[85] examined the effect of PN in 40 patients with acute pancreatitis, who developed pancreatic pseudocyst. Sixty-eight percent of patients showed pseudocyst regression and clinical improvement. However, 35% of the patients developed catheter-related complications.

PN has not been shown to influence mortality and morbidity, despite its effect of decreasing pancreatic secretions. PN is also associated with metabolic, infectious, and hepatic complications. Central line sepsis associated with PN is significantly higher in patients with pancreatitis.[37,48,63,87] The hyperglycemia noted in these patients may also contribute to the higher rate of catheter-related infections, mortality, and morbidity. Therefore, the risks associate with PN, including metabolic complications and catheter sepsis, do not justify its use when EN is a reasonable alternative.

The American Society for Parenteral and Enteral Nutrition (A.S.P.E.N.) practice guidelines for pancreatitis are given in Table 14.4.[7] The practice guidelines are based on graded evidence. The practice guidelines recommend nutrition screening of pancreatitis patients with

---

TABLE 14.4

A.S.P.E.N. Practice Guidelines for Pancreatitis (Adults)

1. Patients with pancreatitis are at nutrition risk and should undergo nutrition screening to identify those who require formal nutrition assessment with development of a nutrition care plan (B)
2. Specialized nutrition support (SNS) should not routinely be used in patients with mild to moderate acute pancreatitis (B)
3. SNS should be used in patients with acute or chronic pancreatitis to prevent or treat malnutrition when oral energy intake is anticipated to be inadequate for 5 to 7 days (B)
4. Enteral nutrition (EN) is the preferred route of SNS in patients with pancreatitis and should be attempted before initiating parenteral nutrition (PN) (A)
5. PN should be used in patients with pancreatitis if SNS is indicated and EN is not tolerated (B)
6. Intravenous lipid emulsions are safe in acute pancreatitis provided triglyceride levels are monitored and remain below 400 mg/dl (B)

Grading of evidence used to support each statement:

(A) There is good research-based evidence to support the guideline (prospective, randomized trials)

(B) There is fair research-based evidence to support the guideline (well-designed studies without randomization)

(C) The guidelines are based on expert opinion and editorial consensus

Source: From A.S.P.E.N. *J. Parenter. Enteral Nutr.*, 26, 68SA, 2002.

assessment of those at risk. The guidelines also promote use of specialized nutrition support only in patients presenting with malnutrition or severe pancreatitis, who cannot consume food orally for more than 5 to 7 days. EN is preferred over PN unless EN is not tolerated.

COMPLEMENTARY AND ALTERNATIVE THERAPIES FOR PANCREATIC HEALTH

Current research efforts are examining the effects of specific nutrients (glutamine, arginine, short-chain fatty acids, nucleotides) in maintaining immune function and the gut mucosal barrier. The addition of trophic hormones (CCK, bombesin, neurotensin, growth hormone, and epidermoid growth factor) may also contribute to the maintenance of gut mucosal integrity.[88] Probiotic therapy is investigated for its role in reducing sepsis and maintaining GI integrity during pancreatitis.[89]

Omega-3 Fatty Acids

The use of immune-enhancing agents in inflammatory conditions has been investigated in numerous studies. Practical application of the research has been hampered by protocols that combine omega-3 fatty acids with other immune-enhancing nutrients in various populations. Foitzik et al.[90] evaluated omega-3 fatty acids and their anti-inflammatory properties in rats with severe induced acute pancreatitis. A goal of the study was to modulate the systemic inflammatory response syndrome (SIRS) that occurs in acute pancreatitis by blocking proinflammatory cytokines. Providing an increased content of omega-3 fatty acids in the diet may displace omega-6 fatty acids within the cell membrane, thereby favoring production of less inflammatory eicosanoids. The rodents with severe acute pancreatitis, who received an omega-6 to omega-3 ratio of 2:1 compared to 7:1, had increased production of anti-inflammatory cytokines and improved renal and respiratory function. This may be indicative of successful modulation of SIRS. Human clinical trials are needed to further evaluate their findings. Studies using fish oil (rich in omega-3 fatty acids) preparations and enriched oral supplements have shown weight stabilization in pancreatic patients.[91,92]

Amino Acids

Glutamine is a nonessential amino acid that can be synthesized by numerous tissues in the body. It has been proposed that glutamine is "conditionally essential" in some stress states such as pancreatitis. Glutamine may be beneficial to the bowel as a trophic agent and important for the preservation and maintenance of bowel mucosa following insult. Ockenga et al.[93] found that the addition of glutamine to PN was associated with a decrease in inflammatory markers and reduced length of PN therapy in acute pancreatitis patients.

Although research has shown some benefits of omega-3 fatty acids, arginine, and glutamine in decreasing the rate of complications by altering cytokine production, other studies have shown risks. Bertolini[94] reported increased mortality in septic patients supplemented with arginine. The Canadian guidelines[95] advise against the use of immune-enhancing agents in septic patients. In contrast, Zaloga[96] has reported that arginine is safe for septic patients. Clinicians must monitor patients closely when providing these nutrients, particularly when given in pharmacological doses.

Herbal Remedies

Mistletoe extract and gemcitabine are currently under study by the National Institutes of Health[97] for the treatment of solid organ tumors, such as pancreatic cancer. European mistletoe extract, *Viscum album* L. has been used in Europe to treat cancers. Data on efficacy and safety are currently inconclusive due to variability in preparations, concentrations, study populations, and study designs. In addition, there is a paucity of data on the potential toxicity of mistletoe and its interactions with chemotherapeutic medications.[97]

Orris root is a member of the Iridaceae family and is used for "gland stimulating."[98] It is used for a plethora of ailments including halitosis, migraine, bronchial asthma, loss of appetite, bowel sluggishness, and ailments of the gallbladder, liver, and pancreas. There is not enough evidence concerning its safety, especially when applied topically versus consumed after peeling and drying. If consumed as fresh juice or root, orris root can cause mucosal irritation, abdominal pain, vomiting, and bloody diarrhea. Topically, it can cause severe skin and mucosal irritation. There are insufficient reliable data on the effectiveness of orris root. Orris root is often found in conjunction with other herbs in homeopathic dilutions or teas.

Jambolan seed is from the Myrtaceae family.[98] Among its many reported benefits are treatment of diabetes, diseases of the pancreas, gastric and pancreatic complaints, nervous disorders, and exhaustion. There are insufficient data addressing the reliability, safety, and effectiveness of jambolan seed. Jambolan seed is consumed as a powdered seed or a liquid extract.

Goat's Rue is of the Fabaceae or Leguminosae family.[98] It is used for supportive therapy for diabetes and as a diuretic. It is often combined with other herbs to stimulate the pancreas and adrenal gland. There are insufficient data on its safety and effectiveness. Fatal toxicity has been reported in grazing animals, but no adverse reactions have been reported in humans. There is a potential for hypoglycemia, particularly when combined with other herbs or treatments for hyperglycemia. Goat's Rue is consumed as a tea.

Prebiotics and Probiotics

The GI tract glands, mucosa, and mucosa-associated lymphoid system contain 70% of the human immune system.[99] The GI tract contains ten times more microbes than eukaryotic cells located in the entire body. Conditions such as overuse of antibiotics and underconsumption of whole grains, fruits, and vegetables contribute to alterations in the normal intestinal flora. Western society is plagued by poor nutritional and behavioral patterns that contribute to health risks. Overconsumption of fat and sugar, reduced intake of whole grains, fruits, and vegetables, stress, and inactivity contribute to obesity and development of metabolic syndrome. An intake of five to eight servings of fresh fruits and vegetables are recommended daily. This amount is impractical for critically ill patients, but there are some intensive care units that utilize juicing machines to improve fruit and vegetable intake in critically ill patients.[99]

Contamination and infection of pancreatic tissue during acute bouts of pancreatitis can contribute to increased mortality. It is hypothesized that the treatment with probiotics with or without prebiotics may decrease the incidence of tissue colonization by non-coli Gram-negative bacteria. However, all lactic acid bacteria, the bacteria primarily used for probiotic therapy, are not equal in action or effectiveness. There are insufficient data to support routine use of probiotics in critically ill patients.[95] Fiber-fermentation lactic acid bacteria are often more effective than the lactic acid bacteria found in yogurt. Enteral products that contain prebiotics (inulin and fructooligosaccharides) are available, although there are insufficient data to recommend the exact dosage required to achieve positive outcomes.

SUMMARY

The pancreas is responsible for many nutritionally related functions. Not all patients with acute or chronic pancreatitis will require nutrition intervention. Thorough nutrition assessment and evidence-based practice should be utilized to provide nutrition management. Specialized nutrition support is generally not initiated in adequately nourished patients with mild to moderate acute pancreatitis. Oral diet should be resumed as pain and elevated pancreatic enzymes resolve. Patients with severe acute pancreatitis often require specialized nutrition support. The enteral route should be the first choice of nutrition supplementation. When PN is indicated, a mixed fuel solution is well-tolerated as long as serum triglycerides are <400 mg/dl and glycemic control is maintained. There is insufficient evidence at this time to recommend supplementation with immune-enhancing agents, pre- or probiotics, or herbal products.[95]

ENDOCRINE PANCREAS AND DIABETES MELLITUS

ENDOCRINE FUNCTION OF THE PANCREAS

The endocrine component consists of cells that secrete pancreatic hormones such as insulin and glucagon into the venous system, draining the pancreas for action at distant tissue sites. The endocrine cells in the pancreas produce peptide hormones that have local, regional, and systemic effects. The endocrine and exocrine functions of the pancreas, though closely related, operate independently of one another. Clusters of cells, called islets, synthesize and secrete hormones. Islets are composed of pancreatic polypeptides (alpha, beta, and delta) and enterochromaffin cells.

Alpha cells secrete glucagon. Glucagon is responsible for gluconeogenesis. Alpha cells are stimulated by hypoglycemia, hyperinsulinemia, catecholamines, and exercise. Glucagon stimulates glycogenolysis in the liver and is a major regulatory hormone of glucose homeostasis.

Glucose stimulates the production and release of insulin from beta cells. During fasting, healthy individuals' baseline insulin levels are very low. Insulin levels rise to approximately 600 to 800% over baseline in response to a glucose challenge.[100] In addition to regulating glucose levels, insulin is also active in mobilizing amino acids to peripheral tissue and in suppression of lipolysis. In the absence of glucose, amino acids and lipids can stimulate insulin release.

Insulin is a 51 amino acid sulfur-containing polypeptide that is translated from mRNA as preproinsulin. There are two amino acid strands, which are linked together by disulfide bonds. Within the endoplasmic reticulum (ER) of the beta cell, preproinsulin is converted to proinsulin and stored. Within the ER, proinsulin is exposed to endopeptidases, which convert proinsulin to C-peptide and insulin. Stimulated beta cells secrete both insulin and C-peptide. Insulin travels in the bloodstream to target cells where it acts on its receptor. The function of C-peptide is unknown.

Glucose disposal into tissue is via a mechanism involving the insulin receptor and glucose transporter complexes. The insulin receptor contains extra-, trans-, and intracellular domains and is expressed in most tissues. Insulin binding to its receptor initiates signaling, which promotes a cascade of reactions involving phospholipid second messengers and insulin receptor substrate proteins. Insulin signaling is a process, which facilitates translocation of glucose transporter proteins from intracellular vesicles to the cell membrane, and ultimately results in glucose uptake by the cell. Insulin signaling also regulates expression of genes involved in glucose and lipid metabolism, for example glucokinase (GK), hormone-sensitive lipase, lipoprotein lipase, tumor necrosis factor-alpha (TNF-α), and peroxisome proliferator-activated receptor-gamma (PPAR-γ).[101] In addition to regulating glucose uptake by cells, insulin is also a growth hormone and promotes accumulation of protein in muscle and fat in adipose tissue. Insulin, via interaction with leptin, also regulates appetite.[102]

Impaired insulin production, secretion, or action results in hyperglycemia and diabetes. Type 1 diabetes is a condition of insulin deficiency caused by autoimmune damage to the beta cells. Type 1 diabetes accounts for about 5% of all cases of diabetes. Type 2 diabetes is a complex disorder involving impaired insulin signaling and action and accounts for >90% of all diabetes cases. In type 2 diabetes, initially insulin levels are elevated. Hyperglycemia results from impaired insulin signaling and action. Over time beta cells fail and insulin levels become deficient. Obesity increases the risk of developing type 2 diabetes. Nutritional intake impacts both obesity and diabetes, and plays an important role in prevention and treatment.

Diabetes affects 150–170 million persons worldwide. Of the 13–18 million persons in the United States who have diabetes, one third to one half of them are undiagnosed. Still, there are over 2000 new cases diagnosed everyday. The prevalence of diabetes in the United States is 1.5% among persons aged 18–44 years, 6% among persons aged 45–64 years, and 11% among persons aged ≥65 years.[103–105] The lifetime risk of type 2 diabetes is about 40% among children with one diabetic parent. Rare genetic forms of diabetes include maturity-onset diabetes of the young (MODY), severe insulin resistance caused by insulin receptor defects, familial lipodystrophy, latent autoimmune diabetes of adults (LADA), and others. Secondary causes of diabetes include pancreatitis, hemochromatosis, excess growth hormone, excess cortisol and glucocorticoid use, drugs, surgery, and pancreatic agenesis.[103,105]

The delta cells secrete somatostatin and vasoactive intestinal peptide. Somatostatin is responsible for regulating intestinal motility. In the pancreas, somatostatin can inhibit the release of either glucagon or insulin and aid in maintaining blood glucose in a very narrow range. Vasoactive intestinal peptide induces glycogenolysis and hyperglycemia (indirectly by stimulating corticotropin) and stimulates gastric fluid secretion. Enterochromaffin cells secrete serotonin and gastrin and perhaps other substances yet to be identified. Recent research shows that islets also produce ghrelin, a hormone involved in appetite regulation and energy homeostasis.[106,107]

TUMORS OF THE PANCREAS AND TREATMENT

Adenocarcinoma originates from the cells of pancreatic ducts. Endocrine tumors of the pancreas originate from hormone-producing cells. Adenocarcinoma is more common. Endocrine tumors are rare, the prevalence in the U.S. population is approximately 1 per 100,000 per year. Endocrine tumors can occur sporadically or as part of multiple endocrine neoplasia type 1 (MEN 1). MEN 1 involves tumors of the pituitary, parathyroids, and pancreas. The pancreatic tumors can produce abnormal amounts of any of the islet hormones, including insulin, glucagon, vasoactive intestinal peptide, pancreatic polypeptide, and somatostatinoma. Surgical resection of the tumor is primary treatment. Chemotherapy may be effective for some types of tumors. A fish oil-enriched nutritional supplement has been shown in short-term studies to improve cancer cachexia and pancreatic cancer cachexia outcomes.[108]

Pancreatic tumors can be associated with gastrin hypersecretion, severe peptic ulcer disease, and secretory diarrhea. This syndrome is called Zollinger Ellison syndrome.[109] Primary treatment with proton pump inhibitors and histamine blockers. Surgery may be indicated in some cases.

DIABETES

Diabetes is the most common consequence of pancreatic dysfunction in the United States and is a burgeoning epidemic worldwide. It is estimated that 25% of the U.S. population meets the diagnostic criteria for the metabolic syndrome, a precursor to type 2 DM, whose constituents include impaired fasting glucose, elevated blood pressure, high triglyceride and HDL cholesterol levels, and expanded waist circumference. Ninety percent of diabetes cases are type 2 diabetes, only 5 to 10% are type 1 diabetes. Key concerns for health practitioners are the

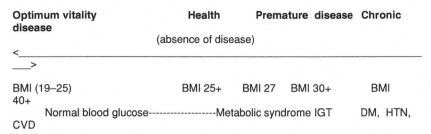

Optimum vitality disease	Health	Premature disease	Chronic
	(absence of disease)		

<____
___>

BMI (19–25)   BMI 25+   BMI 27   BMI 30+   BMI 40+

Normal blood glucose-------------------Metabolic syndrome IGT   DM, HTN, CVD

FIGURE 14.2 Wellness–illness continuum and type 2 diabetes. (From Travis, J., *The Wellness Workbook*, Ten Speed Press, Berkley, CA, 1981.)

prevention of diabetes, early intervention and effective treatment when impaired glucose tolerance (IGT), prediabetes or diabetes (DM) have been identified. Progression to diabetes among those with prediabetes is not inevitable: weight loss and increased activity can normalize glucose levels or delay the onset of diabetes.[110,111] Maintaining goal levels for blood glucose, lipid and blood pressure in persons with diabetes can prevent or delay the onset of diabetic complications including early heart disease and stroke, limb amputations, vision loss, and kidney disease.[112–114]

The integrative nutrition practitioner may view health or disease as a continuum (optimum health at one end, health in the middle, and premature disease on the other end of the continuum — see Figure 14.2). Thus, the continuum of care related to the pancreas may include prevention of diabetes, therapy or treatment (of IGT, DM, metabolic syndrome, or reactive hypoglycemia), and finally the prevention of diabetic complications. From an integrative perspective, lifestyle or other factors that compromise the integrity of the host (person) are viewed as promoters of disease or disease progression (see Figure 14.3). The

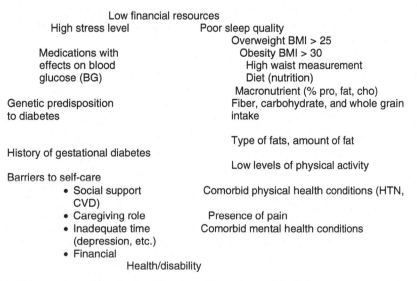

FIGURE 14.3 Factors that effect the health status of a person with diabetes.

greater the environmental, genetic and lifestyle influences, and stressors on the individual, the more likely diabetes and diabetic complications may occur.

Diabetes self-management training (DSMT) is the baseline standard of care and includes nutrition as part of the skills training for people with diabetes.[116] DSMT utilizes the following seven key areas of self-care:

1. Diet or nutrition
2. Exercise or activity
3. Medications
4. Home glucose monitoring
5. Annual eye or fasting lipids or podiatry or microalbumin
6. Stress management
7. Problem solving

MEDICAL NUTRITION THERAPY FOR DIABETES

Assessment

Patient history is the first step in therapeutic intervention: an assessment focused more on the person than on the disease. Each person is a unique system: the state of health and path to well-being and self-care is greatly influenced by nature, nurture, self-efficacy, and genes. Intervention based on a comprehensive history includes anthropometrics, diet history, exercise, medications, social and health history, and supplement review (Table 14.5). Additionally, the following should be taken into consideration:

- Growth charts are an important part of assessment among children with type 1 diabetes.
- For selected individuals, body composition to determine fat percent and lean may be useful as motivation or to track progress with weight management or exercise programs.
- For individuals with type 1 diabetes, men or women over 40 years with type 2 diabetes or patients with diabetes who have been treated with steroids, a dual energy x-ray absorptiometry (DEXA) bone scan may be useful, as these patients are at an increased risk of osteoporosis.
- Micronutrients assessment (amount and sources of vitamins, minerals, with special attention to food sources of antioxidants, magnesium and especially in the newly diagnosed patient, chromium).
- Alcohol: quantity, timing, drug–nutrient interactions, blood glucose (BG) effects, micronutrient implications.
- Sodium and potassium content of foods such as fruits and vegetables and food preparation measures influencing nutrient retention (such as steaming versus boiling).[117]

It is useful to have the client bring in a detailed 3-day food record, including timing of food intake and medication use.

Past medical history — Seek to rule out primary causes of the condition or factors that may be contributing to the development of prediabetes or diabetes such as steroid use, severe infections, etc. Refer for further medical care if indicated before implementing a nutrition plan.

Weight history — Review age of onset and pattern of obesity or weight gain, dieting, and weight history.

TABLE 14.5
Components of Patient Assessment

Anthropometrics	Current anthropometrics: Height, weight, waist measurement, BMI, central adiposity, (optional) body composition	Implications: Waist measures >35 in. (88 cm) for women or >40 in. (102 cm) for men indicates metabolic syndrome and diabetes risk
	History: Previous BMI range	
Diet	Current food intake: Macronutrient amounts and types (quality): amount and type of fiber, glycemic load; micronutrient, phytochemical and fluid intake. Eating times	Individualize dietary recommendations and teaching to prioritize greatest physiological need with patient concerns or goals and lifestyle preferences
	History: Past dietary patterns and weight loss diets and methods	
	Presence or absence of compulsive or emotional, night or binge eating	May benefit from: carbohydrate counting, group education, regular follow-up
Exercise	Current patterns of exercise regarding frequency, intensity, duration. Preferences and barriers to exercise. Frequency of hypoglycemia in proximity to exercise	Exercise testing recommended; special footware may be needed. Review hypoglycemia, ID bracelet, and sports nutrition guidelines
	History of injury or illness, etc. that may alter exercise	
	Pedometer use	
Supplements	Evaluate current supplements	Evaluate excesses or deficiencies
	Discuss supplement questions	
Medications	List all current medicines and dosages including: • Blood glucose control • Hyperlipidemia • Hypertension • Angiotensin receptor blocker (ACE and ARB)	Ensure patient is eating in recommended proximity to type of DM glucose control medications
	Medication compliance	Assess food medication interactions
Laboratory tests	Current A_{1c}, fasting lipid profile, microalbumin, and other pertinent laboratories; also home glucose monitoring to include postprandial (2 h) blood glucose testing	Goals: LDL cholesterol <100 mg/dl, <70 mg/dl if established heart disease or high-risk A_{1c} < 6.5%
	Assess glycemic and lipid history, etc.	

Family history — Identify first-degree relatives with diabetes, obesity, or cardiovascular disease. The integrative practitioner listens to family history; awareness of past family experiences with diabetes may influence disease risk and the patients' adjustment to disease.

If osteoporosis, celiac disease, or gluten sensitivity is suspected comorbid condition with diabetes, especially for patients with type 1, it is recommended that practitioners ask about risk and predisposing factors and suggest discussing testing (including biopsy for celiac disease) if indicated.[118]

For all patients with type 2 diabetes, atherogenic changes equal to those who have had a prior myocardial infarction are likely, and all pertinent nutrition therapy for preexisting cardiovascular disease prevails. Controlling blood lipids and blood pressure are the two primary factors that reduce cardiovascular disease in diabetes.

As with any health condition, asking about (and listening for) other addictions is important. Since self-treatment is the key to good diabetes management, other addictions can undermine good care.

Psychosocial and stress history — Stress hormones interfere with the normal action of insulin; so depressive symptoms, history of depression, high chronic stress levels all may need primary evaluation concurrent with nutrition treatment.

Laboratory evaluation — A variety of laboratory tests beyond the standard biannual or quarterly HbA$_{1c}$, annual microalbumin, and annual fasting lipid profile may help identify the direction for future care. These tests may also be useful:

> Complete blood count (CBC) — anemias
>
> White blood cells (WBC) — high WBC indicates an inflammatory response
>
> Mean corpuscular hemoglobin (MCH), mean corpuscular volume (MCV) — one indicator of folate and B12 levels
>
> C-Reactive protein (CRP) — plasma CRP levels have been shown to predict the development of type 2 diabetes in several diverse populations[119]
>
> Homocysteine, Lp(a) — cardiovascular risk
>
> Thyroid panels — evaluation of concurrent autoimmune conditions, weight balance
>
> Saliva pH — some practitioners value assessment of acidity, alkalinity
>
> Micronutrient levels — folate, B12, B6, etc.
>
> Additional tests that are considered more functional laboratory tests can be quite useful. Nutritionists may order these tests, under the supervision of a medical doctor

> Examples:
>
> 1. Insulin levels, oral glucose tolerance tests
> 2. ELISA testing for delayed food sensitivity
> 3. Gluten intolerance (anti-tTB or tissue transglutaminase test is the most current, historically the antigliadin antibody assay)
> 4. Comprehensive digestive stool analysis, to assess digestive functioning
> 5. Adrenal profile, to assess cortisol and dehydroepiandrosterone (DHEA) status
> 6. Comprehensive thyroid panels (including ultrasensitive TSH and free T$_4$)

Other assessment tools such as food records and blood glucose logbooks are recommended in diabetes care. Psychological evaluation such as the Beck Depression Inventory, especially if patient is in chronic pain (such as with neuropathy), sleep is compromised, or they exhibit undue distress, sadness, or low self-esteem during an office visit. Depression is a frequent comorbid condition with type 2 diabetes and if untreated can adversely influence patient's ability to conduct self-care. Motivational interviewing, stage-of-change and readiness assessments are also recommended to identify patient's readiness and barriers to change.

Nutritional Management Recommendations

Key goals for diabetes nutrition management (type 1 and type 2) are to:

- Normalize blood glucose to reduce the risk for complications of diabetes[120]
- Normalize lipids and lipoprotein profiles to reduce risk for micro- and macrovascular disease, especially coronary artery and cerebral vascular disease[121]
- Normalize blood pressure
- Promote or achieve a good quality of life

Integrative nutrition therapy goals for type 2 may also include:

- Reduction of inflammatory markers[122]
- Use of lifestyle measures (diet and exercise) to minimize need for medication or to "reverse" diabetes[123]
- Weight control

American Diabetes Association (ADA) evidence-based guidelines for nutrition care serve as the basis for medical nutrition therapy. The practitioner may also recommend whole foods, botanicals, or nutritionally dense functional foods as part of the nutrition strategy.

- *Food plan*: Meals and snacks for weekdays and weekends. Carbohydrate counting, the plate method, or exchange system may be utilized to regulate blood glucose, lipids, and weight
- *Exercise plan*: Encouraging patient to reach toward the goal of 30–60 min for 5 or more days per week. Instruct about hypoglycemia prevention and treatment. Encourage or require exercise testing before starting an exercise program, depending on patient's risk status
- An integrative practitioner may also incorporate other methods of health and nutrition management for the client with diabetes including treatment for emotional or compulsive eating (such as Solution Method TM approaches), support groups, and other mind–body therapies[124,125]

TYPE 1 DIABETES

In addition to standard care for type 1 diabetes, nutritional factors that may potentiate destruction of islet cells are important to explore:

- Food allergy or immune response
- Milk (casein)
- Gluten (wheat, oats, barley, rye)

Autoimmune conditions such as celiac disease (gluten sensitivity) occur more frequently in people with type 1 diabetes than in the general population. Restricting gluten reduces the damage from celiac disease, and in children results in a return to healthful digestion or absorption, reductions in anemia, and resumption of normal growth patterns. Finland has "the highest incidence of diabetes and cow's milk consumption in the world," so cow's milk has been investigated as a possible etiologic factor in the development of type 1 diabetes.[126] In 410 sibling pairs with diabetes, children with type 1 diabetes had higher levels of cow's milk protein antibodies with their genetically matched sibling controls, and "these high levels of antibodies are independent risk markers" for type 1 diabetes.[127] The Childhood Diabetes in Finland Study Group found that early introduction of dairy products (before age of 2 months) was associated with an increased risk of type 1 diabetes.[128] The routine inclusion of these allergy evaluations in type 1 diabetes is still controversial and not yet supported by strong evidence (Textbox 14.1).

Textbox 14.1 Impaired Glucose Tolerance, Metabolic Syndrome

Many of the same recommendations and patient experiments (trials) as noted for type 2 diabetes may be pertinent for patients with IGT or for those seeking to avoid diabetes.[129] The effectiveness of macronutrient, fiber, and micronutrient manipulation for diabetes prevention (effects on insulin signaling) and delaying the onset of diabetes are the topics of current study.[130] Costacou and Mayer-Davis[131] have recently completed a review of the role of nutrition in prevention in type 2 diabetes. Wang et al.[132] confirmed a relationship between saturated fat lipid levels and risk for developing type 2 diabetes. In a prospective investigation of 2909 middle-aged adults over 9 years, "the incidence of developing diabetes was significantly associated with a high proportion of saturated fatty acids in plasma cholesterol esters (CE) and phospholipid (PL)" and plasma lipids correlated with dietary intake assessed by food-frequency questionnaire.[132] "All types of dietary fat (except omega-3 fatty acids) may have an adverse effect on insulin sensitivity. Saturated fat may have the greatest effect."[133]

Patients in a randomized, controlled 5-week crossover design trial on a low-glycemic index diet decreased the total body fat mass (without causing weight loss) and decreased leptin, lipoprotein lipase, and hormone-sensitive lipase levels in human abdominal adipose tissue.[134] For this study, carbohydrate foods with a GI < 45% were classified as low glycemic index, foods with a GI > 60 were recommended in the high-GI period. The GIs ascribed to foods were taken from published data or (for the special cereals and LGI cookies) were provided by the suppliers.[135]

Practical guidelines for treating patients with IGT include obtaining a healthy weight as well as improving metabolic indices such as blood pressure, cholesterol levels, etc. Encouraging use of whole grain foods rather than refined carbohydrates, awareness of carbohydrate quality and quantity or carbohydrate counting, and use of exercise to enhance glucose utilization are other disease-prevention strategies.

TYPE 2 DIABETES

Medical nutrition therapy for type 2 diabetes seeks to improve the underlying condition of insulin resistance. Since there may be a 10-year delay between insulin resistance and the clinical diagnosis of IGT or type 2 DM, early intervention with lifestyle changes (nutrition and exercise) is important. In the obese individual with insulin resistance, the pancreas (beta cells) may secrete excess insulin to overcome insulin resistance.[136] Including exercise early in diabetes treatment reduces insulin resistance and may improve liver function and normalize glucagon release. Controlling carbohydrate quantity reduces postprandial hyperglycemia and may prevent hyperinsulinemia and overstimulation by the pancreas, preserving beta cell function.

The diabetes care plan is built on a strong foundation of diet, exercise, and other aspects of self-care. Dietary changes for patients with diabetes may include one or several of the following factors.

Modulate Carbohydrate (Amount, Type, Timing) to Achieve BG Goals

The current ADA recommendation for carbohydrate does not specify a specific percent of calories, but does recommend that "carbohydrate and monounsaturated fat together should provide 60 to 70% of energy intake."[137] Carbohydrate sources such as whole grains, fruits, vegetables, and low-fat dairy are recommended. "Consistency with day-to-day carbohydrate intake" for individuals on fixed daily insulin regimens, and carbohydrate distribution over the day or matching to medications and patient lifestyle are recommended aspects of care.[138]

"A number of factors influence glycemic responses to foods, including the amount of carbohydrate, type of sugar (glucose, fructose, sucrose, lactose), nature of the starch (amylose, amylopectin, resistant starch), cooking and food processing, and food form, as well as other food components (fat and other substances that alter the rate of digestion — lectins, phytates, tannins, and starch protein and starch–lipid combinations)."[139] In type 1 and some type 2 patients, carbohydrate counting is a useful strategy that can give mealtime flexibility when used in conjunction with insulin, etc.

Using the Glycemic Index

The glycemic index is a method of classifying foods according to their potential for elevating blood glucose. Use of the glycemic index and glycemic load in medical nutrition therapy for diabetes is controversial. "In diabetic patients, evidence from medium-term studies suggests that replacing high-glycemic-index carbohydrates with a low-glycemic-index forms will improve glycemic control and, among persons treated with insulin, will reduce hypoglycemic episodes."[140] "Choosing low-GI foods in place of conventional or high-GI foods has a small but clinically useful effect on medium-term glycemic control in patients with type 2 diabetes."[141] The ADA evidence-based nutrition recommendations note that "there is no clear trend in outcome benefits" as a treatment for diabetes and "the ability of individuals to maintain these diets long-term (and therefore achieve glycemic benefit) has not been established."[142] Jarvi et al.[143] showed a low-GI diet "normalized" one of the measures of fibrinolysis, plasminogen activator inhibitor-1, and remained unchanged on the high-GI diet.

Fiber Intake

Increasing fiber, "particularly of the soluble type, above the level recommended by the ADA, improves glycemic control, decreases hyperinsulinemia, and lowers plasma lipid concentrations in patients with type 2 diabetes."[144] Soluble fibers (such as pectin, gums, and mucilages found in apples, beans, and oats) dissolve in water, forming a gel that alters GI transit and glucose absorption rate, and bind cholesterol, and thus are particularly beneficial for diabetes. Insoluble fibers (such as wheat bran and cellulose) are insoluble in water, beneficial for laxation, and contribute to the recommended goal of 25 g/day or more of fiber for adults.

Increase Consumption of Vegetables with Some Fruits and Vegetables

The enhanced satiety of plant foods (fruits and vegetables) may curb hunger and contribute to weight loss.[145] Phytochemicals in plant food are cardioprotective and promote health for vision, bones, and other aspects of total health.

Vitamins

"Persons with diabetes should be educated about the importance of consuming adequate amounts of vitamins and minerals from natural food sources as well as the potential toxicity of megadoses of vitamin and mineral supplements."[146] A low-dose multivitamin or mineral supplement may be advised for those with chronic disease including diabetes.[147,148] The ADA's *Clinical Nutrition Principles and Recommendations in Diabetes* note that supplementation "can be beneficial" if deficiencies of vitamins and minerals are identified, citing evidence-based research on use of single, multiple, low-potency and high-dose supplements on diabetes and some of the complications such as heart disease.[149] In a recent randomized controlled trial of 130 community-dwelling adults with type 2 diabetes, those on supplementation with a multivitamin reported significantly fewer infections ($p < .001$) than the placebo group. Several multivitamin formulations have been shown to reduce elevated CRP levels.[150] Several diabetes-specific multivitamin mineral (MVI) brands of different quality are available.

Vitamin supplementation to include good food or other sources of folate and B12 is recommended for people over 65 years. Adequate folate and B12 maintain normal levels of homocysteine and prevent subclinical vitamin B12 deficiency or pernicious anemia. Supplementing with a minimum of 2.4 mcg of B12 in synthetic form is recommended for people over 65 years. Biotin, a micronutrient active in the TCA cycle, "stimulates glucose-induced insulin secretion in pancreatic beta cells and accelerates glycolysis in the liver and pancreas" by regulating hepatic and pancreatic GK "at both transcriptional and translational levels."[147] "Efficient GK activity is required for normal glucose-stimulated insulin secretion, postprandial hepatic glucose uptake, and suppression of hepatic glucose output and gluconeogenesis by elevated plasma glucose". Ensuring adequate dietary intake or supplements is recommended. Hepatic GK activity is subnormal in diabetes.[148]

Minerals

Chromium

Chromium picolinate or glucose tolerance factor (GTF) chromium supplementation may be useful for a short-term period of 6–8 weeks in newly diagnosed type 2 diabetes or IGT patients in amounts up to 400 mcg/day in two divided doses. The tolerable upper limit (an aspect of the dietary recommended intake guidelines) for chromium is not established, due in part to a low-toxicity profile, however the adequate intake (AI) for chromium in healthy individuals is 25 to 30 μg/day.[149] The ADA (2004) guidelines note that "At the present, benefit from chromium supplementation in persons with diabetes has not been conclusively demonstrated."[150] Numerous studies show that chromium is beneficial in reducing insulin resistance.[151]

Zinc

Zinc is important to ensure adequate zinc intake by evaluating adequate zinc dietary source (generally meats and seafood). Vegetarians may be deficient in zinc intake; people with extra GI loss of fluids, such as diarrhea, may also need additional zinc through food or supplement. Excess zinc, however, can lower the HDL cholesterol; supplementation at doses higher than the UL is not recommended except for short-term instances of wound healing or immune system support.[156]

Since renal complications frequently occur in later stage diabetes, and the primary excretory route for excess minerals is via the kidney, it is imperative that practitioners check recent kidney function including creatinine clearance before suggesting supplemental minerals or mineral-fortified foods. In the absence of normal kidney function (renal excretion), these minerals including chromium can have unanticipated hypoglycemic or toxic effects.

Magnesium

Magnesium may be protective or preventive in early stages of type 2 DM development in adult patients with normal kidney function.[157,158] Lopez-Ridaura et al.[159] found a significant inverse association between low magnesium intake and risk of developing diabetes in a cohort of 127,000 individuals, who were followed for 18 years. Magnesium deficiency may play a role in insulin resistance, carbohydrate intolerance, and hypertension. The UL for magnesium is

350 mg/day for healthy individuals. Magnesium is abundant in natural, unprocessed foods such as green leafy vegetables, whole grains, and beans. In individuals with healthy kidneys (normal kidney function), diarrhea may be a consequence of excess supplemental magnesium intake. As with other supplements, it is especially important to determine safe and effective intake for patients with renal insufficiency or renal failure.

Potassium

For potassium, the ideal recommendation is supplementation via high potassium fruits and vegetables prepared via methods that conserve potassium (raw, steamed, etc.). Potassium loss may be "sufficient to warrant dietary supplementation in patients taking diuretics."[160] KCl as salt substitute or other forms of supplemental or even dietary potassium needs to be limited or stopped, when there is a reduction of urine output (kidney failure).

Phytonutrients

Nutritionally dense foods are recommended on a regular basis to provide supplemental levels of useful nutrients in whole food form. Hundreds of "phyto" (plant) chemicals have been identified with cardiovascular- and cancer-protective properties (see Table 14.6). It is important to gain nutrition via a whole foods diet versus supplementing a poor diet with vitamin or mineral or other supplements alone.

Botanicals

Table 14.7 includes various botanicals and their potential uses in diabetes care or diabetes complications. It should be noted that purity of formulas containing these botanicals is not Food and Drug Administration (FDA) regulated, because impurities and variable amounts of the active ingredient may be present; use of herbal remedies as key strategies to treat blood glucose is not advised at this time. In the future, as purified products become available, use of botanicals may produce safer, more reliable results. While not listed as a contraindication for each botanical, it should be noted that those with demonstrated hypoglycemic effect could cause hypoglycemia if consumed with hypoglycemic medications. Botanicals consumed as food or seasoning (e.g., garlic, bitter melon, turmeric) can be consumed safely.

TABLE 14.6
Attributes of Whole Foods and Risk for Disease

Whole Food	Actions or Attributes	Refs.
Beans	Low glycemic index, soluble fiber, cholesterol reduction, magnesium-rich food	161
Onion	Quercetin, dietary flavenoid (antioxidant), phenolic compounds, hypoglycemic effect	162, 163
Blueberries	Antioxidant	
Salmon, wild, and other fatty fish	Omega-3 fatty acids (antiarrhythmic properties, antithrombogenic, hypotriglyderidemic), reductions in sudden cardiac death	164, 165, 166
Nuts	Source of unsaturated fats, fiber, and magnesium; improves lipid profile	167
Oats and oat bran	Contains beta-glucan, a source of soluble fiber: improves glycemic control, reductions in LDL cholesterol	168, 169, 166

TABLE 14.7
Indications and Contraindications for the Use of Botanicals in Diabetes

Botanical Name	Effects	Contraindications	Evidence
Momordica charantia (bitter melon) (karela — common Indian name)	The juice of the unripe fruit is a hypoglycemic agent with insulin-like properties when injected in animals and humans[167]	Reports of coma, convulsions in children; reduced fertility (mice); favism-like syndrome, and headaches from the juice extract. Consumed as food in the Indian or Asian diet, no toxicity has been reported. May cause digestive discomfort[168]	Most small studies, done in India or in the United States in animal models
Gymnema	Protective effect on the pancreas, postulated to promote regeneration of islet cells.[173] "Increases activity of key enzymes of insulin-dependent glucose utilization pathways, such as phosphorylases and gluconeogenic enzymes" in animal models.[174,175] Chewing *Gymnema* interferes with perception of sweet taste[176]	No significant toxicities are reported. Nausea has been reported in patients who take more than 3 g/day. "Because of the possibility of hypoglycemia when *Gymnema* is used with insulin or other diabetes agents, doses for existing diabetes therapies may have to be adjusted with the addition of *Gymnema*. This product should not be used without medical supervision"[177]	
Coccinia indica	Juice of the leaf contains an amylase and B-sitosterol.[178] Hypoglycemic effects when given orally to type 2 patients with diabetes	No adverse side effects noted in randomized controlled trials (RCTs), controlled clinical trials, or prospective trials[179]	
Opuntia streptacantha (prickly pear) (nopal)	"Nopal leaves, stems, and fruits have some post-meal blood glucose lowering effect" in small human and animal trials[180]	No reported side effects	

Panax quinquefolius (American ginseng)	Hypoglycemic effects shown in animal models and human clinical trials[181]	"May elevate blood pressure; not recommended for people with HTN or CVD"; sources sometimes adulterated[182]
Cinnamon	Decreases fasting glucose, triglyceride, LDL-cholesterol, and total cholesterol in people with type 2 diabetes[183]	Generally regarded as safe (GRAS) food
Curcuma longa (turmeric)	Reductions in LDL and VLDL cholesterol (oral doses) in animal models of diabetes[185]; antioxidant; enhanced wound healing when applied topically to animals[186]	Constituent of curry, the turmeric root has been used in food (spice) for many years
Gamma-linolenic acid (GLA) (evening primrose; borage oil; black currant seed oil)	GLA is an omega-6 fatty acid. Supply of this essential fatty acid, some studies shows, aids in neuropathic pain.[187] "Diabetes appears to decrease the body's ability to make it's own GLA"[188]	For people with epilepsy, large doses of GLA may counteract some seizure medications
Galega officinalis (Goat's Rue)	Used in medieval Europe as a treatment for diabetes. The drug metformin was derived from this plant[189]	
Trigonella (fenugreek seeds)	Mild hypoglycemic effect; high in soluble fiber. Decreases absorption of glucose by slowing transit time. Also fenugreek seed lowers cholesterol and triglycerides in normal and diabetic animals and humans[190]	Induces lactation in breastfeeding women. "Mild gastro-intestinal discomfort in high doses"[191]

		RCT with 60 adults with type 2; cinnamon reduced serum glucose, triglyceride, LDL and total cholesterol[184]

NUTRITIONAL MANAGEMENT OF DIABETIC COMPLICATIONS

Heart Disease

Heart disease is the leading complication of diabetes; blood pressure and lipid control level goals are more stringent than for nondiabetes populations.[192] Lipid control lifestyle strategies such as weight reduction, increasing beans, and other forms of soluble fiber, decreasing saturated fats and *trans*-fatty acids, have less reliance on heavily processed and unlabeled restaurant food. Diet therapy for blood pressure management includes the DASH diet with emphasis on a total of six to seven servings of nonstarchy vegetables and two to three servings of fruits, on weight reduction, and on an improved potassium-to-sodium ratio. Since restaurant food and processed foods including snack foods are the two greatest sources of dietary sodium, the skills of smart shopping, menu preparation, and fixing healthful food at home are important steps to conserving potassium, minimizing sodium, and managing blood pressure.

Neuropathy

Optimal blood glucose control is the key strategy for prevention of diabetic peripheral neuropathy.[193] A variety of other nutrients such as the essential fatty acid (gamma-linolenic acid [GLA]) and the antioxidant (alpha-lipoic acid [ALA]) have been tested both in animals and humans as agents to improve neuoropathic sensory symptoms in diabetic patients with neuropathy.[194] In the randomized controlled SYDNEY trial, a racemic ALA was delivered intravenously at 600 mg daily for 5 days/week to 60 patients with type 2 diabetes and neuropathy. Results in the intervention group (compared to placebo) showed significant reductions in neuropathic sensory symptoms such as pain, improvement of the total symptom score, nerve conduction, and global assessment of efficacy.[195] Currently intravenous ALA is not FDA approved or available in the United States.

SUMMARY

Disordered blood glucose regulation, both in the case of DM and the metabolic syndrome, has become epidemic problems with enormous public health repercussions. Along the spectrum from metabolic syndrome to overt diabetes, ideal blood glucose management includes diet and exercise (lifestyle strategies) as first-line and integral parts of self-care. A wholesome diet should be supplemented with phytonutrient-rich food choices and where indicated, vitamin or mineral supplements. A meal-planning system such as carbohydrate quality or counting with reductions in saturated fat is recommended. Although the botanical supplements that have hypoglycemic activity are numerous, due to the lack of large randomized controlled trials with these botanicals and variance in product standardization and purity, use of botanicals for first-line care is not advised at this time. Precisely because select botanicals do have hypoglycemic effects, individuals should be advised for safety reasons to inform their physician if they choose to experiment with botanical medicines. If patients have not participated in the 10-h Diabetes Self-Management Training (DSMT) classes that Medicare and most insurance companies support, it is recommended that patients be encouraged to attend. The focus of DSMT is integrative and encourages patient or client empowerment and self-responsibility in caring for diabetes. Early education can delay or prevent the development of diabetes or diabetes complications.

PANCREAS CASE STUDY

G.M. is a 54-year-old female initially seen by an endocrinologist for hot flashes and a rash on her torso. She had been taking oral glucocorticoid steroids for the rash, which resolved after treatment. She has experienced significant weight gain over the past 4 years. Her weight at age of 50 years was 116 lb. She currently weighs 200 lb. She denies polyuria, polydipsia. She is walking 15 min daily.

Past medical history: Hyperlipidemia and prior total abdominal hysterectomy

Food allergies: Peanuts, no known drug allergies

Family history: Unknown

Social history: Married, two teenage children. Stopped tobacco 16 years ago. She is an office manager and sits most of the day. Drinks two to three alcoholic drinks weekly

Medications: Premarin, Claritin D

Physical examination: Height 5′2″, weight 200 lb, blood pressure 120/98, BMI 36 kg/m, pulse 70 beats per minute

Others: Examination of the head, neck, heart, lungs is normal; waist circumference is 95 cm (37 in.)

Laboratory examination: normal nonfasting chemistry including glucose 119, cholesterol 230 mg/dl, TG 98, HDL 95, LDL 115, normal liver enzymes

Assessment: G.M. has the following risk factors for the metabolic syndrome: abdominal obesity (waist circumference >88 cm or >35 in.) and BP (>130/85 mmHg).[196] Her weight has increased 84 lb in the last 4 years (an increase of 72% from her usual weight). She does not yet have the other metabolic syndrome risk factors of high triglyceride, high fasting blood glucose, or low HDL. Although her total cholesterol is high, her cholesterol/HDL ratio is good at 2.4. An integrative nutrition assessment would explore the etiology of the weight change and blood pressure including changes in family or socioeconomic, stress level, mood, patterns of eating, activity, and sleep habits. Additionally biochemical assessment of adrenal and thyroid function should be completed to target effective treatment and also prevent further progression of IGT and diabetes.

Treatment plan: (1) Tested A_{1c} = 5.3%. G.M. was asked to perform home glucose monitoring. Results demonstrate more than two fasting glucose readings over 126, which meet the classification for type 2 diabetes. (2) Medical nutrition therapy appropriate to her lifestyle, especially education and goal setting regarding moderation in carbohydrate intake, the DASH diet for hypertension, and dietary modification to yield a 5% or 20-lb weight loss over the next 6 months. These interventions would be expected to reduce her blood pressure and total cholesterol. Implementation would include identifying her stage of change, participatory decision making regarding which behaviors to change, and strengthening conviction and confidence for planned changes. The use of unsaturated fats with a good mix of omega-3 fats such as flax, walnuts and fatty fish, omega-6 fats; and the avoidance of saturated fats would be encouraged for cardiac protection and improving insulin sensitivity. Additionally, substitution of low-glycemic index foods in place of high-glycemic index foods improve fasting glucose and potentially limit postprandial glucose excursions. (3) Graded activity or exercise from her 15 min/day toward the ultimate goal of 60 min or 10,000 steps most days in small reasonable increments. Suggesting use of a pedometer initially to help with self-awareness and motivation. (4) Emotional or group support for weight loss such as Weight Watchers, the Solution Method TM, or a prediabetes group, etc. (5) Use of good health principles are adequate sleep, regular meal timing, etc. (6) Supplementation with a multivitamin and others based on her specific lifestyle factors (such as calcium and vitamin B12).

REFERENCES

1. http://training.seer.cancer.gov (accessed April 2, 2005).
2. Cotran, R.S., *Robbins Pathologic Basis of Disease*, 6th ed., W.B. Saunders, Philadelphia, 1999.
3. Schaffalitzky de Muckadell, O.B. and Fahrenkung, J., Role of secretion in man, in *Gut*, Bloom, S.R., Ed., Churchill Livingstone, Edinburgh, 1978, p. 197.
4. Slaff, J. et al., Protease specific suppression of pancreatic exocrine secretion, *Gastroenterology*, 87, 44, 1984.
5. Levelle-Jones, M. and Neoptolemos, J.P., Recent advances in the treatment of acute pancreatitis, *Surg. Annu.*, 22, 235, 1990.
6. Yousaf, M., McCallion, K., and Diamond, T., Management of severe acute pancreatitis, *Br. J. Surg.*, 90, 407, 2003.
7. A.S.P.E.N. Board of Directors and The Clinical Guidelines Task Force, Guidelines for the use of parenteral and enteral nutrition in adult and pediatric patients, *J. Parenter. Enteral Nutr.*, 26, 68SA, 2002.
8. Ammann, R.W., A clinically based classification system for alcoholic chronic pancreatitis: summary of an international workshop on chronic pancreatitis, *Pancreas*, 14, 215, 1997.
9. Strate, T. et al., Pathogenesis and the natural course of chronic pancreatitis, *Eur. J. Gastroenterol. Hepatol.*, 14, 929, 2002.
10. Izbicki, J.R. et al., Surgical treatment of chronic pancreatitis and quality of life after operation, *Surg. Clin. North Am.*, 79, 913, 1999.
11. Kloppel, G. and Maillett, B., The morphological basis for the evolution of acute pancreatitis into chronic pancreatitis, *Virchows Arch. Pathol. Anat. Histopathol.*, 420, 1, 1992.
12. Ammann, R.W., Heitz, P.U., and Kloppen G., Course of alcoholic chronic pancreatitis: a prospective clinicomorphological long-term study, *Gastroenterology*, 111, 224, 1996.
13. Ammann, R.W. et al., Alcoholic nonprogressive chronic pancreatitis: prospective long-term study of a large cohort with alcohol acute pancreatitis (1976–1992), *Pancreas*, 9, 365, 1994.
14. Yen, S., Hsieh C.C., and Mac Mahon, B., Consumption of alcohol and tobacco and other risk factors for pancreatitis, *Am. J. Epidemiol.*, 116, 407, 1982.
15. Yadav, D. and Pitchumoni C.S., Issues in hyperlipidemic pancreatitis, *J. Clin. Gastroenterology*, 36, 54, 2003.
16. Lowenfels, A.B. et al., Pancreatitis and the increased risk of pancreatic cancer, *N. Engl. J. Med.*, 328, 1433, 1993.
17. Levy, P. et al., Mortality factors associated with chronic pancreatitis. Undimensional and multidimensional analysis of a medical–surgical series of 240 patients, *Gastroenterology*, 96, 1165, 1989.
18. Bomman, P.C. and Beckington, I.J., Chronic pancreatitis, *Br. J. Med.*, 322, 660, 2001.
19. Ranson, J.H.C., The role of surgery in the management of acute pancreatitis, *Ann. Surg.*, 211, 382, 1990.
20. Ranson, J.H.C. et al., Prognostic signs and the role of operative management in acute pancreatitis, *Surg. Gynecol. Obstet.*, 139, 69, 1974.
21. Bradley, E.L., 3rd, Summary of the international symposium on acute pancreatitis, Atlanta, GA, September 11–13, 1992, *Arch. Surg.*, 128, 484, 1993.
22. Larvin, M. and McMahon, M.J., APACHE II score for assessment and monitoring of acute pancreatitis, *Lancet*, 2, 201, 1989.
23. Wilson, C., Heath, D.I., and Imrie, C.W., Prediction of outcome in acute pancreatitis: a comparative study of APACHE II clinical assessment and multiple scoring system, *Br. J. Surg.*, 77, 1260, 1990.
24. Marulendra, S. and Kirby, D., Nutrition support in pancreatitis, *Nutr. Clin. Pract.*, 10, 45, 1995.
25. Balthazar, E.J., Freeny, P.C., and van Sonnenberg, E., Imaging and intervention in acute pancreatitis, *Radiology*, 193, 297, 1994.
26. Khalid, A. and Whitcomb, D.C., Conservative treatment of chronic pancreatitis, *Eur. J. Gastroenterol. Hepatol.*, 14, 943, 2002.
27. Izbicki, J.R. et al., Complications of adjacent organs in chronic pancreatitis managed by duodenum-preserving resection of the head of the pancreas, *Br. J. Surg.*, 81, 1351, 1994.

28. DiMagno, E.P., Go, V.L., and Summerskill, W.H., Relations between pancreatic enzyme outputs and malabsorption in severe pancreatic insufficiency, *N. Engl. J. Med.*, 288, 813, 1973.
29. Layer, P. and Keller, J., Pancreatic enzymes: secretion and luminal nutrient digestion in health and disease, *J. Clin. Gastroenterol.*, 28, 3, 1999.
30. FitzSimmons, S.C. et al., High-dose pancreatic enzyme supplements and fibrosing colonpathy in children with cystic fibrosis, *N. Engl. J. Med.*, 336, 1283, 1997.
31. MacSweeney, E.J. et al., Relation of thickening of colon wall to pancreatic-enzyme treatment in cystic fibrosis, *Lancet*, 345, 752, 1995.
32. Laugier, R. and Grandval, P., Interventional treatment of chronic pancreatitis, *Eur. J. Gastroenterol. Hepatol.*, 14, 951, 2002.
33. Steer, M.L., Waxman, I., and Freedman, S., Chronic pancreatitis, *N. Engl. J. Med.*, 332, 1492, 1995.
34. Friess, H. et al., Surgical treatment and long-term follow-up in chronic pancreatitis, *Eur. J. Gastroenterol. Hepatol.*, 14, 971, 2002.
35. Meier, R. et al., ESPEN guidelines on nutrition in acute pancreatitis, *Clin. Nutr.*, 21, 173, 2002.
36. Robin, A.P., Campbell, R., and Palani, C.K., Total parenteral nutrition during acute pancreatitis: clinical experience with 156 patients, *World J. Surg.*, 14, 572, 1990.
37. Grant, J.P. et al., Total parenteral nutrition in pancreatic disease, *Ann. Surg.*, 200, 627, 1984.
38. Fuhrman, M.P., Charney, P., and Mueller, C., Hepatic proteins and nutrition assessment, *J. Am. Diet. Assoc.*, 104, 1258, 2004.
39. Van Gossum, A. et al., Lipid associated total parenteral nutrition in patients with severe pancreatitis, *J. Parenter. Enteral Nutr.*, 12, 250, 1988.
40. Shaw, J.H. and Wolfe, R.R., Glucose, fatty acid and urea kinetics in patients with severe pancreatitis: the response to substrate infusion and total parenteral nutrition, *Ann. Surg.*, 204, 665, 1986.
41. Cerra, F.B., Hypermetabolism, organ failure and metabolic support, *Surgery*, 101, 1, 1987.
42. Roth, E. et al., Metabolic disorders in severe abdominal sepsis. Glutamine deficiency in skeletal muscle, *Clin. Nutr.*, 1, 25, 1982.
43. Dutta, S.K. et al., Deficiency of fat-soluble vitamins in treated patients with pancreatic insufficiency, *Ann. Int. Med.*, 97, 549, 1982.
44. Bouffara, Y.H. et al., Energy expenditure during severe acute pancreatitis, *J. Parenter. Enteral Nutr.*, 13, 26, 1989.
45. Mann, S., Westenskow, D.R., and Houtchens, B.A., Measured and predicted caloric expenditure in the acutely ill, *Crit. Care Med.*, 13, 173, 1985.
46. Dickerson, R.N. et al., Resting energy expenditure in patients with pancreatitis, *Crit. Care Med.*, 19, 484, 1991.
47. Havala, T., Shronts, E., and Cerra, F., Nutritional support in acute pancreatitis, *Gastroenterol. Clin. North Am.*, 18, 525, 1989.
48. Sax, H.C. et al., Early total parenteral nutrition in acute pancreatitis: lack of beneficial effects, *Am. J. Surg.*, 153, 117, 1987.
49. McArdle, A.H. et al., Effect of elemental diet on pancreatic secretion, *Am. J. Surg.*, 128, 690, 1974.
50. Cassim, M.M. and Allardyce, D.B., Pancreatic secretion in response to jejunal feeding of elemental diet, *Ann. Surg.*, 2, 228, 1974.
51. Stabile, B.E. and Debas, H.T., Intravenous versus intraduodenal amino acids, fats, glucose as stimulants of pancreatic secretion, *Surg. Forum*, 32, 224, 1981.
52. Wolfe, B.M., Keltner, R.M., and Kaminski, D.L., The effect of an infraduodenal elemental diet on pancreatic secretion, *Surg. Gynecol. Obstet.*, 140, 241, 1975.
53. Kelly, G.A. and Nahrwold, D.L., Pancreatic secretion in response to an elemental diet and intravenous hyperalimentation, *Surg. Gynecol. Obstet.*, 143, 87, 1976.
54. Ragins, H. et al., Intrajejunal administration of an elemental diet at neutral pH avoids pancreatic stimulation, *Am. J. Surg.*, 126, 606, 1973.
55. Guan, D., Ohta, H., and Green, G., Rat pancreatic secretory response to infraduodenal infusion of elemental vs. polymeric defined formula diet, *J. Parenter. Enteral Nutr.*, 18, 335, 1994.
56. Voitle, A., Brown, R.A., Echave, V. et al., Use of an elemental diet in the treatment of complicated pancreatitis, *Am. J. Surg.*, 125, 223, 1973.

57. Feller, J.H. et al., Changing methods in the treatment of severe pancreatitis, *Am. J. Surg.*, 127, 196, 1974.
58. Bodoky, G. et al., Effect of enteral nutrition on exocrine pancreatic function, *Am. J. Surg.*, 161, 144, 1991.
59. Kudsk, K.A. et al., Postoperative jejunal feedings following complicated pancreatitis, *Nutr. Clin. Pract.*, 5, 14, 1990.
60. Parekh, D., Lawson, H.H., and Segal, I., The role of total enteral nutrition in pancreatic disease, *South African J. Surg.*, 170, 642, 1969.
61. Grant, J.P., Davey-McCrae, J., and Snyder, P.J., Effect of enteral nutrition on human pancreatic secretions, *J. Parenter. Enteral Nutr.*, 11, 302, 1987.
62. McClave, S.A. et al., Should patients with acute pancreatitis receive early total enteral nutrition? *Gastroenterology*, 108, A739, 1995.
63. Kalfarentzos, F. et al., Enteral nutrition is superior to parenteral nutrition in severe acute pancreatitis: results of a randomized prospective trial, *Br. J. Surg.*, 84, 1665, 1997.
64. Windsor, A.C. et al., Compared with parenteral nutrition, enteral feeding attenuates the acute phase response and improves disease severity in acute pancreatitis, *Gut*, 42, 431, 1998.
65. DeBeaux, A.C., Plester, C., and Fearon, K.C.H., Flexible approach to nutritional support in severe acute pancreatitis, *Nutrition*, 10, 246, 1994.
66. Caliari, S. et al., Pancreatic extracts are necessary for the absorption of elemental and polymeric enteral diets in severe pancreatic insufficiency, *Gastroenterology*, 28, 749, 1993.
67. Raasch, R.H. et al., Effect of intravenous fat emulsion on experimental acute pancreatitis, *J. Parenter. Enteral Nutr.*, 7, 254, 1983.
68. Fried, G.M. et al., Pancreatic protein secretion and gastrointestinal hormone release in response to parenteral amino acids and lipids in dogs, *Surgery*, 92, 902, 1982.
69. Brennan, M.F. et al., A prospective randomized trial of total parenteral nutrition after major pancreatic resection for malignancy, *Ann. Surg.*, 220, 436, 1994.
70. Van den Berghe, G. et al., Intensive insulin therapy in critically ill patients, *N. Engl. J. Med.*, 345, 1359, 2001.
71. Krinsley, J.S., Effective management of intensive glucose management protocol on the mortality of critically ill adult patients, *Mayo Clin. Proc.*, 79, 992, 2004.
72. Nosworthy, J., Colodny, A.H., and Eraklis, A.J., Pancreatitis and intravenous fat: an association in patients with inflammatory bowel disease, *J. Pediatr. Surg.*, 18, 269, 1983.
73. Lashner, B.A., Kersner, J.B., and Hanauer, S.B., Acute pancreatitis associated with high concentration of lipid emulsion during total parenteral nutrition therapy for Crohn's disease, *Gastroenterology*, 90, 1039, 1986.
74. Stabile, B.E. et al., Intravenous mixed amino acids and fats do not stimulate exocrine pancreatic secretion, *J. Physiol.*, 246, G274, 1984.
75. Bivens, G.P. and Stein, T.A., Pancreatic enzyme secretion during intravenous fat emulsion, *J. Parenter. Enteral Nutr.*, 11, 60, 1987.
76. Silberman, M., Dixon, N.P., and Gisenberg, D., The safety and efficacy of a lipid-based system of parenteral nutrition in acute pancreatitis, *Am. J. Gastroenterol.*, 22, 494, 1982.
77. Seibowitz, A.B., O'Sullivan, P., and Iberti, T.J., Intravenous fat emulsions and the pancreas: a review, *Mt. Sinai J. Med.*, 59, 38, 1992.
78. Bush, A. et al., Hyperlipidemia and pancreatitis, *World J. Surg.*, 4, 307, 1980.
79. Grundfest, S. et al., The effect of intravenous fat emulsions in patients with pancreatic fistula, *J. Parenter. Enteral Nutr.*, 4, 27, 1980.
80. Seidner, D.L. et al., Effects of long-chain triglyceride emulsions on reticuloendothelial system function in humans, *J. Parenter. Enteral Nutr.*, 13, 614, 1989.
81. Kontwiek, S.J. et al., Intravenous amino acids and fat stimulate pancreatic secretion, *Am. J. Physiol.*, 236, E678, 1979.
82. Kirby, D.F. and Craig, R.M., The value of intense nutritional support in pancreatitis, *J. Parenter. Enteral Nutr.*, 9, 353, 1985.
83. Latifi, R., McIntosh, J.K., and Dudrick, S.J., Nutritional management of acute and chronic pancreatitis, *Surg. Clin. North Am.*, 71, 579, 1991.

84. Pistero, P.W.T. and Ranson, J.H.C., Nutritional support for acute pancreatitis, *Surg. Gynecol. Obstet.*, 175, 275, 1992.
85. Jackson, M.W. et al., The limited role of total parenteral nutrition in the management of pancreatic pseudocyst, *Am. Surg.*, 59, 736, 1993.
86. Latifi, R. and Dudrick, S.J., The effects of nutrient substrates in acute pancreatitis, in *Surgical Nutrition: Strategies in Critically Ill Patients*, Latifi, R. and Dudrick, S.J., Eds., 1995, p. 147.
87. Goodgame, J.T. and Fischer, J.E., Parenteral nutrition in the treatment of acute pancreatitis: effect on complications and mortality, *Ann. Surg.*, 186, 651, 1977.
88. Cerra, F.B., Nutrient modulation of inflammatory and immune function, *Am. J. Surg.*, 161, 230, 1991.
89. Olah, A. et al., Randomized clinical trial of specific lactobacillus and fibre supplement to early enteral nutrition in patients with acute pancreatitis, *Br. J. Surg.*, 89, 1103, 2002.
90. Foitzik, T. et al., Omega-3 fatty acid supplementation increases anti-inflammatory cytokines and attenuates systemic disease sequelae in experimental pancreatitis, *J. Parenter. Enteral Nutr.*, 26, 351, 2002.
91. Barber, M.D. et al., The effect of an oral nutritional supplement enriched with fish oil on weight-loss in patients with pancreatic cancer, *Brit. J. Cancer*, 81, 80, 1999.
92. Wigmore, S.J. et al., The effect of polyunsaturated fatty acids on the progress of cachexia in patients with pancreatic cancer, *Nutrition*, 12, S27, 1996.
93. Ockenga, J. et al., Effect of glutamine-enriched total parenteral nutrition in patients with acute pancreatitis, *Clin. Nutr.*, 21, 409, 2002.
94. Bertolini, G. et al., Early enteral immunonutrition in patients with severe sepsis: results of an interim analysis of a randomized multicentre clinical trial, *Intensive Care Med.*, 29, 834, 2003.
95. Heyland, D.K. et al., Canadian clinical practice guidelines for nutrition support in mechanically ventilated, critically ill adult patients, *J. Parenter. Enteral Nutr.*, 27, 355, 2003.
96. Zaloga, G.P. et al., Arginine: mediator or modulator of sepsis? *Nutr. Clin. Pract.*, 19, 201, 2004.
97. http://www.clinicaltrials.gov (accessed December 22, 2003).
98. http://80-www.naturaldatabase.com (accessed December 22, 2003).
99. Bengmark, S., Gut microbial ecology in critical illness: is there a role for prebiotics, probiotics, and synbiotics? *Curr. Opin. Crit. Care*, 81, 145, 2002.
100. Brunzell, J.D., Robertson, R.P., Lerner, R.L. et al., Relationships between fasting plasma glucose levels and insulin secretion during intravenous glucose tolerance tests, *J. Clin. Endocrin. Met.*, 42, 222, 1976.
101. McTernan, P.G., Harte, A.L., Anderson, L.A. et al., Insulin and rosiglitazone regulation of lipolysis and lipogenesis in human adipose tissue *in vitro*, *Diabetes*, 51, 1493, 2002.
102. Wilson, J.D., Foster, D.W., Kronenberg, H.M., and Larsen, P.R., Eds., *Williams Textbook of Endocrinology*, 9th ed., W.B. Saunders, Philadelphia, 1998, pp. 1002–1003.
103. National Institute of Diabetes and Digestive and Kidney Diseases, National Diabetes Statistics Fact Sheet: General Information and National Estimates on Diabetes in the United States, 2003, U.S. Department of Health and Human Services, National Institutes of Health, Bethesda, MD, 2003. Rev. ed. U.S. Department of Health and Human Services, National Institutes of Health, Bethesda, MD, 2004. Available at http://diabetes.niddk.nih.gov/
104. Harris, M.I., Flegal, K.M., Cowie, C.C., Eberhardt, M.S., Goldstein, D.E., Little, R.R., Wiedmeyer, H.-M., and Byrd-Holt, D.D., Prevalence of diabetes, impaired fasting glucose, and impaired glucose tolerance in U.S. adults: The Third National Health and Nutrition Examination Survey, 1988–1994, *Diabetes Care*, 21(4), 518, 1998.
105. Wild, S.H., Roglic, G., Green, A., Sicree, R., and King, H., Global prevalence of diabetes: estimates for the year 2000 and projections for 2030, *Diabetes Care*, 27, 1047, 2004.
106. Kumar, V., *Cotran and Robbins Pathologic Basis of Disease*, 7th ed., W.B. Saunders, Philadelphia, 2005, pp. 1189–1205.
107. Wierup, N., Svensson, H., Mulder, H., and Sundler, F., The ghrelin cell: a novel developmentally regulated islet cell in the human pancreas, *Regul. Pept.*, 15, 107(1–3), 63, 2002.
108. Barber, M., Fearson, K.C., Tisdale, M. et al., Effect of a fish oil-enriched nutritional supplement on metabolic mediators in patients with pancreatic cancer cachexia, *Nutr. Cancer*, 40, 118, 2001.

109. Krejs, G.J., Non-insulin secreting tumors of the gastroenteropancreatic system, in *Williams Textbook of Endocrinology*, Wilson, Foster, Kronenberg, and Larsen, Eds., W.B. Saunders, Philadelphia, 1998, pp. 1663–1667.
110. CDC, National Diabetes Fact Sheet, 2003. Available at www.cdc.gov/diabetes/statistics
111. Wolf, A.M., Conaway M.R., Crowther, J.Q. et al., Translating lifestyle intervention to practice in obese patients with type 2 diabetes: Improving Control with Activity and Nutrition (ICAN) study, *Diabetes Care*, 27, 1570, 2004.
112. Diabetes Control and Complications Trial Research Group (DCCT), The effect of intensive treatment of diabetes on the development and progression of long-term complications in insulin-dependent diabetes mellitus, *NEJM*, 329, 977, 1993.
113. Stratton, I.M., Adler, A.I., Andrew, H. et al., Association of glycaemia with macrovascular and microvascular complications of type 2 diabetes (UKPDS 35): prospective observational study, *BMJ*, 321, 2000.
114. Adler, A.I., Stratton, I.M., and Andrew, W., Association of systolic blood pressure with macrovascular and microvascular complications of type 2 diabetes (UKPDS 36): prospective observational study, *BMJ*, 412, 2000.
115. Travis, J., *The Wellness Workbook*, Ten Speed Press, Berkley, CA, 1981.
116. Mensing, C. et al., National standards for diabetes self-management education, *Diabetes Care*, 25(Suppl. 1), S140, 2002.
117. Whelton, P.K. et al., The effects of oral potassium on blood pressure: meta-analysis of randomized controlled clinical trials, *JAMA*, 227, 1624, 1997.
118. Cronin, C.C. et al., High prevalence of celiac disease among patients with insulin-dependent (type 1) diabetes mellitus, *Am. J. Gastroenterol.*, 92, 2210, 1997.
119. Tan, K. et al., C-Reactive protein predicts the deterioration of glycemia in Chinese subjects with impaired glucose tolerance, *Diabetes Care*, 26, 2323, 2003.
120. American Diabetes Association, Nutrition principles and recommendations in diabetes, *Diabetes Care*, 27(Suppl. 1), S36, 2004.
121. American Diabetes Association, Nutrition principles and recommendations in diabetes, *Diabetes Care*, 27(Suppl. 1), S36, 2004.
122. Neff, L.M., Evidence-based dietary recommendations for patients with type 2 diabetes mellitus, *Nutr. Clin. Care*, 6, 52, 2003.
123. Barnard, R.J., Jung, T., and Inkeles, S.B., Diet and exercise in the treatment of NIDDM: the need for early emphasis, *Diabetes Care*, 17, 1469, 1994.
124. Mellin, L., The Solution Method: 2-yr trends in weight, blood pressure, exercise, depression and functioning of adults trained in developmental skills, *J. Am. Diet. Assoc.*, 97, 1133, 1997.
125. Surwit, R.S., *The Mind Body Diabetes Revolution*, Free Press, New York, 2004.
126. Levy-Marchal, C. et al., Antibodies against bovine albumin and other diabetes markers in French children, *Diabetes Care*, 18, 1089, 1995.
127. Saukkonen, T. et al., Significance of cow's milk protein antibodies as risk factor for childhood IDDM: interactions with dietary cow's milk intake and the HLA-DQB1 genotype, *Diabetologia*, 41, 72, 1998.
128. Virtanen, S.M. et al., Early introduction of dairy products associated with increased risk of IDDM in Finnish children. The Childhood in Diabetes in Finland Study Group, *Diabetes*, 42, 1786, 1993.
129. American Diabetes Association (ADA), The prevention or delay of type 2 diabetes, *Diabetes Care*, 25, 746, 2002.
130. Wolever, T.M. and Mehling, C., Long-term effect of varying the source or amount of dietary carbohydrate on postprandial plasma glucose, insulin, triacylglyerol, and free fatty acid concentrations in subjects with impaired glucose tolerance, *Am. J. Clin. Nutr.*, 77, 612, 2003.
131. Costacou, T. and Mayer-Davis, E.J., Nutrition and prevention of type 2 diabetes, *Annu. Rev. Nutr.*, 23, 147, 2003.
132. Wang, L. et al., Plasma fatty acid composition and incidence of diabetes in middle-aged adults: the Atherosclerosis Risk in Communities (ARIC) Study, *Am. J. Clin. Nutr.*, 78, 91, 2003.

133. American Diabetes Association (ADA), Evidence-based nutrition principles and recommendations for the treatment and prevention of diabetes and related complications, *Diabetes Care*, 25(Suppl. 1), S59, 2002.
134. Bouche, C., Rizkalla, S.W., and Luo, J., Five-week, low-glycemic index diet decreases total fat mass and improves plasma lipid profile in moderately overweight nondiabetic men, *Diabetes Care*, 25, 822, 2002.
135. Bouche, C., Five-week, low-glycemic index diet decreases total fat mass and improves plasma lipid profile in moderately overweight nondiabetic men, *Diabetes Care*, 25, 823, 2002.
136. Burke, D. and White, M., IRS proteins and B-cell function, *Diabetes*, 50, S140, 2001.
137. American Diabetes Association (ADA), Evidence-based nutrition principles and recommendations for the treatment and prevention of diabetes and related complications, *Diabetes Care*, 25(Suppl. 1), S52, 2002.
138. American Diabetes Association (ADA), Evidence-based nutrition principles and recommendations for the treatment and prevention of diabetes and related complications, *Diabetes Care*, 25(Suppl. 1), S52, 2002.
139. American Diabetes Association (ADA), Nutrition principles and recommendations in diabetes, *Diabetes Care*, 27(Suppl. 1), S37, 2004.
140. Willett, W., Manson, J., and Simin, L., Glycemic index, glycemic load, and risk of type 2 diabetes, *Am. J. Clin. Nutr.*, 76(Suppl.), 274S, 2002.
141. Brand-Miller, J. et al., Low-glycemic index diets in the management of diabetes, *Diabetes Care*, 26, 2261, 2003.
142. American Diabetes Association (ADA), Evidence-based nutrition principles and recommendations for the treatment and prevention of diabetes and related complications, *Diabetes Care*, 25(Suppl. 1), S51, 2002.
143. Jarvi, A.E. et al., Improved glycemic control and lipid profile and normalized fibrinolytic activity on a low-glycemic index diet in type 2 diabetic patients, *Diabetes Care*, 22, 8, 1999.
144. Chandalia, M., Garg, A., Lutjohann, D. et al., Beneficial effects of high dietary fiber intake in patients with type 2 diabetes mellitus, *NEJM*, 342, 1392, 2000.
145. Tohill, B.C., Seymour, J., Serdula, M. et al., What epidemiologic studies tell us about the relationship between fruit and vegetable consumption and body weight, *Nutr. Rev.*, 62, 365, 2004.
146. American Diabetes Association (ADA), Evidence-based nutrition principles and recommendations for the treatment and prevention of diabetes and related complications, *Diabetes Care*, 25(Suppl. 1), S54, 2002.
147. Barringer, T.A. et al., Effect of a multivitamin and mineral supplement on infection and quality of life. A RCT, Placebo Controlled Trial, *Ann. Intern. Med.*, 138, 365, 2003.
148. Fletcher, R.H. and Fairfield, K.M., Vitamins for chronic disease prevention in adults: clinical applications, *JAMA*, 287, 3127, 2002.
149. American Diabetes Association (ADA), Evidence-based nutrition principles and recommendations for the treatment and prevention of diabetes and related complications, *Diabetes Care*, 25(Suppl. 1), S54, 2002.
150. Church, T.S. et al., Reduction of C-reactive protein levels through use of a multivitamin, *Am. J. Med.*, 115, 702, 2003.
151. Furukawa, Y., Enhancement of glucose-induced insulin secretion and modification of glucose metabolism by biotin, *Nippon Rinsho*, 57, 2261, 1999.
152. McCarty, M.F., High-dose biotin, an inducer of glucokinase expression, may synergize with chromium picolinate to enable a definitive nutritional therapy for type 2 diabetes, *Med. Hypothesis*, 52, 401, 1999.
153. National Academy of Sciences, Dietary Reference Intakes for Vitamin A, Vitamin K, Arsenic, Boron, Chromium, Copper, Iodine, Iron, Manganese, Molybdenum, Nickel, Silicon, Vanadium, and Zinc, 2001, www.nap.edubooks/0309072794/html
154. American Diabetes Association, Nutrition principles and recommendations in diabetes, *Diabetes Care*, 27(Suppl. 1), S36, 2004.
155. Anderson, R.A., Chromium in the prevention and control of diabetes, *Diabetes Metab.*, 26, 22, 2000.

156. Keen, C.L. and Gershwin, M.E., *Annu. Rev. Nutr.*, 10, 415, 1990.
157. Ruy, L.R. et al., Magnesium intake and risk of type 2 diabetes in men and women, *Diabetes Care*, 27, 134, 2004.
158. Song, Y. et al., Dietary magnesium intake in relation to plasma insulin levels and risk of type 2 diabetes in women, *Diabetes Care*, 27, 59, 2004.
159. Lopez-Ridaura, R., Willet, W., Rimm, E.B. et al., Magnesium intake and risk of type 2 diabetes in men and women, *Diabetes Care*, 27, 134, 2004.
160. Shils, M.E. et. al., Eds., *Modern Nutrition in Health and Disease*, 9th ed., Lippincott Williams & Wilkins, Philadelphia, 1999, p. 1381.
161. Jenkins, D., Kendall, C., Marchie, A. et al., Type 2 diabetes and the vegetarian diet, *Am. J. Clin. Nutr.*, 78(Suppl.), 612S, 2003.
162. Chu, Y.F., Sun J., Wu, X., and Liu, R.H., Antioxidant and antiproliferative activities of common vegetables, *J. Agric. Food Chem.*, 50, 6910, 2002.
163. Tjokroprawiro, A., Pikir, B.S., Budhiarta, A.A. et al., Metabolic effects of onion and green beans on diabetic patients, *Tohoku J. Exp. Med.*, 141(Suppl.), 671, 1983.
164. Burr, M., Gilbert, J.F., Holliday, R.M. et al., Effects of changes in fat, fish, and fibre intakes on death and myocardial reinfarction: diet and reinfarction trial (DART), *Lancet*, 334, 757, 1989.
165. Kris-Etherton, P., Harris, W., and Appel, L., Fish consumption, fish oil, omega-3 fatty acids, and cardiovascular disease, *Circulation*, 106, 2750, 2002.
166. Hu, F., Bronner, L., Willett, W. et al., Fish and omega-3 fatty acid and the risk of coronary heart disease in women, *JAMA*, 287, 1815, 2002.
167. Tapsell, L., Gillen, L., Patch, C. et al., Including walnuts in a low-fat/modified-fat diet improves HDL cholesterol-to-total cholesterol ratios in patients with type 2 diabetes, *Diabetes Care*, 27, 2777, 2004.
168. Kabir, M., Oppert, J., Vital, H. et al., Four-week low-glycemic index breakfast with a modest amount of soluble fibers in type 2 diabetic men, *Metabolism*, 51, 819, 2002.
169. Tappy, L., Gugolz, E., Wursch, P. et al., Effects of breakfast cereals containing various amounts of beta-glucan fibers on plasma glucose and insulin responses in NIDDM subjects, *Diabetes Care*, 19, 831, 1996.
170. Jenkins, J., Kendall, C., Faulkner, D. et al., A dietary portfolio approach to cholesterol reduction: combined effects of plant sterols, vegetable proteins, and viscous fibers in hypercholesterolemia, *Metabolism*, 51, 1596, 2002.
171. Agency for Healthcare Research and Quality (AHRQ), *Ayurvedic Interventions for Diabetes Mellitus: A Systematic Review*, AHRQ, Rockville, MD, 2001, p. 17.
172. Shane-McWhorter, L., Biological complementary therapies: a focus on botanical products in diabetes, *Diabetes Spectrum*, 14, 201, 2001.
173. Agency for Healthcare Research and Quality (AHRQ), *Ayurvedic Interventions for Diabetes Mellitus: A Systematic Review*, AHRQ, Rockville, MD, 2001, p. 15.
174. Agency for Healthcare Research and Quality (AHRQ), *Ayurvedic Interventions for Diabetes Mellitus: A Systematic Review*, AHRQ, Rockville, MD, 2001, p. 15.
175. Shanmugasundaram, K.R., Panneerselvam, C., Samudram, P. et al., The insulinotropic activity of *Gymnema sylvestre*, R. Br. An Indian medical herb used in controlling diabetes mellitus, *Pharm. Res. Commun.*, 13, 475, 1981.
176. Shanmugasundaram, K.R., Panneerselvam, C., Samudram, P. et al., The insulinotropic activity of *Gymnema sylvestre*, R. Br. An Indian medical herb used in controlling diabetes mellitus, *Pharm. Res. Commun.*, 13, 15, 1981.
177. Shane-McWhorter, L., Biological complementary therapies: a focus on botanical products in diabetes, *Diabetes Spectrum*, 14, 200, 2001.
178. Agency for Healthcare Research and Quality (AHRQ), *Ayurvedic Interventions for Diabetes Mellitus: A Systematic Review*, AHRQ, Rockville, MD, 2001, p. 18.
179. Yeh, G.Y. et al., Systematic review of herbs and dietary supplements for glycemic control in diabetes, *Diabetes Care*, 26, 1278, 2003.
180. International Diabetes Center (IDC), *A Guide to Herbs and Supplements in Diabetes*, Park Nicollet Institute, St. Louis Park, MN, 2003, p. 31.

181. Yeh, G.Y. et al., Systematic review of herbs and dietary supplements for glycemic control in diabetes, *Diabetes Care*, 26, 1278, 2003.

182. International Diabetes Center (IDC), *A Guide to Herbs and Supplements in Diabetes*, Park Nicollet Institute, St. Louis Park, MN, 2003, p. 29.

183. Khan, A., Safdar, M., Ali Khan, M.M. et al., Cinnamon improves glucose and lipids of people with type 2 diabetes, *Diabetes Care*, 26, 3215, 2003.

184. Khan, A., Safdar, M., Ali Khan, M.M. et al., Cinnamon improves glucose and lipids of people with type 2 diabetes, *Diabetes Care*, 26, 3215, 2003.

185. Babu, P.S. and Srinivasan, K., Hypolipedemic action of curcumin, the active principle of turmeric (*Curcuma longa*) in streptozotocin induced diabetic rats, *Mol. Cell Biochem.*, 166, 169, 1997.

186. Sidhu, G.S., Mani, H., Gaddipati, J.P. et al., Curcumin enhances wound healing in streptozotocin induced diabetic rats and genetically diabetic mice, *Wound Repair Regen.*, 7, 362, 1999.

187. Jamal, G.A. and Carmichael, H., The effect of gamma-linolenic acid on human diabetic peripheral neuropahy: a double-blind placebo-controlled trial, *Diabetes Med.*, 7, 319, 1990.

188. International Diabetes Center (IDC), *A Guide to Herbs and Supplements in Diabetes*, Park Nicollet Institute, St. Louis Park, MN, 2003, p. 25.

189. Oubre, A.Y., Carlson, T.J., and King, S.R., From plant to patient: an ethnomedical approach to the identification of new drugs for the treatment of NIDDM, *Diabetologia*, 40, 614, 1997.

190. Indian Council for Medical Research, Role of fenugreek seeds in diabetes mellitus, *ICMR Bulletin*, 17, 79, 1987.

191. International Diabetes Center (IDC), *A Guide to Herbs and Supplements in Diabetes*, Park Nicollet Institute, St. Louis Park, MN, 2003, p. 26.

192. National Institutes of Health, Detection, evaluation, and treatment of high blood cholesterol in adults (Adult Treatment Panel III), NIH Publication No. 01-3670, 2001, p. 4.

193. Larsen, J.R., Sjoholm, H., Hanssen, K.F. et al., Optimal blood glucose control during 18 years preserves peripheral nerve function in patients with 30 years duration of type 1 diabetes, *Diabetes Care*, 26, 2400, 2003.

194. Jamal, G.A. and Carmichael, H., The effect of gamma-linolenic acid on human diabetic peripheral neuropathy: a double-blind placebo-controlled trial, *Diabetes Med.*, 7, 319, 1990.

195. Amctov, A.S., Barinov, A., Dyck, P.J. et al., The sensory symptoms of diabetic polyneuropathy are improved with alpha-lipoic acid: the SYDNEY trial, *Diabetes Care*, 26, 770, 2003.

196. National Institutes of Health, National Cholesterol Education Program, Detection, Evaluation, and Treatment of High Blood Cholesterol in Adults (Adult Treatment Panel III) Executive Summary, NIH Publication No. 01-3670, 2001, p. 16.

15 Immune System

*Ellyn Silverman, Paul J. Cimoch, David W. Grotto,
Jill Place, and Susan Allen-Evenson*

CONTENTS

IMMUNE SYSTEM BASICS

The immune system is a complex group of cells, molecules, and organs that act together to defend the body against the development of tumor cells and foreign invaders such as bacteria, viruses, and fungi that can cause disease. Optimal health is dependent on the ability of the immune system to recognize and then act against these invaders. Specific factors can affect immune functions such as genetics, age, gender, smoking history, levels of exercise, alcohol consumption, stress, history of vaccinations, early life experiences, and nutritional status.[1]

There are two types of immunity: innate and adaptive. Both components involve various bloodborne factors (complement, antibodies, cytokines, and cells). Innate immunity, also called "nonspecific" immunity, is present at birth and is the body's first line of defense against all invaders. It consists of barriers, such as the skin, or fluids, such as tears, mucus, gastric acid, and saliva. It also protects the body through inflammation of tissues surrounding foreign invaders with white blood cells that takes place shortly after an injury or infection. These innate immune mechanisms make it difficult for infection to enter the body and disseminate, but they cannot prevent disease completely.

If an invader gets past the innate defense, the cells, molecules, and organs of the adaptive immune system develop very specifically tailored defenses against the invader. The immune system calls upon these defenses again whenever this particular invader attacks in the future. The adaptive or "specific" immunity is the second barrier to infection and is acquired throughout life, through immunization or a successful fight against an infection. Adaptive immunity has four distinguishing characteristics:

- It responds only after the invader is present or in the host.
- It is specific. It tailors each of its responses to act only against a particular type of invader.
- It displays memory. The response is better after the initial exposure to an invader even if the next exposure is many years later.
- It does not usually attack normal body components, only those substances it recognizes as foreign.

Adaptive immune responses are reactions to structures on the surface of the invading organism called antigens. Antigens are foreign substances (e.g., protein cells, bacteria, polysaccharides) that stimulate antibody production. The two types of adaptive immune responses are humoral and cell-mediated.

During humoral immune responses, specific proteins called antibodies appear in blood and other bodily fluids. They help to destroy foreign antigens. This type of immune response helps to resist extracellular invaders such as bacteria and toxins. Humoral immune responses can also prevent viruses from entering the cells.

In cell-mediated immune responses, cells that can destroy other cells are activated. They only destroy cells that are infected intracellularly and can reproduce within the cells, such as viruses.

COMPONENTS OF THE IMMUNE SYSTEM

The immune system is made up of complex interactions between the components. Contact between the antigens and the immune system cells occurs in the blood and lymphoid organs, which include the lymph nodes, spleen, and tonsils, as well as specialized areas of the intestine and the lungs. The mature immune cells travel constantly between the blood and lymphoid organs. This recirculation of the immune system cells ensures that the body is continuously monitored for invading substances.

MACROPHAGES

White blood cells are a key factor in the immune system. Macrophages play an integral role in the immune system by surrounding, ingesting, and destroying invading bacteria. This process, called phagocytosis, is part of the inflammatory reaction. Macrophages play an important role in adaptive immunity as antigen-presenting cells (APCs). They attach to invading antigens and deliver them to other components of the adaptive immune system for elimination. Other APCs include dendritic cells and B-lymphocytes.

LYMPHOCYTES

All lymphocytes begin as stem cells in the bone marrow. Lymphocytes mature in two different locations, the bone marrow or the thymus. B-lymphocytes, or B-cells, mature in the bone marrow and make antibodies, which circulate through the blood and other body fluids binding to antigens to help destroy these antigens via the complement system, opsonization, and neutralization.

T-lymphocytes or T-cells mature in the thymus. There are several types of T-lymphocytes. Killer T-lymphocytes are part of cell-mediated immune responses and can directly destroy cells that have specific recognizable antigens on their surface.

T4-helper lymphocytes, a second kind of T-lymphocyte sometimes called CD4 T-lymphocytes, regulate the immune system by controlling the strength and quality of all immune responses. These cells can be thought of as the ruler of the immune system. They orchestrate and coordinate the immune response through a series of messenger molecules called cytokines (e.g., interleukins [IL], interferon [IFN], etc.) T8-suppressor cells, or CD8 T-lymphocytes, downregulate or turn off the immune response. These cells act as a balance to prevent overexpression of the immune response.

ANTIGEN RECEPTORS

Adaptive immunity is specific. Each immune response is tailored to a specific type of invading antigen. Each lymphocyte, as it matures, makes an antigen receptor. This specific surface structure can bind with a matching structure on the invading antigen similar to a lock and key. Lymphocytes have the ability to make billions of different kinds of antigen receptors; however, each individual lymphocyte makes only one kind. When an antigen enters the body, it activates only the lymphocyte with receptors that match it.

ANTIGEN-PRESENTING CELLS

When a foreign invader antigen enters a cell, certain transport molecules within the cell attach themselves to the foreign invaders antigen and transport them to the surface of the cell. They then present this antigen to the T-lymphocytes. APCs include macrophages, dendritic cells, and B-lymphocytes. These transport molecules are made by a group of genes called the major histocompatibility complex (MHC) and are therefore known as MHC molecules. Some of these MHC molecules, called class I MHC molecules, present antigens to killer T-cells. There are other MHC molecules called class II MHC molecules, which present antigens to T4-helper cells.

HUMORAL IMMUNE RESPONSE

The humoral immune response involves a complex series of events after antigens enter the body. First, macrophages take up some of the antigen and attach it to class II MHC molecules, which then present the antigen to the T4-helper cells. The T4-helper cells bind the presented antigen, which stimulates the T4-helper cells to divide and secrete stimulatory molecules called ILs. The cytokines activate the B-lymphocytes that have also bound the antigen. The activated B-lymphocytes then divide and secrete antibodies. Finally, the secreted antibodies bind the antigen and help to destroy it.

ANTIBODIES

Antibodies, Y-shaped proteins called immunoglobins (Ig), are made by the B-lymphocytes. The antibody binds to the antigen at the ends of the arms of the Y. The structure of the base of the Y categorizes antibodies into five main classes: IgM, IgG, IgA, IgD, and IgE. During the humoral immune response, IgM is the first class of antibody made. After several days, other classes appear. Antibodies can sometimes stop an antigen's disease-causing activity simply by neutralizing them. This happens when the antibody binds the antigen and prevents it from interfering with the cell's normal activities. For example, the toxin made by tetanus bacteria binds to nerve cells and interferes with muscle control. Antibodies against tetanus toxin stick to the toxin and cover the part of it that binds to nerve cells, thereby preventing serious disease. All classes of antibodies can neutralize antigens.

Antibodies also help to destroy antigens by getting them ready for ingestion by the macrophages in a process called opsonization. In opsonization, antibodies coat the surface of the antigen, making them more likely to stick to the macrophages and be ingested. Opsonization is especially important in helping the body resist bacterial diseases.

IgM and IgG antibodies are also involved in the complement system. Complement is a group of proteins that cause cells to disintegrate by cutting holes in the cell membrane.

Complement is important in resisting bacteria that are hard to destroy in other ways. The IgM and IgG classes of antibodies work best in the circulatory system, IgA can exit the bloodstream and appear in other bodily fluids; therefore, it is important in preventing infection at mucosal surfaces, such as the intestine and the lung. These sites, where infectious agents typically enter, are making IgA an important player in the resistance of many diseases. IgA is also found in breast milk and helps nursing newborns resist disease.

NUTRIENTS AND THE IMMUNE SYSTEM

The impact of specific nutrients and nutritional status on the immune system is widely known. Extensive research has been done in this area. There have been several reviews of the research that delineate the relationship of single nutrients to immune function. Nutrient availability has the potential to affect almost all aspects of the immune system. The ability of nutrition and diet to enhance or suppress the immune response of healthy persons or to promote optimal health is the topic of much discussion in both scientific and lay literature.

Nutrient status is an important factor contributing to immune competence. Undernutrition impairs the immune system by suppressing immune functions that are fundamental to host protection.[2] Undernutrition that leads to impairment of immune function can be due to insufficient intake of macronutrients or deficiencies in specific micronutrients. Often these conditions occur in combination.

Nutrients that have been demonstrated (in either animal or human studies) as requirements for the immune system to function effectively include: vitamins A, B-6, B-12, C, E, folic acid, zinc, copper, magnesium, iron, coenzyme Q10 (Co-Q10), and selenium. Practically all forms of immunity may be affected by differences in one or more of these nutrients.[1] The most consistent abnormalities are seen in cell-mediated immunity, complement system, phagocyte function, cytokine production, mucosal secretion, antibody response, and antibody affinity.[2] There are also a number of pathological situations in which nutrition plays a primary or secondary determinant of underlying immune impairment. These include obesity, eating disorders, food hypersensitivities, and gastrointestinal (GI) disorders.[2]

From the overview of the immune system, it is clear that deficiencies in one specific nutrient or a combination of nutrients, could affect host defenses negatively in a number of ways. Antigen or cytokine receptor functions on lymphocytes and phagocytic cells can be influenced by nutrients that affect the membrane structure, fluidity, or transmembrane signaling functions. The production of antibodies or cytokines can be altered by the unavailability of protein or by limiting of amino acids. We will now explore a number of the nutrients that have a major effect on our immune system.

MAGNESIUM

Magnesium is an essential mineral in human nutrition with a wide range of biological functions. It ranks second to potassium as an intracellular cation. The adult human body contains approximately 20 to 28 g of which approximately 60% is found in bone, 26% in muscle, and the remainder in soft tissues and body fluids. It is involved in over 300 metabolic reactions and influences the metabolism of many other nutrients. For example, alterations in potassium, calcium, phosphorus, and sodium metabolism are associated with magnesium deficiency.[3] It is necessary for every biological process, including the production of cellular energy, the synthesis of nucleic acids and protein, the electrical stability of cells, muscle contraction, and nerve conduction. Magnesium is particularly involved in B-cell activity and antibody production.[4] Cell proliferation can be suppressed by a deficiency of magnesium by influencing DNA replication and cell-cycle regulation. Evidence reviewed by Kubena and

McMurray[4] indicates that magnesium plays a role in the development, distribution and function of immune cells, and soluble factors that are critical for humoral and cell-mediated immunity.

Magnesium homeostasis is governed by small and large intestinal absorption and renal excretion. Parathyroid hormone (PTH) has a minor role in the control of serum magnesium.[5] Magnesium is found in many foods, and the usual diet typically includes adequate amounts. Good sources are seeds, nuts, legumes, and milled cereal grains, as well as dark green leafy vegetables, because magnesium is an essential part of chlorophyll. Milk is a moderately good source. However, magnesium is lost during the refining of wheat cereals.

Deficiency and Toxicity Information

Signs and symptoms of magnesium deficiency include anorexia, nausea and vomiting, diarrhea, muscle spasms, confusion, tremor, loss of coordination, cardiac arrhythmias, muscle cramps, and hypertension. Magnesium deficiency can cause hypokalemia. Certain drugs may cause magnesium deficiency including thiazide diuretics, loop diuretics, cisplatin, and cyclosporine. A low magnesium intake is now considered to be a potential risk factor for hypertension.[6]

Excess magnesium can cause an inhibition in bone calcification; however, it is unlikely that excesses from dietary or supplemental sources will lead to toxicity. Supplementation is contraindicated in patients with renal failure. It is also contraindicated in those patients with high-grade atrioventricular (AV) blocks unless those patients have an artificial pacemaker.[7] Pregnant women and nursing mothers should avoid magnesium doses greater than 350 mg/day in supplement form unless prescribed by their healthcare provider.

Recommended Dietary Intake and Dosage

The recommended dietary allowance (RDA) for magnesium was increased in 1997. This was the first time recommendations were made for males and females beginning at puberty. There are several forms of magnesium used for nutritional supplementation. These include magnesium oxide, magnesium gluconate, magnesium citrate, magnesium hydroxide, magnesium pidolate, and other amino acid and oligopeptide chelates of magnesium. Typical doses range from 100 to 350 mg/day for correction of deficiency. Taking the supplement with food will decrease the likelihood of diarrhea.

VITAMIN A

Vitamin A refers to a group of fat-soluble substances that are structurally related to and possess the biological activity of the parent substance called all-trans retinol or retinol.[8] There are three preformed compounds that exhibit metabolic activity: the alcohol (retinol), the aldehyde (retinal or retinaldehyde), and the acid (retinoic acid). These active forms of vitamin A exist only in animal products.

Vitamin A plays an important role in immune function by maintaining the skin surface and by helping mucous membranes resist invasion by microorganisms.[9] It is vital for cellular differentiation, growth, reproduction, maintenance of epithelial surfaces, and vision.[9] Vitamin A stimulates and enhances numerous immune processes, including induction of antitumor activity, enhancement of white blood cell function, and increased antibody response.[9] Vitamin A, specifically retinoic acid, acts as a hormone that affects gene expression.

Within the cell, cellular retinol-binding protein (CRBP) transports retinoic acid to the nucleus. In the nucleus, retinoic acid and 9-cis-retinoic acid bind to retinoic acid receptors (RARs) or retinoid receptors (RXRs) on the gene. Subsequent interactions allow the stimulation or inhibition of transcription of specific genes, thus affecting protein synthesis and many body processes. A few of these processes are morphogenesis in embryonic development and epithelial cell function. Vitamin A is also essential in glycoprotein synthesis. Glycoproteins are important for normal cell surface function such as cell aggregation and cell recognition. This role in glycoprotein synthesis may also account for the importance of vitamin A in cell growth because it may increase glycoprotein synthesis for cell receptors that respond to growth factors. There is some evidence in the literature that indicates higher blood levels of carotenoids reduce the risk for several chronic diseases. The only clear function of the carotenoids is a provitamin A.[10] Carotenes have demonstrated a number of immune-enhancing effects in recent studies.[11]

Vitamin A must be hydrolyzed in the stomach and small intestine by proteases, which are combined with vitamin A. In addition, retinyl esters must be hydrolyzed in the small intestine by lipases to retinol and free fatty acids. Once in the intestinal mucosal cells, retinol is bound to a CRBP and reesterified into retinyl esters. Carotenoids and retinyl esters are incorporated into chylomicrons for transport into the lymph and eventually the bloodstream or may be cleaved into retinol. The liver plays a major role in transport and storage of vitamin A. Chylomicron remnants deliver retinyl esters to the liver. Retinol in the liver has three metabolic fates: (1) it may be bound to CRBP, (2) it may be reesterified to form retinyl esters for storage, and (3) it may be bound to retinol-binding protein (RBP). Approximately 50 to 80% of the vitamin A in the body is stored in the liver. This storage capacity is particularly important during periods of low dietary intake when a person is vulnerable for a deficiency.[12] Certain carotenoids, such as beta-carotene, alpha-carotene, and beta-cryptoxanthin are dietary precursors of vitamin A.[8] These are found in plant products. The absorption of carotenoids varies greatly (from 5 to 50%) and is affected by other dietary factors such as the digestibility of the proteins complexed with the carotenoids and the level and type of fat in the diet. Fat-soluble vitamins need dietary fat to be absorbed efficiently.

Deficiency and Toxicity Information

Vitamin A deficiency can result in night blindness, xerosis of the conjunctiva and cornea, keratinization of the lung, GI tract, growth retardation, increased susceptibility to infections and death. A deficiency leads to failures in systemic functions. Children are particularly vulnerable to the effects of vitamin A deficiency. This is a serious health concern in many developing nations. Vitamin A supplementation is usually well tolerated, however, there have been reports of severe sensory neuropathy with certain conditions where there is an inadequate intake of food high in vitamin A, such as malabsorption syndromes. These syndromes include cystic fibrosis, Whipple's disease, Crohn's disease, ulcerative colitis, short bowel syndrome, pancreatic disease, and chronic liver disease.

Doses of vitamin A above 5000 IU are contraindicated in pregnant women and those with hypervitaminosis A. High intakes may cause acute or chronic toxicity. Symptoms include dry rough skin, cracked lips, sparse course hair, and alopecia of the eyebrows.

Recommended Dietary Intake and Dosage

The vitamin A content of foods is measured as retinol activity equivalents (RAE). One RAE equals the activity of 1 μg of retinol. Dietary reference intakes (DRIs) have been determined for vitamin A and are expressed in micrograms (μg) per day. The DRIs for adults are based on levels that provide adequate blood levels and liver stores and are adjusted for differences in average body size. No DRIs have been established for carotenoids. Supplementation has not been shown to be beneficial or harmful. The two principal forms of vitamin A supplements are retinyl acetate and retinyl palmitate. Usually supplementation preparations include a combination of these forms and doses higher than 5000 IU are rarely exceeded in these formulas.

Vitamin C

The term vitamin C applies to substances that possess antiscorbutic activity and include two compounds and their salts: L-ascorbic acid (ascorbic acid) and L-dehydroascorbic acid. Ascorbic acid is the main dietary form of vitamin C. It is an essential nutrient and a water-soluble vitamin. It is important for immune function due to its antioxidant properties. Vitamin C functions in oxidation–reduction reactions and is synthesized by plants and most animals from glucose and galactose. Many different immune-enhancing effects have been demonstrated, including enhancing white blood cell response and function, increasing IFN levels, increasing the secretion of thymic hormones, and improving the integrity of the linings of mucous membranes.[11] It serves as a biochemical redox system involved in many electron transport reactions, including those involved in the synthesis of collagen and carnitine and other metabolic reactions. Vitamin C promotes resistance to infection through its involvement with the immunologic activities of leukocytes, the production of IFN, the process of inflammatory reaction, and the integrity of the mucous membranes.[13] The value of large doses of vitamin C to cure the common cold has been reported; however, the results of the studies are conflicting. It may be helpful in other chronic diseases characterized by oxidative damage to biological molecules. Its oxidative properties are well established and this activity may be helpful in the prevention of some cancers and cardiovascular disease. Vitamin C may also be helpful in protecting against some of the lipid oxidation caused by smoking. Several studies have shown that vitamin C, either alone or in combination with other nutrients, significantly inhibits low-density lipoprotein cholesterol (LDL-C) oxidation.[8] This is most consistent when vitamin C is combined with vitamin E and beta-carotene. It may work by sparing or recycling of vitamin E.

Vitamin C is synthesized by plants and most animals from glucose and galactose. Some species of animals including humans lack the enzyme L-gulonolactone oxidase and therefore cannot biosynthesize the factor. These species of animals absorb vitamin C by active transport and passive diffusion in the small intestine. Vitamin C is transported in the plasma as the reduced form of ascorbic acid. It is taken up by the cells through a glucose transporter and a specific active transport system. The vitamin is concentrated primarily as ascorbic acid and dehydroascorbic acid in many vital organs such as the brain, adrenal glands, and eyes. It is renally excreted.

Vitamin C is expressed quantitatively in milligrams (mg). The recommended dosage for healthy adults is 200 mg/day, which is enough to maximize plasma and lymphocyte levels. The best sources are fruits, vegetables, and organ meats. The amount of actual vitamin C in foods is dependent on their ripeness and the amount of processing that occurs to them. Ascorbic acid is easily destroyed by oxidation, and it is often extracted and discarded in cooking water due to its water solubility.

Deficiency and Toxicity Information

Acute vitamin C deficiency results in scurvy. This deficiency leads to lesions in the mesenchymal tissues and results in impaired wound healing, edema, hemorrhages, and weakness in bone, cartilage, teeth, and connective tissues. Vitamin C toxicity is rare, but can cause GI disturbances and diarrhea. It is the most widely supplemented vitamin in the United States.[14] Those with preexisting kidney stone disease or history of renal insufficiency should exercise caution when using more than the RDA amounts of vitamin C. Those persons with hemochromatosis, thalassemia, or sickle cell anemia might have problems from high doses of vitamin C due to its modulation of iron absorption and transport.

When used in high doses of 3 g or more per day orally, GI distress was the most noted symptom. These included diarrhea, nausea, vomiting, and flatulence.

Recommended Dietary Intake and Dosage

Although as little as 10 mg of vitamin C can prevent scurvy, this level does not provide acceptable reserves of the vitamin. It is also recommended that smokers increase their intake to at least 300 mg/day for antioxidant protection.

FOLATE

Folate refers to pteroylmonoglutamic acid and its derived compounds. It is a member of the B-vitamin family and is also referred to as folic acid. Folic acid is a synthetic form of folate and is used for food fortification and nutritional supplements. Folate participates in several key biological processes including the synthesis of DNA, RNA, and proteins. It is necessary for DNA replication and repair, the maintenance or the integrity of the genome, and is involved in the regulation of gene expression. The principal biochemical function of folate is the mediation of one-carbon transfer reactions. 5-Methyltetrahydrofolate donates a methyl group to homocysteine in the conversion of homocysteine to L-methionine. This is an important reaction in the regulation of serum homocysteine levels. It is also an important factor in the lowering of neural tube defect risks and possibly other birth defects. It may also have antiatherogenic, anticarcinogenic, neuroprotective, and antidepressant actions.[15,16]

Dietary folates are absorbed only as the monoglutamate form of folic acid, 5-methyltetrahydrofolic acid, and 5-formyltetrahydrofolic acid. Absorption of folic acid occurs by active transport mainly in the jejunum, but can also be absorbed by passive transport when ingested in large amounts. Absorption requires hydrolysis to monoglutamate forms by conjugases in the brush border and intracellular mucosa because folate in foods is present in polyglutamate. This hydrolysis is an inefficient way for folate to be absorbed; therefore, only about one-half of the folate found in food is absorbed. Folate is taken up in the intestinal mucosal cell and is reduced to FH4 (tetrahydrofolic acid), which is either transferred to the portal circulation or converted to 5-methyl-FH4 before entering the circulation.

Folates exist in various foods of plant and animal origin. Liver, mushrooms, spinach, asparagus, and broccoli are good sources. Lean beef, whole wheat bread, potatoes, orange juice, and dried beans are also good sources. Analysis of the folate content of foods is complex and difficult. There are typical losses due to storage, cooking, or processing at high temperatures.

Deficiency and Toxicity Information

A deficiency in folate can lead to impaired biosynthesis of DNA and RNA. It is responsible for reduced cell division, therefore affecting the cells, which most rapidly reproduce such as the red blood cells, leukocytes, and epithelial cells of the stomach, intestine, vagina, and uterine cervix. The role of folate in embryogenesis is especially important and a deficiency during pregnancy can cause an increased risk of neural tube defects.[17]

No adverse effects of high oral doses of folate have been reported in animals. The use of folic acid doses above 1 mg/day may precipitate or exacerbate the neurological damage of vitamin B-12 deficiency.

Recommended Dietary Intake and Dosage

The principal form of supplementary folate is folic acid. A typical daily dose is 400 μg. Use of doses of ≥ 1 μg/day requires a prescription.

Vitamin E

Vitamin E exerts good immune-enhancing activity, as it enhances both arms of immunity (antibody-related or humoral and cell-mediated immunity).[18] Vitamin E has a specific role in protecting the body against the damaging effects of free radicals, or reactive oxygen, that are encountered in the environment. There are two active classes of vitamin E: tocopherols and the less active tocotrienols. The vitamers of each series are named according to the position and the number of methyl groups on their ring systems.[19]

Vitamin E is absorbed in the upper small intestine by micelle-dependent diffusion. Vitamin E is a fat-soluble vitamin and its use depends on the presence of dietary fat and adequate biliary and pancreatic function. Its absorption is highly variable and can range from 20 to 70%. The absorbed vitamin E is incorporated into chylomicrons and transported into the general circulation via lymph. Vitamin E is delivered to the liver and is incorporated into very low-density lipoproteins (VLDL).

Vitamin E is the most important lipid-soluble antioxidant in the cell. It is located in the lipid portion of the cell membrane and it protects unsaturated phospholipid membranes from oxidative degradation from highly reactive oxygen species and other free radicals.

It can reduce such radicals into harmless metabolites by donating hydrogen to them. This is called radical scavenging. The antibody function of vitamin E is important in protecting the body against, and treating conditions related to, oxidative stress, such as aging, arthritis, [20] cancer,[21] cardiovascular disease,[22] cataracts, diabetes, and infection. It may also play a protective part in preventing Alzheimer's disease.[23] Vitamin E appears to inhibit platelet adhesion, aggregation, and platelet release reactions. Among prospective cohort studies examining the possible role of vitamin E in cardiovascular disease, The Nurses' Health Study has yielded some significant findings. In a cohort of 87,000 of these nurses, all who were free of cardiovascular disease at the beginning of the study, there was a 34% reduction in cardiovascular disease among those women in the highest versus the lowest quintile of vitamin E intake after adjustment for age, smoking, and other relevant variables. Dietary intake alone did not show this significant inverse relationship, but total intake (diet plus supplementation) did.[24]

Several animal and human studies have shown that vitamin E can improve the immune response in aged animals and humans. *In vitro*, alpha-tocopherol increases mitogenic response of T-lymphocytes from aged mice.[8] The mechanism of this response by vitamin E is not well understood. It has been suggested that vitamin E itself may have mitogenic activity independent of its antioxidant activity.

Alpha-tocopherol was reported to have potent activity against human immunodeficiency virus (HIV)-1.[25] High levels of oxidative stress is thought to contribute to HIV-1 pathogenesis, as well as the pathogenesis of other viral infections. The role vitamin E has on HIV virus may be in part due to its antioxidant activity since it affects membrane integrity and fluidity. HIV is a membraned virus. The alteration of this membrane fluidity may interfere with its ability to bind cell-receptor sites, therefore decreasing its infectivity. It is unclear, however, how much vitamin E it would take to have this effect.

Tocopherols, especially the oils, are synthesized only by plants. Nearly two thirds of the vitamin E in the typical American diet is supplied by salad oils, margarines, and shortenings, about 11% by fruits and vegetables, and about 7% by grains and grain products.[26] The richest sources of the vitamin are found in unrefined edible vegetable oils, such as wheat germ, sunflower, safflower, cottonseed, canola, and olive oils. As vitamin E is insoluble in water it is not lost in cooking in water, but can be destroyed by deep fat frying.

Deficiency and Toxicity Information

In general, clinical manifestations of vitamin E deficiency target the neuromuscular, vascular, and reproductive systems. Symptoms in humans are uncommon and usually occur only in patients with lipid malabsorption or lipid transport abnormalities, such as cystic fibrosis, primary biliary cirrhosis, chronic pancreatitis, short bowel syndromes, and Crohn's disease. Vitamin E is one of the least toxics of all vitamins. Humans are able to tolerate high intakes, at least 100 times the nutritional requirements. The UL for vitamin E in adults is 1000 mg/day. In very high doses, vitamin E can decrease the body's ability to use other fat-soluble vitamins. Fecal excretion is the major route of excretion of oral vitamin E. Those persons on warfarin or other blood-thinning medications should be cautious when using doses greater than 100 mg daily due to its affect on an increased clotting time. Supplementation of doses higher than the RDA should be avoided during pregnancy. High doses should be stopped approximately 1 month before surgery to decrease bleeding complications.

Recommended Dietary Intake and Dosage

Vitamin E is quantified in terms of alpha-tocopherol equivalents. There are several forms of vitamin E commercially available. For the purpose of defining DRIs, the National Research Council restricted vitamin E activity to only one of the homologs of the tocopherol family, alpha-tocopherol. The new RDA for both men and women is 15 mg of alpha-tocopherol per day. Recommended doses for supplementation range from 100 to 400 mg daily.

Vitamin B-6

Vitamin B-6 is the general term for numerous 2-methyl-3, 5-dihydroxymethylpyridine derivatives exhibiting the biologic activity of pyridoxine, the alcohol derivate. The biologically active analogs are the aldehyde pyridoxal and the amine pyridoxamine. All three compounds are converted to the metabolically active coenzyme from pyridoxal phosphate (PLP), which is primarily involved in the metabolism of amino acids.

The metabolically active form of vitamin B-6 is PLP. It is a coenzyme for numerous enzymes involved in practically all reactions in the metabolism of amino acids. It is also involved in aspects of the metabolism of neurotransmitters, glycogen, sphingolipids, heme, and steroids. The PLP is able to react with α-amino groups of the amino acid and stabilize the other bonds on the bound carbon. Therefore vitamin B-6 is essential for various amino acid transaminases, decarboxylases, racemasis, and isomerases. It is needed for the biosynthesis of the neurotransmitters serotonin, epinephrine, norepinephrine, and γ-aminobutyric acid, the vasodilator and gastric secretagogue histamine, and the porphyrin precursors of heme.

Vitamin B-6 is also required for the metabolic conversion of tryptophan to niacin, the release of glucose from glycogen, the biosynthesis of myelin sheaths of nerve cells, and in the modulation of steroid hormone receptors. Vitamin B-6 has antineurotoxic activity and may have activity in a number of inborn errors of metabolism including pyridoxine-dependent seizures in infants, and homocystinuria. Needs for vitamin B-6 increase with increasing intake of protein. Adequate vitamin B-6 status seems to be maintained when the vitamin is consumed in an approximate ratio of 0.016 mg/g of protein.[27]

Vitamin B-6 is absorbed by passive diffusion of the dephosphorylated forms primarily in the jejunum and ileum. The absorption is driven by phosphorylation to form PLP and then by protein binding of each of these metabolites in the intestinal mucosa and blood. The muscle is the largest site of storage containing 80 to 90% of the total body stores.

Vitamin B-6 is widely found in foods. It is found in large quantities in meats, whole grain products (especially wheat), vegetables, nuts, and fortified soy meat products. Much of the vitamin B-6 found in many foods is bound to protein. The vitamin B-6 derived from animal sources tends to be superior in bioavailability.

Deficiency and Toxicity Information

Vitamin B-6 deficiency can lead to metabolic abnormalities due to insufficient production of PLP. The symptoms of a deficiency are dermatologic and neurologic in nature. These include weakness, sleeplessness, peripheral neuropathy, cheilosis, glossitis, stomatitis, and impaired cell-mediated immunity. Deficiency is a rare occurrence in the United States. However, certain medications such as isonicotine hydrazine (INH), penicillamine, cycloserine ethionamide, and theophylline may decrease the absorption and efficacy of vitamin B-6. Vitamin B-6 supplementation is used in the prophylaxis and treatment of vitamin B-6 deficiencies due to the use of the antituberculosis drug, INH. Since INH reacts nonenzymatically with pyridoxal-5′-phosphate to form a metabolically inactive hydrazone, this can lead to the deficient levels of the vitamin. It is recommended that a vitamin B-6 supplement be prescribed concurrently with INH.

Toxicity occurrence is relatively low, although high doses (several grams per day) have produced sensory neuropathy marked by changes in gait and peripheral sensation.[28] Pregnant and nursing mothers should avoid doses of vitamin B-6 greater than 2 to 20 mg daily. It is usually well tolerated; however, there have been reports of severe sensory neuropathy with intakes of 500 mg or greater per day.

Both animal and human studies have demonstrated that vitamin B-6 deficiency affects cellular and humoral responses of the immune system. Vitamin B-6 deficiency results in altered lymphocyte differentiation and maturation, reduced delayed-type hypersensitivity (DTH) responses, impaired antibody production, decreased lymphocyte proliferation, and decreased IL-2 production, among other immunological factors.[29] The risk of vitamin B-6 deficiency is greater in persons with altered immune response such as the elderly, those with uremia and those with HIV. Supplementation of the vitamin in those who are vitamin B-6-deficient has not shown immune-enhancing or immunomodulatory effects to date.

Recommended Dietary Intake and Dosage

Vitamin B-6 is found in nutritional supplements mostly in the form of pyridoxine hydrochloride. It is available in most multivitamins as well as stand-alone form. Typical doses of pyridoxine range from 2 to 20 mg/day. For the management of premenstrual syndrome, it is recommended to increase the dose to 50 to 100 mg/day.

Vitamin B-12

The term vitamin B-12 refers to a family of cobalamin compounds containing the porphyrin-like, cobalt-centered corrin nucleus. The most active of the B-12 compounds are cyanocobalamin and hydroxocobalamin. It is the most complex vitamin chemically of all of the vitamins. Vitamin B-12 works in close partnership with folate in the synthesis of the building blocks for DNA and RNA synthesis. Vitamin B-12 is metabolically active only as derivatives that have either a 5′-deoxyadenosine or methyl group attached covalently to the corrin ring cobalt atom. These conversions are accomplished by vitamin B-12 coenzyme synthetase and 5-methyl-FH4, homocysteine methyltransferase, respectively.

Vitamin B-12 functions in two coenzyme forms: adenosylcobalamin and methylcobalamin. In these forms, the vitamin plays an important role in the metabolism of propionate, amino acids, and single carbons. These processes are vital for normal metabolism of all cells, especially those of the GI tract, bone marrow, and nervous tissue. There is some preliminary indication that vitamin B-12 may be helpful in inhibiting a precancerous condition in the lungs of smokers, which it may help to ameliorate the symptoms of some neuropsychiatric disorders and that it might be useful in some capacity for people with chronic fatigue syndrome and HIV disease.[30]

Vitamin B-12 is bound by protein to food and needs to be released by pepsin in the stomach. Vitamin B-12 then combines with R-proteins (cobalophilins) in the stomach and moves into the small intestine, where the R-proteins are hydrolyzed and intrinsic factor (IF), a specific binding protein for B-12 binds the cobalamin. The majority of vitamin B-12 is absorbed by this active transport and IF is essential to the process. After absorption, cobalamin binds to the plasma R-proteins known as transcobalamins (TCs). One of these TCs, TC-II, is the main transporter protein for newly absorbed cobalamins as they circulate to peripheral tissues.[31] Vitamin B-12 is secreted in the bile and reabsorbed via the enterohepatic circulation. Vitamin B-12 is synthesized by bacteria, but the vitamin produced from the microflora in the colon is not absorbed. The richest sources of the vitamin are the liver and kidney of animals that are the source of the food (such as the cow), as well as, milk, eggs, fish, cheese, and muscle meats. Plant foods are not a source of vitamin B-12. There is speculation that fermented foods contain sufficient B-12 to meet their needs. However, this theory is not supported by analysis.[32] Since vitamin B-12 in food is found bound to protein, approximately 70% of its activity is retained during the cooking process. However, an appreciable amount can be lost when milk is pasteurized or evaporated.

Deficiency and Toxicity Information

Vitamin B-12 deficiency can cause impaired cell division and it is thought to be important in immune function. Vitamin B-12 is particularly utilized in the rapidly dividing cells of the bone marrow and intestinal mucosa and a deficiency leads to arrested synthesis of DNA. The reduction in mitotic rate results in abnormally large cells and a characteristic megaloblastic anemia. The anemia of B-12 deficiency is related to the fact that inadequate B-12 leads to a secondary folate deficiency. Vitamin B-12 deficiency has also been associated with Alzheimer's disease. The most common cause of vitamin B-12 deficiency is malabsorption of the vitamin due to lack or inadequate secretion of IF. This type of deficiency can result from aging[33] or autoimmune incapacitation of IF. Long-term consumption of strict vegan diets without supplemental vitamin B-12 typically leads to very low circulating levels of the vitamin. A deficiency can also occur as a result of a total gastrectomy or bariatric surgery, which interferes with the production of IF. Bacterial overgrowth of the small intestine can also lead to lower levels of vitamin B-12.

Symptoms of vitamin B-12 deficiency include a lemon-yellow tint to the skin and eyes resulting from concurrent anemia and jaundice from ineffective erythropoiesis, smooth, beefy, red tongue, neurologic disorders, and psychiatric manifestations such as impaired mentation and depression. The best assessment of vitamin B-12 levels is made by measuring blood levels of the metabolites methylmalonic acid (MMA) and homocysteine, which are B-12 dependent. This, however, is an expensive testing procedure. Serum B-12 levels are not a good indicator of vitamin status.[8] There is no apparent B-12 toxicity reported. Cyanocobalamin should not be supplemented in patients with Leber's optic atrophy. This is a congenital disorder associated with chronic cyanide intoxication.

Recommended Dietary Intake and Dosage

The principal form of vitamin B-12 used in nutritional supplements is cyanocobalamin. A general dosage range is between 3 and 30 μg daily. Absorption decreases generally with age.

Due to this fact, the Food and Nutrition Board advises that those persons older than 50 years of age should consume foods fortified with B-12 or take a vitamin B-12-containing nutritional supplement to meet the RDA (2.4 μg).

SELENIUM

Selenium is an ultratrace mineral, which is found in small amounts in the body. It is necessary to maintain levels of glutathione peroxidase (GSH-Px), an enzyme containing selenium. GSH-Px acts together with other antioxidants and free radical scavengers to reduce cellular peroxides and free radicals into water and other harmless molecules. Selenium as seleno-methionine or selenocysteine is found widely distributed in the body. Cellular glutathione peroxidase (CGSH-Px) has been found in almost all cells and extracellularly as well. Seleno-protein P, another selenium-containing molecule, may act as a free radical scavenger and in the transported form of selenium. Vitamin E and selenium may reinforce each other's antioxidant action against oxidative damage. They act together to keep cells healthy. This may play a role in cancer prevention.[34]

Absorption of selenium occurs in the upper segment of the small intestine. When the intake of selenium increases, there is an increased excretion in the urine. Assessment of selenium status is done by measuring selenium GSH-Px in serum platelets, and erythrocytes or in whole blood.

The selenium concentration found in foods depends on the selenium content of the soil and water where the food was grown. Major food sources include Brazil nuts, seafood, kidney, liver, meat, and poultry. Fruits and vegetables are not good sources of selenium.

Deficiency and Toxicity Information

Selenium deficiency takes years to develop. It is a rare deficiency. However, in China and Mongolia, selenium deficiency has been reported. In the Keshan Province of China, a form of cardiomyopathy has been reported. The disease, Keshan disease, affects mainly women and children. Another selenium deficiency disease is known as Kashin–Beck disease and is common in preadolescent and adolescent children. The soil selenium content is low where these two diseases are prevalent. Some of the symptoms are symmetrical stiffness, swelling, and pain in the interphalangeal joints of the fingers. Osteoarthritis also develops in their elbows, knees, and ankles.[35]

The only reported selenium toxicity is reported in China.[36] Signs of toxicity, referred to as selenosis, include skin and nail changes, tooth decay, and GI distress.

Recommended Dietary Intake and Dosage

The RDAs for selenium were redefined in 2000. These levels are 55 μg/day for women, men and adolescents (ages 14 to 18). The children's range is from 20 to 30 μg/day. The RDA for pregnancy is 60 μg/day and during lactation it increases to 70 μg/day.

COPPER

Copper is a normal part of blood. It is an established essential micronutrient. It has many tissue-related functions and therefore carries a risk of deficiency.[37] Copper is found in large concentrations in the liver, muscle, brain, heart, and kidney. Skeletal muscle contains approximately 40% of all the copper in the body. It is a component of many enzymes and manifestations of deficiency are attributable to enzyme failures. Copper has a well-documented role in oxidizing iron before it is transported in the plasma. Lysyl oxidase, a copper-containing enzyme, is essential to the lysine-derived cross-linking of collagen and elastin, and connective tissue strength.[38] Copper also has a role in mitochondrial energy production and protects against oxidants and free radicals. It helps to promote the synthesis of melanin and catecholamines.

Copper absorption occurs in the small intestine. Entry at the mucosal surface is completed by facilitated diffusion, and it exits across the basolateral membrane primarily by active transport. There is some evidence to suggest that the amount of copper absorbed is regulated by the mucosal cells. The net absorption of copper varies from 25 to 60%. Fiber and phytate may slightly inhibit copper absorption as they do with several minerals. Approximately 90% of the copper in serum is incorporated into ceruloplasmin and the rest is loosely bound to albumin, transcuprein, and other proteins. It is transported in the blood to the tissues, primarily bound to albumin. Ceruloplasmin is a functional protein that acts as an enzyme in the erythrocyte-forming cells of the bone marrow. The copper bound to albumin may serve as a temporary storage site. Copper is secreted from the liver as a component of bile, which is the major route of excretion for copper. Small amounts of copper are found in urine, sweat, and menstrual fluid.

Copper is found widely in food which includes animal products (except for milk) and most diets provide between 0.6 and 2 mg/day. Good sources of copper are shellfish, organ meats, muscle meats, chocolate, nuts, cereal grains, dried legumes, and dried fruit.

Deficiency and Toxicity Information

Copper deficiency can be identified by a decrease in serum copper and ceruloplasmin levels. Copper-containing enzymes in blood cells have not been identified.[39] A deficiency in copper is characterized by anemia, neutropenia, and skeletal abnormalities, especially demineralization of the bone. There are other changes that occur such as dyspigmentation and defective elastin formation. Death may occur due to a failure of erythropoiesis, as well as cerebral and cerebellar degradation. Neutropenia and leukopenia are the best early indicators of copper deficiency in children. The classic cases of copper deficiency were reported in the 1960s among malnourished Peruvian infants with diarrhea who were fed diluted cow's milk.[40] As large amounts of copper are stored in the liver, deficiency develops slowly as the nutrient's stores become depleted. It is a rare deficiency, probably because copper accumulates in the liver throughout life in most individuals.[41]

Menkes' syndrome, also known as "Kinky–Hair" syndrome, is a sex-linked recessive defect that results in copper malabsorption, increased urinary copper loss, and abnormal intracellular copper transport, all leading to an abnormal distribution of copper among organs and within the cells. Infants with this syndrome have retarded growth, defective keratinization of hair, hypothermia, degenerative changes in aortic elastin, and progressive mental deterioration. These infants usually do not survive more than a few months.[42]

A toxic level of copper can come from excessive supplementation or the use of copper salts in agriculture. Liver cirrhosis develops as well as abnormalities in red blood cell formation.

The amount of copper found in the serum increases during pregnancy and with the use of oral contraceptives. It also increases in concentration in patients with acute and chronic infections, liver disease, and pellagra. Wilson's disease is a genetic disorder, which leads to a degeneration of liver synthesis of ceruloplasmin and manifests itself as an accumulation of copper within the body, especially in the eyes. A strict vegan diet may help patients with Wilson's disease due to the low levels of copper in fruits and vegetables.

Recommended Dietary Intake and Dosage

Copper supplementation is available in several forms, including cupric oxide, copper gluconate, copper sulfate, and copper amino acid chelates. Typical doses range from 1.5 to 3.0 mg/day.

Zinc

Zinc has been known to be an essential mineral since the 1960s.[43,44] It is primarily an intracellular ion, functioning in association with more than 300 different enzymes of various classes. Almost all of it is bound to protein. It participates in reactions involving either synthesis or degradation of major metabolites such as carbohydrates, lipids, protein, and nucleic acids. It is important due to its role as a component of several proteins and its function as an intracellular signal in brain cells. Zinc is involved in the stabilization of protein and nucleic acid structure and the integrity of subcellular organelles, as well as in transport processes, immune function, and expression of genetic information. Zinc is found in large quantities in the nucleus where it stabilizes the structures of RNA and DNA. It is required for the activity of RNA polymerases, which are important in cell division. It has a role in chromatin proteins involved in transcription and replication of RNA. Since it is found in the crystalline structure of bone, and at the zone of demarcation, it is thought that zinc is needed for the formation of bone enzymes and adequate osteoblastic activity.

There is also a correlation between zinc and the immune system. It has been shown to promote the destruction of foreign particles and microorganisms, act as a protectant against free radical damage, is required for proper white blood cell function, and is a necessary cofactor in activating serum thymic factor — a thymus hormone with profound immune-enhancing properties.[45]

Zinc absorption and excretion are controlled by poorly understood homeostatic mechanisms. Absorption of zinc involves two pathways: (1) a saturable carrier mechanism operating most efficiently at low zinc intakes when luminal zinc concentrations are low, and (2) a passive mechanism involving paracellular movement when zinc intakes and luminal concentrations are high. Solubility by zinc in the gut lumen is critical to its absorption. The absorption of zinc is affected not only by the level of zinc in the diet, but also by the presence of certain interfering substances, especially phytates.[46]

Approximately 80% of the daily intake of zinc for most Americans is provided by meat, fish, poultry, ready-to-eat breakfast cereals, milk, and milk products.[47] Oysters and other shellfish, liver, and dry beans are also good sources. The content of typical diets ranges between 10 and 15 mg/day. Women usually take in less due to their lower caloric intake.

Deficiency and Toxicity Information

The clinical signs of zinc deficiency were first reported in young boys in Iran and Egypt. The symptoms included short stature, hypogonadism, mild anemia, and low plasma zinc levels.[44] The deficiency was caused by a diet high in unrefined cereals and unleavened breads, which contain high levels of fiber and phytate, both of which bind zinc in the intestine and prevent absorption. Other symptoms are hypogeusia, delayed wound healing, alopecia, and a diverse range of skin lesions. Zinc deficiency can be acquired as the result of malabsorption, starvation, or increased losses from urine excretion. Persons with alcoholism may also have altered zinc metabolism.[48] A zinc deficiency can cause various immunologic deficits. It can lead to thymic atrophy, lymphopenia, reduced lymphocyte proliferation response to mitogens, a selective decrease in T4-helper cells, decreased natural killer (NK) cell activity, and a decreased thymic hormone activity. It can also impair IL-2 production.

Pregnant and lactating women should avoid zinc doses higher than RDA amounts (15 to 19 mg/day). Doses of zinc up to 30 mg daily are generally well tolerated. The most common adverse reactions include GI affects such as nausea, vomiting, and a metallic taste. High doses of zinc may be immunosuppressive.[48]

Recommended Dietary Intake and Dosage

There are several supplementary forms including zinc gluconate, zinc oxide, zinc aspartate, zinc iodinate, and zinc citrate. A typical dose is about 15 mg daily.

IRON

Iron is an essential mineral. Its function relates to its ability to perform in oxidation and reduction reactions. It is a reactive element that interacts with oxygen and forms intermediates with the potential to damage cell membranes or degrade DNA. Iron has to be bound to proteins to prevent its potentially harmful oxidative effects. Iron has a role in red blood cell function, myoglobin activity and has numerous other interactions in heme and nonheme enzyme functions. It performs in the blood and is involved in the respiratory transport of oxygen and carbon dioxide. It is an important component of the cytochromes involved in the process of cellular respiration and energy (ATP) generation. The function of iron is paramount in the formation of hemoglobin, which is synthesized in immature red blood cells in the bone marrow. Hemoglobin works in two ways: (1) iron-containing heme combines with oxygen in the lungs and then releases the oxygen in the tissues, and (2) it picks up carbon dioxide in the tissues and then releases it in the lungs. Myoglobin is also a heme-containing protein and serves as an oxygen reservoir within muscle. Iron is only lost from the body through bleeding and in very small amounts through defecation, sweat, and the normal loss of hair and skin. Approximately 200 and 1500 mg of iron is stored in the body as ferritin and hemosiderin. Thirty percent of iron is stored in the liver, and another 30% in the bone marrow. The rest is found in the spleen and liver. Approximately 50 mg/day can be taken from iron stores. The amount of ferritin circulating in the body can be closely correlated with total body iron stores. The determination of ferritin levels is an excellent tool for the evaluation of iron status.

Iron is also important in the normal function of the immune system.[49] An adequate iron concentration is essential for changes in the immune response. Iron is a required fuel for bacteria. If an overload occurs it may result in an increased risk of infection or worsening of infection. Iron deficiency can affect hormonal and cellular immunity.

The best sources of dietary iron are liver, followed by seafood (oysters and fish), kidney, heart, lean meat, and poultry. Dried beans and vegetables are the best plant sources. Milk and milk products are devoid of iron. The foods that supply the greatest amounts of iron in the U.S. diet include ready-to-eat cereals fortified with iron.

Deficiency and Toxicity Information

Iron deficiency is the precursor to iron-deficiency anemia. It is especially prevalent in children and women of childbearing age. Groups that are considered at risk are infants younger than 2 years of age, adolescent females, pregnant women, and older adults. A diet rich in iron and supplements helps with this type of anemia. In later stages of iron-deficiency anemia, the blood becomes hypochromic and microcytic. High-dose supplementation with either ferrous sulfate or ferrous gluconate is taken until levels become more normal. Iron deficiency may be a result of injury, hemorrhage, or illness, such as GI disturbances, which interfere with iron absorption. The diet plays a major role in iron levels in the body. If the diet is low in iron, protein, folate, or vitamin C, the serum iron levels can decrease. Persons with iron-deficiency anemia should be counseled in the adequate intake requirements and how to reach them.

The main cause of iron overload is hereditary hemochromatosis. This overloading of iron storage is seen in patients with sickle cell disease, or thalassemia major who need frequent transfusions. Iron overload is linked to a specific gene that favors excessive iron absorption.

Iron supplementation may be contraindicated for either older (postmenopausal) women or older men due to the association of increased risks for heart disease and cancer. Increased intake of iron over the RDA may contribute to an enriched oxidative environment in the body that favors oxidation of LDL-C and arterial vessel damage.

Recommended Dietary Intake and Dosage

DRIs have been established for iron. The RDAs have increased in recent years for post-menopausal women and adolescent females. Full-term infants are born with a reserve of iron from maternal transfer through the placenta. Premature infants have limited reserves of iron since iron and other minerals are transferred from mother to baby during the last trimester. Constipation is one prevalent GI side effect of iron supplementation.

CONCLUSION

The immune system has multiple components functioning in a complicated series of processes. All the various components have an interrelated part in the balance of a well-functioning immune response. Any changes to this balance can cause an altered state of wellness or disease. Micronutrients, antioxidants, macronutrients, and nutrition status all play a critical role in a healthy-functioning immune system. Alternative and integrative medical practices have been discussed along with traditional medical science to help address problems with the immune system. It is important for the consumer to beware, since the science is still evolving in this area. There are many who prey on immune compromised individuals, sometimes with the best of intentions, yet the scientific validity of their claims may be suspect. People who are affected by an immune system disease are sometimes desperate for relief, a cure, an answer. It is the responsibility of the medical community to provide valid and scientifically based answers to the ongoing questions related to the immune system.

REFERENCES

1. Calder PC, Kew S. The immune system: a target for functional foods? *Br J Nutr*, 2002;88 (Suppl 2):S165–S177.
2. Marcos A et al. Changes in the immune system are conditioned by nutrition. *Eur Clin Nutr*, 2003;57(Suppl 1):S66–S69.
3. Durlach J. The role of magnesium in immunity. *J Nutr Immunol*, 1993;2:107–126.
4. Kubena KS, McMurray DN. Nutrition and the immune system — a review of nutrient–nutrient interactions. *J Am Diet Assoc*, 1996;96(11):1156–1164.
5. Rude RK. Magnesium deficiency: a cause of heterogeneous disease in humans. *J Bone Miner Res*, 1998;13:749–758.
6. Appel IJ et al. A clinical study of the effects of dietary patterns on blood pressure. *N Engl J Med*, 1997;336:1117–1124.
7. Lim R, Herzog WR. Magnesium for cardiac patients: is it a valuable treatment supplement? *Contemp Int Med*, 1998;10:6–9.
8. PDR for Nutritional Supplements. Thompson Healthcare, 2001.
9. Semba RD. Vitamin A, immunity, and infection. *Clin Infect Dis*, 1994;19:489–499.
10. Institute of Medicine, Food and Nutrition Board. *Dietary Reference Intakes. Proposed Definition and Plan for Review of Dietary Antioxidants and Related Compounds*, National Academy Press, Washington, D.C., 1998.
11. Bendich A. Vitamin C and immune responses. *Food Technol*, 1987;41:112–114.
12. Li E, Norris AW. Structure/function of systolic vitamin-A binding proteins. *Annu Rev Nutr*, 1996;16:205–234.

13. Packer L, Fuchs J, Eds., *Vitamin C in Health and Disease*, Marcel Dekker, New York, 1997.
14. Johnston C, Luo B. Comparison of the absorption and excretion of three commercially available sources of vitamin C. *J Am Diet Assoc*, 1994;94:779–784.
15. Kim Y-I. Folate and carcinogenesis: evidence, mechanisms, and implications. *J Nutr Biochem*, 1999;10:66–88.
16. Jacques PF, Selhub J, Boston AG, et al. The effect of folic acid fortification on plasma folate and total homocysteine concentrations. *N Engl J Med*, 1999;340:1449–1454.
17. Butterworth C Jr, Bendich A. Folic acid and the prevention of birth defects. *Annu Rev Nutr*, 1996;16:73–97.
18. Beisel W et al. Single-nutrient effects of immunologic function. *JAMA*, 1981;245:53–58.
19. Horwitt MK. My valedictory on the differences in biological potency between RRR-alpha-tocopherol and all-rac-alpha-tocopheryl acetate. *Am J Clin Nutr*, 1999;69:341–342.
20. Can C et al. Vascular endothelial dysfunction associated with elevated serum homocysteine levels in rat adjuvant arthritis: effect of vitamin E administration. *Life Sci*, 2002;71:401.
21. Malmberg KJ et al. A short term dietary supplementation of high doses of vitamin E increases T helper 1 cytokine production in patients with advanced colorectal cancer. *Clin Cancer Res*, 2002;8(6):1772–1778.
22. Fairfield KM, Fletcher RH. Vitamins for chronic disease prevention in adults: scientific review. *JAMA*, 2002;287:3116–3126.
23. Morris MC et al. Dietary intake of antioxidant nutrients and the risk of incident Alzheimer disease in a biracial community study. *JAMA*, 2002;287:3261.
24. Stampfer MJ, Hennekens CH, Manson JE, et al. Vitamin E consumption and the risk of coronary disease in women. *N Engl J Med*, 1993;328:1444–1449.
25. Baum MK et al. Influence of HIV infection on vitamin status and requirements. *Ann NY Acad Sci*, 1992; 669:165–174.
26. Institute of Medicine, Food and Nutrition Board. *Dietary Reference Intakes for Vitamin C, Vitamin E, Selenium, and Carotenoids*, National Academy Press, Washington, D.C., 2000.
27. Driskell JA. Vitamin B-6 requirements of humans. *Nutr Res*, 1994;14:293–324.
28. Schaumberg HJ et al. Sensory neuropathy from pyridoxine abuse. *N Engl J Med*, 1983;309:445–448.
29. Gridley DS et al. *In vivo* and *in vitro* stimulation of cell-mediated immunity by vitamin B6. *Nutr Res*, 1988;8:201–207.
30. Harriman GR, Smith PD, et al. Vitamin B-12 malabsorption in patients with acquired immune deficiency syndrome. *Arch Intern Med*, 1989;149;2039–2041.
31. Groff JL, Gropper SS. *Advanced Nutrition and Human Metabolism*, 3rd ed., Wassworth/Thomson Learning, Belmont, CA, 1999, p. 584.
32. Specker BL et al. Increase urinary methylmalonic acid excretion in breast-fed infants with vegetarian mothers and identification of an acceptable dietary source of vitamin B-12. *Am J Clin Nutr*, 1988;47:89–92.
33. Carethers M: Diagnosing vitamin B-12 deficiency, a common geriatric disorder. *Geriatrics*, 1988;43:89–112.
34. Clark LC et al. Effects of selenium supplementation for cancer prevention in patients with carcinoma of the skin: a randomized controlled trial. *JAMA*, 1996;276:1957–1963.
35. Sokoloff L. Kashin–Beck disease. Current status. *Nutr Rev*, 1988;46:113–119.
36. Yang GQ et al. Endemic selenium intoxication of humans in China. *Am J Clin Nutr*, 1983;37:872–881.
37. Uauy R et al. Essentiality of copper in humans. *Am J Clin Nutr*, 1998;67(Suppl 5):952S–959S.
38. Rucker et al. Copper, lysyl oxidase, and extracellular matrix protein cross-linking. *Am J Clin Nutr*, 1998;67(Suppl 5):996S–1002S.
39. Milne DB. Copper intake and assessment of copper status. *Am J Clin Nutr*, 1998;67(Suppl):1041S–1045S.
40. Cordano A. Clinical manifestations of nutritional copper deficiency in infants and children. *Am J Clin Nutr*, 1998;67(Suppl): 1012S–1016S.

41. Kelley DS et al. Effects of low-copper diets on human immune response. *Am J Clin Nutr*, 1995;62:412.

42. Buchman Al et al. Copper deficiency secondary to a copper transport defect, a new copper metabolic disturbance. *Metabolism*, 1994;43:1462–1469.

43. Halsted JA et al. Zinc deficiency in man — the Shiraz experiment. *Am J Med*, 1972;53:277–283.

44. Prasad AS et al. Zinc metabolism in patients with the syndrome of iron deficiency anemia, hepatosplenomegaly, dwarfism, and hypogonadism. *J Lab Clin Med*, 1963;61:537–549.

45. Dardenne M et al. Contributions of zinc and other metals to the biological activity of serum thymic factor. *Proc Natl Acad Sci*, 1982;79:5730–5733.

46. Fairweather-Tait SJ. Zinc in human nutrition. Nutr Res Rev, 1998;1:23.

47. Suber AF et al. Dietary sources of nutrients among US adults, 1989–1991. *J Am Diet Assoc*, 1998; 98:537–547.

48. King JC et al. Zinc. In Shils ME et al., Eds., *Modern Nutrition in Health and Disease*, 8th ed., Vol. 1, Lea and Febiger, Philadelphia, 1994.

49. Beard JL. Iron biology in immune function, muscle metabolism and neuronal functioning. *J Nutr*, 2001;131:568–580.

CLINICAL APPLICATION: GRAVES' DISEASE

David W. Grotto

DESCRIPTION

Graves' disease is an example of an autoimmune condition where an immune attack is specifically directed against the thyroid gland. Thyroid eye disease (TED) is the most frequent extrathyroidal manifestation of Graves' disease and in most instances it is mild and nonprogressive, but in 3 to 5% of cases it is severe. Less frequently, Graves' also appears as alterations of the pretibial skin (the skin on the front of the lower leg).

It occurs in less than one quarter of 1% of the population and is more prevalent among females in their middle decades, eight times more than males. Typically, it occurs in middle age but can also occur in children, adolescents, and in the elderly. It is not a communicable disease although it has been known to occur between husbands and wives. Though the disease is not curable, it is a completely treatable.[1]

The mechanism by which Graves' disease occurs is unknown, although it is likely it develops in genetically prone individuals. Antibodies target the thyrotropin receptor (TSH-R) and promote the development of glandular overactivity. It was once thought that NK T-cells may be involved in the pathogenesis of Graves' disease but recent research has not supported this theory.[2] Susceptibility loci within immune response genes have been identified. In addition, several environmental factors have been proposed for involvement in the development of autoimmune thyroid disease and may initiate genetic expression of the disease.

Polychlorinated biphenyls (PCBs) can alter thyroxin levels and result in symptoms of thyroid disorders.[3] Drinking water that was contaminated with organic hydrocarbons resulted in blocked activity of thyroid hormones.[4] Several other pollutants have been found to block the metabolism of thyroid hormones.[5]

Infections and stress play a part as Graves' disease may have its onset after an external stressor. To date, there lacks substantial evidence to support causality and a significant component of the genetic predisposition to this disease remains unclear as the Graves' gene in DNA has not yet been identified.[6]

CONVENTIONAL TREATMENT

Antithyroid Drugs

Antithyroid drugs are used primarily to treat Graves' hyperthyroidism. Specifically, thionamides, propanolol, and iodide are the drugs of choice; however, lithium carbonate and perchlorate are used as well. These drugs have specific mechanisms, effectiveness, and potential side effects that are of important consideration in choosing an appropriate treatment course for a patient.

Thionamides

The thionamide group of drugs acts mainly to inhibit the production of thyroid hormones. Carbimazole (CBZ), propylthiouracil (PTU), and methimazole (MMI) are the three most frequently used drugs. There is no firm evidence that the side effects are greater in any particular drug. However, carbimazole has to be added to the list of drugs capable of inducing acute pancreatitis, and it is recommended to discontinue this medication as soon as there is evidence of pancreatic dysfunction.[7] About 40% of patients treated with thionamides as definitive therapy for Graves' disease enter sustained remission after an initial course.

Propanolol

Propanolol is the most commonly used β-blocking drugs and acts mainly to inhibit the adrenergic effects of Graves' disease for symptomatic control. In addition, it also has some effect on inhibiting the conversion of T4 to more potent T3. β-Blocking drugs mostly play an adjuvant role in therapy and are commonly used to control symptoms of hyperthyroidism until first-line therapies (thionamides or radioiodine) take hold. They have been used before to prepare patients with mild hyperthyroidism for surgery. It is contraindicated in patients with obstructive airway disease or cardiac failure and used with precaution in diabetics.

Iodine

At different dosages, iodine has paradoxical effects on the thyroid as it can cause hypo- or hyperthyroidism. Rapid improvement in thyrotoxic symptoms typically occurs within 2 to 7 days. Iodides usually are initiated after onset of thionamide therapy and are avoided if treatment with radioactive iodine seems likely. The major side effects of iodides are hypersensitivity and reversible iodism if iodine treatment is stopped. Iodism causes a metallic taste in the mouth, mucous ulcers, acneiform rash, and swollen salivary glands.

In summary, antithyroid drugs require no surgery or use of radioactive materials. However, disadvantages include prolonged treatment and the failure rate after a course of 1.5 to 2 years is at least 50%. It is also impossible to predict which patient is likely to go into remission and some goiters enlarge and become vascular during treatment. Though rare, dangerous drug reactions like agranulocytosis or aplastic anemia can occur.

Radioiodine Therapy

Radioiodine (I-131) destroys part or all of the thyroid gland and renders it incapable of overproducing thyroid hormone. It is the treatment of choice for recurrent Graves' disease after subtotal thyroidectomy or after antithyroid drugs become ineffective. It is the treatment of first choice in the elderly, but radioactive iodine is not routinely given to children and adults in their reproductive years. The major concerns are its genetic effects and the possible induction of malignancy. All evidence to date indicates that radioiodine given in typical doses does not increase the risk of leukemia, thyroid carcinoma, or other tumors. However, in one study, a small but definite increase in thyroid and small bowel cancers was seen in individuals who received radioactive iodine to treat hyperthyroidism.[8]

Presurgery

Patients are rendered euthyroid with antithyroid drugs (thionamides) before treatment in order to reduce the likelihood of a "thyroid storm." Although this is very rare, a risk of it happening is present as a surge of thyroid hormones are released from the gland when cellular death occurs. Thyroid storm may occur in poorly prepared patients.

Surgery

Surgical treatment was the earliest treatment for Graves' disease introduced by Kocher who by 1889 had performed over 350 operations with a low mortality rate of 2.4%. Until the early 1940s, surgery was the only definitive treatment. It still remains an effective and valuable therapy, as the cure rate is both rapid and high if the total goiter is removed. Today, due to the safety and simplicity of radioiodine, plus the availability of antithyroid medications, it is used less frequently. Disadvantages include recurrence of thyrotoxicosis occurs in 5 to 10% of cases, postoperative thyroid insufficiency occurs in 20 to 45% of cases, and in less than 0.5% of cases, parathyroid insufficiency occurs. Possible side effects of surgery include bleeding, respiratory obstruction, recurrent laryngeal nerve paralysis, and hypothyroidism (this usually occurs within 2 years, and figures of 20 to 45% have been reported), parathyroid insufficiency, thyrotoxic crisis (storm), and wound infection.[9–12]

Nonsevere TED requires only supportive measures, such as eye ointments, sunglasses, and prisms. By contrast, severe TED requires aggressive treatment, either medical (high-dose glucocorticoids, orbital radiotherapy) or surgical (orbital decompression). The choice of treatment relies on the assessment of both TED severity and activity. Removal of controllable risk factors, especially cigarette smoking, is important to improve the course and the therapeutic outcome. Novel promising treatments, to be verified in large series of patients, include somatostatin analogs and cytokine antagonists. Skin symptoms of Graves' disease may be treated with glucocorticoid creams and ointments.[13]

INTEGRATIVE APPROACHES

Malnutrition is thought to be linked with the incidence of Graves' disease. Fasting and anorexia nervosa, both of which are associated with nutrient depletion and deficiencies, also decrease thyroid function.[14] It was found that young, Japanese woman, who were diagnosed with the disease had low levels of vitamin D.[15] Vitamin E and Co-Q10 were measured in a study of hyperthyroid patients before treatment and the presence of oxidative stress and decreased antioxidant metabolites were found. The authors suggested that supplementation with antioxidant agents during periods of hyperthyroidism is warranted.[16] Poor iron status results in lowered thyroid function.[17] Low thyroid function results in poor utilization of fats in the maintenance of skin integrity.[18] Selenium deficiency may be attributed to the inability of conversion of thyroxin to T3.[19] Overall, high dosages of certain vitamin or mineral combinations, given under the supervision of a trained physician, can help alleviate hyperthyroidism.[20]

Alternative treatment includes consumption of certain foods that help naturally suppress thyroid hormone production. Some types of foods are reputed to be goitrogenic such as members of the Brassica family (which includes cauliflower, Brussels sprouts, cabbage, and broccoli) and also kohlrabi, sweet potatoes, almonds, peaches and peanuts, and possibly soy. The Brassica family interferes with the metabolism of thyroid hormones only when they are consumed in high amounts.[21]

An ongoing debate is the role of soy and its possible mechanism in blocking the production of thyroid hormone or possibly the effectiveness of thyroid medication. Soy in infant formulas was attributed to the development of thyroid disorders and was found to occur more frequently among infants who consumed soy formula than in those who consumed breast milk.[22-24] Soy is also known to interfere with iodine absorption in the gut. Thyroxin levels have been observed to rise in adults who consume soy and there may be compounds in soy that affect thyroid activity, but this has not been deemed conclusive at this time.

Various botanical combinations have been studied in Japan and China. Evaluation of a traditional Chinese blend called Jiayanxiao (JYX) in combination with Tapazole on thyrotoxic exophthalmos showed effectiveness in elevating vision, decreasing palpebral fissure altitude, lowering degree of exophthalmos, and lowering serum T3 in comparison with the placebo group.[25] Some Chinese herbs could induce cell apoptosis when used in combination with antithyroid drugs in treating Graves' disease.[26]

Foods to avoid include wheat, dairy products, sugar, saturated fats, caffeine, and artificial sweeteners. An ideal diet would have adequate, but not excess protein, fresh fruit, brown rice, millet, and lightly steamed vegetables. It is also important to avoid any food allergens as allergic reactions heighten the autoimmune response. The thyroid controls metabolism and tendencies to gain weight may be of concern. Reducing caloric intake while increasing fresh fruits and vegetables for their antioxidant, nutrient, and energy is optimal. Swelling is frequently a problem for Graves' patients and sodium restriction is suggested therefore, avoiding salt and high-sodium canned and frozen foods are recommended.[27]

According to Elaine Moore, author of *Graves' Disease, A Practical Guide*, McFarland, who has also been diagnosed with Graves' disease a number of homeopathic preparations have been successfully used such as kelpsan, Coffea, Pulsatilla, Thyroidinum, and *Natrum muriaticum* have been used in the treatment of hyperthyroidism. She has also found that herbals including *Lycopus virginicus* (bugleweed), *Melissa* (lemon balm), *Leonurus cardica* (motherwort), and *Lithospermum* may help to provide benefit.[28]

Many integrative therapies such as acupuncture exercise, meditation, and various mind–body therapies may provide comfort measures and relief. Stress reduction and dietary changes are integral steps in any healing plan. Stress reduction technique methods include biofeedback, meditation, tai chi, yoga, and prayer therapy. Stress directly reduces the number of immune system cells, which would curb autoantibody production, and stress is a well-known trigger of autoimmune disease. Ayurvedic medicine, craniosacral therapy, and acupuncture have also been used successfully.[29] However, patients in one study with Graves' ophthalmopathy who received acupuncture twice a week during 2 months showed no significant change in eye muscle volume, Hertel measure, palpebral aperture, intraocular pressure, Hess chart, or improvement of the irritative conjunctival symptoms.[30]

REFERENCES

1. http://www.ngdf.org/faq.htm.
2. Luo W, Guo H, Aosai F, Yano A. Role of natural killer T cells in Graves' disease. *Chin Med J Engl*, 2002;115(8):1183–1185.
3. McKinney JD, Pedersen LG. Do residue levels of polychlorinated biphenyls (PCBs) in human blood produce mild hypothyroidism? *J Theor Biol*, 1987;129(2):231–241.
4. Gaitan E, Cooksey RC, Matthews D, Presson R. *In vitro* measurement of antithyroid compounds and environmental goitrogens. *J Clin Endocrinol Metab*, 1983;56:767–773.
5. Muir T, Zegarac M. Societal costs of exposure to toxic substances: economic and health costs of four case studies that are candidates for environmental causation. *Environ Health Perspect*, 2001;109(Suppl 6):885–903.

6. Becker W, Schicha H. The thyroid. *Eur J Nucl Med Mol Imaging*, 2002;29(Suppl 2):S417–S424.
7. Marazuela M, Sanchez de Paco G, Jimenez I, Carraro R, Fernandez-Herrera J, Pajares JM, Gomez-Pan A. Acute pancreatitis, hepatic cholestasis, and erythema nodosum induced by carbimazole treatment for Graves' disease. *Endocrinol J*, 2002;49(3):315–318.
8. Jayne AF, Patrick M, Michael S, Joan B, Peter B. Cancer incidence and mortality after radioiodine treatment for hyperthyroidism: a population-based cohort study. *Lancet*, 1999;353:2111–2115.
9. Arem R. *The Thyroid Solution*, Ballantine Books, New York, 1999.
10. "Graves' Disease." Produced by The Thyroid Foundation of America, Inc. and The American Thyroid Association, Inc.
11. Lahita RG, *Textbook of the Autoimmune Diseases*, Lippincott Williams & Wilkins, Philadelphia, 2000.
12. Dayan CM, Leech NJ. Controversies in the management of Graves' disease. *Clin Endocrinol*, 1998;49:273–280.
13. Streetman DD, Khanderia U. Diagnosis and treatment of Graves disease. *Ann Pharmacother*, 2003;37(7–8):1100–1109.
14. Curran-Celentano J, Erdman Jr JW, Nelson RA, Grater SJ. Alterations in vitamin A and thyroid hormone status in anorexia nervosa and associated disorders. *Am J Clin Nutr*, 1985;42:1183–1191.
15. Yamashita H, Noguchi S, Takatsu K, Koike E, Murakami T, Watanabe S, Uchino S, Yamashita H, Kawamoto H. High prevalence of vitamin D deficiency in Japanese female patients with Graves' disease. *Endocrinol J*, 2001;48(1):63–69.
16. Bianchi G, Solaroli E, Zaccheroni V, Grossi G, Bargossi AM, Melchionda N, Marchesini G. Oxidative stress and anti-oxidant metabolites in patients with hyperthyroidism: effect of treatment. *Horm Metab Res*, 1999;31(11):620–624.
17. Beard JL, Borel MJ, Derr J. Impaired thermoregulation and thyroid function in iron-deficiency anemia. *Am J Clin Nutr*, 1990;52:813–819.
18. Ai J, Leonhardt JM, Heymann WR. Autoimmune thyroid diseases: etiology, pathogenesis, and dermatologic manifestations. *J Am Acad Dermatol*, 2003;48(5):641–659.
19. Beckett GJ, Nicol F, Rae PW, Beech S, Guo Y, Arthur JR. Effects of combined iodine and selenium deficiency on thyroid hormone metabolism in rats. *Am J Clin Nutr*, 1993;57:240S–243S.
20. http://www.hmc.psu.edu/healthinfo/h/hyperthyroidism.htm.
21. Heaney RK, Fenwick GR. Natural toxins and protective factors in Brassica species, including rapeseed. *Nat Toxins*, 1995;3(4):233–237.
22. Chorazy PA, Himelhoch S, Hopwood NJ, Greger NG, Postellon DC. Persistent hypothyroidism in an infant receiving a soy formula: case report and review of the literature. *Pediatrics*, 1995;96: 148–150.
23. Jabbar MA, Larrea J, Shaw RA. Abnormal thyroid function tests in infants with congenital hypothyroidism: the influence of soy-based formula. *J Am Coll Nutr*, 1997;16(3):280–282.
24. Fort P, Moses N, Fasano M, Goldberg T, Lifshitz F. Breast and soy-formula feedings in early infancy and the prevalence of autoimmune thyroid disease in children. *J Am Coll Nutr*, 1990;9(2): 164–167.
25. Liao S, Huang Y, Li L. Clinical observation on treatment of thyrotoxic exophthalmos with Jiayanxiao plus Tapazole. *Zhongguo Zhong Xi Yi Jie He Za Zhi*, 1999;19(6):335–336.
26. Zhao J, Gao L, Liu X. Preliminary study on Chinese herb induced apoptosis of thyrocytes in Graves' disease. *Zhongguo Zhong Xi Yi Jie He Za Zhi*, 2000;20(6):433–435.
27. http://www.ngdf.org/Bull01.PDF.
28. Elaine AM, *Graves' Disease, A Practical Guide*, McFarland, 2001.
29. Comparing conventional and holistic healing suggestions for Graves' disease by Elaine Moore. http://www.naturalhealth.org/articles/comparingconventional.htm.
30. Rogvi-Hansen B, Perrild H, Christensen T, Detmar SE, Siersbaek-Nielsen K, Hansen JE. Acupuncture in the treatment of Graves' ophthalmopathy. A blinded randomized study. *Acta Endocrinol (Copenh)*, 1991;124(2):143–145.

CLINICAL APPLICATION: MULTIPLE SCLEROSIS

David W. Grotto

DYSFUNCTION

Multiple sclerosis (MS) is an inflammatory autoimmune disease of the central nervous system (CNS) that results in the presence of multiple sclerotic lesions via demyelination of nerve cell sheaths in the brain and spinal cord. It is estimated that over one million cases occur worldwide and that in the United States alone, this number is thought to exceed 250,000 to 350,000 cases annually.[1] Several studies suggest a possible genetic link to MS whereas approximately one quarter of MS patients have an affected relative.[1,2] In upper geographical latitudes, higher rates of MS appear to occur in up to 50 to 100 cases out of 100,000 populations versus 5 to 10 cases per 100,000 in the lower latitudes. This has spurred research into the theory that latitude may influence the production of vitamin D in the skin. There may be a possible connection in that lower vitamin D levels have found in MS subjects.[3,4]

Before sophisticated imaging technology became available, the "hot bath" test was used as a method of diagnoses as it was discovered that many MS sufferers had intolerance to heat. Today, the diagnostic imaging test of choice for the diagnosis of MS is magnetic resonance imaging (MRI). It can accurately detect what is referred to as "white matter plaques," which is thought to be the result of the autoimmune traits of this potentially debilitating disease. Immune effectors including T-cells invade the brain and attack nerve cells, removing their myelin sheaths while obliterating their axons and remaining components.[5]

Often occurring in early adulthood, most frequent symptoms of MS include numbness, impaired vision, bladder dysfunction and loss of balance, psychological changes, and weakness. The severity of the disease can vary for up to 30 years with periodic episodes of remission, but in many cases it steadily progresses to severe disability and the premature death of approximately 3000 people each year in the United States.[6,7]

It is thought that MS may be initiated by exposure to environmental agents during childhood or early adulthood as suggested by researchers. Viral infections such as nidoviruses, retroviruses, and varicella zoster have shown possible causation. Several viruses including herpes (HHV-6), measles, and even canine distemper have been investigated to determine if they are implicated as a contributing agent; however, to date, no specific virus has been proven to trigger MS. Other environmental factors thought to be linked to MS include toxins such as solvents and pesticides, x-rays exposure, and environmental exposure to domesticated animals such as cats, birds, and dogs.[8-10]

As part of a remission strategy, it is important to avoid the same causative agents of the initial disease that may also act as triggers for relapse. These include exposure to environmental toxins, viral infections, food allergies, stress, pregnancy, and heat exposure. Respiratory infections, sinusitis, and heat exposure alone may account for a considerable amount of relapses.[11,12]

CONVENTIONAL APPROACHES

Historically, drug therapies for MS mostly consist namely of immunosuppressants such as prednisone, cortisone, Cytoxan, and methotrexate, which are fairly effective but may have undesirable side effects. In addition, IFN β-1b has been used since 1993 as a prevention therapy, but often produces severe adverse side effects as well. IFN β-1a and glatiramer acetate are newer approved conventional drugs that have been developed to treat MS and are classified as "partially effective" for use in relapsing types of MS.[13] In addition, European trials indicate a role for intravenous immunoglobulin in reducing relapses; however, many of these therapies are quite costly and as mentioned earlier, not without their share of debilitating side effects. In light of the limitations of these conventional drug therapies alone for MS, an integrative approach is well worth investigating.[14,15]

INTEGRATIVE APPROACHES

Diet

There have been some dietary factors implicated in the progression of MS including food allergies and intolerances, digestive malfunctions, including malabsorption and dysbiosis, and a high-animal fat diet.[16] Dr. Roy Swank demonstrated that MS subjects who followed a diet that consisted of 20 g or less of fat (less than 15 g of saturated fat), lived longer and generally had less deaths than did those who consumed higher amounts of fat. Dr. Swank also demonstrated in his research that 95% of the patients who were placed on his diet before developing clinical impairment of the disease did not have significant progression of MS during the 35-year period.[17–19]

Also of concern is the possible link between diets containing gluten and dairy products as potential allergens and the prevalence of MS.[20,21] Malabsorption syndrome may be rampant in the MS population. A study of 52 MS patients found that 42% had fat malabsorption, 41% had difficulties fully digesting meat, 27% had abnormal absorption capacity, and 12% did not absorb vitamin B-12.[22] Dr. Paris Kidd discussed this type of malabsorption and a condition known as "dysbiosis" which he feels may be corrected using digestive enzymes and probiotics as part of an overall approach.[16] In addition, an optimal diet including reduced animal fat intake, increased intakes of vegetables, and cold-water marine fish and avoidance of allergenic foods may be ideal for the MS patient.[23–25]

Supplements

Recently, dietary supplements have been recommended for all adults according to a study in the *Journal of the American Medical Association*; however, dietary supplementation for MS patients may require a more sophisticated approach.[26] In addition, the incorporation of antioxidants, omega-3 fatty acids, and a variety of other nutrients including phytonutrients may hold some benefit.[27]

Fatty acids, specifically linoleic acid (LA), gamma-linolenic acid (GLA), and omega-3 types may affect severity of MS symptoms. A meta-analysis of 181 patients concluded that LA at 20 g/day reduced disability, severity, and the duration of relapses, especially in patients with early disease with minimal disability. Though a small study, the researchers concluded that GLA from primrose oil improved peripheral blood flow and handgrip strength in participants overall. Increased omega-3 fatty acid intake has demonstrated improvement in patients diagnosed with other autoimmune diseases such as rheumatoid arthritis (RA) and Crohn's disease. A review of blood work from several MS patients has revealed low docosahexaenoic acid (DHA) and eicosapentaenoic acid (EPA) levels; additionally one small trial showed some improvement in symptoms of MS from fish oil supplementation.[27–31]

Oxidative stress may be indicated in many immune dysfunctions and is most certainly increased in MS. Serum levels of vitamin E have been shown to be low in MS patients and lipid peroxidation markers increased in cerebrospinal fluid (CSF), especially during periods of disease progression. The enzyme GSH-Px, which is known to reduce peroxides, is markedly decreased in red and white blood cells, and the CSF of MS patients. One study gave a high-dose mixed antioxidant supplement containing selenium, vitamins E, and C to the subjects daily for 5 weeks. GP activity increased up to five times and fell within the normal range without additional side effects.[27,32–34]

A total of 100 MS patients received a traditional Tibetan herbal formula known as Adaptrin, previously known as Padma 28. Of these patients, 50 experienced overall improvement in addition to increased muscle strength and improved bladder function. In other investigations of herbal remedies, a double-blind, placebo-controlled 7-day trial examining the effects of ginkgo biloba failed to reduce MS exacerbations.[35,36]

Vitamin deficiencies are also prevalent in the MS patient. As mentioned earlier, vitamin D decreases with increasing latitude. Most MS patients have vitamin D deficiency and this alone can lead to lower bone mass and a higher risk of fracture. This can be exacerbated by the osteopenic side effects of glucocorticoids widely used in MS therapy.[3,37] Vitamin B-12 is a key nutrient factor supporting myelin formation. And its deficiency is a recognized cause of CNS demyelination. B-12 levels were lower in the CSF of MS patients; if not always lower in the serum.[38] A Japanese study administered 60 mg of methylcobalamin by mouth to patients for 6 months. Improvements in sensory nerve potentials were observed, however no motor nerve improvement was demonstrated.[39]

Therapies

In MS patients, raising histamine may help to block autoimmunity. Elaine DeLack, a registered nurse who was diagnosed with MS, developed a histamine cream called Procarin. It was given to 55 MS patients through a clinic in Kent Washington and was found to be effective in 67% of the cases. Areas of improvement included activities of daily living, grip strength, sense of balance, fatigue, bladder control, and cognitive functioning.[40]

Exercise has been advocated as a mainstay to reduce stress and relapse events in the MS patient. A study found a synergistic benefit when using osteopathic manipulation therapy combined with maximal-effort exercise. Significant improvements in strength and ambulatory levels were discovered in female patients with MS using this combination. Improvements in activities of daily living were also demonstrated.[41]

Hyperbaric oxygen therapy (HBO2T) involves exposure to oxygen at pressures higher than normal air given in multiple sessions repeated typically on a daily basis. Most of the randomized trials to date generally have included a course of 20 treatments at pressures between 1.75 and 2.5 atm abs daily for 60 to 120 min over 4 weeks and were compared against a placebo regimen. None of these studies, however, have compared the efficacy of HBO2T against conventional therapies. Though there may be possible therapeutic effects in selected subgroups of patients to prolonged courses of HBO2T at more modest pressures, there is little controlled evidence that HBO2T results in any benefit for patients with MS. However, all of these trials lasted less than 2 months. The Federation of Multiple Sclerosis Therapy Centers in the United Kingdom HBOT protocol involves indefinite long-term treatment, preferably on a weekly basis, following the initial intense treatment period of 4 weeks. Results of this protocol suggest HBOT may benefit MS.[42]

Clinical trials have shown that cannabis, specifically Delta (9)-tetrahydrocannabinol, and nabilone may provide relief from spasticity, pain, tremor, and nocturia in patients with MS (eight trials) or spinal cord injury (one trial). There is also supporting clinical research in animal studies. The theory is that cannabinoid-induced reductions in tremor and spasticity are mediated by cannabinoid receptors, both CB (1) and CB (2). However, research is lacking whether increased endocannabinoid production occurs in MS. Further research is needed to find ways of achieving consistency in drugs that provide therapeutic effects without unwanted effects.[43]

REFERENCES

1. Anderson DW, Ellenberg JH, Leventhal CM, et al. Revised estimate of the prevalence of multiple sclerosis in the United States. *Ann Neurol*, 1992;31:333–336.
2. Willer CJ, Ebers GC. Susceptibility to multiple sclerosis: interplay between genes and environment. *Curr Opin Neurol*, 2000;13:241–247.
3. Hayes CE, Cantorna MT, DeLuca HF. Vitamin D and multiple sclerosis. *Proc Soc Exptl Biol Med*, 1997;216:21–27.
4. Murray MT, Pizzorno JE. Multiple sclerosis. In Murray MT, Pizzorno JE, Eds., *Encyclopedia of Natural Medicine*, Prima Health, Rocklin, CA, 1998, pp. 666–676, 900–901.
5. Waxman SG. Multiple sclerosis as a neuronal disease. *Archs Neurol*, 2000;57:22–24.
6. Perlmutter D. BrainRecovery.com. *Powerful Therapy for Challenging Brain Disorders*. The Perlmutter Health Center, Naples, FL, www.brainrecovery.com, 2000.
7. Gaby AR. Commentary: multiple sclerosis. *Nutr. Healing*, 1997;4:1–11.
8. Ross RT, Cheang M, Landry G, et al. Herpes zoster and multiple sclerosis. *Can J Neurol Sci*, 1999;26:29–32.
9. Bergstrom T. Herpesviruses — a rationale for antiviral treatment in multiple sclerosis. *Antiviral Res*, 1999;41:1–19.
10. Landtblom AM, Flodin U, Karlsson M, et al. Multiple sclerosis and exposure to solvents, ionizing radiation, and animals. *Scand J Work Environ Health*, 1993;19:399–404.
11. Sibley WA, Bamford CR, Clark K. Clinical virus infections and multiple sclerosis. *Lancet*, 1985;1:1313–1315.
12. Ingalls TH. Triggers for multiple sclerosis. *Lancet*, 1986;ii:160.
13. Noseworthy JH. Progress in determining the causes and treatments of multiple sclerosis. *Nature*, 1999;399:A40–A47.
14. Clegg A et al. Disease-modifying drugs for multiple sclerosis: a rapid and systematic review. *Health Technol Assess*, 2000;4(9):1–101.
15. Weinshenker BG. The natural history of multiple sclerosis. *Neurol Clin*, 1995;13:119–146.
16. Kidd PM. Multiple sclerosis, an autoimmune inflammatory disease: prospects for its integrative management. *Altern Med Rev*, 2001;6(6):540–566.
17. Swank RL, Dugan BB. Effect of low saturated fat diet in early and late cases of multiple sclerosis. *Lancet*, 1990;336:37–39.
18. Swank RL. Multiple sclerosis: twenty years on a low fat diet. *Arch Neurol*, 1970;23:460–474.
19. Swank RL. A prospective discussion of past international nutrition catastrophes — indications for the future. *Nutrition*, 1997;13:344–348.
20. Hewson DC. Is there a role for gluten-free diets in multiple sclerosis? *Hum Appl Nutr*, 1984;38A:417–420.
21. Butcher PJ. Milk consumption and multiple sclerosis — an etiological hypothesis. *Med Hypotheses*, 1986;19:169–178.
22. Gupta JK, Ingegno AP, Cook AW, et al. Multiple sclerosis and malabsorption. *Am J Gastroenterol*, 1977;68:560–565.
23. Bates D, Cartlidge NEF, French JM, et al. A double-blind controlled trial of long-chain $N-3$ polyunsaturated fatty acids in the treatment of multiple sclerosis. *J Neurol Neurosurg Psychiatry*, 1989;52:18–22.
24. Ehrentheil OF. Role of food allergy in multiple sclerosis. *Neurology*, 1952;2:412–426.
25. Wright JV. Multiple sclerosis. *Nutr Healing*, 1997;4:1–12.
26. Fletcher RH, Fairfield KM. Vitamins for chronic disease prevention in adults: clinical applications. *JAMA*, 2002;287:3127–3129.
27. Cendrowski W. Multiple sclerosis and MaxEPA. *Br J Clin Pract*, 1986;40:365–367.
28. Cunnane SC, Ho SY. Essential fatty acid and lipid profiles in plasma and erythrocytes in patients with multiple sclerosis. *Am J Clin Nutr*, 1989;50:801–806.
29. Dworkin RH, Bates D, Millar JHD, et al. Linoleic acid and multiple sclerosis: a reanalysis of three double-blind trials. *Neurology*, 1984;34:1441–1445.

30. Simpson LO, Shand BI, Olds RJ. Dietary supplementation with Efamol and multiple sclerosis. *New Zealand Med J*, 1985;98:1053–1054.
31. Nordvik I, Myhr KM, Nyland H, Bjerve KS. Effect of dietary advice and *n*−3 supplementation in newly diagnosed MS patients. *Acta Neurol Scand*, 2000;102:143–149.
32. Shukla VKS, Jensen GE, Clausen J. Erythrocyte glutathione peroxidase deficiency in multiple sclerosis. *Acta Neurol Scand*, 1977;56:542–550.
33. Jimenez-Jimenez FJ, de Bustos F, Molina JA, et al. Cerebrospinal fluid levels of alpha-tocopherol in patients with multiple sclerosis. *Neurosci Lett*, 1998;249:65–67.
34. Mai J, Sorensen PS, Hansen JC. High dose antioxidant supplementation to MS patients. *Biol Trace Elem Res*, 1990;24:109–117.
35. Korwin-Piotrowska T, Nocon D, Stankowska-Chomicz A, et al. Experience of PADMA 28 in multiple sclerosis. *Phytother Res*, 1992;6:133–136.
36. Brochet B, Guinot P, Orgogozo JM, et al. Double blind placebo controlled multicentre study of ginkgolide B in treatment of acute exacerbations of multiple sclerosis. *J Neurol Neurosur Psychiatr*, 1995;58:360–362.
37. Nieves J, Cosman F, Herbert J, et al. High prevalence of vitamin D deficiency and reduced bone mass in multiple sclerosis. *Neurology*, 1994;44:1687–1692.
38. Reynolds EH. Multiple sclerosis and vitamin B12 metabolism. *J Neuroimmunol*, 1992;40:225–230.
39. Kira J, Tobimatsu S, Goto I. Vitamin B12 metabolism and massive-dose methyl vitamin B12 therapy in Japanese patients with multiple sclerosis. *Intern Med (Tokyo)*, 1994;33:82–86.
40. Gillson G, Wright JV, DeLack E, Ballasiotes G. Transdermal histamine in multiple sclerosis: Part 1. Clinical experience. *Altern Med Rev*, 1999;4:424–428.
41. Yates HA, Vardy TC, Kuchera ML, Ripley BD, Johnson JC. Effects of osteopathic manipulative treatment and concentric and eccentric maximal-effort exercise on women with multiple sclerosis: a pilot study. Department of Manipulative Medicine, Kirksville College of Osteopathic Medicine, MO 63501–1443, USA. hyates@kcom.edu.
42. Bennett M, Heard R. Treatment of multiple sclerosis with hyperbaric oxygen therapy. *Undersea Hyperbaric Med*, 2001;28(3):117–122.
43. Pertwee R. Cannabinoids and multiple sclerosis. *Pharmacol Ther*, 2002;95(2):165–174.

CLINICAL APPLICATION: CANDIDIASIS

David W. Grotto

DESCRIPTION

Candida albicans is a commensal organism that normally colonizes the GI tract and sometimes the skin in healthy individuals. In abnormal conditions, yeast overgrowth of *C. albicans* can occur and unlike other systemic mycoses, it is endogenous and not generally acquired from the surrounding environment. The diversity of infections attributed to *C. albicans* is considerable varying from milder conditions such as oral and genital thrush to fatal, systemic superinfections in patients who are already seriously ill with other diseases. Most people have an occasional bout with a candidal infection at one time or another in their lives; however, a steady increase in the frequency of invasive fungal infections has been observed in the past two decades, particularly in immunosuppressed patients. In recipients of bone marrow transplants, *C. albicans* and *Aspergillus fumigatus* remain the primary pathogens.[1]

Interest in *Candida* infections, and in *C. albicans* in particular, has increased in recent years as fatal infections have become more prevalent and new *Candida*-based pathologies have been recognized. A fairly substantial amount of alternative practitioners have based their practice on the notion that chronic allergy to *Candida* can trigger a plethora of common illnesses.[2]

Infections due to *Candida* account for about 80% of all major systemic fungal infections. *Candida* is now the fourth most prevalent organism found in bloodstream infections and is the most common cause of fungal infections in immunocompromised people. The frequency of nosocomial candidiasis has risen at least fivefold in the 1980s, making it one of the most common hospital-acquired infections. Although often a benign, self-limited problem, it may be associated with excess mortality of $\geq 40\%$ (i.e., deaths attributable to candidiasis rather than to underlying diseases) and prolongation of hospitalizations.

Oral candidiasis (thrush) commonly affects patients with acquired immune deficiency syndrome (AIDS) or with other causes of compromised T-cell-mediated immune defense mechanisms and occasionally affects others. Candidiasis involving the esophagus, trachea, bronchi, or lungs is a defining opportunistic infection in AIDS. Mucocutaneous candidiasis frequently complicates AIDS, but hematogenous dissemination is unusual until immunocompromise becomes profound. Vaginal candidiasis commonly affects women, including those with normal immunity, especially after antibiotic use. Neutropenic patients receiving cancer chemotherapy are at high risk for developing life-threatening disseminated candidiasis. Candidemia and especially hematogenous endophthalmitis are frequent nosocomial infections in nonneutropenic patients who have prolonged hospitalizations; infection is often related to multiple traumas or surgical procedures, multiple courses of broad-spectrum antibacterial therapy, and total parenteral nutrition. Intravenous (IV) lines and the GI tract are the usual portals of entry. Endocarditis may occur in relation to IV drug abuse, valve replacement, or intravascular trauma. Fungemia may lead to meningitis as well as to focal involvement of skin, subcutaneous tissues, bones, joints, liver, spleen, kidneys, eyes, and other tissues.

Because *Candida* strains are commensals, their culture from sputum, the mouth, the vagina, urine, stool, or skin does not necessarily signify an invasive, progressive infection. A characteristic clinical lesion must also be present, histopathologic evidence of tissue invasion documented, or other causes excluded. Positive cultures of blood, CSF, pericardium or pericardial fluid, or tissue biopsy specimens provide definitive evidence that systemic therapy is needed. Histopathologic appearance of typical combined yeasts, pseudohyphae, and hyphae in tissue specimens also is diagnostic. However, antifungal therapy often is started presumptively. Various serologic assays to detect antibodies or antigens have been developed, but none has sufficient specificity or sensitivity to be useful for rapid diagnosis or diagnostic exclusion in seriously ill patients.

CONVENTIONAL TREATMENT

Conditions such as neutropenia, malnutrition, or uncontrolled diabetes can predispose one to disseminated candidiasis and all forms can be potentially serious, progressive, and even fatal. Potent antifungal medications delivered via IV, such as amphotericin B, alone or in combination with flucytosine, are typically recommended for the severely ill and immunocompromised patients. In nonneutropenic patients, fluconazole is often used as it has been shown to be as effective as amphotericin B in both neutropenic and nonneutropenic patients. Research is lacking to support optimal treatment regimens for other forms of disseminated candidiasis; however, the majority of experts still recommend amphotericin B over high-dose fluconazole though its effectiveness may be the same.[3]

In somewhat milder forms of candidiasis optimal treatment protocols vary:

- Cutaneous candidiasis can be effectively treated with a variety of antifungal powders and creams.

- In oral thrush, topical, antifungal medications such as nystatin (Mycostatin, Nilstat), which seldom has significant side affects, and clotrimazole are most often used. For more severe cases, ketoconazole (Nizoral) (which has an incidence of hepatitis of about 1 in 10,000) or fluconazole (Diflucan) can be taken once a day by mouth. For milder cases, a suspension of nystatin can be swished in the mouth and swallowed, or a clotrimazole lozenge can be dissolved in the mouth. *Candida* esophagitis can be treated with ketoconazole, itraconazole (Sporanox), or fluconazole (most effective medication in patients with HIV/AIDS).
- Vaginal yeast infections can be treated with prescription and over-the-counter antifungal medications that are administered directly into the vagina as tablets, creams, ointments, or suppositories.

The Food and Drug Administration (FDA) produced a frequently asked question (FAQ) sheet on tips on fighting vaginal infections that included the following advice:

- Wear loose, natural-fiber clothing, and underwear with a cotton crotch.
- Limit wearing of panty hose, tights, leggings, nylon underwear, and tight jeans.
- Do not use deodorant tampons and feminine deodorant sprays, especially if you feel an infection beginning.
- Dry off quickly and thoroughly after bathing and swimming — do not stay in a wet swimsuit for hours.
- It is better not to have sex in your teens, but if you are sexually active, always use a latex condom.[4]

INTEGRATIVE APPROACHES

The most well-known physicians who have promoted the concept of "candidiasis hypersensitivity" have been C. Orian Truss, M.D., author of book called *The Missing Diagnosis*[5] and William G. Crook, M.D., author of *The Yeast Connection*.[6] They felt this syndrome existed primarily from overuse of antibiotics but also due to several other predisposing conditions. The following reviews their proposed predisposing factors and symptoms associated with candidiasis including from the book *Conquering Yeast Infections: The Non-Drug Solution* by S. Colet Lahoz, RN, MS, L.Ac.[7]:

Predisposing Factors

- Broad-spectrum antibiotics destroy the healthful bacteria that control the *Candida* population.
- Chemical preservatives in food also support *Candida* overgrowth.
- Immunosuppression resulting from steroid drugs, chemotherapy agents, prolonged illness, stress, alcohol abuse, smoking, lack of exercise, lack of rest, and poor nutrition.
- Female gender are more susceptible due to sustained high levels of estrogen which impair immune system function, *C. albicans* is stimulated by progesterone which are elevated during pregnancy and in the second half of each menstrual cycle and from synthetic progestins found in oral contraceptives. The female anatomy lends itself to the ready migration of *C. albicans* from the rectum to the genitourinary system.
- High-refined carbohydrate, low-fiber diets feed yeast.
- Allergies to foods and airborne chemicals. If ELISA-ACT testing reveals food allergies, those foods need to be avoided during the recovery period.

Symptoms

Fatigue, especially after eating	Poor digestion (constipation or diarrhea, gas, bloating, cramps, heartburn, nausea, gastritis, colitis, etc.)	Carbohydrate cravings	*Irritability*
Mood swings	Headaches	Migraines	Inability to concentrate
Poor memory	Confusion dizziness	MS-like symptoms (slurred speech, loss of muscle coordination, vision affected)	*Depression*
Anxiety	Paranoia	Urinary tract and vaginal infection and inflammation (urgency, burning)	Menstrual difficulties
Impotence	Infertility	Prostatitis	Rectal itch
Cold and flu symptoms	Allergies including hay fever	*Asthma*	Chest pain
Habitual coughing	Sore throat	Earaches	Athlete's foot
Jock itch	*Skin rash*	Hives	Psoriasis
Ringworm	Rough skin on sides of arms, which gets worse at certain times of the month or under increased stress	Early childhood diagnosis of hyperactivity, aggressiveness, cradle cap, diaper rash, thrush, chronic ear infection, tonsillitis, and colic	*Feel bad all over*
Arthritis-like symptoms	White coating on tongue upon rising[6]		

Darkfield microscopy, blood tests for *Candida* antibodies, stool analysis, and electrodermal screening are diagnostic tools used by alternative physicians to arrive at a diagnosis of candidiasis. However, in a review of 100 chronic fatigue patients, no differences were found in historical, physical, or laboratory findings among those who believed their problem was attributed to yeast and those who did not.[8] Little data exists to support the accuracy of these tests.

Many alternative physicians feel that there is ample clinical and anecdotal evidence that those who have been diagnosed with candidiasis overall do better when they follow a diet absent of sugar, yeast-containing substances, and wheat. Strict adherence to these guidelines is imperative as even the slightest transgression may bring back unwanted symptoms in their opinion. In addition, alternative practitioners usually advocate eliminating dairy products due to their allergy potential and lactose-sugar content for combating *C. albicans*.

There exists promising research indicating administration of selected microorganisms (probiotics) and substances that help them implant in the gut (prebiotics) may be beneficial in the prevention and treatment of certain intestinal infections, and possibly in the treatment of vaginal infections. Placebo-controlled studies demonstrated that these agents have been used successfully to prevent antibiotic-associated bacterial infections and *Candida vaginitis*. There is a high level of evidence for positive effects of some prebiotics to alleviate constipation, treat hepatic encephalopathy, alleviation of antibiotic-associated intestinal disorders, and gastroenteritis. Positive trials have suggested preventive effects against intestinal colonization with specific gut pathogens including *Clostridium difficile* and *Helicobacter pylori*.[9]

The author of *Alternative Medicine: The Definitive Guide* lists several recommendations by various complementary and alternative medicine (CAM) physicians that they interviewed on candidiasis in their book. Here is an overall summary of their recommendations:

- Avoid all sugar
- Use a rotation diet if allergies are suspected
- Eliminate all foods containing yeast
- Avoid caffeinated beverages
- Include vitamin B complex, C, E, A, beta-carotene, selenium, calcium, and zinc
- Incorporate plant enzymes
- Probiotics such as *Lacto acidophilus* and *Bifidobacterium bifidum* for intestinal flora
- Herbs such as berberine, golden seal, Oregon grape, and barberry
- Antifungal herbs such as garlic, chamomile, aloe vera, ginger, cinnamon, rosemary, licorice, oil of oregano, and tea tree oil
- Hydrogen peroxide therapy
- Ayurvedic medicine and acupuncture[10]

The Life Extension Foundation also lists several similar recommendations on their Web site for controlling candidiasis:

- Bifido bacteria can dramatically increase the quantity of beneficial bacteria in the gut. Acidophilus bacteria also can help to fight *Candida* in the upper intestinal tract.
- Garlic, biotin, caprylic acid has a direct yeast-killing effect in the intestine.
- Fiber can help to remove yeast and fungus from the intestines.
- Goldenseal (*Hydrastis canadensis*) best taken as an infusion such as a teabag or 4 g, three times a day in capsule form.
- Oil of oregano comes in an enteric-coated capsule taken on an empty stomach, one capsule three times a day. Both have antifungal properties.
- Intravenous vitamins, particularly vitamin C, during the recovery period.
- Nystatin.
- Diflucan.
- Shark liver oil has demonstrated an antifungal effect in laboratory studies. Shark liver oil capsules, containing 200 mg of alkyl glycerol, can be taken in doses of five capsules a day for up to 30 days.
- Sucrose and fructose should be avoided, since these types of sugars can cause yeast overgrowth.
- 150 ml of yogurt enriched with live *L. acidophilus* is associated with an increased colonization of friendly bacteria in the rectum and vagina. This results in reduced episodes of bacterial vaginitis. Women with chronic vaginal *Candida* infections often use yogurt. This should not be used for treating yeast syndrome or for those with known milk sensitivity.
- Tea tree oil (*Melaleuca alternifolia*) against a wide range of fungal isolates including species of *Candida*. Studies indicate that controlled doses of tea tree oil may be used as an effective topical treatment for dermatological *Candida* infection and paronychia.
- Supplemental hydrochloric acid and pancreatic enzymes if indicated.[11]

Warnings are given to those who strictly follow these regimens as often they will report "feeling worse" after following the nutritional regimen for only 2 to 4 weeks. This is attributed to a probably result of yeast die off and the ill effect of toxin release. Therefore, it is highly recommended to include ample fluid, fiber, and medical supervision when embarking on anti-yeast-promoting diet. CAM physicians may also suggest a 2-week trial of proper dietary interventions before undertaking treatment with antifungal agents.

Proponents of "candidiasis hypersensitivity" most often prescribe the antifungal drug nystatin. In a double-blind trial, nystatin did no better than a placebo in relieving systemic or psychological symptoms of "candidiasis hypersensitivity syndrome."[12] Also used is ketoconazole, which as mentioned earlier can cause liver toxicity and has been responsible for several deaths.

Dr. Steven Barrett, the author of *Chemical Sensitivity: The Truth about Environmental Illness*, argues that there is little scientific evidence to support the concept of candidiasis hypersensitivity. He references the position of The American Academy of Allergy, Asthma, and Immunology:

- The concept of candidiasis hypersensitivity is speculative and unproven.
- Its basic elements would apply to almost all sick patients at some time because its supposed symptoms are essentially universal.
- Overuse of oral antifungal agents could lead to the development of resistant germs that could menace others.
- Adverse effects of oral antifungal agents are rare, but some inevitably will occur; and neither patients nor doctors can determine effectiveness (as opposed to coincidence) without controlled trials.
- Because allergic symptoms can be influenced by many factors, including emotions, experiments must be designed to separate the effects of the procedure tested from the effects of other factors.[13]

REFERENCES

1. Rolston K. Overview of systemic fungal infections. *Oncology (Huntingt)*, 2001;15(11 Suppl 9):11–14.
2. Odds FC. *Candida* infections: an overview. *Crit Rev Microbiol*, 1987;15(1):1–5.
3. http://www.yeastinfectionresource.com/yeast/key-clinical-issues.asp.
4. http://www.fda.gov/fdac/features/396_yst.html.
5. Truss CO. *The Missing Diagnosis*, The Missing Diagnosis, Inc., Birmingham, 1983.
6. Crook WG. *The Yeast Connection: A Medical Breakthrough*, Professional Books, Jackson, Tenn., 1983, 1984, 1986.
7. Colet Lahoz S. *Conquering Yeast Infections: The Non-Drug Solution*. Pentland Press, North Carolina, 1996.
8. Renfro L et al. Yeast connection among 100 patients with chronic fatigue. *Am J Med*, 1989; 86:165–168.
9. Marteau P, Boutron-Ruault MC. Nutritional advantages of probiotics and prebiotics. *Br J Nutr*, 2002;87(Suppl 2):S153–S157.
10. Goldberg B. *Alternative Medicine. The Definitive Guide*, 2nd ed., Celestial Arts, Berkeley, 2002.
11. http://www.lef.org/protocols/prtcl-028.shtml.
12. Dismukes W et al. A randomized double-blind trial of nystatin therapy for the candidiasis hypersensitivity syndrome. *N Engl J Med*, 1990;323:1717–1723.
13. http://www.quackwatch.org/01QuackeryRelatedTopics/candida.html.

CLINICAL APPLICATION: THE COMMON COLD AND INFLUENZA

David W. Grotto

DYSFUNCTION

The common cold (Rhinovirus) refers to a viral infection that takes place mainly in the nasal passages but also occurs in the upper sinuses ears and bronchial tubes. In fact, there are over 100 different varieties of cold viruses with Rhinoviruses attributed to over half of the common colds today.

When a cold virus infects nasal cells, histamine, kinins, ILs, and prostaglandins (PGE2) are released. They cause dilatation and leakage of blood vessels, prompting mucus gland secretion. These mediators activate the common sneeze and cough reflexes and stimulate pain nerve fibers. In turn, they bring on all of the classic symptoms such as sneezing, runny nose, watery eyes, nasal obstruction, sore or scratchy throat, cough, hoarseness, headache, feverishness, chilliness, and overall ill in what we know as the common cold. Colds can last on average for a week or more with milder forms lasting 2 or 3 days and more severe cases lasting for up to 2 weeks.[1,2]

Colds are most contagious during the first 3 days of the onset of symptoms. Rhinoviruses are spread by droplets in the nasal cavity generated by coughing, sneezing, and nose blowing rather than hand-to-hand contact.[3] Apart from a healthy diet and lifestyle program, avoidance of the infected person is still the best method for preventing colds.

CONVENTIONAL TREATMENT

Antihistamines, nonsteroidal anti-inflammatory drugs (NSAIDs), decongestants (vasoconstrictors), cough suppressants (narcotics), and anticholinergics (ipratropium) are the most common medical treatments offered today.

Antihistamines

More recent studies of first generation antihistamines have dispelled older studies that suggested that antihistamines were ineffective in treating the common cold.[4,5] In contrast, they are quite effective in reducing the sneezing and runny nose of colds. However, they are not without their major side effects, namely drowsiness, which can be severe in some people.[6] First generation antihistamines have been found to cause difficulty in urination in men who have enlarged prostate glands and may potentially worsen glaucoma. The newer second generation antihistamines are nonsedating, however, have not demonstrated the same degree of effectiveness for treating symptoms of colds.

Nonsteroidal Anti-Inflammatory Drugs

Apart from pain relief, only a few clinical trials have been published on its use for treating colds. Side effects of NSAIDs include irritation of the GI tract, prolonged bleeding, and reduced kidney function.[7]

Decongestants

Nose drops and sprays create the most rapid, immediate relief for cold. When the decongestant effect of the drug wears off, nasal congestion recurs. Nasal decongestants may burn and irritate the throat and tend to lose their effectiveness over time and result in "rebound" obstruction and mucosal damage. Rapid heart rate, blood pressure elevation, and nervousness have been reported in oral decongestants.[8]

Anticholinergics

Anticholinergics inhibit the action of the parasympathetic nervous system on mucus gland secretion. They are unable to act against histamine rendering them less effective in preventing sneezing but were found to reduce nasal discharge patients with colds. Side effects include difficulty in urination in men with prostate disease and worsening glaucoma.[9]

Cough Suppressants

Cough suppressants, especially those that contain codeine and dextromethorphan, act on the brain to depress the cough reflex center. Several trials have demonstrated their effectiveness in treating chronic coughs but few published studies evaluating their effectiveness in coughs due to colds. Cough suppressants can cause GI discomfort and should not be used in subjects where expectorants are indicated.[10]

COMPLEMENTARY AND ALTERNATIVE MEDICINE TREATMENTS

Home-based remedies for colds and flu are commonly used by many cultures. These remedies appear to be complementary to biomedical treatment (i.e., antipyretics, over-the-counter cold remedies, and fluids). Very few have been found to be potentially hazardous if taken in moderation.[11] The following reviews limited research studies on natural remedies for the common cold.

Echinacea

Eighty adult patients with early symptoms of a cold defined by the modified Jackson score of at least 5 points and experience of rhinorrhea and a subjective sensation of having a cold were used in a study evaluating the effectiveness of a standardized Echinacea product. In the treatment group the median time of illness was 6 days compared to 9 days in the control group. It was determined that Echinacea was clinically effective in alleviating symptoms more rapidly than placebo in patients with a common cold.[12] Earlier results from 12 clinical studies published from 1961 to 1997 concluded that Echinacea was beneficial for treating the common cold. Results, however, were questionable as the study design appeared to have "flaws." Five more recent trials have been published since 1997 showing mixed results; namely two demonstrated Echinacea lacked efficacy for treating and preventing URTI symptoms, and three concluded that it was effective in reducing the frequency, duration, and severity of common cold symptoms. These results have been subject to criticism due to small study size and not using commercially available, standardized dosage forms. Although evidence for Echinacea's efficacy is inconclusive, it appears to be safe.[13]

Garlic

One hundred and forty-six volunteers were randomized to receive a placebo or an allicin-containing garlic supplement, one capsule daily, over a 12-week period. The active-treatment group had significantly fewer colds than the placebo group (24 versus 65, $P < 0.001$). The placebo group, in contrast, recorded significantly more days challenged virally (366 versus 111, $P < 0.05$) and a significantly longer duration of symptoms (5.01 versus 1.52 days, $P < 0.001$).[14]

Vitamin C

One hundred and sixty-eight subjects participated in a randomized study to evaluate vitamin C's effectiveness in combating colds versus a placebo. For the duration of the 2-month period, the treatment group had significantly fewer colds (37 versus 50, $P < 0.05$), fewer days challenged virally (85 versus 178), and a significantly shorter duration of severe symptoms (1.8 versus 3.1 days, $P < 0.03$).[15] Four hundred volunteers took upwards of 3 g of vitamin C daily for 18 months. It was found that doses of vitamin C in excess of 1 g daily taken shortly after onset of a cold did not reduce the duration or severity of cold symptoms compared with a vitamin C dose less than the minimum recommended daily intake. However, the study's reliance on respondents' self-diagnosis of symptom severity and onset may be a weakness in the study design.[16] Thirty trials of variable quality before the year 2000 revealed long-term daily supplementation with vitamin C in large doses did not appear to prevent colds. However, several of the trials did suggest modest benefit in reducing duration of cold symptoms.[17]

The role of dietary and supplemental vitamin C, vitamin E, and beta-carotene effects on the incidence of common cold episodes was examined in a cohort of 21,796 male smokers. Participants were queried three times per year for 4 years on common cold episodes. Dietary vitamins C and E and beta-carotene had no meaningful association with common cold incidence. Long-term vitamin E and beta-carotene supplementation had no overall effect. Vitamins C and E and beta-carotene had no overall association with the incidence of common cold episodes.[18]

Zinc

Of ten published randomized controlled trials, only five reported that zinc lozenges reduced the duration of cold symptoms. The reasons for the different results among these trials include differences in doses, salts, and formulations of zinc lozenges; differences in study design; and difficulty in truly blinding study participants.

Fifty participants were entered in a study within 24 h of developing cold symptoms. It was found that a zinc acetate lozenge formulation was more effective than the placebo in decreasing the duration and severity of cold symptoms, cough, and nasal discharge. Due to its distinctive taste, twice as many zinc-treated subjects correctly identified their lozenges at the end of the study, suggesting that blinding may be difficult to achieve.[19]

Not only are the zinc lozenges easy to identify, many people complain of the bitter aftertaste of them so other routes of delivery certainly warrant investigation for effectiveness. In a study of 91 volunteers, intranasal zinc gluconate for prevention of experimental rhinovirus infection and illness was reviewed. Of the 41 who were treated, zinc treatment appeared to have no effect on total symptom score, rhinorrhea, nasal obstruction, or the proportion of infected volunteers who developed clinical colds.[20] However, a multisite study of 213 patients evaluated the product Zicam, a nasal gel for its efficacy as a treatment for the common cold. The study was conducted over a 5-month period. One hundred and eight patients received zinc therapy within the first 24 h of reported symptoms, and 105 reviewed placebo. At study's end, the duration of symptoms was 2.3 days (± 0.9) in the zinc group and 9.0 days (± 2.5) in the control group — a statistically significant difference ($P < 0.05$).[21]

Homeopathy

Very little clinical research exists in the evaluation of the efficacy of homeopathic remedies in fighting the common cold. A few European clinical tests have investigated their merit. One test was carried out on 170 West German army soldiers suffering from common cold. The randomized test was double-blinded. The purpose was to compare the effectiveness of a combination homeopathic preparation (Gripp-Heel) with that of acetylsalicylic acid (ASA). No significant difference was determined with respect to changes in clinical findings, subjectively assessed complaints, or length of time the patients were unable to work.[22]

Another study examined 53 outpatients suffering from common cold who were again randomly assigned to either ASA or the homeopathic drug Eupatorium perfoliatum D2 in a controlled clinical trial. The efficacy of the drugs was assessed on day 1, 4, and 10 of the infection by symptom checklists and physical examinations. Neither subjective complaints nor body temperature or laboratory findings showed any significant differences between groups, which was taken as evidence that both drugs were equally effective.[23]

AYURVEDIC APPROACH

The following is an example of an Ayurvedic approach to the treatment of the common cold. An anti-Kapha (phlegm) diet should be taken. It should be warm, light, and simple. Dairy products, according to Ayurveda, are Kapha promoting and should be avoided. Lemon and ginger juice can be taken with warm water and honey three times a day. A good formula can be made with equal parts basil, sandalwood, and peppermint, 2 to 3 tsp put them in a cup of water, bring to boil, and then have it up to three times a day. Sitopaladi powder is an extremely effective remedy for common colds and problems of sinus congestion. The dose is 1 to 5 g with honey, three times a day. Sweating is very helpful. One simple method is to induce sweating is to drink a hot cup of tea, and lie down in the bed and take some blanket and let the body sweat for 15 to 20 min.

INFLUENZA

DESCRIPTION

Influenza, most commonly known as "the flu" or "grippe" refers to many strains of viral illness that are more intense than a common cold that usually include fever, muscle ache, headache, and fatigue. There are two types of influenza: types A and B, which infect the throat, nose, lungs, bronchial tubes, and middle ear. Some kinds of flu have cold-like symptoms with sore throat or respiratory involvement; others affect the digestive tract, with diarrhea, nausea, or vomiting. The common cold generally lasts up to a week, but the influenza virus typically lasts for up to 12 days, and a persistent cough can continue for some time after that.

Millions of people in the United States — about 10 to 20% of U.S. residents will get the flu each year. An average of about 20,000 people per year in the United States die from the flu, and 114,000 per year have to be admitted to the hospital as a result of influenza.[24]

CONVENTIONAL TREATMENT

Although it is thought that a flu shot is the best way to prevent the flu, there are antiviral drugs that can be used to help prevent and treat influenza. The four available drugs are:
- amantadine
- rimantadine
- zanamivir
- oseltamivir

Treatment with any of these drugs can shorten the time a person infected with influenza feels ill by approximately 1 day, if the treatment is started within the first 2 days of illness. However, common side effects can include nervousness, anxiety, difficulty in concentrating, lightheadedness, and GI side effects like nausea and loss of appetite, delirium, hallucinations, agitation, and seizures. Decreased respiratory function and bronchospasm have been reported with use of zanamivir. Zanamivir is generally not recommended for use in persons with underlying lung disease such as asthma and chronic obstructive pulmonary disease. Other side effects reported by less than 5% of those who have used this drug are diarrhea, nausea, sinusitis, nasal infections, bronchitis, cough, headache, and dizziness.[25]

The elderly or those with compromised immune function are more susceptible to influenza infection. Because the "flu bug" can be life-threatening in these populations, a flu vaccine is often recommended. In a small study of subjects aged 65 years and older, investigators looked at the effect of nutrition on antibody response to an influenza vaccine. A 7-month nutritional supplementation program containing energy, vitamins, and minerals, including enhanced levels of antioxidants resulted in a significantly larger mean fold increase upon vaccination in the supplement group (2.76 ± 0.66) compared to the placebo group (1.91 ± 0.66). Antioxidants may have a beneficial effect on antibody response to influenza vaccination in the elderly population.[26]

Homeopathic remedies may offer some relief for influenza sufferers. Though there is little clinical data to support its purported benefit, the following homeopathic remedies are often used in a CAM practice setting.

Aconitum Napellus

Indication
A flu that comes on suddenly and intensely — with fever, anxiety, constricted pupils, and strong thirst — is likely to respond to this remedy. The person may feel fearful or agitated, and the fever can alternate with chills. Symptoms are often worst around midnight. Exposure to cold wind or a shock of some kind often precedes the illness.

Apis Mellifica

Indication
This remedy may be helpful if a person has dry fever that alternates with sweating, facial flushing, and a very sore throat with swollen tonsils. Pain may extend to the ears, and the eyelids may be swollen. Exposure to cool air and cold applications may bring relief. Despite the fever, thirst usually is low. The person can be very irritable, disliking interference.

Arsenicum Album

Indication
A person who needs this remedy during flu feels chilly and exhausted, along with an anxious restlessness. The person may be thirsty, but often only takes small sips. If the digestive system is involved, nausea with burning pain, or vomiting and acrid diarrhea may occur. If the flu is respiratory, a watery, runny nose with sneezing paroxysms and a dry or wheezing cough are often seen. The person's head usually feels hot, while the rest of the body is chilly.

Belladonna

Indication
Sudden, intense symptoms — including fever, red face, hot skin, and extreme sensitivity to light and jarring — suggest a need for this remedy. The person may have a very red sore throat, a pounding headache, a nagging cough, or other throbbing and inflammatory symptoms. Despite high fever, the person's hands and feet may feel cold, or chills and heat may alternate.

Bryonia

Indication
When a person is very grumpy and feels miserable with the flu, wanting only to lie still and be left alone, this remedy is likely to be useful. Headache, muscle aches, and cough or stomach pain may be the major symptoms. Everything feels worse from even the slightest motion. The person's mouth usually is dry, with a thirst for long cold drinks.

Eupatorium Perforliatum

Indication
Flu with deep pain occurring in the legs or back ("as if the bones would break") often responds to this remedy. Pain may be felt in the eyeballs, with a heavy sensation in the head. Illness often begins with chills and thirst, followed by high fever. Chills may be felt in the back and legs, and the aching in the bones is worse from motion. The person feels "wiped out" and miserable.

Ferrum Phosphoricum

Indication
This remedy may be helpful during flu with fever, headache, rosy cheeks, and a feeling of weariness. Sensitive eyes, a short hard cough, strong thirst, and vomiting after eating are other indications. This remedy is often helpful in early stages of flu or fever, even if symptoms are not especially clear.

Gelsemium

Indication
Symptoms of fatigue and aches that come on gradually, increasing over several days, may indicate a need for this remedy. The face feels heavy, with droopy eyes and aching. A headache may begin at the back of the neck and skull, and the person may feel chills and heat running up and down the spine. Anxiety, trembling, dizziness, perspiration, and moderate fever are other indications for *Gelsemium*.

Nux Vomica

Indication
When this remedy is indicated in influenza, the person may have high fever, violent chills, strong nausea, and cramping in the digestive tract (or a painful cough and constricted breathing if the flu is respiratory in nature). Headache usually occurs, along with oversensitivity to sound, bright light, and odors. A person who needs Nux Vomica is often very irritable, feeling worse from exertion and worse from being cold in any way.

Oscillococcinum (also called *Anas barbariae*)

Indication
Oscillococcinum is one of the common names used for a remedy that is widely used for prevention and treatment of flu in the United States and Europe. Research suggests that it has strong antiviral effects.

Phosphorus

Indication
When this remedy is needed during flu, the person has a fever with an easily flushing face, and feels very weak and dizzy. Headache, hoarseness, sore throat, and cough are likely. If the focus is digestive, stomach pain, and nausea or vomiting usually occur. A person who needs this remedy often has a strong anxiety, wanting others to be around to offer company and reassurance. Strong thirst, with a tendency to vomit when liquids warm up in the stomach, is a strong indication for phosphorus.

Rhus Toxicodendron

Indication

A person who needs this remedy during flu feels extremely restless. Fever is accompanied by bone and muscle aches. Sore throat, red tongue, a teasing cough, and nausea and bloating are other likely symptoms. Soreness and stiffness may be felt all over, with improvement from hot showers or from getting up and pacing. A person who needs *Rhus tox* usually feels worse when waking up, after lying in bed, or from keeping still too long. Rubbing and stretching can relieve symptoms. Warmth and movement are equally effective.

Sulfur

Indication

This remedy may be useful if a flu is very long-lasting or has some lingering symptoms — often after people have neglected to take good care of themselves. Symptoms, either digestive or respiratory, will often have a hot or burning quality. The person may feel hot and sweaty, with low fever and reddish mucous membranes. Heat aggravates the symptoms, and the person often feels worse after bathing.[27,28]

Naturopathic approaches often combine homeopathic remedies with other CAN interventions. The California Association of Naturopathic Physicians suggests the following strategies for preventing and treating influenza:

- At the first sign of illness, rest to prevent progression of the illness.
- Maintain a healthy lifestyle. Get 8 h of sleep, relax often, eat moderately, drink plenty of pure water, and decrease consumption of alcohol, coffee, and sugar.
- Viruses are often passed by touch. Wash your hands frequently and avoid shaking hands with those who are already sick.
- Eat very lightly at first sign of feeling badly. It is especially useful to cut back to only fruits and vegetables. Follow your body's inclination. If you are hungry, eat more and if not, eat less.
- Switch from coffee to tea for its antibacterial and antiviral action; eating garlic liberally for its antibacterial, antiviral, and antifungal activity; and adding yogurt to your diet as it sets up a beneficial situation in the colon.
- Useful early homeopathic prevention includes the use of oscillococcinum or other flu products. Ferrum phos cell salt for early stages of feverish conditions.
- As a preventive measure, take a good high potency multivitamin–mineral from a health food store, naturopathic physician, or other natural health practitioner, daily, with at least 1000 mg vitamin C, 50,000 IU vitamin A (unless pregnant), 400 IU vitamin E, 15 mg zinc, and 25 + mg of the B vitamins.
- Drink one quart of pure water for every 50 lb of body weight. Avoid all other fluids, coffee, tea, and sodas.
- Take a long, hot bath with a teaspoon of added eucalyptus or thyme oil (unless you are taking homeopathic medicines). Towel-dry and then pop into bed for a deep rest.[29]

Reports of greater psychological stress may also influence intensity of symptoms of influenza. In a study of 55 volunteers who had been injected with influenza A virus, investigators measured the severity of their respiratory symptoms, the amount of mucus production, and levels of IL-6 after 7 days. Subjects had completed questionnaires that measured their levels of psychological stress before their inoculation. Researchers discovered that the subjects who reported greater psychological stress before being inoculated responded to infection with more intense symptoms, greater mucous production, and higher concentrations of IL-6 in their nasal secretions.[30]

There are many reports of psychological morbidity in spousal caretakers of patients with dementia. Fifty spousal caretakers of dementia patients were compared in a study to 67 controls of similar socioeconomic status and were measured for anxiety and depression levels along with salivary cortisol concentrations. Participants received an influenza vaccine and IgG antibody titers to each strain were measured. Mean scores of emotional distress were significantly higher in caretakers at each time point than in controls (all $P < 0.0003$). Mean salivary cortisol concentrations were higher in caretakers than controls at all three assessments. Sixteen percent of 50 caretakers and 39% of 67 controls had a fourfold increase in at least one of the IgG titers ($P = 0.007$). Elderly caretakers of spouses with dementia have increased cortisol levels, poorer antibody response to influenza vaccine and may be more vulnerable to infectious disease than the population of a similar age.[31]

REFERENCES

1. Gwaltney JM. The common cold. In *Principles and Practices of Infectious Diseases*, 5th ed., Churchill Livingstone, New York, 2000, pp. 651–656.
2. Gwaltney JM, Hendley J, Simon G, Jordan WS. Rhinovirus infections in an industrial population. II. Characteristics of illness and antibody response. *JAMA*, 1967;202:494–500.
3. Jennings LC, Dick EC. Transmission and control of Rhinovirus colds. *Eur J Epidemiol*, 1987;3(4):327–335.
4. Doyle WJ et al. A double-blind, placebo-controlled clinical trial of the effect of chlorpheniramine on the response of the nasal airway, middle ear and eustachian tube to provocative Rhinovirus challenge. *Pediatr Infect Dis J*, 1988;7:229–238.
5. Gwaltney JM, Paul J, Edelman DA, O'Connor RR, Turner RB. Randomized controlled trial of clemastine fumarate for treatment of experimental Rhinovirus colds. *Clin Infect Dis*, 1996;22:656–662.
6. Babe KS, Serafin WE. Histamine, bradykinin, and their antagonists. In Goodman and Gilman's *The Pharmacological Basis of Therapeutics*, 9th ed., McGraw-Hill, New York, 1996, pp. 581–600.
7. Graham NM, Burrell CJ, Douglas RM, Debelle P, Davies L. Adverse effects of aspirin, acetaminophen, and ibuprofen on immune function, viral shedding, and clinical status in Rhinovirus-infected volunteers. *J Infect Dis*, 1990;162:1277–1282.
8. Hoffman BB, Lefkowitz RJ. Catecholamines, sympathomimetic drugs, and adrenergic receptor antagonists. In Goodman and Gilman's *The Pharmacological Basis of Therapeutics*, 9th ed., McGraw-Hill, New York, 1996, pp. 199–248.
9. Hayden FG, Diamond L, Wood PB, Korts DC, Wecker MT. Effectiveness and safety of intranasal ipratropium bromide in common colds: a randomized, double-blind, placebo-controlled trial. *Ann Int Med*, 1996;125:89–97.
10. Freestone C, Eccles R. Assessment of the antitussive efficacy of codeine in cough associated with common cold. *J Pharmacy Pharmacol*, 1997;49:1045–1049.
11. Pachter LM, Sumner T, Fontan A, Sneed M, Bernstein BA. Home-based therapies for the common cold among European American and ethnic minority families: the interface between alternative/complementary and folk medicine. *Arch Pediatr Adolesc Med*, 1998;152(11):1083–1088.
12. Schulten B, Bulitta M, Ballering-Bruhl B, Koster U, Schafer M. Efficacy of *Echinacea purpurea* in patients with a common cold. A placebo-controlled, randomized, double-blind clinical trial. *Arzneimittelforschung*, 2001;51(7):563–568.
13. Giles JT, Palat CT, Chien SH, Chang ZG, Kennedy DT. Evaluation of *Echinacea* for treatment of the common cold. *Pharmacotherapy*, 2000;20(6):690–697.
14. Josling P. Preventing the common cold with a garlic supplement: a double-blind, placebo-controlled survey. *Adv Ther*, 2001;18(4):189–193.

15. Van Straten M, Josling P. Preventing the common cold with a vitamin C supplement: a double-blind, placebo-controlled survey. *Adv Ther*, 2002;19(3):151–159.

16. Audera C, Patulny RV, Sander BH, Douglas RM. Mega-dose vitamin C in treatment of the common cold: a randomised controlled trial. *Med J Aust*, 2001;175(7):359–362.

17. Douglas RM, Chalker EB, Treacy B. Vitamin C for preventing and treating the common cold. *Cochrane Database Syst Rev*, 2000;(2):CD000980.

18. Hemila H, Kaprio J, Albanes D, Heinonen OP, Virtamo J. Vitamin C, vitamin E, and beta-carotene in relation to common cold incidence in male smokers. *Epidemiology*, 2002;13(1):32–37.

19. Prasad AS, Fitzgerald JT, Bao B, et al. Are zinc acetate lozenges effective in decreasing the duration of symptoms of the common cold? *J Fam Pract*, 2000;49(12):1153.

20. Turner RB. Ineffectiveness of intranasal zinc gluconate for prevention of experimental Rhinovirus colds. *Clin Infect Dis*, 2001;33(11):1865–1870.

21. Hirt M, Nobel S, Barron E. Zinc nasal gel for the treatment of common cold symptoms: a double-blind, placebo-controlled trial. *Ear Nose Throat J*, 2000;79(10):778–780, 782.

22. Maiwald VL, Weinfurtner T, Mau J, Connert WD. Therapy of common cold with a homeopathic combination preparation in comparison with acetylsalicylic acid. A controlled, randomized double-blind study. *Arzneimittelforschung*, 1988;38(4):578–582.

23. Gassinger CA, Wunstel G, Netter P. A controlled clinical trial for testing the efficacy of the homeopathic drug Eupatorium perfoliatum D2 in the treatment of common cold. *Arzneimittelforschung*, 1981;31(4):732–736.

24. http://www.cdc.gov/ncidod/diseases/flu/fluinfo.htm.

25. Morbidity and Mortality Weekly Report (MMWR), April 12, 2002/Vol. 51/No. RR-3.

26. Wouters-Wesseling W, Rozendaal M, Snijder M, Graus Y, Rimmelzwaan G, De Groot L, Bindels J. Effect of a complete nutritional supplement on antibody response to influenza vaccine in elderly people. *J Gerontol A Biol Sci Med Sci*, 2002;57(9):M563–M566.

27. www.homeopathic.com/ailments/new/Influ.htm.

28. www.healthnotes.com.

29. http://www.mercola.com/2000/dec/31/naturopathic_advice.htm.

30. Cohen S, Doyle WJ, Skoner DP. Psychological stress, cytokine production, and severity of upper respiratory illness. *Psychosom Med*, 1999;61(2):175–180.

31. Vedhara K, Cox NK, Wilcock GK, Perks P, Hunt M, Anderson S, Lightman SL, Shanks NM. Chronic stress in elderly caretakers of dementia patients and antibody response to influenza vaccination. *Lancet*, 1999;353(9153):627–631.

CLINICAL PERSPECTIVES: RHEUMATOID ARTHRITIS

Susan Allen-Evenson

As awareness of CAM increases more and more patients are taking responsibility for their own healthcare. Just as the name implies, CAM offers an array of complementary and alternative approaches to conventional medical treatments. Why would not a patient be eager to try therapies that may increase the effectiveness of their standard treatment? In fact, many are pleased to discover that in some cases CAM can offer alternate therapies with fewer side effects that are equally as effective, if not more so, than what conventional medicine can provide. Many CAM therapies are backed by sound science although continuing research is always needed. However, as CAM moves closer into the mainstream, patients are afforded a broad variety of experienced and credentialed CAM practitioners who further underscore the soundness of the therapies.

It has been reported that as much as 40% of rheumatology patients visit a complementary medicine practitioner in the course of their disease.[1] One distinct advantage to working with a CAM practitioner verses a conventional one is that patients are offered an extremely thorough and comprehensive initial assessment. It is not uncommon for a patient in a CAM setting to have an initial appointment that lasts anywhere from 1 to 3 h, sometimes more. In order to treat the patient from a CAM perspective, health is assessed via physical, biochemical, and mental or emotional perimeters. Diet and lifestyle are considered as equally important factors in the assessment. "Treat the patient, not the disease" is often the CAM practitioner's motto. A patient's overall biochemical balances and physiologic functions are measured to determine possible relationships to disease. This is what CAM practitioners commonly refer to as functional illness, the state in which there is not yet a diagnosable disease but clearly the patient is compromised or debilitated in some way. The CAM practitioner realizes that patient-centered healthcare is the most successful treatment approach. When the patient is invested in their health, they ultimately realize a better outcome.

As with many conditions, CAM therapies for RA focus on possible causes rather than simply treating symptoms. While it is widely accepted that RA is an autoimmune condition, what triggers the autoimmune response is still a mystery. Thus far, investigation has centered on a genetic predisposition, GI dysfunction, altered hepatic detoxification, food allergies and diet, and pathogenic microorganisms.[2–4] Even if these are not actual causes of RA, it is generally accepted in the CAM community that many of these factors will at the very least exacerbate the condition and are worth further investigation.

Once diagnosis for RA is made, conventional medicine offers classic allopathic therapies involving anti-inflammatory as well as immune suppressing drugs. While drugs do offer some relief, many patients are left with devastating side effects. Aspirin and other NSAIDs provide relief of pain and swelling but produce serious GI side effects such as bleeding and bowel permeability thus creating or increasing one of the suspect causes of RA. Corticosteroids and other immune suppressing drugs are also used with a variety of often debilitating side effects including nausea and vomiting, diarrhea, acne, weight gain, or significant weight loss (depending on the drug), blurred vision, loss of hair, increased rate of infections, weakness, and fatigue.

While CAM practitioners look to address underlying factors known to be involved with the disease process (intestinal permeability, food allergies, circulating immune complexes (CICs), free radicals, immune dysfunction, etc.) their initial approach is to offer the patient relief for pain and inflammation while supporting joint regeneration. However, unlike conventional treatment modalities, this treatment is done with diet and an array of natural alternatives, many of which have little or no side effects. After consulting both conventional and CAM practitioners it is ultimately up to the patient to decide if natural therapies should be used as an alternative to traditional pharmaceuticals or in conjunction with them. Whatever the decision, diet should be considered a vital component to any therapy for control of inflammation.

Saturated fats, because of their arachidonic acid content, promote the production of inflammatory PGE2, and other proinflammatory mediators like thromboxanes, and leukotrienes. Therefore, in RA and other inflammatory conditions, fat intake is often limited to 20% of calories. For the same reason, fat-containing animal proteins and dairy products are limited as well. In fact, research shows that vegetarian diets significantly improve inflammatory symptoms of RA.[5–9] This is presumably because they decrease the availability of arachidonic acid while simultaneously supplying linoleic and linolenic acids. Additionally, avoidance of hydrogenated oils further helps to tip the scales toward a positive balance of fatty acids.

Many double-blind trials have shown that the omega-3 fatty acids in fish oil, EPA, and DHA help relieve symptoms of RA.[4,10–12] Fish oil, because of its anti-inflammatory activity, is commonly used in the treatment of allergies and other inflammatory conditions. It is for this reason, RA patients are told to eat more cold-water fish. This is a notable exception to the vegetarian protocol typically recommended. Fish containing the highest amounts of omega-3s are mackerel, tuna, salmon, and halibut.

Because it is difficult to get an effective amount of fish oil from fish alone and especially because it is possible that toxins and mercury levels would accumulate to undesirable levels if fish were eaten daily, patients are advised to supplement the diet with fish oil capsules. Then again, fish oil supplements present their own set of problems. Not only can fish oil supplements contain impurities but also it has been shown that many commercially available fish oils contain very high levels of lipid peroxides that greatly stress antioxidant defense mechanisms.[4,13,14] This oxidation mostly occurs due to the processing of the oil that makes the oil unstable. Patients should be careful to choose a brand of natural stable fish oil that has solid clinical evidence of its effectiveness. It should also be free of contamination as proven with repeat independent assays. It is very important that fish oil be processed to prevent oxidation. In addition, mixed tocopherols and other natural antioxidants such as rosemary further stabilize the product. Lastly, good fish oil should not have a "fishy" odor, nor should it produce GI side effects.

An acidic pH of the body can also cause increased pain and inflammation. For this reason RA patients are encouraged to reduce their intake of foods and beverages that leave the body more acidic following ingestion. These foods include sugar, most grains, coffee, alcohol, and again a culprit, animal proteins including dairy. Further, the patient is encouraged to increase consumption of alkalizing foods including vegetables like broccoli, cauliflower, and sea vegetables, lentils, sweet potato, and fruits like pineapple, watermelon, nectarines, and raspberries. It is important to clarify the distinction between what is considered a healthy food and what is the metabolic response to that food. Foods can be healthy or not, independent of their effect on the body's pH balance. Patients can easily monitor their pH level by testing their first morning's urine. Test strips (pH papers) are inexpensive and usually obtainable at drug stores.

There are many natural anti-inflammatory substances that the CAM practitioner has available for use with RA patients. Most commonly overlooked, yet quite effective, are proteolytic enzymes given between meals (to be discussed later). More commonly used substances include curcumin (turmeric), boswellia, ginger, and a topical analgesic containing natural menthol.

Curcumin is the active principle of turmeric, a yellow spice typically used in curry dishes. Curcumin exerts excellent anti-inflammatory and antioxidant effects.[15–17] A preliminary double-blind study found that 400 mg curcumin three times per day was as effective as certain drug therapies for people with RA.[18] While drug therapies carry potential for significant side effects, curcumin has no apparent side effects.

Boswellia, a traditional Ayurvedic herbal remedy, has been shown to have beneficial effect on pain and stiffness, as well as improved joint function.[19,20] It appears that boswellia has anti-inflammatory action much like that of NSAIDs. But unlike NSAIDs, long-term use is generally considered safe and does not lead to the irritation or the ulceration of the stomach. Boswellia gum extract is often recommended at 400 to 800 mg three times per day or less if used in combination with other natural anti-inflammatory agents.

Ginger is also known to reduce joint stiffness. Its ability to inhibit the formation of inflammatory mediators along with its strong antioxidant activities and protease component suggests a possible benefit in inflammatory conditions.[21,22] A recent double-blind, placebo-controlled study found that a specific patented combination of ginger and greater galangal (EVEXT.77) at only 255 mg twice a day provided a significant reduction in knee pain and stiffness.[23] This combination taken with meals appears to be even more effective than ginger alone and like other natural substances mentioned, does not involve the same side effects of NSAIDs.

Topical anti-inflammatories are an important answer for pain relief to the RA patient; however, most provide very little benefit other than a cooling sensation. In addition, many topicals contain toxins such as camphor. Topical analgesic derived from natural sources such as menthol (versus camphor) should be used so as not to contribute to the toxic burden. With the addition of other ingredients such as methylsulfonylmethane (MSM), white willow bark, ginger root oil, and aloe vera, a topical also provides support to the joint tissue while providing anti-inflammatory relief.

In the treatment of RA it is important to support the joint tissue and tissue repair processes. One of the best natural substances that is clinically shown to repair degenerated tissues is a stabilized glucosamine sulfate (GS) at 1500 mg daily or 20 mg/kg daily if one is obese or on diuretics.[24,25] GS is highly hydroscopic, meaning it attracts and absorbs water very easily. Alone, the GS molecule is likely to be oxidized leading to its eventual degradation. The most effective GS supplement is stabilized with sodium and chloride. The resulting, nonhydroscopic substance is stable at normal temperature and relative humidity. Chondroitin sulfate has been shown to work synergistically with GS; however, if its molecular weight is greater than 16.000 Da then absorption is minimal or none.[26] MSM, a bioavailable form of sulfur, is also often combined with GS because of its joint support and pain-relieving properties.

As anti-inflammatory and joint support therapies are initiated, the CAM practitioner focuses much attention on the gut or bowel function. Without proper digestion, absorption, and elimination, it is not likely that the nutritional benefit of foods will be realized. Any disruption of these processes could potentially cause substantial and progressive health problems throughout the body.[3,27,28] Therefore restoring the integrity and proper function of the gut appears to be critical for a successful outcome with the RA patient. The CAM practitioner uses a highly specific test such as a Comprehensive Stool Analysis and Parasitology to assess gut function as well as to identify possible imbalances in intestinal flora, pathogenic bacteria, or parasites. An additional test may also be warranted to confirm an intestinal barrier function problem.

Individuals with RA often have increased intestinal permeability to dietary and bacterial antigens. Moreover, they may experience alterations in bacterial flora leading to what is commonly termed "dysbiosis." Research has shown that the severity of RA symptoms is associated with the degree of bacterial overgrowth in the small intestines.[3,29–33] Once the pathogens are identified, the CAM practitioner has an arsenal of natural substances to decrease or "kill off" pathogenic organisms such as bacteria, candida, or parasites. Natural substances include grapefruit seed extract, oils of oregano and thyme, garlic, berberine, *Artemisia annua*, and black walnut hull.

The balancing of intestinal ecology is important for overall gut health.[34,35] It is for this reason that directly following the treatment to decrease pathogens, the gut is recolonized with "friendly" bacteria, the most common being *Lactobacillus acidophilus* and *B. bifidum*. These probiotic supplements often include fructooligosaccharides (FOS) as a growth factor to help promote the recolonization effort. Some practitioners will recommend the initiation of probiotics at the onset of treatment. However, as FOS could potentially promote the growth of the pathogens, probiotics containing FOS should not be recommended during the treatment phase.

As previously mentioned, intestinal barrier function is often compromised in RA patients. Increased intestinal permeability is often viewed as the cause of producing high amounts of CICs in the bloodstream. CICs are routinely elevated in RA patients and are thought to be factors that contribute to the pathogenesis of RA.[4,36] CICs develop from bowel inflammation associated with maldigestion and food allergies, plus dietary factors. There are many bowel irritants known. Examples include large undigested protein molecules, allergenic foods, and inflammatory PGE2-promoting foods (as mentioned earlier).

To help reduce increased levels of circulating CICs, and alleviate painful and often debilitating inflammation, CAM practitioners investigate the possibility of allergies or so called "hypersensitivities" to food. Problematic foods or food additives, drinks, chemicals, and airborne allergens can be identified through a variety of testing methods. The potential drawback to this testing is that it can be costly and occasionally the results are not 100% reliable. A diet journal is a less costly method of identification. Here, the patients keep track of everything they eat and drink while noting what is suspected to aggravate or trigger symptoms. The main problem with the food diary is that it is a very tedious exercise. Moreover, these results may not always be reliable either as reactions from food sensitivity can sometimes occur up to 24 to 72 h after ingestion. This makes it extremely difficult to pinpoint the actual offending substances that are worsening the symptoms. Also, these types of observational diaries are often inadequate for assessing chemical and airborne sensitivities.

Nonetheless, elimination of allergic foods and other offenders has been shown to offer significant benefit to some individuals with RA.[4,37–40] The most common allergic foods associated with RA are wheat, corn, dairy products, beef, and the nightshade family foods that include tomato, potato, eggplants, peppers, and tobacco. By whatever means, once the offenders are identified, the patient then avoids these for a period of 1 to 3 months, three being more standard. After the avoidance period, the foods, food additives, and drinks are slowly introduced back into the diet one at a time every 3 to 4 days. If a flare-up ensues at any time, what was most recently added is removed again for another period of 3 to 6 months and then introduced again. Often the patient finds that there is an amount that can be tolerated before symptoms develop. It is not uncommon to find that a small amount maybe once a week is not a problem but ingesting it more often or in a higher amount will bring on symptoms.

Research has shown that a fasting variation to the previous protocol provides some RA patients significant relief from their symptoms.[4,5,41–43] This version has the patient fast for 7 to 10 days, consisting of herbal teas, garlic, vegetable broth, decoction of potatoes and parsley, and the following juices: carrots, beets, and celery. After the fast, a new food item is reintroduced every second day. If an increase in symptoms is noted during the 48-h period, it is omitted for at least 7 days before it is tried again. If the food causes symptoms again, it is removed from the diet permanently. The results of the study using this protocol further support the positive results reflected in other studies where for many patients, short-term fasting followed by a vegetarian diet substantially reduced disease activity.[4,5,44–46]

Being careful to always go back to underlying issues, the CAM practitioner will look for the link between foods or food allergies and inflammation. Invariably, they will find themselves returning to gut function. Knowing that large protein molecules trigger inflammation in the bowel, the problem can often be traced back to protein digestion either as it occurs in the stomach or in the small intestines or often both. By improving digestion of proteins, the CAM practitioner will not only resolve bowel inflammation caused by large protein molecules but will also allow for the many additional benefits associated with proper protein digestion.

It is very common for impaired protein digestion to be associated with hypochlorhydria, or the inefficient production of hydrochloric acid in the stomach. This condition of hypoacidity is most commonly associated with advanced age but is also seen in younger individuals under chronic and severe stress. Several studies have shown that with increasing age, the ability to secrete gastric acid decreases.[27,28,47] More specifically, low stomach acidity has been found in more than half of those aged 60 or older. Research has linked hypoacidity to RA and other autoimmune disorders.[48,49] Correction of hypochlorhydria therefore deserves strong consideration as part of the treatment modality.

Common sign and symptoms of hypoacidity are bloating, belching, and flatulence immediately after meals along with indigestion, undigested food in the stools, and multiple food allergies. Hypochlorhydric patients can also have weak, peeling or cracked fingernails, itching around the rectum, acne, and chronic candida infections. Since gastric acid analysis testing is not widely available, if hypoacidity is suspected, a clinical trial of HCL supplements is often suggested.

As an aside, adequate protein digestion improves many biochemical functions in the body. One particular function of interest is that of the thyroid gland.[50,51] Thyroid hormone production is dependent on the amino acid tyrosine. One has to ask if it is just a coincidence that many RA patients also present with hypothyroid. Many CAM practitioners choose to link impaired protein digestion, and the potential for tyrosine insufficiency as one of the causes of a hypothyroid condition. In that respect they may choose to recommend short-term supplemental tyrosine while gut function is restored and then reassess the thyroid rather than to immediately start conventional hypothyroid medication.

A secondary, but equally important part of protein digestion involves the pancreas and occurs in the small intestine. Proteolytic enzymes are produced by the pancreas and secreted into the small intestine to complete protein digestion that was initiated in the stomach. Again, the elderly seem to be the group who most experience mild pancreatic insufficiency.[27,28] Symptoms are very similar to hypochlorhydria; however, pancreatic function is more easily assessed with the comprehensive stool analysis test referred to earlier. Pancreatic enzyme products are an effective treatment for pancreatic insufficiency and are widely used.[4,52] Full strength (10X), undiluted enzymes are preferred over lower potency products. The addition of other proteolytic enzymes such as bromelain, papain, and chymotrypsin makes for an extremely effective supplement. To aid in digestion, enzymes should be taken immediately before a meal. However, if also taken between meals, pancreatic enzymes have the added benefit of reducing CICs in the bloodstream as well as providing anti-inflammatory benefits.[53]

Recent research shows a possible relationship role for altered hepatic detoxification ability in RA and other autoimmune conditions.[2,54] Reduced hepatic function is likely caused by toxins from environment or internally caused toxins, especially those from the gut. CAM practitioners may choose to assess hepatic function with a hepatic detoxification profile test. Additionally, urine toxic elements testing will help to identify specific toxins that may be problematic. Supporting healthy liver detoxification as well as healthy liver cells is a key element in the treatment of RA. Standardized milk thistle extract has been clinically shown to support detox while also improving liver cells including the specialized macrophages of the liver, the Kupffer cells. Kupffer cells help to reduce CICs as well as macromolecules that may have penetrated the intestinal barrier.[55,56]

Autoimmune conditions are characterized by the altered ratio of highly activated lymphocytes and weakly activated lymphocytes. Pentacyclic oxindole alkaloid (POA) cat's claw has been reported in the *Journal of Rheumatology* and is also one of the most often used natural agents for RA in Austria where it is produced. POA cat's claw is clinically shown to have immune modulatory effects that help to normalize altered lymphocyte ratios in autoimmune conditions.[57,58] Cat's claw contains both POA and tetracyclic oxindole alkaloids (TOA), however any presence of TOA will antagonize the immune modulating effects of POA. Research demonstrates clinical success with TOA free cat's claw. In addition, there is also research supporting the use of low molecular weight thymus extract for normalizing the immune response.[59]

Indeed, it is important for patients with autoimmune conditions to have immune modulation, not stimulation. To better support the immune system and prevent free radical damage, a diet rich in fresh fruits and vegetables cannot be overstated in the dietary treatment of RA. Antioxidant nutrients, such as selenium, zinc, and vitamin C, are clinically shown to be reduced in many RA patients.[4,6–8,60–63] The best sources of selenium are Brazil nuts, fish, and grains. Foods rich in zinc include oysters, whole grains, nuts, and seeds. Vitamin C rich sources include broccoli, Brussels sprouts, cabbage, citrus fruits, tomatoes, and berries.

To ensure adequate antioxidant intake and immune support, patients are advised to supplement their diet with an iron-free multivitamin or mineral supplement with perhaps even an additional antioxidant nutrient combination. Because of its anti-inflammatory action, an additional amount of buffered vitamin C is often recommended for a total intake of 1000 to 3000 mg daily. The iron-free recommendation comes from the fact that in RA, although serum iron levels are usually low, iron-binding capacity is also low. Therefore supplemental iron is often useless and may actually promote further free radical damage.[4,64] In RA iron supplementation is not indicated unless there is an anemia that is due specifically from blood loss.

Attention to adrenal function may be warranted especially for those patients who have been on corticosteroid medications. Lifestyle factors such as lack of exercise, poor diet, and stress can also deplete adrenal function. The CAM practitioner can better assess adrenal function with laboratory tests that measure cortisol levels and dehydroepiandrosterone (DHEA). DHEA can be supplemented if it is low.[65,66] If additional support is needed, there are several natural substances such as ginseng, pantothenic acid, and vitamin C that can be given to maintain proper adrenal function.

RA patients can benefit from a variety of stress reduction techniques such as meditation and exercises like yoga, swimming, tai chi, and chi gong. In addition, the CAM approach to the treatment of RA may include adjunct therapies such as massage therapy, acupuncture, emotional freedom technique (EFT), chiropractic, and biofeedback.[3] When combined with treatments as described above, these therapies provide RA patients with a comprehensive treatment protocol that better ensures a successful outcome.

Some may consider the extra time and extra visits often necessary for CAM treatments a drawback. Another unfortunate issue is the reluctance of insurance companies to cover these therapies leaving CAM virtually unavailable for much of the population who simply cannot afford it. Nevertheless, with public demand and healthcare reform this should eventually change.

The main reasons patients turn to complimentary medicine in the first place are the failure of conventional drugs to bring about significant relief of symptoms and the concern about potential drug side effects.[1,3,4,67,68] It appears CAM's many benefits far outweigh the downsides. With CAM approaches, patients appreciate better relationships with their healthcare providers and the opportunity they have to become personally empowered to help manage their own health. Furthermore, patients may experience the added benefit of improving other related conditions because of CAM's unique "total" approach to health. Ultimately, with CAM, patients can achieve successful outcomes overall. Furthermore, these outcomes are achieved usually with fewer complicating side effects while providing insight into underlying causes of ill health where conventional medicine has fallen short.

REFERENCES

1. Vecchio PC. Attitudes to alternative medicine by rheumatology outpatient attenders. *J Rheumatol*, 1994;321:145–147.
2. McKinnon RA, Newbert DW. Possible role of cytochrome P450 in lupus erythematosus and related disorders. *Lupus*, 1994;3(6):473–478.
3. The Burton Goldberg Group. *Alternative Medicine: The definitive Guide*, Future Medicine Publishing, Fife, WA, 1994, pp. 531–532.
4. Murray, MT. The natural approach to rheumatoid arthritis. *Am J Nat Med*, 1996;3(1):8–21.
5. Peltonen R et al. Changes of fecal flora in rheumatoid arthritis during fasting and one-year diet. *Br J Rhematol*, 1994;33:638–643.
6. Darlington LG, Ramsey NW. Clinical review: review of dietary therapy for rheumatoid arthritis. *Br J Rheumatol*, 1993;32:507–514.
7. Buchanan HM, Preston EJ, Brooks PM, et al. Is diet important in rheumatoid arthritis? *Br J Rheumatol*, 1991;30:125–134.
8. McCrae F, Veerapen K, Dieppe P. Diet and arthritis. *Practitioner*, 1986;230:359–361.
9. Shapiro JA et al. Diet and rheumatoid arthritis in women: a possible protective effect of fish consumption. *Epidemiology*, 1996;7:255–263.

10. Cleland LG et al. Clinical and biochemical effects of dietary fish oil supplements in rheumatoid arthritis. *J Rheumatol*, 1988;15:1471–1475.

11. Van der Temple H et al. Effects of fish oil supplementation in rheumatoid arthritis. *Ann Rheum Dis*, 1990;49:76–80.

12. Nielsen GL et al. The effects with dietary supplementation with $n-3$ polyunsaturated fatty acids in patients with rheumatoid arthritis: a randomized, double-blind trial. *Eur J Clin Invest*, 1992;22:687–691.

13. Shukla VKS, Perkins EG. The presence of oxidative polymeric materials in encapsulated fish oils. *Lipids*, 1991;26:23–26.

14. Fritshe KL, Johnston PV. Rapid autoxidation of fish oil in diets without added antioxidants. *J Nutr*, 1988;118:425–426.

15. Ammon HPT, Wahl MA. Pharmacology of *Curcuma longa*. *Planta Medica*, 1991;57:1–7.

16. Miyase T et al. Natural antioxidants: antioxidant compounds isolated from rhizome of *Curcuma longa* L. *Chem Pharmacol Bull*, 1985:33:1725–1728.

17. Satoskar RR, Shah SJ, Shenoy SC. Evaluation of anti-inflammatory property of curcumin (diferuloyl methane) in patients with prospective inflammation. *Int J Clin Pharmacol Ther Toxicol*, 1986;24:651–654.

18. Deodhar SD, Sethi R, Srimal RC. Preliminary studies on antirheumatic activity of curcumin (diferuloyl methane). *Ind J Med Res*, 1980;71:632–634.

19. Singh GB, Singh S, Bani S. Anti-inflammatory actions of boswellic acids. *Phytomedicine*, 1996;3:81–85.

20. Etzel R. Special extract of *Boswellia serrata* (H15) in the treatment of rheumatoid arthritis. *Phytomedicine*, 1996;3:91–94.

21. Kiuchi F et al. Inhibition of prostaglandin; and leukotriene biosynthesis by gingerols and diarylheptanoids. *Chem Pharmacol Bull*, 1992;40:387–391.

22. Srivastava KC, Mustafa T. Ginger (*Zingiber officinale*) in rheumatism and musculoskeletal disorders. *Med Hypothesis*, 1992;89:342–348.

23. Altman RD, Marcussen KC. Effects of a ginger extract on knee pain in patients with osteoarthritis. *Arthr Rheum*, 2001;44(11):2531–2538.

24. Gaby AR. Natural treatments for osteoarthritis. *Altern Med Rev*, 1999;4:330–341.

25. Muller-Fassbender H et al. Glucosamine sulfate compared to ibuprofen in osteoarthritis of the knee. *Osteoarthritis Cartilage*, 1994;2:61–69.

26. Adebowale AO et al. Analysis of glucosamine and chondroitin sulfate content in marketed products and the $CaCO_2$ permeability of chondroitin sulfate raw materials. *JAMA*, 2000;3:37–44.

27. Vellias B, Bala D, Albarda JL. Effects of aging process on digestive functions. *Compr Ther*, 1991;17(8):46–52.

28. Russell RM. Changes in gastrointestinal function attributed to aging. *Am J Clin Nutr*, 1992;55:1203S–1207S.

29. Ebringer A et al. Klebsiella antibodies in ankylosing spondylitis and proteus antibodies in rheumatoid arthritis. *Br J Rheumatol*, 1988;27:72–85.

30. Allan RN. Extra-intestinal manifestations of inflammatory bowel disease. *Clin Gastroenterol*, 1983;12:617–632.

31. Henriksson AE, Blomquist L, Nord CE, et al. Small intestinal bacterial overgrowth in patients with rheumatoid arthritis. *Ann Rheum Dis*, 1993;52(7):503–510.

32. Segal AW, Isenberg DA, Hajirousou V, et al. Preliminary evidence for gut involvement in the pathogenesis of rheumatoid arthritis. *Br J Rheumatol*, 1986;25:162–166.

33. Zaphiropoulos GC. Rheumatoid arthritis and the gut. *Br J Rheumatol*, 1986;25:38–40.

34. Macfarlane GT, Cummings JH. Probiotics and prebiotics; can regulating the activities of intestinal bacteria benefit health? *BMJ*, 1999;318:999–1003.

35. Madsen K. The use of probiotics in intestinal disease. *Can J Gastroenterol*, 2001;15:817–822 (Abstract).

36. Husby S, Jensenius JC, Svehag SE. Passage of undegraded dietary antigen into blood of healthy adults. *Scand J Immunol*, 1985;22:88–92.

37. Panush RS. Delayed reactions to foods. Food allergy and rheumatoid arthritis. *Ann Allergy*, 1986;56:500–503.

38. Van de Laar MAFJ, Ander Korst JK. Food intolerance and rheumatoid arthritis in a double blind, controlled trial of the clinical effects of elimination of milk allergens and azo dyes. *Ann Rheum Dis*, 1992;51:298–302.

39. Jenkins R, Rooney P, Jones D, et al. Increased intestinal permeability in patients with rheumatoid arthritis. A side effect of oral nonsteroidal anti-inflammatory drug therapy? *Br J Rheumatol*, 197;26:103–107.

40. Smith MD, Gibson RA, Brooks PM. Abnormal bowel permeability in ankylosing spondylitis and rheumatoid arthritis. *J Rheumatol*, 1985;12:299–305.

41. Hafstrom I, Ringertz B, Gyllenhammar H, et al. Effects of fasting on disease activity, neutrophil function, fatty acid composition, and leukotriene biosynthesis in patients with rheumatoid arthritis. *Arthr Rheum*, 1988;31:585–592.

42. Hicklin JA, McEwen LM, Morgan JE. The effect of diet in rheumatoid. *Clin Allergy*, 1980;10:463–467.

43. Kroker GF, Stroud RM, Marshall R, et al. Fasting and rheumatoid arthritis. A multicenter study. *Clin Ecol*, 1984;2:137–144.

44. Kjeldensen-Kragh J et al. Controlled trial of fasting and one-year vegetarian diet in rheumatoid arthritis. *Lancet*, 1991;338:899–902.

45. Skoldstam L, Larson L, Lindstrom ED. Effects of fasting and lacto vegetarian diet in rheumatoid arthritis. *Scand J Rheumatol*, 1979;8:249–255.

46. Peltonen R et al. Changes in faecal flora in rheumatoid arthritis during fasting and one-year vegetarian diet. *Br J Rheumatol*, 1994;33:638–643.

47. Henrikson K, Uvnab-Moberg K, Nonl CE, et al. Grastrin, gastric acid secretion, and gastric microflora in patients with rheumatoid arthritis. *Ann Rheum Dis*, 1986;45:475–483.

48. De Witte TJ et al. Hydrochloridria and hypergastrinemia in rheumatoid arthritis. *Ann Rheumatic Dis*, 1979;38:14–17.

49. Peltonen R, Nenonen M, Helve T, et al. Faecal microbial flora and hypergastrinemia in rheumatoid arthritis. *Annals*, 1979;38:14–17.

50. Krupsky M et al. Musculoskeletal symptoms as a presenting sign of long-standing hypothyroidism. *1st J Med Sci*, 1987;23:1110–1113.

51. Hoohberg MC et al. Hypothyroidism presenting as a polymyositis-like syndrome. *Arthr Rheum*, 1976;10:1363–1366.

52. Horger I. Enzyme therapy in multiple rheumatic diseases. *Therapiewoche*, 1983;33:3948–3957.

53. Ransberger K. Enzyme treatment of immune complex diseases. *Arthr Rheum*, 1986;8:16–19.

54. Brown TA, Russel MW, Mestecky J. Elimination of intestinally absorbed antigen into the bile by IgA. *J Immunol*, 1984;132:780–782.

55. Socken DJ et al. Secretory component-dependant hepatic transport of IgA antibody-antigen complexes. *J Immunol*, 1981;127:316.

56. Russel MW et al. Immunoglobulin A mediated hepatobiliary transport constitutes a natural pathway for disposing of bacterial antigens. *Infect Immunol*, 1983;42:1041–1048.

57. Mur E et al. Randomized double blind trial of an extract from the pentacyclic alkaloid-chemotype of *Uncaria tomentosa* for the treatment of rheumatoid arthritis. *J Rheumatol*, 2002;29:678–681.

58. Wurm M et al. Pentacyclic oxidole alkaloids form *Uncaria tomentosa* induce human endothelial cells to release a lymphocyte proliferation regulating factor. *Planta Medica*, 1998;65:701–704.

59. Kouttab NM, Prada M, Cazzola P. Thymomodulin: biological properties and clinical applications. *Med Oncol Tumor Pharmacother*, 1989;6:5–9.

60. Tarp U et al. Selenium treatment in rheumatoid arthritis. *Scand J Rheumatol*, 1985;14:264–268.

61. Pandley SP, Bhattacharya SK, Sundar S. Zinc in rheumatoid arthritis. *Ind J Med Res*, 1985;81:818–820.

62. Mullen A, Wilson CWM. The metabolism of ascorbic acid in rheumatoid arthritis. *Pract Nutr Sci*, 1976;35:8A–9A.

63. Levin M. New concepts in the biology and biochemistry of ascorbic acid. *New Engl J Med*, 1986;314:892–902.

64. Nishiya K, Matsueda H, Shirakami T, et al. Serum and urinary ferritin levels in patients with rheumatoid arthritis. *Acta Med Okayama*, 1985;39:321–328.
65. Van Vollenhoven R, Engleman EG, McGuire JL. Dehydroepiandrosterone in systematic lupus erythematosus. Results of a double-blind, placebo-controlled, randomizes clinical trial. *Arthr Rheum*, 1995;38:1826–1831.
66. Van Vollenhoven RF et al. An open study of dehydroepiandrosterone in systemic lupus erythematosus. *Arthritis Rheum*, 1994;37:1305–1310.
67. Scott DL, Symmons DP, Coulton BL, et al. Long-term outcome of treating rheumatoid arthritis. Results after 20 years. *Lancet*, 1989;I:1108–1111.
68. Sigthorsson G, Tibble J, Hayllar J, Menzies I, Macpherson A, Moots R, Scott D, Gumpel MJ, Bjarnason I. Intestinal permeability and inflammation in patients on NSAIDs. *Gut*, 1998;43: 506–511.

CLINICAL APPLICATION: IMMUNE-ENHANCING POWER OF MUSHROOMS

Jill Place

The healing power of mushrooms has been recognized for thousands of years, but scientists have only been able to isolate their immune-enhancing components for about 30 years. Only about 50 of the over 30,000 varieties of mushrooms and other fungi have been found to have immune-enhancing properties, and very few of those have been extensively studied. These few may be so effective in stimulating and modulating the immune system that one scientific review dubbed them "immunoceuticals.[1]" Research also suggests that mushrooms may increase insulin response,[2] lower blood pressure,[3] improve lipid profiles,[4] and be effective in the prevention or treatment of liver disorders.[5] These effects may or may not have immune or autoimmune components.

IMMUNOCEUTICAL STRUCTURE

Most immunoceutical mushroom extracts are chemically classified as beta-D-glucan high-molecular-weight polysaccharides or beta-D-glucan-bound proteins, also called proteoglycans. Proteoglycans appear to have greater immune-enhancing activity than their beta-D-glucan cousins.[6] Beta-D-glucan polysaccharides include *Grifola* and Maitake D-fraction from *Grifola frondosa*, lentinan from *Lentinus edodes*, and schizophyllan from *Schizophyllum commune*. Proteoglycans include polysaccharide Krestin (PSK), also called Krestin, and polysaccharopeptide (PSP), both of which are isolated from *Coriolus versicolor*. Other immunoceutical fungi studied in the medical literature include Hakumokuji (*Tremella fuciformis*), Tochukaso (*Cordyceps sinensis*), Choreimaitake (*Polyporus umbellatus*), and Reishi (*Ganoderma lucidum*).

Mushroom extracts may be drawn from several stages in the life cycle. A mushroom begins this cycle when spores are generated from a mature fruiting body. The spores then germinate and form the true body of the mushroom, mycelial threads that then anchor their growth in several mediums from dead wood to living organisms. After the mycelium matures it sprouts a new fruiting body that we commonly recognize as a mushroom. Some extracts, such as the Maitake D-fraction (*G. frondosa*) come from the fruiting bodies of the fungus, while extracts derived from *L. edodes* and the proteoglycans PSK and PSP, come from the cultured mycelia. A few extracts, including some distilled from *G. lucidum*, are derived from the dormant spores, the germinating spores, the sporoderm-broken germinating spores, and the lipids extracted from the germinating spores.[7] Both the form of the extract and the chemical structure influence the potency and efficacy of the mushroom preparation.

MECHANISMS OF IMMUNOCEUTICAL ACTION

Although the immune-enhancing mechanisms of fungi extracts are not totally clear, these polysaccharides and polysaccharide–protein complexes possibly enhance cell-mediated immune responses and act as biological response modifiers.[8] The cells of the immune system are regulated through the release of various cytokines. Fungi extracts may increase the activity of immune-stimulating cytokines, such as IL-2, and inhibit immunosuppressive cytokines, such as NF-kappa B, thereby stimulating immune system activity.[9]

When the immune system is mobilized, many different types of immune cells are called to action. Proteoglycans may help dendritic cells to mature and be stimulated to better recognize and target foreign material such as tumors and other cancerous cells.[10] Increased activity of macrophages, other phagocytes, and NK cells may be directly stimulated or influenced indirectly through antioxidant enzymes and enzyme cascades.[11,12] Overproduction of superoxide radicals (O_2^-) or superoxide dismutase (SOD) abnormalities exist in many diseases. Proteoglycans derived from *C. versicolor* may be able to mimic the actions of SOD and therefore protect macrophages and other cells against (O_2^-)-damage.[13–17] Beta-D-glucans such as grifolan from *G. frondosa* may also upregulate nitric oxide synthase and nitric oxide (NO) production. NO is an important effector molecule on antimicrobial and antitumor effects of macrophages.[18,19] Krestin may also influence the production of GSH-Px, another important antioxidant enzyme.[20] Other fungi such as *G. lucidum* and *G. tsugae* also exhibit antioxidant properties.[21]

Immunoceuticals and Cancer

Polysaccharides isolated from fungi, especially PSK and PSP, are the most studied of any natural cancer compound. More than 50 human studies have been conducted on PSK–PSP. These studies strongly suggest that these extracts increase postoperative and posttreatment survival in humans.[9] These effects may be mostly due to stimulation of the immune system and inhibition of immunosuppression through the mechanisms previously discussed. All human studies conducted with these extracts were done during chemotherapy or radiotherapy treatment. Most of this research suggested that treatment and PSK and PSP resulted in greater survival rates than treatment alone.[22–26] PSK seems to be most effective for cancers of the stomach, esophagus, nasopharynx, colon, rectum, and lung, and PSP appears to be most beneficial for stomach, esophageal, and lung cancer.

PSK–PSP as well as other polysaccharides may also inhibit cancer progression in animals.[9] About 40 animal studies were done on PSK–PSP. Several pointed to the mechanisms of reduced tumor-induced immunosuppression[27] and increased NK cell activity.[28] Boik pointed out that the effects of PSK were tumor-specific, greater on smaller tumors, and had to do with the tumor's sensitivity to NK cell activity.[9,29]

Other mushroom extracts,[30–32] such as those from *L. edodes*,[33–35] *G. lucidum*,[36,37] *S. commune*, *Trametes versicolor*, *Inonotus obliquus*, *Flammulina velutipes*, *Sclerotinia sclerotioru*, *C. sinensis*,[38–40] and the Maitake D-fraction of *G. frondosa*[41–45] have been researched in *in vitro* and animal studies and in limited human studies. Much of this research points to the immunomodulatory effects of these extracts as the main mechanism for possible inhibition of cancer progression.

A few nonfungi high-molecular-weight polysaccharides may also be capable of directly killing cancerous cells and suppressing tumor growth through immunomodulatory mechanisms. These include Astragalus, and Eleutherococcus, familiarly known as Siberian ginseng. These are among the most commonly used Chinese herbs and are frequently used in China to treat cancer patients. A few of the handful of human studies are cited here.[46–49]

Immunoceuticals and Other Disease States

A few research studies suggest that nonpolysaccharide fractions of *G. lucidum*, the highly oxygenated lanosterols and triterpenes that include ganoderic acid alpha, ganoderic acid beta, lucidumol A, ganoderiol F, and ganodermanontriol from the fruiting body and spores showed significant anti-HIV-1 protease activity.[50,51] A two-phase placebo-controlled trial with asymptomatic AIDS patients showed that the beta-D-glucan lentinan can increase levels of CD4 cells and decrease levels of a marker of viral replication, the p24 antigen.[52] Maitake D-fraction may also be valuable as a direct inhibitor of HIV as well as an immune stimulant.[53]

Extracts of *C. sinensis* may also be helpful in treating immunomodulatory nephropathy[54] and systemic autoimmune diseases such as lupus.[55]

Dosages and Forms of Administration

Many polysaccharide extracts, such as those from shiitake and schizophyllan, are too large in molecular weight to be orally bioavailable. They are administered intravenously, intramuscularly, intraperitoneally, or intratumorally. Some cancer studies with PSK proved most effective with a combination of preoperative intratumoral treatment and postoperative oral treatment. Others, such as extracts of *Coriolus*, Reishi, and Maitake can be taken orally as a tea, decoction, powder, or capsule. Much of the research seems to indicate that the safest form is a soluble tea or decoction. This form has been used for a thousand years in China and Japan. Combinations of herbs and polysaccharides such as *Shi Quan Da Bu Tang* and *Bu Zhong Yi Qi Tang* have also been used quite successfully in Traditional Chinese Medicine and may be more effective than single preparations. PC-SPES, an herbal mixture containing *G. lucidum*, showed that it could lower PSA levels in prostate cancer in several studies until it was recalled because of contamination of its raw ingredients.[56] Combinations may be better in three ways: (1) they can be more effective against cancer when combined with other natural compounds that stem immune invasion and metastases,[9] (2) they can target a broader range of cancer cells as some polysaccharides are tumor-specific, and (3) combinations can achieve a daily desired dose, approximately 2 to 6 g of crude mushroom, 1 to 2 g of powder, and 1 ml of tincture, without risking the possible toxicity due to large amounts of a single preparation. Therapeutic IV doses for cancer patients of up to 0.5 to 2 mg/kg in high-risk surgical patients are not uncommon.

Contraindications

Orally, most beta-D-glucans are well tolerated. Because they are immunostimulants, they may decrease the effects of immunosuppressants. They should be avoided in pregnancy and lactation, as there is little reliable information about safety. Because Reishi seems to have anticoagulant effects, taking it with anticoagulant and antiplatelet drugs might increase bruising and bleeding, and use with antihypertensives might increase the risk of hypotension. Theoretically, Reishi might increase the risk of bleeding in people with thrombocytopenia. There has been one isolated study where shiitake caused rash, GI discomfort, and eosinophilia,[57] but too large an amount (4 g) of powder (not the most desirable form) possibly caused toxicity. Shiitake has also caused hypersensitivity pneumonitis due to spore inhalation,[58,59] and contact dermatitis in mushroom workers.[60,61] IV beta-D-glucans may cause chills and fever, redness, joint and lower back pain, swelling, headache, diarrhea, dizziness, flushing, hypotension, hypertension, vasodilation, nausea, vomiting, leukocytosis, hives, and excessive urination.[62]

CONCLUSION

There is an overwhelming amount of research that beta-D-glucan and proteoglycan polysaccharides alone or in combination with other polysaccharides and herbs may be efficacious in boosting immune response and aiding those with cancer, AIDS, and other immune disorders. Much of the research, however, has been with single preparations. And most of the cancer research has not produced profound anticancer effects. Perhaps the next step might be with placebo-controlled double-blind trials and combinations of polysaccharides, herbs, and other natural compounds that might create these profound effects, and a greater body of research in the Western medicine arena.

REFERENCES

1. Kidd PM. The use of mushroom glucans and proteoglycans in cancer treatment. *Altern Med Rev*, 2000;5:4–27.
2. Horio H, Ohtsuru M. Maitake (*Grifola frondosa*) improve glucose tolerance of experimental diabetic rats. *Nutr Sci Vitaminol (Tokyo)*, 2001;47(1):57–63.
3. Kabir Y, Yamaguchi M, Kimura S. Effect of shiitake (*Lentinus edodes*) and Maitake (*Grifola frondosa*) mushrooms on blood pressure and plasma lipids of spontaneously hypertensive rats. *J Nutr Sci Vitaminol (Tokyo)*, 1987;33(5):341–346.
4. Fukushima M, Ohashi T, Fujiwara Y, Sonoyama K, Nakano M. Cholesterol-lowering effects of Maitake (*Grifola frondosa*) fiber, shiitake (*Lentinus edodes*) fiber, and enokitake (*Flammulina velutipes*) fiber in rats. *Exp Biol Med (Maywood)*, 2001;226(8):758–765.
5. Lee EW, He P, Kawagishi H, Sugiyama K. Suppression of D-galactosamine-induced liver injury by mushrooms in rats. *Biosci Biotechnol Biochem*, 2000;64(9):2001–2004.
6. Sakagami H, Aoki T. Induction of immunopotentiation activity by a protein-bound polysaccharide, PSK (review). *Anticancer Res*, 1991;19:65–96.
7. Liu X, Yuan JP, Chung CK, Chen XJ. Antitumor activity of the sporoderm-broken germinating spores of *Ganoderma lucidum*. *Cancer Lett*, 2002;182(2):155–161.
8. Ooi VE, Liu F. Immunomodulation and anti-cancer activity of polysaccharide–protein complexes. *Curr Med Chem*, 2000;7(7):715–729.
9. Boik J. *Natural Compounds in Cancer Therapy*. Oregon Medical Press, Princeton, MN, 2001.
10. Tomochika H, Gouchi A, Okanobu K, et al. The effect and distribution of a protein-bound polysaccharide preparation, PSK (Krestin), intratumorally injected prior to surgery into gastric cancer patients. *Acta Med Okayama*, 1989:43:289–297.
11. Adachi Y, Okazaki M, Ohno N, Yadomae T. Enhancement of cytokine production by macrophages stimulated with $(1{\rightarrow}3)$-beta-D-glucan, grifolan (GRN), isolated from *Grifola frondosa*. *Biol Pharm Bull*, 1994;17(12):1554–1560.
12. Wang HX, NG TB, Liu WK, Ooi VE, Chang ST. Polysaccharide–peptide complexes from the cultured mycelia of the mushroom *Coriolus versicolor* and their culture medium activate mouse lymphocytes and macrophages. *Int J Biochem Cell Biol*, 1996;28(5):601–607.
13. Pang ZJ, Chen Y, Zhou M. Polysaccharide Krestin enhances manganese superoxide dismutase activity and mRNA expression in mouse peritoneal macrophages. *Am J Chin Med*, 2000;28(3–4): 331–341.
14. Kobayashi Y, Kariya K, Saigenji K, Nakamura K. Suppressive effects on cancer cell proliferation of the enhancement of superoxide dismutase (SOD) activity associated with the protein-bound polysaccharide of *Coriolus versicolor* QUEL. *Cancer Biother*, 1994;9(2):171–178.
15. Wei WS, Tan JQ, Guo F, Ghen HS, Zhou ZY, Zhang ZH, Gui L. Effects of *Coriolus versicolor* polysaccharides on superoxide dismutase activities in mice. *Zhongguo Yao Li Xue Bao*, 1996;17(2):174–178.
16. Nakamura K, Matsunaga K. Susceptibility of natural killer (NK) cells to reactive oxygen species (ROS) and their restoration by the mimics of superoxide dismutase (SOD). *Cancer Biother Radiopharm*, 1998;13(4):275–290.

17. Kariya K, Nakamura K, Nomoto K, Matama S, Saigenji K. Mimicking of superoxide dismutase activity by protein-bound polysaccharide of *Coriolus versicolor* QUEL, and oxidative stress relief for cancer patients. *Mol Biother*, 1992;4(1):40–46.

18. Ohno N, Egawa Y, Hashimoto T, Adachi Y, Yadomae T. Effect of beta-glucans on the nitric oxide synthesis by peritoneal macrophage in mice. *Biol Pharm Bull*, 1996;19(4):608–612.

19. Asai K, Kato H, Hirose K, Akaogi K, Kimura S, Mukai S, Inoue M, Yamamura Y, Sano H, Sugino S, Yoshikawa T, Kondo M. PSK and OK-432-induced immunomodulation of inducible nitric oxide (NO) synthase gene expression in mouse peritoneal lymorphonuclear leukocytes and NO-mediated cytotoxicity. *Immunopharmacol Immunotoxicol*, 2000;22(2):221–235.

20. Pang ZJ, Chen Y, Zhou M, Wan J. Effect of polysaccharide krestin on glutathione peroxidase gene expression in mouse peritoneal macrophages. *Br J Biomed Sci*, 2000;57(2):130–136.

21. Mau JL, Lin HC, Chen CC. Antioxidant properties of several medicinal mushrooms. *J Agric Food Chem*, 2002;50(21):6072–6077.

22. Chu KK, Ho SS, Chow AH. *Coriolus versicolor*: a medicinal mushroom with promising immunotherapeutic values. *J Clin Pharmacol*, 2002;42(9):976–984.

23. Fukushima M. Adjuvant therapy of gastric cancer: the Japanese experience. *Semin Oncol*, 1996;23(3):369–378.

24. Iino Y, Yokoe T, Maemura M, et al. Immunochemotherapies versus chemotherapy as adjuvant treatment after curative resection of operable breast cancer. *Anticancer Res*, 1995;15(6B):2907–2911.

25. Ogoshi K, Satou H, Isono K, et al. Immunotherapy for esophageal cancer. A randomized trial in combination with radiotherapy and chemotherapy. *Am J Clin Oncol*, 1995;18(3):216–222.

26. Torisu M, Hayashi Y, Ishimitsu T, et al. Significant prolongation of disease-free period gained by oral polysaccharide K (PSK) administration after curative surgical operation of colorectal cancer. *Cancer Immunol Immunother*, 1990;31(5):261–268.

27. Matsunaga K, Morita I, Iijima H, et al. Competitive action of a biological response modifier, PSK, on a humoral immunosuppressive factor produced in tumor-bearing hosts. *J Clin Lab Immunol*, 1990;31(3):127–136.

28. Suo J, Tanaka N, Hizuta A, Yunoki S, Orita K. Suppression of natural killer cell activity by liver metastasis of cancer and restoration of killer activity by oral administration of a Basiodomycotes-derived polysaccharide, PSK. *Acta Med Okayama*, 1994;48(5):237–242.

29. Algarra I, Collado A, Garrido F. Protein-bound polysaccharide PSK abrogates more efficiently experimental metastases derived from H-2 negative than from H-2 positive fibrosarcoma tumor clones. *J Exp Clin Cancer Res*, 1997;16(4):373–380.

30. Borchers AT, Stern JS, Hackman RM, Keen CL, Gershwin ME. Mushrooms, tumors, and immunity. *Proc Soc Exp Biol Med*, 1999;221(4):281–293.

31. Wasser SP, Weis AL. Therapeutic effects of substances occurring in higher Basiodomycotes mushrooms: a modern perspective. *Crit Rev Immunol*, 1999;19(1):65–96.

32. Jiang SM, Xiao ZM, Xu ZH. Inhibitory activity of polysaccharide extracts from three kinds of edible fungi on proliferation of human hepatoma SMMC-7721 cell and mouse implanted S180 tumor. *World J Gastroenterol*, 1999;5(5):404–407.

33. Wang GL, Lin ZB. The immunomodulatory effect of lentinan. *Yao Xue Xue Bao*, 1996;31(2):86–90 [Article in Chinese].

34. Liu M, Li J, Kong F, Lin J, Gao Y. Induction of immunomodulating cytokines by a new polysaccharide–peptide complex from culture mycelia of *Lentinus edodes*. *Immunopharmacology*, 1998;40(3):187–198.

35. Yamamoto Y, Shirono H, Kono K, Ohashi Y. Immunopotentiating activity of the water-soluble lignin rich fraction prepared from LEM — the extract of the solid culture medium of *Lentinus edodes* mycelia. *Biosci Biotechnol Biochem*, 1997;61(11):1909–1912.

36. Wang SY, Hsu ML, Hsu HC, Tzeng CH, Lee SS, Shiao MS, Ho CK. The anti-tumor effect of *Ganoderma lucidum* is mediated by cytokines released from activated macrophages and T lymphocytes. *Int J Cancer*, 1997;70(6):699–705.

37. Wang SY, Hsu ML, Hsu HC, Tzeng CH, Lee SS, Shiao MS, Ho CK. The anti-tumor effect of *Ganoderma lucidum* is mediated by cytokines released from activated macrophages and T lymphocytes. *Chin Med J (Engl)*, 1992;105(2):97–101.

38. Bok JW, Lermer L, Chilton J, Klingeman HG, Towers GH. Antitumor sterols from the mycelia of *Cordyceps sinensis*. *Phytochemistry*, 1999;51(7):891–898.

39. Chiu JH, Ju CH, Wu LH, Lui WY, Wu CW, Shiao MS, Hong CY. *Cordyceps sinensis* increases the expression of major histocompatibility complex class II antigens on human hepatoma cell line HA22T/VGH cells. *Am J Chin Med*, 1998;26(2):159–170.

40. Xu RH, Peng XE, Chen GZ, Chen GL. Effects of *Cordyceps sinensis* on natural killer activity and colony formation of B16 melanoma. *Chin Med J (Engl)*, 1992;105(2):97–101.

41. Suzuki I, Itani T, Ohno N, Oikawa S, Sato K, Miyazaki T, Yadomae T. Effect of a polysaccharide fraction from *Grifola frondosa* on immune response in mice. *J Pharmacobiodyn*, 1985;8(3):217–226.

42. Sanzen I, Imanishi N, Takamatsu N, Konosu S, Mantani N, Terasawa K, Tazawa K, Odaira Y, Watanabe M, Takeyama M, Ochiai H. Nitric oxide-mediated antitumor activity induced by the extract from *Grifola frondosa* (Maitake mushroom) in a macrophage cell line, RAW264.7. *J Exp Clin Cancer Res*, 2001;20(4):591–597.

43. Suzuki I, Itani T, Ohno N, Oikawa S, Sato K, Miyazaki T, Yadomae T. Antitumor activity of a polysaccharide fraction extracted from cultured fruiting bodies of *Grifola frondosa*. *J Pharmacobiodyn*, 1984;7(7):492–500.

44. Kodama N, Komuta K, Nanba H. Can Maitake MD-fraction aid cancer patients? *Altern Med Rev*, 2002;7(3):236–239.

45. Suzuki I, Hashimoto K, Oikawa S, Sato K, Osawa M, Yadomae T. Antitumor and immunomodulating activities of a beta-glucan obtained from liquid-cultured *Grifola frondosa*. *Chem Pharm Bull (Tokyo)*, 1989;37(2):410–413.

46. Zee-Chang RK. Shi-quan-da-bu-tang (ten significant tonic decoction), SQT. A potent Chinese biological response modifier in cancer immunotherapy, potentiation, and detoxification of anticancer drugs. *Meth Find Exp Clin Pharmacol*, 1992;14(9):725–736.

47. Zhang R, Qian J, Yang G, et al. Medicinal protection with Chinese herb-compound against radiation. *Aviat Space Environ Med*, 1990;61:729–731.

48. Bohn B, Nebe CT, Birr C. Flow-cytometric studies with *Eleutherococcus senticosus* extract as an immunomodulatory agent. *Arnneimittelforschung*, 1987;37(10):1193–1196.

49. Kupin VI, Polevaia EB. Stimulation of the immunological reactivity of cancer patients by eleutherococcus extract. *Vopor Onkol*, 1986;32(7):21–26 [in Russian].

50. el-Mekkawy S, Meselhy MR, Nakamura N, Tezuka Y, Hattori M, Kakiuchi N, Shimotohno K, Kawahata T, Otake T. Anti-HIV-1 and anti-HIV-1-protease substances from *Ganoderma lucidum*. *Phytochemistry*, 1998;49(6):1651–1657.

51. Min BS, Nakamura N, Miyashiro H, Bae KW, Hattori M. Triterpenes from the spores of *Ganoderma lucidum* and their inhibitory activity against HIV-1 protease. *Chem Pharm Bull (Tokyo)*, 1998;46(10):1607–1612.

52. Gordon M, Bihari B, Goosby E, et al. A placebo-controlled trial of the immune modulator, lentinan, in HIV-positive patients: a phase I/II trial. *J Med*, 1998;29(5–6):305–330.

53. Nanba H, Kodama N, Schar D, Turner D. Effects of Maitake (*Grifola frondosa*) glucan in HIV-infected patients. *Mycoscience*, 2000; 41:293–295.

54. Lin CY, Ku FM, Kuo YC, Chen CF, Chen WP, Chen A, Shiao MS. Inhibition of activated human mesangial cell proliferation by the natural product of *Cordyceps sinensis* (H1-A): an implication for treatment of IgA mesangial nephropathy. *J Lab Clin Med*, 1999;133(1):55–63.

55. Yang LY, Chen A, Kuo YC, Lin CY. Efficacy of a pure compound H1-A extracted from *Cordyceps sinensis* on autoimmune disease of MRL lpr/lpr mice. *J Lab Clin Med*, 1999;134(5):492–500.

56. de la Taille A, Hayek OR, Burchardt M, Burchardt T, Katz AE. Role of herbal compounds (PC-SPES) in hormone-refractory prostate cancer: two case reports. *J Altern Complement Med*, 2000;6(5):449–451.

57. Levy AM, Kita H, Phillips SF, Schkade PA, Dyer PD, Gleich GJ, Dubravec VA. Eosinophilia and gastrointestinal symptoms after ingestion of shiitake mushrooms. *J Allergy Clin Immunol*, 1998;101(5):613–620.

58. Murakami M et al. Decreased pulmonary perfusion in hypersensitivity pneumonitis caused by Shiitake mushroom spores. *J Intern Med*, 1997;241(1):85–88.

59. Matsui S et al. Hypersensitivity pneumonitis induced by Shiitake mushroom spores. *Intern Med*, 1992;31(10):1204–1206.
60. Nakamura T. Shiitake (*Lentinus edodes*) dermatitis. *Contact Dermatitis*, 1992;27(2):65–70.
61. Ueda A et al. Allergic contact dermatitis in shiitake (*Lentinus edodes* (Berk) Sing) growers. *Contact Dermatitis*, 1992;26(4):228–233.
62. Beta-glucan monograph. Stockton, CA: Natural Medicines Comprehensive Database; 1995–2002: posted at http://wwww.naturaldatabase.com/monograph.asp?mono_id=1041&hilite=1

CASE STUDY

Ellyn Silverman and Paul J. Cimoch

This patient is a 27-year-old Caucasian heterosexual male who was diagnosed with the AIDS after presenting with *Pneumocystis carinii* pneumonia (PCP) in the summer of 2002. Patient had been very healthy and doing well until the summer of 2002, when he developed respiratory symptoms. He was treated with several courses of antibiotics as an outpatient without any improvement. He subsequently started having high fevers, weight loss, malaise, and shortness of breath. Chest x-ray revealed bilateral pneumonia and patient was hospitalized. Patient identified as having PCP and was treated with IV Bactrim. After a hospitalization during which he almost required intubation and mechanical ventilation, the patient was able to be discharged after 3 weeks. Initial immune system parameters revealed a CD4$^+$ T-helper lymphocyte count of 10 cells/mm^3 with a viral load greater than 750,000 copies/ml. Patient is 6′ tall and his usual body weight was 176 lb. Upon admission he weighed 160 lb and before discharge from the hospital he weighed 152 lb. Before becoming our patient, he was taking a multivitamin, vitamin C and vitamin E supplementation. He was started on antiretroviral therapy during his hospitalization with Combivir and Sustiva.

Patient was subsequently seen at the Center for Special Immunology (CSI) after his acute care hospitalization. He was still on high doses of oral Bactrim and his antiviral agents. He was complaining of severe fatigue, malaise, anorexia, and occasional nausea. We stopped his antiviral agents because of his symptomatology and treated him with antiemetics. Initial evaluation by the Registered Dietitian revealed a caloric intake of about 1200 kcal/day with a total protein intake of about 55 g. Initial bioelectric impedance analysis (BIA) revealed a body cell mass (BCM) of 36% of his weight with a body fat (BF) of 15% and a body mass index (BMI) of 19.7. With the help of the dietitian, the patient was started on a high calorie, high protein, small frequent meals diet in addition to using Marinol for appetite stimulation and nausea. Micronutrient and antioxidant assessments were performed through a SpectraCell laboratory analysis and hormonal levels were checked.

Indeed, the patient was subsequently found to have hypogonadism. He was immediately started on testosterone replacement therapy with AndroGel topically twice a day. His SpectraCell nutrient analysis revealed deficiencies of folate, B-12, calcium, and the antioxidants Co-Q10, selenium and glutathione. Total antioxidant function (TAF) was 36% (normally greater than 75%). The patient was started on oral supplementation with a broad-spectrum multivitamin (with enhanced B-vitamin levels), *N*-acetylcysteine (NAC), alpha-lipoic acid, and Co-Q10.

With these interventions the patient started to feel better and immediately gained back 9 lb within the first 6 weeks. BIA at that time revealed a BCM of 38% of his body weight with a BF of 16%. Caloric intake had improved by 3-day diet analysis to 2800 kcal/day with a protein intake of 126 g/day.

After completing an extended course of antibiotic therapy for his PCP and finally having a clear chest x-ray, he was restarted on antiretroviral therapy with Trizivir and Kaletra. He tolerated this therapy reasonably well with some initial nausea, headaches, loose stools, and malaise, although these symptoms gradually abated over 2 to 4 weeks. Viral load a month after being on antiviral therapy had dropped to 36,000 copies/ml and after 2 months was down to 2600 copies/ml. CD4$^+$ T-lymphocyte counts, however, had only improved to 29 cells/mm^3.

We continued to follow the patient monthly with frequent reassessments by the Registered Dietitian. He was instituted on a progressive exercise program and referred to physical therapy for strengthening and conditioning. After 6 months of interventions, patient's weight was up to 173 lb, although his BCM was only 39% of his body weight. Total and free testosterone levels were physiologic. At this time we instituted an anabolic cycle with the oral agent Oxandrin, 10 mg twice a day for 16 weeks. During this time, the patient gained 9 lb of BCM and his BIA showed his BCM to be 43% of his body weight and his BMI had increased to 24.12.

Despite oral micronutrients and antioxidants, a repeat SpectraCell analysis after 6 months on supplement therapy continued to show a low TAF at 40%. As such, he was administered weekly infusions of glutathione (100 mg), alpha lipoic acid (100 mg), and selenium (200 mcg). After weekly infusions for a month, and then monthly infusions for 5 months, patient's repeat SpectraCell analysis showed a TAF of 72% and correction of his other micronutrient deficiencies. His BCM was maintained off the anabolic agents and clinically he was feeling extremely well with good energy, vitality, and well-being.

Immune system assessments after 9 months showed a viral load, which was below the limits of detection (less than 50 copies/mg) with a CD4$^+$ T-lymphocyte count of 92 cells/mm.^{3} He continues to tolerate the antiviral therapy well and continues with a three times per week exercise program in addition to being monitored by the Registered Dietitian every 3 months.

16 Renal Nutrition

Margaret Furtado and Carlos DaSilva

CONTENTS

INTRODUCTION

In order to appreciate the paramount importance of nutritional issues in the management of renal patients, we will start with a brief overview of renal physiology.

The kidneys are two bean-shaped small organs, about 4 in. (10 cm) long and about 2.5 in. (6.4 cm) wide located near the vertebral column at the small of the back. The left kidney lies a little higher than the right kidney (see Figure 16.1). The kidneys are responsible for the near constant composition of internal body fluids in spite of wide variations of solute and fluid intake among different individuals or same individuals in different circumstances. This is a function essential to life that permits enzymatic processes, neural impulses, cardiac contractility and electric impulses, blood pressure control, and tissue perfusion to proceed unabated in spite of climatic variations and environmental challenges.

REVIEW OF NORMAL RENAL PHYSIOLOGY

Receiving about 20% of the cardiac output and endocrine/paracrine regulation by a myriad of hormones and autacoids, the kidneys are responsible for the constancy of the internal environment (see Figure 16.2).

SODIUM AND WATER

The control of the extracellular volume and blood pressure levels depend on the ability of healthy kidneys to regulate total body water and sodium through the effects of hormones and hemodynamic variations imposed by changes in sodium balance. For example, if a large, sudden increase in salt intake is maintained there will be an initial positive balance of sodium and water that will trigger hormonal changes (e.g., suppression of renin, angiotensin, and aldosterone, increase in atrial natriuretic peptide) and hemodynamic changes with mild volume expansion with increased natriuresis. This will ensure subsequent achievement of a new steady state when excretion matches the intake after a few days. This mild volume expansion is usually not noticeable, but in some individuals, may be associated with development of hypertension (salt-sensitive subjects) through an initially elevated cardiac output

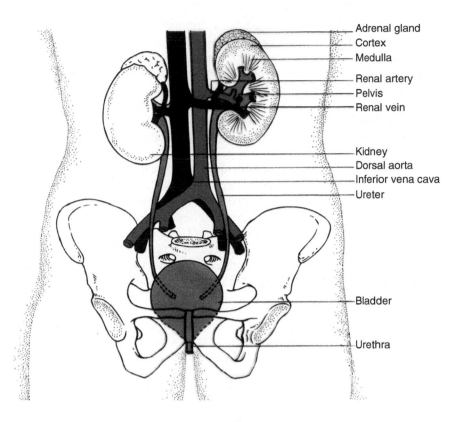

FIGURE 16.1 Anatomy of the Kidneys.

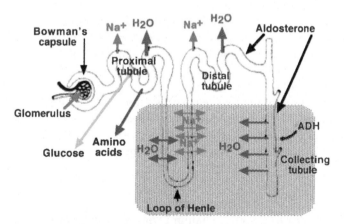

FIGURE 16.2 Overview of physiology of fluid and electrolyte balance in the kidneys.

and subsequent persistent elevation of peripheral vascular resistance. The converse is true for salt restriction in the diet, with initial negative balance of sodium and water, and subsequent achievement of a new steady state mediated through hormonal and hemodynamic adaptations. This leads to the correction of hypertension in salt-sensitive subjects.[1]

The reason that sodium and water are so interconnected has to do with the fact that sodium is the major extracellular cation and changes in sodium concentration have a transient impact on serum osmolality, sensed by osmoreceptors in the hypothalamus; and effective circulating volume, as sensed by baroreceptors in the central circulation and the juxtaglomerular apparatus in the kidneys.

When faced with increased osmolality, the osmoreceptors increase the release of antidiuretic hormone (ADH) and hypothalamic receptors trigger increased thirst sensation, thus enhancing free water retention by the kidneys and correction of serum osmolality. This mild volume expansion will suppress aldosterone, renin, angiotensin, and stimulate release of atrial natriuretic peptide with gradual increase in the sodium excretion to achieve neutral balance. In other words, if salt intake is increased, the result is volume expansion and not hypernatremia. If severe salt restriction is achieved, or salt losses occur (e.g., by the use of potent loop diuretics) the result is volume depletion and usually not hyponatremia.

Potassium

The renal regulation of potassium excretion is so efficient that it is almost impossible to produce hyperkalemia by increasing oral intake in the presence of healthy kidneys. Even large increases in potassium intake can be handled by normally functioning kidneys. Increased potassium excretion due to a multifaceted response will ensue. Elevated aldosterone levels, increased delivery of sodium to distal parts of the nephron, and increased number and function of Na,K-ATPases in the basolateral membranes of collecting duct cells, as well as increase in basolateral membrane surface, termed potassium adaptation, will increase the capacity of renal potassium excretion enormously.[2]

The kidneys are not as efficient in conserving potassium. When faced with severe potassium restriction or gastrointestinal (GI) losses, hypokalemia may ensue before maximum potassium retention is achieved by the kidneys.

The development of hyperkalemia in the setting of acute or advanced chronic renal failure (CRF) can be life-threatening. It affects the resting electric potential of the myocardial cells, and predisposes one to the development of fatal arrhythmias. This is a frequent indication for emergent hemodialysis (HD) and the reason for potassium restriction when diseased kidneys cannot provide neutral potassium balance.

Hypokalemia can ensue in the first few weeks after starting diuretic therapy.[3] Potassium levels should be monitored and supplementation or addition of potassium-sparing diuretics added to the medical regimen, especially in patients with poor oral intake and using digitalis preparations, because hypokalemia predisposes to digitalis toxicity.

Calcium, Phosphorus, and Bones

The 1-hydroxylation step of 1,25 (OH) vitamin D happens in the proximal tubular cells and is impaired with renal parenchymal damage and inhibited by hyperphosphatemia. The active 1,25 (OH) vitamin D is an inhibitory factor for parathyroid hormone (PTH) release while hypocalcemia and hyperphosphatemia are direct stimuli for parathyroid cells to release PTH.

Failing kidneys with decreased glomerular filtration rate (GFR) lead to phosphate retention. Increase in serum phosphate will determine an elevated calcium and phosphorus product and deposition of calcium in bones and soft tissues with detrimental health effects.[4]

Hypocalcemia, hyperphosphatemia, and vitamin D deficiency act in concert in the genesis of secondary hyperparathyroidism due to renal insufficiency,[5] and a phosphate-restricted diet and phosphate binders are used in patients with renal failure to prevent this type of osteodystrophy.

ACID–BASE BALANCE

Through the reabsorption of filtered bicarbonate and reclamation of bicarbonate used to buffer endogenous acid formation during metabolism, the kidneys play a very important part in the maintenance of acid–base equilibrium. The net acid excretion should be equal to the acid load generated by the metabolism, and depends on the ammoniagenesis by proximal tubular cells and proton pump function in the distal parts of the nephron. Both of these processes are impaired with the progression of kidney disease. Consumption of endogenous bone buffers to counteract the acid accumulation seen with failing renal function compounds the problem, and accounts for stunted growth in children and worse osteodystrophy in adults.[8]

It is good practice during pre-chronic kidney disease (CKD) care to monitor bicarbonate levels and replace base equivalents to maintain levels between 20 and 22 meq/l.[8] Sodium bicarbonate salts can be used for this aim. Previous concerns that increased sodium load would cause worsening hypertension or edema have not been confirmed. It seems that sodium bicarbonate behaves differently from sodium chloride in this respect. Citrate as a base equivalent should be used cautiously because it increases aluminum absorption and accumulation with decreased renal function.[9,10]

METABOLIC IMPACT OF AZOTEMIA

The uremic milieu is blamed for many of the signs and symptoms observed in patients with advanced renal insufficiency. It is thought that a constellation of different toxins is responsible for these effects.[11] Urea can be one of these toxins, which can be used as a marker, but does not explain all of the deleterious effects of azotemia.

The phagocytic activity of white blood cells, the antibody production after antigenic challenge and integrity of integument are subnormal or impaired in patients with CKD. Therefore, susceptibility to infections is increased, and the ability to fight infections is compromised.

There is increased protein catabolism, which is accentuated by chronic metabolic acidosis and poor oral intake. Susceptibility to hyper- and hypoglycemia increases due to insulin resistance and increased half-life of both oral hypoglycemic agents and insulin, which is commonly seen with decreased renal function. Accelerated atherosclerosis is seen due to frequent association with hypertension and dyslipidemia; retention of homocysteine[12,13] and increased levels of asymmetrical dimethylarginine (ADMA),[14] and increased inflammation. The advanced age of patients with advanced kidney disease and prolonged periods of azotemia also play a role.

COMMON CAUSES OF CHRONIC RENAL FAILURE

In simple terms, renal diseases can be classified as predominantly glomerular, tubulo-interstitial, vascular, or affecting the collecting system. Most of these diseases can be further classified as secondary, when a systemic disease or exposure is known to be causal, or as primary, when the proximate factors that caused the pathologic findings are currently unknown.

GLOMERULAR DISEASES

By far, the most common secondary form of glomerular disease is diabetic nephrosclerosis, also known as Kimmestiel–Wilson glomerulosclerosis. Other forms of secondary glomerular disease include postinfectious glomerulonephritis, systemic lupus erythematosus (SLE), amyloidosis, hepatitis C-related cryoglobulinemia, and membrano-proliferative glomerulonephritis.[16] IgA nephropathy is the most common form of glomerulonephritis worldwide. At the present time, its etiology is unknown, but the pathogenesis may be related to abnormal glycosylation of IgA molecules that deposit in the glomerular mesangium. Ongoing studies to assess the role of fish oil for therapy of this disease should help to clarify controversial results obtained in different studies.

Other examples of secondary glomerular diseases include membranous nephropathy and minimal changes disease. These may be associated with solid tumors and Hodgkin's lymphoma, respectively. Human immunodeficiency virus (HIV) nephropathy, and other forms of focal and segmental glomerulosclerosis, are common in African Americans, and are a frequent cause of end-stage renal disease (ESRD) in urban centers.

TUBULO-INTERSTITIAL DISEASES

This type of kidney lesion may be acute, such as an allergic reaction to beta lactamic antibiotics like nafcillin or chronic, such as a consequence of lead exposure (saturnine gout), chronic lithium exposure, analgesic nephropathy, and immune-mediated diseases like Sjogren's syndrome and sarcoidosis.

Ingestion of Chinese herbal tea as part of a slimming regimen may cause chronic interstitial nephritis. Aristolochic acid has been proposed as the possible component of Chinese herbal tea that caused hundreds of cases of ESRD and urothelial cancers in Belgium during the last decade.[17,18]

Chronic pyelonephritis due to reflux or urinary diversion procedures may also evolve into chronic interstitial nephritis and eventual progressive loss of renal function.

Genetic diseases that affect the tubules as well as the interstitium include adult polycystic kidney disease, Fabry's disease, and primary hyperoxaluria.

VASCULAR DISEASES

This is an important group of kidney diseases that may be divided into large vessel disease, usually atherosclerotic vascular disease, and small vessel diseases, including vasculitis-like antineutrophil cytoplasmic antibody (ANCA)-associated glomerulonephritis, SLE, and vaso-occlusive diseases such as scleroderma, accelerated hypertension, cholesterol atheroemboli, antiphospholipid antibody syndrome, and sickle cell disease.

The combination of abdominal obesity, dyslipidemia, insulin resistance, and hypertension has been termed "Syndrome X"[19] and is related to accelerated coronary artery disease and atherosclerosis. The increase in the aging population in the Unites States has resulted in an increase in survivors of vascular events (e.g., acute myocardial infarction and strokes), but late development of ischemic nephropathy with inexorable progression to ESRD. Aggressive lipid management, increased physical activity and weight loss, associated with tight control of blood pressure, may help to curb the prevalence of Syndrome X.

COLLECTING SYSTEM DISEASE

Intrarenal and extrarenal obstruction are often preventable or treatable causes of renal failure. Intrarenal tubular obstruction by crystals is seen with high doses of sulfonamide, indinavir, or uric acid in the tumor lysis syndrome.

Extrarenal obstruction is more often caused by calculi. However, fragments of a necrotic papilla, clots or retroperitoneal fibrosis, are alternative reasons for decline in renal function due to "postrenal" or obstructive factors.

TABLE 16.1
Stages of Chronic Kidney Disease

Stage	Description	GFR (ml/min/1.73 m^2)
1	Kidney damage with normal of ↑ GFR	≥90
2	Kidney damage with mild ↓ GFR	60–89
3	Moderate ↓ GFR	30–59
4	Severe ↓ GFR	15–29
5	Kidney failure	<15 (or dialysis)

Chronic kidney disease is defined as either kidney damage or GFR <60 ml/min/1.73 m^2 for ≥3 months. Kidney damage is defined as pathologic abnormalities or markers of damage, including abnormalities in blood or urine tests or imaging studies.

DEFINITION AND CLASSIFICATION OF STAGES OF CHRONIC KIDNEY DISEASE

CKD is a major public health problem. Improving outcomes for people with CKD requires a coordinated worldwide approach to prevention of adverse outcomes through defining the disease and its outcomes, estimating disease prevalence, identifying earlier stages of disease and antecedent risk factors, and detection and treatment for populations at risk for adverse outcomes.[20]

The presence of CKD should be established, based on the presence of kidney damage and level of kidney function (GFR), irrespective of diagnosis. Among patients with CKD, the stage of disease should be assigned based on the level of kidney function, according to the K/DOQI CKD classification (see Table 16.1).[20]

Identifying the presence and stage of CKD in an individual is not a substitute for accurate assessment of the cause of kidney disease, extent of kidney damage, level of kidney function, comorbid conditions, complications of decreased kidney function, or risks for loss of kidney function or cardiovascular disease in that patient. Defining stages of CKD requires "categorization" of continuous measures of kidney function, and the "cut-off levels" between stages are inherently arbitrary. Nonetheless, staging of CKD will facilitate application of clinical practice guidelines, clinical performance measures, and quality improvement efforts to the evaluation and management of CKD.[20]

ACUTE RENAL FAILURE

CAUSES AND CLINICAL SCENARIOS

Acute renal failure (ARF) may be caused by trauma, dehydration, exogenous nephrotoxins, shock resulting in ischemia, and sepsis. Acute tubular necrosis (ATN), also known as acute intrinsic renal failure, is the major cause of ARF.[15] Patients developing ARF as a result of critical illness, sepsis, or major trauma may be at especially high nutritional risk, since they may have an accelerated rate of protein degradation, resulting in lean body mass losses. Deleterious effects of this process may include poor wound healing and increased infection and mortality rates. The principles of nutritional therapy for ARF patients are similar to those for patients with other catabolic clinical states. However, the multiple metabolic consequences of acute uremia must be considered when an ARF patient requires nutritional support. These not only affect fluid, electrolyte, and acid–base balance, but also the metabolism of amino acids, proteins, carbohydrates, and lipids.[15]

NUTRITIONAL NEEDS

Protein

The recommended protein intake for patients with ARF is 0.6 g/kg/day, for the nondialyzed, nonhypercatabolic patient whose GFR falls to less than 10 ml/min.[16] Those ARF patients on HD should increase protein intake to 1.2 g/kg/day, with at least 50% coming from high biological value (HBV) protein. Patients undergoing peritoneal dialysis (PD) should receive 1.2 to 1.3 g/kg/day of protein, with at least 50% as HBV protein.[20]

Calories

Caloric requirements for ARF patients may vary, although the usual recommendation is for 35 kcal/kg/day, depending on the degree of hypermetabolism present.[20] Nausea, anorexia, or poor compliance with an oral diet may warrant enteral tube feeding therapy. Those patients with a malfunctioning GI tract may require parenteral nutrition.

Vitamins and Minerals

It is imperative to monitor serum electrolytes closely in all ARF patients. Serum potassium and phosphate levels are often elevated, at least initially, and serum sodium may be lowered in nondialyzed patients with compromised urinary output (oliguria) and hypotonic fluid intake. Those patients with ATN, the major cause of ARF, may experience salt and water overload during the oliguric phase. There may be salt and water depletion during the diuretic or recovery phase of the disease. The oliguric or anuric patient undergoing HD may still require a sodium restriction of 2000 to 3000 mg/day and a potassium restriction of 1500 to 3000 mg/day.[20]

Fluids

Fluid recommendations for ARF patients with compromised urinary output (e.g., oliguria) should be based upon urinary output plus the addition of 500 ml fluid (approximate) to replace estimated insensible losses. Additional fluid may need to be added for those patients with fever, diarrhea, or other conditions, resulting in increased fluid losses. It is recommended that anuric patients be allowed a baseline fluid goal of 1000 ml/day if receiving HD therapy 3 days/week.[20,21]

NUTRITIONAL NEEDS AND MANAGEMENT OF PRE-CHRONIC KIDNEY DISEASE PATIENTS (NOT ON DIALYSIS)

PROTEIN

For individuals who have CRF, which is characterized by a GFR < 25 ml/min, who are not undergoing dialysis, the institution of a low-protein diet, providing 0.60 g protein/kg/day should be considered.[20,22] For those who will not or cannot accept such a rigid restriction, or if unable to maintain an adequate energy intake with this level, an intake of up to 0.75 g protein/kg/day may be prescribed. At least 50% of protein ingested should be of HBV protein.[22]

Evidence suggests that dietary protein restriction can slow the rate of progression of renal failure and the time until end-stage renal failure.[24,25] In addition, low-protein diets may ameliorate uremic symptoms and some of its metabolic complications.[25,26]

CALORIES

The recommended dietary energy intake for individuals with CRF who are not undergoing dialysis is 35 kcal/kg/day for those younger than 60 years of age, and 30 to 35 kcal/kg/day for those individuals 60 years of age and older.[22]

FAT

Since CRF patients may be consuming significantly less protein than that recommended for dialysis patients, additional fat may be necessary in order to provide adequate calories. If the patient does not present with hyperlipidemia, fat calories can be increased, particularly adding monounsaturated fats.[20] Lipid profiles (cholesterol, low-density lipoprotein [LDL], high-density lipoprotein [HDL], triglyceride) should be monitored regularly.

SODIUM

Renal sodium excretion falls with the progression of renal failure. Sodium intake may need to be limited in order to prevent sodium retention, edema, hypertension, and congestive heart failure. The diet may need to be restricted to 2000 to 3000 mg sodium/day.[20]

POTASSIUM

A dietary potassium restriction is often necessary, since the kidneys usually diminish their capacity to excrete excess potassium. High potassium foods are often discouraged at this stage (see Table 16.2) while low potassium foods are generally not restricted (see Table 16.3).

CALCIUM AND PHOSPHORUS

Among patients with CRF, restriction of dietary phosphorus is often recommended, since the kidney is the major organ for maintaining phosphorus homeostasis. A phosphorus restriction between 800 and 1200 mg/day is usually recommended for patients displaying evidence of hyperphosphatemia (see Table 16.4).[20]

FLUIDS

Fluid balance may be evidenced if the urinary output equals the daily fluid intake. If the patient becomes fluid-overloaded or edematous, a fluid restriction or the initiation of a loop diuretic agent or both may be necessary. It is usually necessary to use larger doses of loop diuretics to obtain the same effect in patients with impaired renal function.[20]

VITAMINS AND IRON

CRF patients may need to supplement their diet due to protein and mineral restrictions. Renal formulations of vitamins, which provide specific levels of B-complex vitamins and ascorbic acid, may be ideal to meet the patient's needs without the risks of fat-soluble vitamin toxicity (e.g., vitamin A toxicity). The kidney's progressive inability to convert vitamin D into its active form may necessitate the prescription of vitamin D in its active form or a vitamin D analog. Patients receiving erythropoietin (EPO) therapy for anemia often require iron supplementation.[20,22]

TABLE 16.2
High Potassium Fruits and Vegetables

High Potassium Vegetables	High Potassium Fruits
Artichokes	Apricots
Asparagus	Avocados
Bamboo shoots	Bananas
Beans (kidney, lima, pinto, navy)	Cantaloupes
Broccoli	Dates
Chard, swiss	Dried fruits
Greens	Figs
Kohlrabi	Honeydew melon
Mushrooms	Mangos
Parsnips	Nectarines
Potatoes	Oranges
Spinach	Papayas
Squash (acorn, butternut)	Passion fruit
Sweet potatoes	Plantains
Pumpkin	Prunes
Tomatoes (juice also)	Raisins

Note: Although potatoes are high in potassium, they may be allowed on low potassium diets if soaked properly. The potatoes must be peeled, diced into small pieces, and soaked in a large amount of water for 4 h or more (50% or more potassium is removed).

TABLE 16.3
Low Potassium Fruits and Vegetables

Low Potassium Vegetables	Low Potassium Fruits
Bean sprouts	Apples, applesauce
Cabbage	Blackberries
Cauliflower	Blueberries
Corn	Cranberries
Cucumbers	Fruit cocktail
Green beans	Grapes
Eggplant	Lemon
Escarole	Lime
Green peppers	Pears
Kale	Persimmon
Lettuce	Raspberries
Mustard greens	Strawberries
Onions	Tangerines
Radishes	Watermelon
Zucchini	

TABLE 16.4
High and Low Phosphorus Foods

High Phosphorus Foods	Low Phosphorus Foods
Beans (all except green)	Bagel (white)
Bran	Bread (French)
Cheese, hard varieties	Bread (pita, white, Italian)
Chocolate	Cheese, cream
Ice cream	Egg white
Ice milk	Farina
Lentils	Gelatin
Milk (all varieties)	Pasta (white)
Pasta (wheat)	Popcorn
Peas, dried	Pretzels
Peanuts	Rice, white
Peanut butter	Rice milk
Soybeans	Sherbet
Tofu	Sorbet
Walnuts	Sour cream
Wheat flour	Sprite
Yogurt	Sugar

Note: High protein foods, such as meats, poultry, fish, seafood, are generally high in phosphorus, but are encouraged (within recommended guidelines) due to HBV protein and importance of adequate protein in the diet.

CHRONIC RENAL FAILURE

HEMODIALYSIS AND NUTRITION

Numerous studies have documented that 20 to 60% of HD patients are malnourished.[21,23–25] The etiology of malnutrition in dialysis patients is multifactorial. Evidence appears to indicate that toxins that accumulate with renal failure suppress appetite and contribute to nutritional decline once patients are on maintenance dialysis.[25,26]

Uremic patients have a reduction in their food intake that starts in the pre-CKD period and correlates with the decline in GFR. Chronic inflammation, which contributes to malnutrition, is associated with suboptimal dietary intake. Experimental studies have shown that chronic inflammation impairs the synthesis of albumin, which is one of the most powerful prognostic indicators of morbidity and mortality in dialysis patients.[24,25] Recent epidemiologic studies have suggested that both increased serum levels of leptin and inflammation may reduce nutrient intake and contribute to the development of protein energy malnutrition.[25,26] Leptin is a peptide hormone produced by the "ob" gene of the adipocytes, may regulate satiety and eating behaviors.[27] An inappropriate elevation of circulatory leptin has been found in uremic patients due to decreased plasma clearance.[27] It has been speculated that this event may be one factor that mediates anorexia and wasting in the CRF population.[26,27]

Nutritional Needs for Chronic Kidney Disease Patients on Hemodialysis

Protein
The recommended dietary protein intake (DPI) for clinically stable maintenance HD patients is 1.2 g/kg/day. At least 50% of the dietary protein should be of HBV.[22]

Calories

The recommended daily energy intake for maintenance HD patients is 35 kcal/kg/day for those who are less than 60 years or age, and 30 to 35 kcal/kg/day for individuals 60 years or older. Since older age may be associated with reduced physical activity and lean body mass, a daily energy intake of 30 to 35 kcal/kg/day for older patients with more sedentary lifestyles has been suggested.[22]

Fats

Patients with CKD may be at higher risk for hyperlipidemia, in part due to dysfunction of lipoprotein lipase, resulting in increased LDL and triglyceride levels, while HDL levels may be normal or low.[24] Nutrition education of these patients often involves counseling regarding low-fat, low-cholesterol diet plans, which simultaneously allow for recommended protein and caloric needs. Lipid-lowering agents may be necessary if diet alone cannot normalize the patient's lipid profile.

Sodium and Fluid

HD patients are often advised to restrict sodium to 2000 to 3000 mg/day, with a fluid allowance of 1000 ml/day plus the amount of urinary output (often estimated to be 500 ml/day). Excessive ingestion of sodium may increase thirst and the risk for pulmonary edema and congestive heart failure. HD patients with excessive weight gains between treatments may need to further restrict sodium and fluid intake.[20]

Potassium

Potassium recommendations may vary, but a general recommendation is for daily levels in the diet ranging from 1500 to 3000 mg/day.[20] Potassium intake should be individualized to maintain normal serum potassium levels between 3.5 and 6.0 meq/l (predialysis levels). Patients on HD are often asked to avoid high potassium foods (see Table 16.2) in order to lower the risk for hyperkalemia.

Calcium and Phosphorus

Phosphorous excretion decreases as renal function deteriorates. Unfortunately, dialysis only removes approximately 1000 mg of phosphorus per treatment, which is insufficient to control serum phosphorus levels for most maintenance HD patients. Therefore, it is imperative that these patients monitor phosphorus intake in their diet by limiting high phosphorus foods (see Table 16.2). In addition, most patients on HD require the addition of a phosphorus binder, such as calcium or non-calcium-based binders. The goal of nutritional therapy is to achieve and maintain a serum phosphorus level of approximately 3.5 to 5.5 mg/dl.[20,22]

Vitamins and Iron

HD patients generally receive supplementation of folic acid (1 mg/day), pyridoxine (10 mg/day), the dietary reference intake (DRI) for other B-complex vitamins, and ascorbic acid (60 to 100 mg/day) due to probable existing dietary deficiencies of these vitamins and losses occurring during the dialysis treatment.[20] Maintenance HD patients may also require supplements containing the active form of vitamin D, which can be administered either orally or parenterally. Within the past decade, vitamin D analogs which may result in less phosphorus and calcium absorption than calcitriol have been developed. The emergence of these analogs (e.g., doxercalciferol and paricalcitol) may allow for better control of hyperparathyroidism with fewer deleterious effects resulting from hyperphosphatemia and hypercalcemia.[22] Iron supplements for patients on HD usually are necessary if they are also receiving EPO therapy for anemia.

PERITONEAL DIALYSIS AND NUTRITION

Protein

The recommended DPI for clinically stable PD patients is 1.2 to 1.3 g/kg/day, with at least 50% of the dietary protein of HBV. Protein losses into peritoneal dialysate are almost invariably higher than those seen during HD, averaging approximately 5 to 15 g/24 h. During episodes of peritonitis, dialysate protein losses may be considerably higher.[22]

Calories

The recommended daily energy intake for maintenance PD patients is 35 kcal/kg/day for individuals less than 60 years of age, and 30 to 35 kcal/kg/day for individuals 60 years of age or older.[22]

Fats

PD patients, along with HD patients, have a higher incidence of hyperlipidemia. In addition, PD patients may be at higher risk for hypertriglyceridemia due to constant infusions of dextrose into the peritoneal cavity.

Sodium and Fluid

Since most PD patients perform their treatments daily, sodium and fluid allowances are usually quite liberal. In general, sodium recommendations may be approximately 3000 to 4000 mg/day.[20] Fluid allowance is often suggested to range between 2000 and 2500 ml/day, plus 500 ml/day for insensible losses.[20] Patients with good residual renal function and on diuretic therapy with increased urinary output, may not need to limit fluid intake while on daily PD therapy.

Potassium

Patients on PD are often capable of maintaining normal serum potassium levels without a potassium restriction, since daily PD treatments remove a significant amount of potassium. A potassium supplement may be necessary.

Mineral Needs for Peritoneal Dialysis Patients

Calcium and Phosphorus
Because PD, like HD, only removes a relatively small amount of phosphorus, PD patients must also control their calcium and phosphorus levels via the use of phosphorus binders and low phosphorus diets.

Vitamins and Iron
Vitamin and iron needs for PD patients are similar to those for HD patients. As with HD patients, vitamin A (retinol) should be avoided, since the serum concentration is elevated (hypervitaminosis A). This is due to increased levels of retinol-binding protein, which in turn is catabolized by the kidney. Vitamin C should be restricted to 100 to 150 mg/day, since higher doses can lead to the accumulation of oxalate.[20]

TRANSPLANTATION AND NUTRITION

Nutritional Needs

Protein
The recommended daily protein intake for transplanted patients may vary, but the general goal is between 1.3 and 2.0 g/kg/day. Various factors, such as stress, metabolic needs, graft function, and physical activity may determine which end of the protein range patients may fall within. High doses of corticosteroids and the stress of surgery may precipitate protein catabolism.[20]

Calories
The recommended caloric intake for renal transplant patients is 30 to 35 kcal/kg/day, based on dry weight or usual body weight (UBW).[20,22] Sufficient calories, in addition to adequate protein intake, are imperative in the postoperative period, where wound healing is promoted. In addition, the patient's body is fighting organ rejection, infection, and other possible insults, all of which may increase energy needs. However, since increasing appetite is commonly seen with corticosteroid therapy, weight maintenance, once the patient is at a desirable weight, is the long-term goal.

Carbohydrates
A restricted-carbohydrate diet may be necessary, since high-dose corticosteroid therapy may result in hyperglycemia. Those patients who develop diabetes or glucose intolerance may require a calorie-restricted diet in order to better reach and maintain a desirable body weight.

Fat
Immunosuppressive therapy, as well as obesity, may precipitate or exacerbate hyperlipidemia, often seen after renal transplantation. Many patients may benefit from a low-fat, low-cholesterol diet in order to decrease the risks of hyperlipidemia. A lipid-lowering agent may be necessary.

Sodium and Fluid
The particular level of sodium restriction must be individualized. Most renal transplant patients, provided they do not present with edema or hypertension, may enjoy a more liberal sodium intake. If the patient has significant edema postoperatively, then sodium intake may be restricted to approximately 2000 mg/day.[20] In general, a fluid restriction is not necessary, unless ATN or rejection of the transplanted kidney occurs.

Potassium
The use of calcineurin inhibitors (cyclosporine, tacrolimus) may result in hyperkalemia, and may warrant a potassium restriction, even among those patients with good function from the transplanted kidney. Rejection of the kidney or ATN may necessitate a potassium restriction.[20]

Calcium and Phosphorus
If the transplanted kidney is functioning well, neither dietary phosphorus nor phosphorus binders are needed. In fact, low phosphorus levels may be seen due to increased phosphorus excretion and bone uptake. Therefore, a high-phosphorus diet or phosphorus supplementation or both may be necessary for some posttransplant patients. Since corticosteroid therapy interferes with calcium absorption, the use of calcium supplements may be necessary.[20]

Vitamins and Iron

The posttransplant patient may continue on renal vitamins, at least temporarily, especially if dietary restrictions are imposed in order to treat rejection or ATN. Iron therapy may also be needed if EPO administration is needed to treat anemia.

Table 16.5 provides a summary of the nutrition management recommendations for patients requiring dialysis and not.

NEPHROTIC SYNDROME

This syndrome may have many etiologies, and is characterized by the presence of large quantities of protein (>3.0 to 3.5 g/day) in the urine. In all of these cases, however, this proteinuria is due to damage to the glomerular basement membrane, which results in its increased permeability to protein. Individuals with nephrotic syndrome often present with poor appetite, muscle wasting, and protein malnutrition secondary to these large protein losses. This syndrome (when it is linked with a decrease in serum albumin resulting in decreased plasma oncotic pressure) is also characterized by edema or swelling. It is very common, among these patients, to see either elevations in serum cholesterol or triglycerides (or both). A high-protein diet may worsen albumin excretion through the damage of the glomerular membrane. Therefore, a moderate protein restriction (0.8 to 1.0 g/kg/day) is recommended early in the diagnosis of nephrotic syndrome.[20,22] This restriction may reduce the amino acid load to the glomerulus, perhaps diminishing the quantity of albumin crossing the damaged glomerular membrane.[20] Caloric needs for weight maintenance are estimated to be 35 kcal/kg/day. Because these patients are often edematous, dry weight should be used for this calculation. Controlling edema through sodium restriction (often prescribed 2000 mg/day) and appropriate use of diuretic therapy are essential in the management of nephrotic syndrome.[16]

NEPHROLITHIASIS (KIDNEY STONES)

Among patients with kidney stones, the goal of nutrition therapy is to eliminate the diet-related risk factors for stone formation, and to prevent the growth of existing stones. First, and most importantly, a high fluid intake is an essential component of diet therapy for patients with nephrolithiasis.[20] An increase in daily urine output to 2 liters or more is needed to maintain dilute urine and reduce the concentration of stone-forming substances.[6,7] Although hypercalciuria is the most common metabolic abnormality seen among individuals with whom calcium stones are formed, most cases are not attributed to variations in dietary calcium. In fact, a very low-calcium diet may increase the absorption and subsequent excretion of oxalate, which promotes formation of calcium oxalate stones in susceptible individuals.[20] Maintaining a calcium intake in the range of 600 to 800 mg/day should prevent hyperoxaluria and long-term negative calcium balance.[20]

CHALLENGES IN THE MANAGEMENT OF PHOSPHORUS AND BONE DISEASE

RENAL OSTEODYSTROPHY

Currently, approximately 60% of HD patients have phosphorus levels greater than 5.5 mg/dl and 40% have Ca × P greater than 60. It has been recommended that target levels should become 9.2 to 9.6 mg/dl for calcium, 2.5 to 5.5 mg/dl for phosphorus, less than 55 for Ca × P product, and 100 to 200 pg/ml for intact PTH.[30] Attainment of these goals may assist in the

TABLE 16.5
A Summary of the Nutrition Management Recommendations for Patients Requiring Dialysis and Not Requiring Dialysis

Nutrients	CRF (No Dialysis)	HD	PD	Transplant
Calories (kcal/day)	30–35	30–35	30–35	30–35
Protein (g/kg/day)	0.6–0.75 (at least 50% HBV protein)	1.2 (at least 50% HBV protein)	1.2–1.3 (at least 50% HBV protein)	1.3–2.0 (increased needs with stress of surgery or corticosteroid use)
Fat	Varies; if lipid profile within normal limits (WNL): increase fat to provide kcal (monounsaturated)	Low-fat, low-cholesterol (if increased lipid profile)	Low-fat, low-cholesterol (if increased lipid profile)	Low-fat, low-cholesterol (often have increased lipid profile)
Fluid	Urinary output + 500 ml for losses	1000 ml/day (+ urine output/losses)	2000–2500 ml/day (+ urine/losses)	Restriction usually not needed, (unless ATN or kidney rejection)
Na^+	2000–3000 mg/day	2000–3000 mg/day	3000–4000 mg/day	Usually liberal (unless + edema or HTN: 2000 mg/day, if so)
K^+	1500–3000 mg/day	1500–3000 mg/day	Liberal (may even need K^+ supplement)	Usually liberal (cyclosporin may increase K^+)
Ca^{2+}	Needs vary (check PO_4)	Needs vary (check PO_4)	Needs vary (check PO_4)	Calcium supplement may be necessary
PO_4	12–15 mg/g protein (maximum 1200 mg/day)	12–15 mg/g protein (maximum 1200 mg/day)	12–15 mg/g protein (maximum 1200 mg/day)	Liberal (low PO_4 levels may be seen due to increased excretion)
Vitamins	Avoid vitamin A (often on B-complex and vitamin C)	Avoid vitamin A (take B-complex and vitamin C)	Avoid vitamin A (take B-complex and vitamin C)	Daily multivitamin (MVI) may be helpful if dietary restrictions

Source: From Morrison, G. and Hark, L., *Medical Nutrition and Disease*, Blackwell Science, Cambridge, MA, 1996, pp. 305–320.

prevention of uremic calcification, cardiac death, and vascular disease. This is important to consider, since cardiovascular disease accounts for nearly 50% of all deaths in dialysis patients, and the incidence of cardiovascular death is dramatically higher than that seen in the general population.[30] In addition, calcification of cardiac tissue has been reported in nearly 60% of dialysis patients upon autopsy.[31-33] Electron beam computed tomography (EBCT) can be used to detect different calcification stages in a variety of tissues, and is a sensitive tool for detecting calcified coronary artery plaques, as well as cardiac and valvular calcifications. HD patients have high calcium scores on EBCT imaging, and these are associated with elevations in $Ca \times P$ product. In a recent study, patients with calcification were found to have had twice the daily calcium intake from calcium-based phosphate binders than patients without calcification.[34] One of the possible adverse effects of calcium-based phosphate binders is hypercalcemia, which may in turn result in arterial calcifications.[35-37] However, whether or not calcium-based phosphate binders definitively increase calcification remains controversial. As many patients in the above referenced studies had prolonged periods of severe hyperparathyroidism and underwent parathyroidectomy, factors that obviously confound the interpretation of cardiovascular outcomes. Strategies to reduce cardiac risk in HD patients may include the use of a dialysate low in calcium, use of vitamin D analogs that are less hypercalcemic, and use of calcium-free phosphate binders. One such calcium-free phosphate binder, sevelamer hydrochloride, has been associated with improved lipid profiles, a consideration for patients at risk for coronary artery disease.[38]

ADVANTAGES AND DISADVANTAGES OF PHOSPHORUS BINDERS

- Calcium-containing phosphorus binders are effective, but add to excess calcium load, and may contribute to increased incidence of hypercalcemia.
- Aluminum-containing phosphorus binders are very effective, but recognition of aluminum toxicity has severely restricted their use.
- Aluminum-free, calcium-free phosphorus binders may be effective without toxicity or excess calcium load; may increase the risk of acidemia.

CONTROVERSIAL THERAPIES FOR END-STAGE RENAL DISEASE PATIENTS

L-CARNITINE

Carnitor (L-Carnitine) is a naturally occurring substance required in mammalian energy metabolism. It has been shown to facilitate long-chain fatty acid entry into cellular mitochondria, therefore delivering substrate in all tissues except the brain. L-Carnitine has been approved as a drug in a number of European and other international countries for use in multiple conditions, such as myocardial ischemia, renal dialysis, and other types of carnitine deficiency or abnormal metabolic states.[39-41] In the United States, the oral form of carnitine was approved in 1985 for the indication of primary carnitine deficiency. In 1993, both the intravenous (IV) and oral forms were approved by the Food and Drug Administration (FDA) for the additional indication of secondary carnitine deficiency primarily due to inborn errors of metabolism. One study strongly suggested a contribution of carnitine deficiency to cardiac dysfunction,[39] while another study found that administration of L-carnitine ameliorated cardiac function.[40] It is also thought that carnitine may improve the response to exogenous EPO in refractory patients. This was in accordance with yet another study which found that the maximum oxygen consumption in HD patients increased with administration of L-carnitine.[41] However, the question of deleterious effects of long-term elevated carnitine levels in continuously supplemented patients remains open.[42] Although the substance has a low order of acute toxicity according to the usual criteria[43] there are reports that long-term high-dose administration tends to promote abnormalities in platelet aggregation.[44,45]

Further research is needed to better ascertain the long-term effects and overall efficacy of L-carnitine supplementation in the renal population.

INTRADIALYTIC PARENTERAL NUTRITION AND INTERMITTENT PARENTERAL NUTRITION

For ESRD patients who are unable to tolerate and do not respond to oral or enteral nutrition, including enteral tube feedings, intradialytic parenteral nutrition (IDPN) for HD patients, or intermittent parenteral nutrition (IPN) for PD patients, may allow for effective treatment of malnutrition while patients receive their dialysis treatment.[46] Previously published studies support the use of IDPN for selected maintenance HD and PD patients who are malnourished, have malabsorption due to short bowel syndrome or chronic pancreatitis and are failing conservative treatment.[47–50] However, other reports have found the data supporting the use of IDPN to be weak,[51] or best limited to patients who are unable to tolerate oral or enteral protein-rich foods or formulas designed to meet daily protein requirements.[52] Table 16.6 illustrates the advantages and disadvantages of IDPN.

At the present time, Medicare criteria are extremely restrictive regarding payment for IDPN or IPN or both, and many private insurance companies have declined to pay for these therapies, feeling they are unnecessary and ineffective. In addition, evidence that tube feedings have failed is required for most diagnoses.[46]

USE OF APPETITE STIMULANTS (MEGACE, MARINOL, AND OTHERS)

Megace is the brand name of megestrol acetate, a synthetic substance derived from the female hormone, progesterone. The drug is primarily marketed for the treatment of breast cancer, which has spread to other parts of the body. Another possible use of Megace is to stimulate appetite in order to produce weight gain. The actual way Megace works in appetite stimulation is unclear.[53] Researchers in Italy demonstrated that Megace is effective in producing weight gain in patients with advanced HIV disease.[54] Some studies seem to indicate that the drug plays a role in fat synthesis in the body.[55] At present, there have not been any documented studies looking at the use of Megace with renal patients. Therefore, research is needed in this area in order to better understand the implications of Megace supplementation in patients with renal disease.

Marinol (dronabinol) is a well-known pharmaceutical appetite stimulant prescribed for HIV. Chemically, it is a pure version of the most well-known active ingredient in marijuana

---

TABLE 16.6

Advantages and Disadvantages of IDPN

Advantages of IDPN (compared to tube feeding or total parenteral nutrition [TPN])
- No need for a dedicated enteral feeding tube or vascular access
- Ultra-filtration during dialysis (which reduces the risk of fluid overload)
- No demands on the time or effort of the patient

Disadvantages of IDPN
- Provision of insufficient calories and protein to support long-term daily needs (e.g., IDPN given during dialysis for only 3 days/week)
- Does not change patient's food behavior
- Does not encourage patient to eat more healthy meals
- Therapy is expensive[18]

called delta-l-tetrahydrocannabinol (THC). Unlike marijuana, Marinol is an oral drug that can be prescribed by a physician in three different dosages. Marinol has recently been approved to treat nausea in cancer.[56] In studies, Marinol treatment significantly improved appetite in people with HIV, while trends toward improved body weight and mood, and decreases in nausea and vomiting were seen.[57]

Corticosteroids were the first agents to undergo placebo-controlled, double-blind evaluation for possible use in cancer cachexia. The first such trial, conducted in the 1970s by Moertel and colleagues at the Mayo Clinic, demonstrated that corticosteroids can stimulate appetite in patients with advanced, incurable cancer. Several subsequent placebo-controlled trials, using various steroid preparations and doses, have confirmed these results.[58]

Although anecdotal reports of improved nutritional intake can be achieved with the use of these agents (e.g., Megace, Marinol, corticosteroids) and others, particularly in patients with superimposed HIV disease or cancer or both, there are no randomized, double-blinded, controlled studies to corroborate their use in ESRD patients.

GROWTH HORMONE AND ANDROGENS

The exogenous administration of growth hormone (or its analog) has been shown to influence bowel adaptation by enhancing mucosal hyperplasia following extensive intestinal resection in animals. In addition, IGF-1, which is regulated by the growth hormone, has been shown to increase the weight and length of the small and large intestine.[59] One study found that combined administration of growth hormone, glutamine, and a modified diet enhanced nutrient absorption from the remnant bowel after massive intestinal resection.[60] These changes occurred in a group of patients who had previously failed to adapt to the provision of enteral nutrients. Anabolism has been observed during administration of recombinant growth hormone and insulin-like growth factor-1 in malnourished maintenance dialysis patients.[61] Although more research is needed, it is possible that these supplements may provide an avenue for improving the overall outcomes for renal patients with GI disorders and malabsorption (see Textbox 16.1 and Textbox 16.2).

Textbox 16.1   Star Fruit — Renal Patients, Beware!

Patients with renal failure, even those not yet undergoing dialysis, can develop severe and potentially fatal neurologic complications after eating star fruit.[62] Clinical symptoms and outcomes of uremic patients ingesting star fruit are quite variable, and may progress to death.[63] In a study of 32 uremic patients with intoxication by star fruit,[63] it was determined that the most common symptoms were persistent and intractable hiccups, vomiting, variable degrees of disturbed consciousness, decreased muscle power, limb numbness, paresis, insomnia, paresthesias, and seizures. Although star fruit is high in potassium, there was no detection of any alteration in serum potassium levels among the uremic patients with star fruit intoxication.[63] At present, there are no reports of star fruit intoxication in people with normal renal function. However, Chang et al.[64] found that certain uremic patients failed to develop neurologic symptoms following star fruit ingestion. Patients who were promptly treated with HD, including those with severe intoxication, recovered without sequelae. Patients with severe intoxication who were not treated or treated with PD did not survive.[63] The authors concluded that HD, especially on a daily basis, is the ideal treatment for star fruit intoxication. PD is of no use as a treatment, especially when changes in mental status are detected.[63]

Textbox 16.2   Focus on Star Fruit — Origin and Uses

Star fruit (*Averrhoa carambola*) is believed to have originated in Ceylon and the Moluccas, but it has been cultivated in Southeast Asia and Malaysia for many centuries. It is commonly grown in southern China, Taiwan, and India. The fruit was introduced in southern Florida before 1887.[65,66] It is very popular in the Philippines and Australia, and moderately so in some of the South Pacific islands. There are some subspecies in the Caribbean islands, in Central America, and in topical West Africa. It is also common in Brazil, where it is served as a fresh beverage, or as an industrialized juice, as it is also served throughout the world. It is widely used in restaurants for decorative purposes. In India, ripe fruit is administered to halt hemorrhages and to relieve bleeding hemorrhoids. In Brazil, carambola, or star fruit, is used as a popular remedy for "urinary problems."[65]

CASE STUDY 1

M.S. is a 75-year-old, African American female HD patient. She has been on HD for approximately 3 years, and has always had fairly normal laboratory work. However, over the past 2 months, Mrs. M.S's labs have changed:

- (Predialysis) labs 2 months ago: BUN 60, creatinine 8.5, K^+ 4.6, calcium 9.4, PO_4 6.1, albumin 4.0, CO_2 25; Kt/Vd 1.5
- (Predialysis) labs now: BUN 21, creatinine 3.7, K^+ 3.9, calcium 8.5, PO_4 3.2, albumin 2.9, CO_2 15; Kt/Vd 1.03

Over the course of the past 2 months, she has experienced anorexia, and her oral intake has deteriorated to <1000 kcal/day and <30 g of protein/day (per registered dietitian [RD] assessment).

How can you explain these changes in her blood test results?
How could her anorexia be improved?

Answer:

The combination of low pre-HD blood urea nitrogen, decreased albumin, potassium, and phosphorus is very suggestive of poor nutritional intake. Her decreased Kt/Vd (a measurement of dialysis dose) suggests that the efficiency of her renal replacement therapy has decreased and this may be a factor to explain her anorexia.

The response to this life-threatening scenario should include a multidisciplinary effort to improve efficiency of HD sessions (usually by increasing the time of each session, but also by increasing the membrane surface of dialyzer, testing the access for recirculation and arranging for its revision if elevated). A thorough review of patient's dietary habits and an assessment for underlying depression will also be in order.

CASE STUDY 2

J.T. is a 54-year-old Taiwanese man on PD for 3 years, presenting to the University Hospital Emergency Department with the following symptoms: sudden-onset limb numbness, muscle weakness, intractable hiccups, and seizures. Lab reports found the following: BUN 104, creatinine 8.7, K^+ 5.2, calcium 9.2, PO_4 5.7, albumin 3.9, CO_2 22, Kt/Vd 2.1.

What could be a possible cause of patient's current symptoms?

Does the patient's cultural background increase the likelihood of this assumption?

What is the best course of action for Mr. J.T. while in the hospital?

Answer:

This is a typical presentation for star fruit (*A. carambola*) toxicity in patients with advanced renal disease. The consumption of this fruit is more common in patients from Southeast Asian descent and the toxin is poorly removed by PD.

The best course of action would be insertion of temporary access and proceeding with emergent HD therapy.

REFERENCES

1. Weinberger, M.H., Salt sensitivity of blood pressure in humans, *Hypertension*, 27:481, 1996.
2. Rabinowitz, L., Aldosterone and potassium homeostasis, *Kidney International*, 49:1738, 1996.
3. Rose, B.D. and Post, T.W., *Clinical Physiology of Acid–Base and Electrolyte Disorders*, 5th ed., McGraw-Hill, New York, 2001, pp. 453–456.
4. Ganesh, S.K., Stack, A.G., and Levin, N.W., Association of elevated serum PO_4, $Ca \times PO_4$ product, and parathyroid hormone with cardiac mortality risk in chronic hemodialysis patients, *Journal of the American Society of Nephrology*, 12:2131, 2001.
5. Llach, F., Secondary hyperparathyroidism in renal failure. The trade-off hypothesis revisited, *American Journal of Kidney Diseases*, 25:663, 1995.
6. Parivar, F., Low, R.K., and Stoller, M.L., Influence of diet on urinary stone disease, *Journal of Urology*, 155:432, 1996.
7. Borghi, L., et al. Comparison of two diets for the prevention of recurrent stones in idiopathic hypercalciuria, *New England Journal of Medicine*, 346:77, 2002.
8. Bushinsky, D.A., The contribution of acidosis to renal osteodystrophy, *Kidney International*, 47:1816, 1995.
9. Molitons, B.A., Froment, D.E., Mackenzie T.A., et al. Citrate: a major factor in the toxicity of orally administered aluminum compounds, *Kidney International*, 36(6):949–953, 1989.
10. Nolan, C.R., Califano, J.R., and Butzin, C.A., Influence of calcium acetate or calcium citrate on internal aluminum absorption, *Kidney International*, 38(5):937–941, 1990.
11. Vanholder, R., Desmet, R., Glorieux, G., et al. Review of uremic toxins: classification, concentration and interindividual variability, *Kidney International*, 63(5):1934–1943, 2003.
12. Morris, R.C. and Sebastian, A., Alkali therapy in renal tubular acidosis; who needs it? *Journal of the American Society of Nephrology*, 13:2186, 2002.
13. Malinow, M.R., Bostom, A.G., and Krauss, R.M., Homocyt(e)ine, diet and cardiovascular disease. A statement for health care professions from the Nutrition Committee, American Heart Association, *Circulation*, 99:178, 1999.
14. Bostom, A.G. and Culleton, B.F., Hypercysteinemia in chronic renal disease, *Journal of the American Society of Nephrology*, 10:891, 1999.
15. Zoccali, C., Bode-Boger, S.M., and Mallamaci, F., Plasma concentration of asymmetrical dimethyl-arginine and mortality in patients with end stage renal disease: a prospective study, *Lancet*, 358:2131, 2001.
16. Stefiman-Breen, C. and Johnson, R.J., Hepatitis C virus-associated glomerulonephritis, *Advances in Internal Medicine*, 43:79, 1998.
17. Yang, C.S., et al. Rapidly progressive fibrosing interstitial nephritis associated with Chinese herbal drugs, *American Journal of Kidney Diseases*, 35:313, 2000.
18. Nortier, J.L., Martinez, M.C., and Schmeiser, H.H., Urothelial carcinoma associated with the use of Chinese herb (*Aristolochia fangchi*), *New England Journal of Medicine*, 342:1686, 2000.
19. Steinberg, H.O., Chaker, H., and Leaming, R., Obesity/insulin resistance is associated with endothelial dysfunction. Implications for the syndrome of insulin resistance, *Journal of Clinical Investigation*, 97:2001, 1996.

20. Morrison, G. and Hark, L., *Medical Nutrition and Disease*, Blackwell Science, Cambridge, MA, 1996, pp. 305–320.
21. Druml, W., Nutritional Management of acute renal failure, *American Journal of Kidney Diseases [Online]*, 37(1 Supplement 2):S89–S94, 2001.
22. NKF-K/DOQI *Clinical Practice Guidelines for Nutrition in Chronic Renal Failure*, National Kidney Foundation, New York, 2001, pp. 41–105.
23. Dwyer, J.T., et al. The Hemodialysis (HEMO) pilot study: nutrition program and participant characteristics at baseline, *Journal of Renal Nutrition*, 8:11–20, 1998.
24. Acchiardo, S.R. and Smith, S.O., Effects of nutrition on morbidity and mortality in hemodialysis patients, *Dialysis & Transplantation*, 29:614–619, 2000.
25. Mehrotra, R. and Kopple, J.D., Nutritional management or maintenance dialysis patients: why aren't we doing better? *Annual Review of Nutrition*, 21:343–379, 2001.
26. Paskalev, D.N., et al. Some medical aspects of nutritional therapy in elderly chronic renal failure patients, *Dialysis & Transplantation*, 31(9):607–614, 2002.
27. Nordfors, L., et al. Low leptin gene expression and hyperleptinemia in chronic renal failure, *Kidney International*, 54(4):1267–1275, 1998.
28. Maroni, B.J. and Mitch, W.E., Role of nutrition in prevention of the progression of renal disease, *Annual Review of Nutrition*, 17:435–455, 1997.
29. Mitch, W.E. and Maroni, B.J., Nutritional complications in the treatment of patients with chronic uremia, *Mineral and Electrolyte Metabolism*, 24(4):285–289, 1998.
30. Block, G.A. and Port, F.K., Re-evaluation of risks associated with hyperphosphatemia and hyperparathyroidism in dialysis patients: recommendations for a change in management, *American Journal of Kidney Diseases*, 35(6):1226–1237, 2000.
31. Braun, J., et al. Electron beam computed tomography in the evaluation of cardiac calcifications in chronic dialysis patients, *American Journal of Kidney Diseases*, 27:394–401, 1996.
32. Kuzela, D.C., et al. Soft tissue calcification in chronic dialysis patients, *The American Journal of Pathology*, 86:403–424, 1977.
33. Ribeiro, S., et al. Cardiac valve calcification in haemodialysis patients: role of calcium-phosphate metabolism, *Nephrology Dialysis Transplantation*, 13:2037–2040, 1998.
34. Raggi, P., Detection and quantification of cardiovascular calcifications with electron beam tomography to estimate risk in hemodialysis patients, *Clinical Nephrology*, 54(4):325–333, 2000.
35. Guerin, A.P., et al. Arterial stiffening and vascular calcifications in end-stage renal disease, *Nephrology Dialysis Transplantation*, 15(7):1014–1021, 2000.
36. Collins, A.J., et al. Hospitalization risks between Renagel phosphate binder treated and non-Renagel treated patients, *Clinical Nephrology*, 54(4):334–341, 2000.
37. Block, G.A., Prevalence and clinical consequences of elevated Ca × P product in hemodialysis patients, *Clinical Nephrology*, 54(4):318–324, 2000.
38. Llach, R., Hyperphosphatemia in end-stage renal disease patients: pathophysiological consequences, *Kidney International*, 56 (Supplement 73):31–37, 1999.
39. Lasagna, L. and Schreiner, G., Role of L-carnitine in treating renal dialysis patients, *Dialysis & Transplantation*, 23(4):178, 1994.
40. Van Es, A., et al. Amelioration of cardiac function by L-carnitine administration in patients on haemodialysis, *Contributions to Nephrology*, 98:28–35, 1992.
41. Ahmad, S., et al. Multicenter trial of L-carnitine in maintenance hemodialysis patients. II. Clinical and biochemical effects, *Kidney International*, 38:912–918, 1990.
42. Rosenthal, A.F., Free and total serum carnitine: shall the analyses begin? *Dialysis & Transplantation*, 31(8):570–574, 2002.
43. Medical Economics. Carnitor. *Physicians' Desk Reference*, 56th ed., 2002, pp. 3242–3245.
44. Kalinowski, M., et al. Effects of L-carnitine on erythropoiesis and blood platelet aggregation in patients with chronic renal failure treated with hemodialysis, *Pol Merkuriusz Lek*, 6:76–78, 1999.
45. Wechsler, A., et al. High dose of L-carnitine increases platelet aggregation and plasma triglyceride levels in uremic patients on hemodialysis, *Nephron*, 38:120–124, 1984.
46. Schwebke, L.M. and Lazarus, J.M., the importance of parenteral nutrition options for the malnourished ESRD patient, *Focus on NUTRITION*, 1998, pp. 26–30.

47. Wolfson, M. and Jones, M., Intraperitoneal nutrition, *American Journal of Kidney Diseases*, 33(1): 203–204, 1999.
48. Chertow, G.M., et al. Laboratory surrogates of nutritional status after administration of intraperitoneal amino acid-based solutions in ambulatory peritoneal dialysis patients, *Journal of Renal Nutrition*, 5(3):116–123, 1995.
49. Chertow, G.M., et al. The association of intradialytic parenteral nutrition administration with survival in hemodialysis patients, *American Journal of Kidney Diseases*, 24(6):912–920, 1994.
50. Capelli, J.P., et al. Effect of intradialytic parenteral nutrition on mortality rates in end-stage renal disease care, *American Journal of Kidney Diseases*, 23(6):808–816, 1994.
51. Foulks, C.J., An evidence-based evaluation of intradialytic parenteral nutrition, *American Journal of Kidney Diseases*, 33(1):186–192, 1999.
52. Chertow, G.M., Modality-specific nutrition support in ESRD: weighing the evidence, *American Journal of Kidney Diseases*, 33(1):193–197, 1999.
53. Torres, G., Megace to stimulate appetite, *Gay Men's Health Crisis Treatment Issues*, 5(9), 1991.
54. VII International Conference on AIDS, Abstracts #W.B. 2392, #M.B. 2198, # M.B. 2233, Florence, Italy, June 1991.
55. Tchekmedyian, N.S., Hickman, M., and Heber, D., Treatment of anorexia and weight loss with megestrol acetate in patients with anorexia and AIDS, *Seminars in Oncology*, 18:35–42, 1991.
56. Vergel, N. and Mooney, M., Appetite stimulation: medicinal marijuana, Marinol, and Megace, http://www.medibolics.com, Issue # 7, 1998.
57. Beal, J.E., et al. Dronabinol as a treatment for anorexia associated with weight loss in patients with AIDS, *Journal of Pain and Symptom Management*, 10:89–97, 1995.
58. Loprinzi, C., *Anorexia and Cachexia. Cancer Management: A Multidisciplinary Approach*, 5th ed., PRR, Melville, NY, 2001.
59. Byrne, T.A., Nompleggi, D.J., and Wilmore, D.W., Advances in the management of patients with intestinal failure, *Transplantation Proceedings*, 28(5):2683–2690, 1996.
60. Byrne, T.A., et al. Growth hormone, glutamine, and a modified diet enhance nutrient absorption in patients with severe short bowel syndrome, *Journal of Parenteral and Enteral Nutrition*, 19(4):296–302, 1995.
61. Fouque, D., Causes and interventions for malnutrition in patients undergoing maintenance dialysis [Review], *Blood Purification*, 15(2):112–120, 1997.
62. Reuters Health, Star fruit warning: eating star fruit may be fatal in uremic patients, *American Journal of Kidney Diseases*, 35:189–193, 2000.
63. Neto, M.M., et al. Intoxication by star fruit (*Averrhoa carambola*) in 32 uraemic patients: treatment and outcome, *Nephrology, Dialysis, Transplantation*, 18(1):120–125, 2003.
64. Chang, J.M., Hwang, and Kuo, H.T., Fatal outcome after ingestion of star fruit (*Averrhoa carambola*) in uremic patients, *American Journal of Kidney Diseases*, 35:189–193, 2000.
65. Morton, J.F., *Fruits of Warm Climates*, Flair Books, Miami, FL, 1987, pp. 125–128.
66. Margen, S., *The Wellness Encyclopedia of Food and Nutrition*, Health Letter Association, New York, 1992, pp. 271–282.

17 Respiratory Health

Jennifer Doley, Richard Berry, and Mary Marian

CONTENTS

INTRODUCTION

Oxygen, vital to life, and carbon dioxide, deadly to cells, are released when energy in the food we eat is metabolized. The pulmonary system transports needed oxygen to the organ systems and expunges carbon dioxide from the body. It is therefore imperative that a properly functioning pulmonary system be maintained to ensure good health. This chapter will examine the normal pulmonary system and show how lung disease or dysfunction can hamper the exchange of oxygen and carbon dioxide.

A brief review of the function of the lungs is warranted. By contraction of the large muscular organ, the diaphragm, air is pulled into the pulmonary system through the air passages, ultimately reaching the air sacs or alveoli at the end of the bronchial trees. Here oxygen diffuses from the alveoli to the blood in the pulmonary capillaries, while carbon dioxide is released from the pulmonary capillaries to the alveoli, to be exhaled through the breath upon relaxation of the diaphragm. Any dysfunction of the alveoli, bronchioles, major bronchi, or the diaphragm that causes a decrease in the amount of oxygen exchanged results in a reduction of oxygen reaching the blood, and therefore body organs. We will review a number of pulmonary disease processes.

There is an increasing interest in the relationship between nutrition and lung health. Epidemiological studies suggest that dietary habits may have an influence on lung function and the development of common respiratory diseases such as asthma, chronic obstructive pulmonary disease (COPD), and lung cancer. Nutrition also plays a vital role in maintaining health and well-being for individuals with cystic fibrosis (CF). Additionally, the presence and progression of many respiratory diseases can have a significant and adverse effect not only on nutritional status but also on morbidity and mortality. Medications commonly used in the treatment of pulmonary disease, such as bronchodilators and corticosteroids, can also have an adverse impact on nutritional status and quality of life. In an effort to stem the side effects related to the treatment or the disease itself, many individuals with pulmonary conditions are turning to complementary and alternative medicine (CAM). Therefore, it is important for the health care professional to have a thorough understanding of the role which nutrition plays in respiratory health, as well as the treatment of common respiratory ailments.

CHRONIC OBSTRUCTIVE PULMONARY DISEASE

As the name implies, obstructive pulmonary disease results from an obstruction to the flow of air through the pulmonary system. In this category are emphysema, bronchitis, asthma, bronchiolectasis, CF, and airway stenosis or narrowing.[1]

It is estimated that 14 million Americans are affected with COPD.[2] COPD is defined as a condition in which there is chronic obstruction to airway flow due to chronic bronchitis or emphysema. COPD is classified as Type A and Type B; Type A has an emphysema predominance and Type B has a bronchitis predominance.[1,2] Emphysema and chronic bronchitis are specific diseases and should be treated as such. In emphysema, the alveoli no longer have a normal grape-like appearance but are damaged, resulting in impairment of air exchange. Chronic bronchitis is defined clinically as a chronic, productive cough on most days for 3 months of 2 consecutive years; obstruction results from narrowing of the airway lumen with mucosal thickening and excess mucous.[3] It is important to note that the acute exacerbation of chronic bronchitis causes the majority of office visits each year for problems related to COPD.[4] With bronchodilators and in the absence of infection, obstruction may not be severe but is nevertheless still present. Other pulmonary diseases such as CF, bronchiectasis, and bronchiolitis may be associated with airway obstruction, but are not considered a part of COPD.

One of the major causes of COPD is tobacco smoke. Smokers have ten times the risk of dying of emphysema and chronic bronchitis than nonsmokers. Smoking also increases the risks of developing COPD in people with a deficiency of a chemical called alpha-1-antitrypsin. Passive smoking, or second-hand smoke, is also implicated as a carcinogen and can lead to severe COPD as well.[5] People who are, therefore, exposed to second-hand smoke are at an increased risk for developing lung cancer and chronic bronchitis. Air pollution caused by oxidants (oxides of nitrogen, hydrocarbons, and sulfur dioxide) also has a significant role in the development of COPD. The obstruction of airflow in COPD can result from many causes, including airway collapse during expiration, mucosal thickening or inflammation, edema as seen in asthma, and hypertrophy of the mucosal glands as seen in bronchitis. In chronic cases, there is a loss of the elastic recoil of the lungs, which normally prevents collapse of the airway during expiration. Chronic bronchitis patients tend to retain carbon dioxide and can eventually develop complications of the cardiovascular system including cor pulmonale.[6]

Diagnosis is made by history and physical examination, chest x-ray, pulmonary function tests, and arterial blood gases.[7] History and physical examination frequently reveal cigarette smoking, chronic productive cough, dyspnea, and lung findings suggestive of infection including ronchi and rales. Other common findings are obesity and peripheral edema. Patients usually present with COPD in the fifth or sixth decade of life.[2] If a young person exhibits these COPD symptoms, the possibility of alpha-1-antitrypsin deficiency must be considered high in the differential.

The treatment of COPD entails elimination of precipitating factors such as smoking, and exposure to second-hand tobacco and environmental pollutants. Obstructive symptoms are addressed by giving sprays or chemicals to open up the bronchi. The patient may be given steroids to reduce inflammation and fluids, and, in some cases, antibiotics to eradicate an infectious process.[5] The most important treatment in COPD is smoking cessation.[1,2,7-9] The use of nicotine patches or other modalities to assist in the treatment of nicotine addiction should be used as a mainstay measure. Patients who have low oxygenation while resting should also be supplied with supplemental oxygen, as it may prolong life, reduce hospitalizations, and improve the patient's quality of life. In severe COPD patients, the rate of survival is directly proportional to the use of supplemental oxygen.[2]

Type A patients should be offered a trial of bronchodilator therapy during exacerbations. In moderate to severe COPD, ipratropium has a longer duration. Theophylline is considered a third-line agent and is used in patients who fail bronchodilator therapy.[2] Corticosteroids are usually given to patients with frequent exacerbations and to those who fare poorly with conventional therapy, however, steroid use has increased in recent years, with good results.[2,9] Although the use of antibiotics is sometimes the mainstay of patients with acute COPD, the efficacy of antibiotic use is not clear.[1,2]

Type B COPD, or emphysema, is characterized by enlargement of the air space and destruction of the walls of the alveoli. Patients with emphysema are usually thin and carbon dioxide retention is seen in the late stages of the disease. It is important in the work-up of individuals with emphysema and COPD to take an alpha-1-antitrypsin level, which may be replaced, thus slowing the worsening of the disease process. Treatment options for Type B COPD are significantly less than those for Type A. In emphysema, the process by which air is exchanged from the alveoli to the capillaries is significantly reduced. It is, therefore, important for early diagnosis to be made and early intervention is essential for longevity.[6]

MEDICAL NUTRITION THERAPY

Malnutrition is very common in patients with COPD, with a reported incidence ranging from 35–60%.[10,11] Furthermore, poor nutritional status is associated with an increased incidence of morbidity and mortality.[12,13] Patients with weight loss generally have severe disease. Foley et al.[14] recently found that weight loss and body composition abnormalities are independent predictors of morbidity and mortality. Additionally, compromised nutritional status adversely affects functional capacity and quality of life. Weight loss in patients with COPD is linked with decreased lung function, dyspnea, respiratory infections, decreased peripheral muscle function, and reduced respiratory muscle strength.[15–17] Malnourished patients also reportedly have a lower forced expiratory volume (FEV_1) and forced vital capacity (FVC) values, higher carbon dioxide partial pressure values, and lower arterial pH values.[18] The loss of skeletal muscle mass experienced by a significant percentage of patients with COPD results in limited exercise capacity and a poorer overall health status, resulting in a negative impact on prognosis.

While a number of factors have been shown to promote tissue catabolism, no single mechanism has been clearly identified as a primary contributor for weight loss (see Table 17.1). Shortness of breath, copious production of respiratory secretions, and persistent cough all can diminish appetite as well as energy for eating. Since it is difficult to breathe and eat at the same time, the extremely dyspneic patient may be unable to coordinate breathing with swallowing in an efficient manner.[18] As the patient puts forth a greater effort for breathing, intake is commonly compromised.

Studies investigating total resting and energy expenditures in the COPD population have yielded mixed results.[19,20] A number of studies have found that patients with COPD are typically hypermetabolic.[20,21] Conversely, Tang et al.[20] recently reported that total energy expenditure (TEE) in underweight patients with COPD was no different than patients with normal weight. Factors associated with elevations in TEE include increased work for breathing, medication use, and elevated cytokine levels. Elevated levels of tumor necrosis factor-α (TNF-α), and soluble TNF-receptors have been noted in COPD patients with weight loss.[22] Evidence for the involvement of TNF-α-related systemic inflammation in the pathogenesis of tissue depletion has been cited in several studies.[22,23]

Insufficient dietary intake is another component contributing to the alteration in energy balance. Several studies have shown that dietary intake relative to resting energy expenditure (REE) is diminished in weight-losing patients compared with weight-stable COPD patients.[20,24] Increased dyspnea or decreased arterial oxygen saturation during eating and increased dyspnea caused by gastric distention, resulting in a reduction in functional residual capacity are cited factors.[25] Weight loss is particularly common during acute exacerbations of COPD. In addition to poor appetite, negative nitrogen balance has been reported in hospitalized patients with COPD.[25] Protein turnover studies suggest both an increase in protein synthesis and protein breakdown, with the latter predominating.[23] Increased protein breakdown may be related to an increase in circulating cytokines, such as interleukin-6 and TNF-α, and the catabolic effects of corticosteroids used for the treatment of COPD exacerbations.[25]

TABLE 17.1
Factors Associated with Nutritional Depletion in COPD

Poor appetite due to
Disease-specific symptoms
  Copious secretions
  Cough
  Fatigue
Elevated resting and total energy expenditure due to
Increased energy and oxygen costs
Catabolic intermediary metabolism
Effects of medications (especially β_2-agonists)
Systemic inflammatory environment
Inadequate dietary intake

Nutritional Requirements

All patients with COPD should receive a comprehensive nutrition assessment including a review of weight history, dietary intake, medication and supplement use, laboratory indices, functional abilities, psychosocial interactions, and medical history. In addition to the traditional nutritional assessment parameters such as height and weight, body composition should also be assessed, as COPD patients with a healthy body mass index (BMI) have been found to have lower levels of fat-free mass (FFM) and bone mineral density (BMD).[23] Bolton et al. report that these findings are associated with disease severity.

Nutrition recommendations, goals, and measured outcomes should be incorporated into the overall medical care plan. Requirements for energy can be estimated via the basal energy expenditure (BEE) × 1.3 or through indirect calorimetry measurements.[25] For patients without compromised hepatic or renal function, protein needs can be approximated at 1.5 g/kg/day.[25] The recommendations for micronutrients parallel those set forth by the dietary reference intake (DRI) levels established for adults, however, an increased intake of vitamin C is recommended for individuals using tobacco.

Osteoporosis is fairly common in patients with COPD, with a reported frequency ranging from 36% (osteoporosis) up to 56% (low BMD).[23] Factors contributing to low BMD include physical inactivity, systemic inflammation, inadequate calcium and vitamin D intake, and chronic corticosteroid use.[23] Glucocorticoids are the most common cause of drug-induced osteoporosis. Decreases in BMD reportedly occur in 86% of patients using high-dose steroids for >1 year.[26] Decreases in BMD are also noted in medium (71%) and low-dose (33%) therapies.[26] The prevalence and incidence of osteoporosis is expected to increase as the use of inhaled steroids continues to rise paralleling an increase in the aging population. Steroid-induced osteoporosis is also reportedly underdiagnosed and undertreated.[26] The National Osteoporosis Foundation recommends that all patients receiving chronic glucocorticoid therapies (>1 month) of ≥7.5 mg/day of prednisone or an equivalent drug should be screened for osteoporosis.[26,27]

Strategies that may reduce the prevalence and incidence of osteoporosis include use of the lowest effective steroid doses, smoking cessation, weight-bearing exercise, and adequate consumption of micronutrients associated with BMD such as calcium, vitamin D, magnesium, and vitamin K (see Chapter 8).

Nutrition Support

The use of oral commercially prepared nutrition supplements is commonly employed in an effort to augment calorie and protein intake. Studies of short-term (2–3 weeks) supplementation reported a significant increase in body weight and respiratory muscle function.[12,28] These short-term benefits are thought to result from repletion of muscle water and potassium, as well as small changes in the composition of lean body mass.[29] Fuenzalida et al. assessed the immune response to short-term (21-day) nutritional supplementation in nine patients with severe COPD; refeeding and weight gain were associated with a significant increase in absolute lymphocyte count.[30] Significant improvements in respiratory and peripheral skeletal muscle function, as well as exercise capacity and health-related quality of life, were noted in other studies with the use of oral supplements providing about 1000 kcal/day.[31,32] However, the efficacy of using such supplements is sometimes disappointing primarily due to a compensatory drop in usual food intake. Moreover, none of the clinical trials performed thus far have been of sufficient duration to address whether weight loss is a marker of disease severity or whether interventions resulting in increasing or maintaining weight influence morbidity and mortality. In a recently updated review for the Cochrane Database, Ferreira et al.[33]

examined the evidence from nine studies regarding the role of nutrition support in patients with stable COPD. They concluded that the impact of nutrition on the studied outcomes was small, and that small sample sizes, heterogonous populations, and short-supplementation periods hindered all studies.

A plethora of commercially prepared oral and enteral supplements have been designed for patients with respiratory conditions, though there is little evidence of their efficacy for patients with COPD. These formulas have been developed to provide a greater proportion of nonprotein calories as fat instead of carbohydrate. Theoretically, this may be advantageous because of the potential for a greater CO_2 production resulting in a greater ventilatory load from the metabolism of higher carbohydrate meals. However, subsequent clinical studies have found that CO_2 production significantly increased only when caloric intake was markedly greater than actual needs.[34,35] Furthermore, Akrabawi et al.[35] found that gastric emptying was significantly delayed with the use of a higher fat supplement. High-fat diets may also cause bloating, loose stools, or diarrhea. Additionally, meal-related oxyhemoglobin desaturation may diminish energy intake and contribute to meal-related dyspnea, particularly in individuals with COPD who are hypoxemic at rest.[11]

Evidence supporting the use of enteral nutrition (EN) in patients with COPD is limited. Whittaker et al.[28] investigated the use of enteral feedings for 16 days in malnourished patients with stable COPD. Weight gain and maximal expiratory pressure increased in patients receiving EN. Donahoe et al.[36] evaluated the use of EN for 4 months in patients with COPD and an ideal body weight of $<85\%$. While the EN subjects experienced an average 3.3 kg weight gain, no significant improvements were noted in physiologic outcomes. Lastly, in the Study to Understand Prognoses and Preferences for Outcomes and Risks of Treatments (SUPPORT), EN was associated with significantly reduced survival rates in patients with COPD.[37] Although the control group was not randomized, these results suggest that careful consideration should be given to the potential benefits and risks before using EN in this population, unless the oral route for nutrition is unavailable, as with mechanically ventilated patients.

COMPLEMENTARY AND ALTERNATIVE MEDICINE THERAPIES

Reportedly, 41% of patients who have COPD use CAM therapies.[38] Multivitamins and mineral supplements were the most commonly used CAM modalities, while garlic was the most commonly used herbal supplement.[38] CAM was generally used as adjunct therapy to traditional medicine and not as a replacement for conventional medical care. The primary reasons reported for using CAM therapies include: to counteract the side effects of prescribed medications, improve general well-being and alleviate symptoms related to the disease, and to compensate for dietary deficiencies due to the restriction of certain foods.[38] Moreover, many patients believe that CAM therapies are safe because they tend to be "natural."

Overall, there is a paucity of data from clinical studies evaluating whether CAM therapies may provide any benefits for patients with COPD. However, data from a few small studies investigating the potential use of acupressure, acupuncture, or mind–body therapies are available. Maa et al.[39] found that acupressure, as part of a pulmonary rehabilitation program, was effective in reducing dyspnea when compared with sham acupressure. Wu et al.[40] also reported positive outcomes; acupressure significantly improved pulmonary function, dyspnea scores, 6-min walking distance measurements, state anxiety scale scores, and physiological indicators in patients with COPD compared with those of the sham group. Sliwinski and Kulej[41] found that 64% of patients with COPD taking oral steroids were able to eliminate or significantly reduce their steroid use with prolonged acupuncture. Louie[42] recently reported that guided imagery resulted in a statistically significant increase in partial percentage of oxygen saturation in the treatment group, but found no significant effects on other physiological parameters such as heart rate, upper thoracic surface electromyography, skin conductance, and peripheral skin temperature. Patients with COPD report that efficacy is less important than safety when using CAM therapies.[38] Given the scarcity of studies investigating the risks and benefits of CAM, it is important for health care practitioners to have some basic knowledge about whether CAM modalities may be harmful or helpful in this patient population.

SUMMARY

Weight loss and loss of lean body mass are key indicators of disease progression in patients with COPD and are positively associated with increased morbidity and mortality. Improvements in weight and respiratory muscle strength and reductions in mortality have been reported with nutrition supplementation and anabolic stimulus; however, whether these changes result in improvements of other outcomes, such as quality of life, functional status, and morbidity and mortality remain to be determined. Clinical trials are needed to better determine which patient subgroups may benefit from nutrition and pharmacologic intervention.

PNEUMONIA

Pneumonia occurs when the alveoli or lower lung tissue are infected with bacteria, viral, or fungal pathogens, causing increased inflammation, blockage, and, if not treated, potentially sepsis and eventually death. A detailed discussion of organisms associated with pneumonia is beyond the scope of this text. However, the most common organisms include *Pseudomonas aeruginosa*, *Staphylococci aureus*, *Klebsiella pneumonia*, *Hemophilus influenza*, *Moraxella catarrhalis*, and *Legionella pneumonia*. The following are some characteristics of these organisms and the pneumonias they may cause:

Streptococci pneumonia: *S. pneumonia* is the cause of approximately 90% of all cases of adult pneumonia, especially in immunocompetent individuals.[1] It is most common in infants and the elderly. The sputum in these individuals may be blood-streaked or rusty. Effusions of the lung are common and cavitations of the lung are rare.

S. aureus: *S. aureus* is present in the upper air passageway and nasal passageway in approximately 40% of normal adults. Pneumonia caused by *S. aureus* is uncommon, but is more likely to occur in immunocompromised patients and in patients with severe diabetes mellitus, especially if it is uncontrolled. Patients who are drug abusers and those on dialysis are also at higher risk for developing *S. aureus* pneumonia. In these cases, lung abscesses may be seen and there is usually concomitant high mortality.[1]

P. aeruginosa: *P. aeruginosa* is the organism usually found in patients with CF and bronchiolectasis. Patients with COPD, congestive heart failure (CHF), alcohol abuse, or diabetes mellitus may also be at risk for developing pneumonia caused by this organism. A high mortality rate is seen in cases where early treatment to eradicate this organism is lacking.[1]

K. pneumonia: *K. pneumonia* is most commonly seen in alcoholics, patients with diabetes, and patients with prolonged hospitalization. A lung abscess may develop in these patients, therefore early detection is essential.

H. influenza: *H. influenza* is an unencapsulated organism and may be present in up to 60% of healthy individuals. The unencapsulated strain, however, is the one most likely found in sepsis. Individuals with this pneumonia frequently have COPD or are alcoholics. There have also been *H. influenza* outbreaks in the military.[1]

M. catarrhalis: *M. catarrhalis*, a Gram-negative diplococci, is part of the normal flora in healthy individuals. Most common in the winter months, it can cause sinusitis, otitis, and pneumonia. Patients who have COPD, alcoholism, chronic diabetes, and those who are immunocompromised usually are more likely candidates for this infection. Cavitation of the lungs, as compared with other organisms, is usually rare.[1]

L. pneumonia: *L. pneumonia* is a Gram-negative bacillus that thrives in a moist environment. Epidemics have occurred in contaminated air-conditioning coolant towers and also in contaminated hospital showers. Increased risk for this organism includes COPD, smoking, cancer, diabetes mellitus, and immunocompromised patients.

In hospital-acquired, or nosocomial, pneumonia, about 50% of the cases is caused by Gram-negative bacilli, including *S. aureus*, *Streptococcus*, anaerobes, and *Legionella* species. The risk factors for the development of nosocomial pneumonia include shock, coma, prolonged treatment with antibiotics, and prolonged mechanical ventilation.

Early treatment of pneumonia is essential. Broad-spectrum antibiotics should be used in the early days of treatment until the specific organism is identified and antibiotic susceptibility is determined. At that point, specific antibiotics for which the organism is sensitive to can be used for continued treatment. It is important to mention that the misuse, or over use, of antibiotics has lead to the development of many resistant organisms, some of which are not treatable with any known antibiotic. Antibiotics treat bacterial illnesses, and should not be used for viral infections. It is important that health care providers educate patients on the correct use of antibiotics.

CYSTIC FIBROSIS

CF is the most common lethal autosomal recessive disease among Caucasians in the United States, though survival rates have increased markedly in recent years; the median survival age is the early to mid-thirties.[43] Reportedly, CF occurs in blacks in the ratio of 1:17,000, in Asians 1:90,000, and among Caucasians 1:2,000–3,000.[6] The diagnosis of CF is usually made before the age of 10 years. CF is characterized by copious exocrine gland secretion, affecting the lungs, sweat and salivary glands, intestine, pancreas, and liver. Excess mucous secretions, resulting in obstruction of airflow and leading to hypoxia, cause lung dysfunction in CF. Diagnosis of CF is made by identity of the chemical features of CF, a positive family history, and a sweat chloride of 20 meq/l.[6] The pulmonary characteristics of CF may include nasal polyps, progressive cystic bronchiolectasis, significant purulent sputum, coughing up blood, and occasionally collapse of the lungs called pneumothorax. There is an increased incidence of *P. aeruginosa* infection with CF.[6]

Pulmonary treatment of CF includes management of the obstructive lung disease, drainage of purulent secretions, immunization against influenza, and significant hydration. Postural drainage and percussion, or chest physiotherapy (CPT), is also essential in the pulmonary treatment of CF. Gravity, percussion, and vibration are used to loosen thick respiratory mucous secretions so that they may be effectively expelled by coughing.

Oral corticosteroids are used to reduce pulmonary inflammation in CF, however, long-term use, especially in children, is limited due to harmful side effects, including osteoporosis and glucose intolerance. Inhaled corticosteroids are better tolerated with fewer side effects, however, evidence of benefit is lacking and further studies are needed. The incidence of CF-related diabetes is high, up to 28% in patients over the age of 35 years.[43] The CF Foundation has recommended yearly screening for CF-related diabetes after the age of 14 years.[43] The incidence of osteoporosis in all patients with CF is about 10%, with marked increase in risk with increasing age, due to the use of corticosteroids and inadequate intake or malabsorption of the vitamins and minerals essential to bone health.[43]

Other medical treatments may include the anti-inflammatory ibuprofen, which has been used more routinely in children with CF, though risks of renal toxicity must be weighed when deciding dosage and duration of treatment.[44] Azithromycin, with both antimicrobial and anti-inflammatory properties, has been used successfully short term in treating both adults and children with CF, and studies of longer treatment duration are under way.[45] In some cases, lung transplant is an option; currently, 120 to 150 lung transplants per year are performed in the United States on patients with CF.[43]

The gastrointestinal symptoms and management of CF are discussed elsewhere in this text. Management of inflammation is also a key treatment of CF, and is discussed more extensively later.

MEDICAL NUTRITION THERAPY

Individuals with CF are at high risk for malnutrition for a number of reasons. As pancreatic insufficiency is common, malabsorption is a frequent contributor to nutritional complications. Other factors interfere with the intake of adequate nutrition, including shortness of breath, coughing, and anorexia during illness. Malnutrition in CF patients has been directly linked to reduced pulmonary function; wasting results in weakened respiratory muscles and immunity, therefore maintenance of nutritional status is essential for quality of life and improved mortality.[46] The incidence of malnutrition among children with CF is steadily decreasing with improvements in treatment and more aggressive nutritional management. The 2004 weight data in children aged 0 to 18 years show improvements from data collected in 1990; however, the average weight percentile for children with CF ranges from about 15 to 40, depending on age.[43]

Nutrition needs vary depending on the patient's severity of illness, age, activity level, and gender, but calorie and protein needs are an estimated 10–30% higher than the average population. An intake of 120–150% of the recommended daily allowances (RDA) for energy is recommended, due both to increased energy expenditure and nutrition losses due to malabsorption. Higher fat diets (35–40% of calories) are usually recommended to meet these increased calorie needs. Supplementation of fat-soluble vitamins is frequently necessary, as deficiencies are common, even in patients adequately supplemented with pancreatic enzymes. Sodium needs are elevated due to excess sodium excretion in the sweat; sodium intake in the average American diet is usually adequate to meet needs in CF; however, increased salt consumption may be recommended in infants, and in adults during periods of fever, hot weather, or increased physical activity.[46]

Supplementation of antioxidant nutrients has been suggested in patients with CF, as their lungs are exposed to excessive oxidative stress, and plasma levels of antioxidants are often low.[45,46] Rust et al.[47] and Renner et al.[48] demonstrated a reduction in pulmonary exacerbations in children supplemented with 1 mg/kg, up to 50 mg/day, of beta-carotene for 12 weeks. No data are yet available confirming improved pulmonary function with beta-carotene supplementation, although the studied doses appear to be well-tolerated.[47,48] Supplementation of other antioxidants, such as vitamin E, vitamin C, selenium, and vitamin A has also been studied singly and together. While most studies show improvement or normalization of plasma nutrient levels and a reduction in circulating biomarkers of oxidative stress, no change in lung function has been demonstrated. Further research is needed to help ascertain antioxidant effects on quality of life, mortality, and overall pulmonary function.[46]

The fatty acids $(n-3)$ and $(n-6)$ polyunsaturated fatty acids (PUFAs) have a significant effect on inflammatory responses. Fatty acid levels are altered in CF patients; arachidonic acid (AA), a proinflammatory agent when metabolized, is elevated, and docosahexaenoic acid (DHA), an anti-inflammatory agent, is low. Essential fatty acid deficiency may be caused by abnormalities in fatty acid metabolism, as well as malnutrition and fat malabsorption. The $(n-3)$ PUFAs, which include eicosapentaenoic acid (EPA) and DHA, may be supplemented in patients with CF in the form of fish oils.[49] DeVizia et al.[50] and Lawrence and Sorrell[51] reported mild improvements in lung function; studied doses range from 1.28 to 2.7 g of EPA/ day and 0.93 g of DHA/day, with duration of treatment from 6 weeks to 8 months. Side effects are mild, most commonly GI-related, sometimes necessitating increases in pancreatic enzyme doses. Further research is needed to fully understand the potential role fatty acids may play in the treatment of CF.

Addition of nutritional anti-inflammatory and antioxidant compounds in short-term trials has shown positive effects in some pulmonary symptoms and biomarkers of CF; further long-term studies are needed to determine their effect on long-term outcomes such as overall lung function and life expectancy.

COMPLEMENTARY AND ALTERNATIVE MEDICINE THERAPIES

The use of CAM in the treatment of CF is fairly common, as with other chronic medical conditions. Stern et al.[52] reported, of both pediatric and adult CF patients, a 66% prevalence of the use of CAM, which included group prayer, reading religious articles, and chiropractic treatment. Most respondents reported perceived benefits to these modalities.[52] It is important for physicians and other members of the medical team to be able to accurately discuss with their patients the potential benefits, risks, and effectiveness of CAM therapies.

While CPT is a critical part of pulmonary management in CF, it can cause fatigue, increased energy expenditure, oxygen desaturation, and respiratory muscle fatigue. Several modalities have been used to improve the effectiveness of CPT. In a study examining the use of music therapy for infants and toddlers, parents played music specifically chosen by a music therapist during CPT. Results suggested that the children listening to music therapy enjoyed CPT more than control groups. While not directly affecting pulmonary function, researchers suggested that increased enjoyment of such a vital component of CF management would help parents establish a more positive treatment routine.[53] The use of noninvasive ventilation during CPT, via bilevel positive airway pressure (BiPAP) devices, has also shown positive results, such as improved inspiratory muscle function and oxygen saturation, in adults with acute pulmonary exacerbations and in children.[54,55]

Inspiratory muscle training has also been suggested as a method to improve pulmonary function in patients with CF. Several small studies of inspiratory muscle training showed an increase in inspiratory muscle function, diaphragm thickness, improved lung volumes, increased physical work capacity, and improved quality of life.[56,57]

A number of other CAM modalities have been used with CF patients, and while studies are limited in number and small in size, preliminary results are positive. Lin et al.[58] reported that acupuncture was effective in reducing complaints of pain in patients with CF. Anbar[59] examined the use of self-hypnosis by both adults and children with CF and reported that 86% of participants described relief of pain, increased relaxation, and better control of symptoms related to CF. And Hernandez-Reif et al.[60] described a reduction of anxiety in children with CF receiving daily massage therapy. While these studies give no definitive evidence of improved pulmonary function with the use of these therapies, their results are intriguing and indicate further research is warranted.

Recent studies have revealed a defect in the glutathione transport system in CF patients. Glutathione is produced in the body from the amino acids glutamine, glycine, and cysteine. Glutathione functions as an antioxidant, and is found in high concentrations in organs that are exposed to an oxidant-rich atmosphere, such as the cornea and lung. Glutathione levels in CF patients have been found to be markedly low in the epithelial lining fluid of the lungs. This deficiency is seen not as a result of reduced glutathione production, but rather as a result of reduced glutathione efflux from cells. Inhaled buffered glutathione has been studied as a treatment, with positive results; larger studies are warranted. Oral glutathione is considered as well; further studies are needed to determine if glutathione is absorbed intact in the digestive system.[61] At present, the Cystic Fibrosis Foundation does not advocate the use of glutathione in patients with CF, as its effectiveness and safety are unknown, although they are making efforts to design and fund large clinical trials on glutathione.[62]

While some preliminary data suggest potential benefits of CAM modalities in the treatment of CF, such as supplementation of antioxidants and glutathione, and the use of mind–body techniques, there is not yet evidence that these therapies will affect overall morbidity and mortality. Further research is needed in this area.

LUNG CANCER

Any overgrowth of tissue in the lungs, including lung cancer, will decrease the capacity of the lungs to exchange air. About 90–95% of lung cancers in men and about 70–80% of cancers in women result from cigarette smoking.[1] It is, therefore, imperative that those in the health care industry teach their patients the risk of lung cancer with cigarette smoking, the importance of smoking cessation, and that in an ex-smoker the risk for lung cancer declines over approximately 5 years.[6] As previously mentioned, passive smoking, or second-hand smoke, is also associated with an increased risk of lung cancer.[5] There are a number of occupations that increase the risk of lung cancer as well, including those requiring work with iron, arsenic, and methyl ether, and those which involve exposure to radioactive agents and asbestos.

Lung cancer is divided into two types, small cell, occurring almost exclusively in smokers, and non-small cell. Types of non-small cell lung cancer are squamous, adenocarcinoma, and large cell.[5] The location of the tumor can help differentiate the type of cancer; squamous cell cancer tends to occur centrally in the lung, while large cell and adenocarcinomas are usually more peripheral in the lung. Adenocarcinoma is the most frequent physiological subtype of carcinoma in nonsmokers but is also found in smokers. Depending on the position of the cancer, the airway may be compromised early or later in the stage of the illness. Removal of a part of a lung or even the complete lung may be necessary to alleviate the growth of this type of cancer.

NUTRITION AND LUNG CANCER PREVENTION

Diets low in vegetables and fruits are associated with an increased risk for lung cancer, even in the face of tobacco abuse.[63] It is unknown which bioactive compound or compounds in plant foods provide the chemoprotective effects, although there is consistent evidence that a higher intake of antioxidants is inversely associated with a lower risk for lung cancer. Because it had been noted that the intake of beta-carotene had been inversely associated with lung cancer in various populations, this antioxidant was trialed in early intervention studies as a possible chemopreventive agent for lung cancer.[64] However, beta-carotene supplementation has since been associated with an increased risk for mortality as reported in the ATBC Prevention study.[65] This study, which involved male smokers from Finland, found a 16% higher incidence of lung cancer in the group receiving beta-carotene supplementation.[65] The adverse impact associated with high doses may be due to antioxidant-independent mechanisms that are associated with induction of the cytochrome P-450 enzymes and altered normal retinoid signaling.[66] Furthermore, supplementation with other antioxidants such as vitamins A, C, and E has not been shown to offer any benefits in reducing the risk for lung cancer.[67]

On the other hand, diets rich in carotenoids, tomatoes, and tomato-based products may reduce the risk for lung cancer. A lower risk for lung cancer has been observed when the highest quintiles versus the lowest quintiles are compared for consumption of the following phytochemicals: lycopene (reduced by 28%), lutein or zeaxanthin (reduced by 17%), beta-cryptoxanthin (reduced by 15%), total carotenoids (reduced by 16%), and serum beta-carotene (reduced by 19%).[68] Other dietary antioxidants such as flavonoids, especially quercetin, may also reduce the risk of lung cancer.[64] Similar to other antioxidants, flavonoids eliminate free radicals; foods such as apples, onions, and white grapefruits are good sources of flavonoids.

Recently, as part of the Iowa Women's Health Study, Lee and Jacobs[69] followed 34,708 postmenopausal women, aged 55–69 years for 16 years to determine the incidence of lung cancers. During the study period, 700 lung cancers were diagnosed. A review of the dietary data collected at baseline and throughout the study suggested that a high dietary heme iron intake may increase the risk of lung cancer, whereas high dietary zinc may decrease the risk among postmenopausal women who consume high-dose vitamin C supplements.[69] These data are particularly important to smokers, for whom vitamin C supplementation is a common recommendation.

Low selenium levels, especially for men, are also associated with an increased risk for lung cancer, whereas higher levels of selenium appear to provide a protective effect.[70] Epidemiological evidence also suggests a role for dietary phytoestrogens in decreasing lung cancer risk.[71] Individuals in the highest phytoestrogen intake tertiles have a reduction in risk of lung cancer of 24%.[71]

NUTRITION DURING TREATMENT

After diagnosis, cancer patients become very interested in not only treatment options, but also seek information on how to beat cancer and improve outcomes through nutrition, dietary and herbal supplement use, and nutritional complementary therapies. Family, friends, health care providers, health food stores, the media, and the Internet are sources of information. Many times, patients become overwhelmed and confused when inundated with an abundance of conflicting information.

The continuum of cancer survival includes treatment, recovery, and living with advanced cancer. Each stage is associated with different needs and challenges as the presence of cancer and the oncological treatment therapies have a profound effect on nutritional status. Nutrition is an important component of medical care; nutrition goals include the following:

- Prevention or reversal of nutritional deficiencies
- Prevention or improvement in treatment-related symptoms
- Enhanced response to therapy
- Decreased morbidity related to disease and treatment
- Prevention or improvement in functional ability
- Maintenance or improvement in quality of life

Ideally, patients should be screened for nutritional risk before oncological therapy begins. The results of the Eastern Cooperative Oncological Group study[72] revealed that the presence of a 5% or more weight loss from usual body weight prior to initiation of therapy had a negative impact on outcome in terms of quality of life and survival. While anorexia has been reported as the most common problem affecting the ability of patients with cancer to consume adequate oral nutrition, newly diagnosed patients with advanced cancer also complained of abdominal fullness (60%), constipation (58%), taste changes (46%), mouth dryness (40%), nausea (39%), and vomiting (27%) prior to initiation of antineoplastic treatment.[73] Antineoplastic therapies, including surgery, chemotherapy, and radiation, are known contributors to malnutrition. Chemotherapy can result in mucositis, taste changes, early satiety, diarrhea, constipation, anorexia, nausea, and emesis. Radiation therapy when directed toward organs associated with the mechanics of eating or nutrient absorption can lead to esophageal stricture, reflux, gastritis, radiation enteritis, xerostemia, dysphagia, odynophagia, diarrhea, and malabsorption. Each of these treatment-induced effects can promote malnutrition and should be aggressively treated.

Patients identified at moderate and high nutritional risk should receive a comprehensive nutritional assessment, which includes evaluation of anthropometric measurements (including weight history, BMI, and waist-to-hip ratio), nutrition history, physical examination for signs of nutritional deficiencies, and laboratory data (e.g., electrolytes, renal functions, glucose, serum albumin, serum prealbumin, hemoglobin and hematocrit together with mean corpuscular volume (MCV), and mean corpuscular hemoglobin concentration (MCHC)). Assessment of performance status and quality of life should also be considered part of a comprehensive nutritional assessment. Patients identified with malnutrition should receive an individualized plan for nutrition intervention that includes goals for clinical outcomes as well as plans for intervention. This plan should be in concert with not only the medical team's goals but also the patient's or caregiver's wishes. Patients should be reassessed on a regular basis to allow for evaluation of the intervention's success and to determine if the nutrition care plan should be revised based on the patient's clinical status, treatment plan, etc.

Patients diagnosed with lung cancer reportedly experience weight loss moderately (48–61%), while patients with advanced cancer experience malnutrition most frequently.[72] REE is reportedly increased in patients with lung cancer, which is a likely contributor to weight loss.[74] Although higher energy intakes reportedly lead to weight gain, these gains typically increase in fat mass rather than lean body mass.[74] Further studies are needed to determine if anti-inflammatory medications, dietary agents such as (n–3) fatty acids, and exercise might be effective therapies for preserving FFM during chemotherapy.

Although no clinical studies have evaluated the benefits of an increased intake of fruits and vegetables for treatment and recovery of lung cancer, it is reasonable to assume this may be beneficial. In general, individuals with lung cancer should follow the American Cancer Society's dietary recommendations for nutrition during treatment (see Table 17.2).

Use of Supplements during Antineoplastic Therapy

For patients undergoing antineoplastic therapy, whether or not to use dietary or antioxidant supplements is an important issue. Chemotherapy induces a greater level of stress than the cancer itself. During chemotherapy, lipid peroxidation products are increased, thereby

---

TABLE 17.2
Nutrition Recommendations for Dietary Intake during Antineoplastic Therapies

Consume a balanced diet containing a wide variety of colorful, unprocessed, appetizing foods

Consume clean and wholesome foods with reduced levels of additives, preservatives, hormones, antibiotics, and other chemicals

Choose the majority of foods from plant sources

Reduce intake of animal foods — choose lean cuts of meat and poultry, and low fat dairy products

Increase intake of omega-3 fatty acids through the consumption of wild salmon and other cold-water fish, green leafy vegetables, and nuts

Avoid polyunsaturated vegetables oils, margarines, all partially hydrogenated oils and foods that contain trans-fatty acids

Drink green or black tea regularly

Take a multivitamin–mineral supplement daily

Maintain body weight

Be physically active

reducing the free-radical trapping capacity of blood plasma, resulting in diminished plasma levels of antioxidants. This high level of oxidative stress is thought to overcome the oxidative defenses of the cancer cell and its specialized systems that normally decrease lipid peroxidation. Increasing lipid peroxidation reduces or inhibits cancer cell proliferation and interferes with the activity of chemotherapy.[75] This may have an important impact on the response to chemotherapy as individuals with depleted antioxidant levels may fail to respond to treatment.[75] It has been suggested that antioxidants should be supplemented during chemotherapy. Of note, *in vitro* and animal studies have suggested that maintaining micronutrient levels can improve the antitumor activity of chemotherapeutic modalities.[76,77] Several studies have shown that high doses of individual antioxidant micronutrients inhibit the growth as well as promote apoptosis in cancer cells *in vitro*.[78] These antioxidants also reduce the growth of tumors in animal models and certain human tumors (cervical and oral cancers) without affecting the growth of healthy cells.[78] It is also believed that antioxidants may reduce the toxicity associated with chemotherapy.[75]

Radiation therapy causes damage to both normal and cancer cells, primarily through the production of free radicals and, to a lesser extent, direct ionization. It has been postulated that if radiation-modifying agents can either selectively protect normal cells against radiation damage or enhance the effects of radiation on tumor cells but not healthy cells, the efficacy of radiation therapy could be improved. Thus far, however, such agents have been found to be ineffective.[78] Therefore, it has been proposed that antioxidants might be the most useful selective radiation-modifying agents that are nontoxic. Researchers and clinicians are divided on this issue; some believe that antioxidants may protect both cancer and healthy cells, while others believe that antioxidants might improve the efficacy of radiation therapy by increasing tumor response and diminishing the toxic impact on normal cells.[78]

A few case reports have stated that high doses of micronutrients, including antioxidants, have been well tolerated by people receiving radiation therapy and chemotherapy. Although a placebo-controlled clinical trial investigating the use of antioxidants during radiation therapy has not been conducted, a randomized pilot trial using high-dose multiple micronutrients and antioxidants (including vitamins C and E, and natural beta-carotene) for cancer patients receiving radiation and chemotherapy has been completed.[78] It was reported that participants tolerated the antioxidant or micronutrient supplementation without adverse effects and quality of life was improved during radiation therapy.

Based on the clinical data to date, the prevailing recommendation in clinical practice is that antioxidant supplements should not be used during chemotherapy or radiation therapy. Supplements tend to provide nutrients and antioxidants at levels that are 1000 times greater than those found in food. Noncontrolled clinical trials have found no changes in antioxidants levels with supplementation during therapy, and no reduction in toxicity-related symptoms such as mucositis, alopecia, and stomatitis. Studies have also demonstrated that cancer cells readily absorb vitamins and contain higher vitamin C concentrations than the surrounding healthy tissue.[79,80]

COMPLEMENTARY AND ALTERNATIVE MEDICINE THERAPIES

Several surveys of CAM use by cancer patients have found that from 30 to 69% of patients with cancer use one or more CAM therapies as part of their cancer treatment. These therapies include herbal remedies, vitamins, and special diets. Reportedly, most people with cancer do not expect CAM therapies to cure their cancer.[81] Instead, CAM therapies are used to treat symptoms and side effects such as pain, nausea, fatigue, and anxiety that frequently arise due to either the disease or the antineoplastic therapies utilized.

Conventional cancer treatment therapies have generally been studied for safety and effectiveness through a rigorous scientific process that includes clinical trials with large numbers of patients. Until recently, less was known about the safety and effectiveness of complementary and alternative methods. Some CAM therapies have undergone rigorous evaluation, while others have not. With this new evidence, some CAM modalities are now accepted as complementary therapies to help cancer patients feel better as well as improve their quality of life. To gain greater insight into the appropriate use of CAM therapies, the National Cancer Institute and the National Center for Complementary and Alternative Medicine are currently sponsoring various clinical trials to study complementary and alternative treatments for cancer. Current trials that may include patients with lung cancer are investigating shark cartilage, massage therapy, and mistletoe extract. Acupuncture for chemotherapy-related nausea and vomiting; healing touch massage for anxiety, nausea, and lymphedema; and exercise to improve physical function and psychological or physical symptoms have been found to be safe and effective modalities for addressing many of the symptoms related to cancer.[82] An in-depth review of the efficacy of CAM modalities and cancer is beyond the scope of this chapter.

When advising lung cancer patients on the use of CAM modalities, the health care practitioner should consider the following:

- Discuss the evidence that supports efficacy and safety
- Respect the patient's beliefs and choices
- Encourage integrative therapies
- Discourage any therapies that delay conventional treatment with proven efficacy

Additional information regarding the safety and efficacy of CAM therapies and cancer can be obtained from the following Web sites:

- www.quackwatch.org
- cis.nci.nih.gov/fact/
- www.mskcc.org
- mdanderson.org/

Subscriptions: www.herbalgram.org, www.naturaldatabase.com

ADULT RESPIRATORY DISTRESS SYNDROME

Adult respiratory distress syndrome (ARDS) is a potentially fatal disorder of the bronchi, resulting in severely impeded air exchange. It can be caused by a number of incidents, including trauma, shock, aspiration, transfusions, and infections.[6] Mortality may reach as high as 50%, if ARDS is not diagnosed early and treated aggressively.[5] Characteristics of ARDS include diffuse pulmonary infiltrates (although in early stages a chest x-ray may be normal or suggest pneumonia), severe hypoxemia due to shunting and ventilation or perfusion mismatch, and an abnormal or low pulmonary capillary wedge pressure.[6] In ARDS, the cells of the capillary wall become inflamed and swell, resulting in a "leaky" capillary membrane. Protein is deposited in the alveoli, thus decreasing the area in which oxygen can be exchanged. Fibrosis usually develops within days or weeks. Although use of steroids is a common treatment for ARDS, there have been no studies that show a decrease in mortality or morbidity with this mode of treatment.[5,6] As the most common cause of ARDS is sepsis, aggressive broad-spectrum antibiotics should be utilized. Mechanical ventilation with positive airway pressure is usually necessary to decrease mortality.[5]

MEDICAL NUTRITION THERAPY

Nutrition support is essential for ARDS patients, as most require mechanical ventilation. While parenteral nutrition may be necessary in patients with nonfunctional GI tracts or severe hemodynamic instability, EN is the preferred method of nutrition support. The primary focus of nutritional care is to provide adequate calories and protein. Nutrition needs may be elevated depending on the precipitating cause of ARDS, as in trauma and sepsis, but it is also essential to avoid overfeeding patients with respiratory failure, as provision of excess calories has been shown to increase CO_2 production, and therefore increase the burden of work on the lungs. Protein needs are elevated, and may be as high as 1.5–2.0 g/kg.[83]

Modulation of immune function through the use of specialized enteral formulas may also be of benefit in treating patients with ARDS. Fatty acids, particularly EPA and gamma-linolenic acid (GLA), have been shown to downregulate immunity, therefore aiding the reduction in inflammation in patients with inflammatory diseases such as ARDS. ARDS results in an increased production of free radicals, therefore increasing the body's need for neutralizing antioxidants. An enteral formula is available that contains EPA from fish oil, GLA from borage oil, and supplemental amounts of antioxidants in the form of vitamin E, vitamin C, and carotenes. In clinical studies, ARDS patients receiving EPA, GLA, and antioxidants showed improvements in gas exchange and reduced requirements for mechanical ventilation.[84]

Other considerations in enterally feeding ARDS patients include the type of feeding tube, patient positioning, and the use of propofol. Small intestinal feeds may be better tolerated, as critically ill patients frequently have delayed gastric emptying.[85] Patients may be intermittently placed in the prone position, thus increasing the risk of aspiration of enteral formulas; feeding postpylorically may eliminate the need to hold enteral feeds while the patient is proned.[86] Propofol, a short-acting sedative commonly used in vented patients, is delivered in a fat base, and can therefore contribute significantly to the patient's calorie provision. The use of this medication must be monitored closely, and adjustments to the feeding rate made accordingly.

NON-NUTRITION MANAGEMENT

Placing ventilated ARDS patients in the prone position has been shown to improve oxygenation via reduced compression of the lungs by edematous overlying tissue. No studies on proning have demonstrated improved mortality.[87] In addition to proning, kinetic therapy may also be used to treat ARDS. Kinetic therapy is achieved via the use of specialty beds that continuously turn the patient by inflating and deflating areas of the mattress. Kinetic therapy has been shown to help redistribute localized edema and mobilize pulmonary secretions, thus minimizing infection and atelectasis. Further research is needed to determine kinetic therapy's significance in the improvement of oxygenation and gas exchange in ARDS.[88]

Inhaled surfactant is used successfully in infants with respiratory distress syndrome. Surfactant reduces alveolar surface tension, thus preventing alveolar collapse; concentrations of surfactant have been found to be low in patients with ARDS. However, research on its use in adult patients has shown no statistically significant benefit of surfactant use in this population.[87]

Inhaled nitric oxide has also been proposed as a treatment for ARDS; it acts as a vasodilator, helps improve oxygenation, and reduces mean pulmonary arterial pressure. Other potentially beneficial effects include anticoagulation, anti-inflammatory, and antimicrobial qualities. Despite these promising characteristics, however, research results are mixed; improved oxygenation may only occur for a limited time after treatment, and there has been no documented survival benefit.[87]

Prostaglandin E1 also acts as a vasodilator and has anti-inflammatory effects, however, like nitric oxide, studies have shown improvement in oxygenation but no positive effect on mortality. Prostacyclin, another prostaglandin, acts as a vasodilator, platelet aggregation inhibitor, and may increase surfactant protein secretion. Studies have also demonstrated increased oxygenation, but have not shown any improvement in mortality.[87]

SEVERE ACUTE RESPIRATORY SYNDROME

Severe Acute Respiratory Syndrome (SARS) emerged in late 2002 in China and spread worldwide, although a majority of the reported cases are in China.[89] The first case of SARS appeared in a health care worker from the Guangdong province in China, who was hospitalized for pneumonia while visiting Hong Kong, where he eventually died. By March 2003, the disease had spread to Hong Kong, Vietnam, and as far away as Canada. By the end of April 2003, there were over 4300 documented SARS cases and 250 SARS-related deaths in 25 countries worldwide.[89–92] The SARS virus appears to be common in animals and, because of the close proximity of animals to humans in the Guangdong province in China, it appears that the virus was transmitted to humans.

Fatal SARS infections are marked by diffuse alveolar damage, macrophage infiltration, and epithelial cell proliferation.[93] SARS patients can present with a variety of symptoms depending on the stage of infection. Early stage infection indications include a fever, which is seen in 100% of cases, chills (73–100%), headaches (30–70%), myalgias or muscle aches (20–60%), and malaise (70%). Later stage infections are marked by dyspnea (60–80%), diarrhea (20–70%), symptoms of respiratory failure (78%) as well as a dry and unproductive cough, which produces a crackling sound (57–100%).[94] The additional finding of travel within 10 days of onset of symptoms in a locale known to be affected by SARS outbreaks may also indicate infection. Close contact, such as kissing, embracing, sharing eating or drinking utensils, close conversation (less than 3 ft), or direct physical contact with a person known or suspected to be infected by SARS may further suggest possible infection. A diagnosis may be made by the detection of the antibody to SARS-CoV.[95] At present, there is no specific treatment recommended from the Centers for Disease Control (CDC) to treat SARS. Under current federal executive orders revised on April 4, 2003, SARS is considered a detainable communicable disease, which means that the government can legally quarantine potentially infected persons to prevent its spread.[89] When handling such cases, standard precautions such as hand hygiene, as well as airborne and contact precautions should be taken.[95]

ASTHMA

Asthma affects approximately 5% of the U.S. population, and approximately 470,000 annual hospitalizations are attributed to asthma.[8,96] Asthma is characterized by airway inflammation and responsiveness to stimuli, and symptoms include wheezing, difficulty in breathing, chest tightness, and coughing.[2,7] Other conditions may cause wheezing; these diagnoses must be considered in those who do not respond to asthma therapy. There are a number of physiological hallmarks of asthma. These include mucus gland hypertrophy, mucus hypersecretion, epithelial discrimination, widening of the basal membrane, and infiltration of eosinophils.

Asthma usually follows a pattern of periods without symptoms, followed by exacerbations caused by known and unknown stimuli. Asthma attacks are episodes of shortness of breath or wheezing, which may last for minutes, up to an hour, or several days in status asthmaticus. Status asthmaticus is an acute, severe, and prolonged attack, which may be fatal.[96] In the absence of attacks, patients may be completely symptom-free.[7] The associated cough with asthma may be either productive or dry and the severity of symptoms varies greatly among patients. Asthma symptoms are frequently worse at night and in the cooler winter months. Essentials of diagnosis include symptoms of airflow obstruction, worsening symptoms at night, prolonged expiration and wheezing on examination, and reversibility of airflow obstruction.[2] Findings of increased nasal mucosal swelling, increased nasal secretions, and the presence of nasal polyps increase the possibility of asthma.[2]

Bronchial hyperresponsiveness or irritability is generally present in all forms of asthma. It is important for the health care provider to realize that there are a number of irritants that can cause asthma exacerbation. These include perfume, cleaning solutions, smoke, dust, vegetable dust, which includes cotton dust, flour, ground coffee, and a variety of other irritants.[2,7,96,97] Chemicals in plastics including polyvinylchloride, food industry agents including egg proteins, and animal parts such as horse dander and rodent urine have also been implicated in the exacerbation of asthma. Certain medications, including aspirin, have also been implicated in the exacerbation of asthma, and can lead to status asthmaticus. It is therefore important to obtain a complete occupational, social, and medical history in a patient who presents with these symptoms.

The presence of asthma, nasal polyps, and asthma allergy is called the triad syndrome, or Samter syndrome, and was first described in 1922 by Ferdinand Widal et al.[98] It is a well-known syndrome in asthmatics and it is characteristic of bronchial asthma, nasal polyps, and intolerance to aspirin and aspirin-like medications including nonsteroidal anti-inflammatory drugs (NSAIDS). This syndrome is seen primarily in adults, but may occasionally occur in teenagers and children.[98] It is essential in these patients that their health care provider is aware that aspirin and anti-inflammatory medications, such as Motrin, can lead to angioedema and exacerbation of asthma, which if untreated can eventually lead to death.[98,99]

The goals of managing an asthma exacerbation are prompt recognition of the diagnosis, correction of the hypoxemia, and rapid reversal of the airflow obstruction to prevent further decline or future episodes.[2,100] Successful long-term management includes patient education, objective measurements of airflow obstruction, and adherence to a medication plan for daily use and exacerbations.[2] Medications for long-term control may include inhaled corticosteroids, systemic steroids if necessary, and long-acting β_2-agonists.[101] Leukotriene modifiers should be considered for those patients with aspirin-induced asthma or those who are unable to master the metered dose inhaler technique involved with inhalation treatment.[7] Methylxanthines such as theophylline may be most useful for controlling nighttime symptoms but require frequent drug level monitoring. The avoidance of certain medications that may potentially severely affect asthmatic patients also needs to be considered. In addition to avoidance of aspirin and NSAIDS, beta-blockers, used to treat hypertension and coronary artery disease, should also be avoided as they may exacerbate bronchospasms in asthmatics.[97] Education should include avoidance of triggers of airway responsiveness, avoidance of cold air and exercise, and avoidance of aspirin and NSAIDS. Soriano et al.[102] reported that patients who were taught how to use their peak flow meters had a significantly improved asthma control than those who were not. This underscores the necessity of patient education in long-term management.

MEDICAL NUTRITION THERAPY

The prevalence of asthma continues to increase despite the progress that has been made in the treatment options. Medications used for the treatment of asthma, including inhaled corticosteroids and short- and long-acting β_2-agonists, are highly effective in relieving symptoms and disease management, however, side effects and reduced efficacy limit long-term use. Alternative therapies, including dietary manipulation, may be of benefit in reducing the reliance on medications, reducing the costs of care, and promoting positive clinical outcomes such as improvements in functional ability and quality of life.

Increasing evidence suggests that dietary modification has the potential to influence the severity of asthma, and reduce the prevalence and incidence of the disease.[103] Global changes in dietary patterns, as evidenced by the increasing consumption of a Western diet, have paralleled the rise in the prevalence and incidence of asthma. Inflammation is an important part of the pathology of many medical conditions, including asthma. The Western diet, typified by a decreased intake of fruit, vegetables, whole grains, and $(n - 3)$ fatty acids, and an increased consumption of $(n - 6)$ fatty acids, sodium, refined grains and sugar, and red and processed meats, is associated with greater intake of the allergens and proinflammatory foods.[104,105] This type of diet has been cited as a contributing factor to the rising incidence of asthma.[104,106,107]

The available evidence regarding the association between diet and asthma ranges from observational to randomized controlled clinical trials. Although an in-depth discussion of the literature is beyond the scope of this chapter and is available elsewhere, Table 17.3 provides a summary of the antioxidants and PUFAs that may play a role in the development and treatment of asthma.[106,122–124] An inadequate intake of fruits and vegetables results in a deficit of antioxidants and is associated with a reduction in the lung antioxidant defenses, increased airway susceptibility to oxidant damage, resulting in airway inflammation and asthma.

TABLE 17.3
Nutrients That May Play a Role in the Prevalence and Incidence of Asthma

Nutrient	Potential Mechanism	Comments
Antioxidants		
Vitamin A and carotenoids	Needed for normal respiratory epithelial and lung development	Lower levels reported in patients with asthma[108]; beneficial association reported between dietary carotenoid intake and ventilatory function and respiratory symptoms[109,110]
Vitamin C	Intracellular and extracellular antioxidant activity	Dietary vitamin C associated with FEV_1 in adults; epidemiologic studies suggest a beneficial link between vitamin C intake and asthma[111]; no RCTs report a significant improvement in asthma with vitamin C supplementation[112]
Vitamin E	Protects against oxidant-induced membrane injury	Longitudinal data show a high vitamin E intake is associated with a decrease in asthma incidence. The only PRCT to date found no clinical benefit of vitamin E supplementation for 6 weeks in patients with asthma[113]
Selenium	A potent antioxidant, selenium, is an integral part of the body natural antioxidant glutathione peroxidase system	Decreased serum level reports in patients with asthma. Serum levels positively associated with FEV_1 in adults. One completed RCT found improvement in clinical assessments of asthma control in selenium-supplemented group[110]
Flavonoids	Antioxidant properties	Mixed results reported.[104,114] Greater intake of apples associated with a reduction in incidence of asthma; red wine may reduce the severity in some individuals[114]

Continued

TABLE 17.3 (Continued)
Nutrients That May Play a Role in the Prevalence and Incidence of Asthma

Nutrient	Potential Mechanism	Comments
Minerals		
Magnesium	Bronchodilator and smooth muscle relaxant	Mixed results reported.[115,116] IV magnesium sulfate resulted in improved peak expiratory flow rate in acute asthma exacerbations
Sodium	Increase in airway responsiveness and increased smooth muscle contraction	Available data from clinical studies suggest a trend that consumption of a low sodium diet maybe beneficial for patients with asthma[103]
Fatty acids		
Omega-6 fatty acids	Possess proinflammatory properties Increased arachidonic acid production	Observational and intervention study results mixed[107,117]
Omega-3 fatty acids (EPA and DHA)	Possess anti-inflammatory properties	Epidemiological studies suggest that a diet high in omega-3 fatty acids may have a beneficial effect on airway hyperresponsiveness.[105] Results from clinical studies equivocal[118–121]

Fatty acids may play a key role in the promotion of inflammation. Evidence from epidemiological and clinical secondary prevention trials has found that PUFAs have a significant influence on the prostaglandin pathways. These data are consistent with the proposed pathway by which dietary intake of $(n-3)$ PUFA modulates lung disease. The ratio of $(n-6)$ to $(n-3)$ fatty acids in our diet has greatly changed in the past years due to the introduction of processed vegetable oils and food preservation. The traditional Western diet is associated with a 20–25 fold greater amount of $(n-6)$ than $(n-3)$ PUFAs. Some experts recommend a healthier ratio of 5:1 to reduce the risk for many of the diseases associated with fat intake.

Dietary surveillance data report that Americans are still not meeting the national dietary guidelines that have been established to reduce the risk for chronic diseases and inflammatory conditions. The Behavioral Risk Factor Surveillance System Data found that more than 75% of the U.S. population failed to meet the recommended five servings each day of fruits and vegetables.[125] Furthermore, the continued consumption of a diet high in the omega-6 PUFAs, *trans*-fatty acids, refined carbohydrates, and sugars encourages a greater intake of omega-6 fatty acids and promotes inflammation. On the flip side, a diet heavy on vegetables, lean meats, whole grains, and omega-3 fatty acids diminishes the inflammatory process. In order to lessen the inflammatory effect of diet on the body, the anti-inflammatory diet is recommended (see Table 17.4). The anti-inflammatory diet encourages the consumption of fresh, unprocessed foods such as whole grains, fruits, vegetables, plant proteins, and omega-3 fatty acids (see Textbox 17.1 for further discussion of fish oils). Whether dietary supplementation with antioxidants and omega-3 fatty acids (as fish oils) would be beneficial for reducing the incidence of asthma as well as for treatment is not clear (see Table 17.3 for a review of evidence regarding supplementation). Large, well-designed prospective randomized trials are needed to better determine whether dietary supplementation would be beneficial.

TABLE 17.4
Components of the Anti-Inflammatory Diet

Avoid processed foods
   Commercially prepared convenience and fast foods
Increase intake of foods high in omega-3 fatty acids
   Salmon, tuna, sardines, mackerel, herring
   Soy, pumpkins and sunflower seeds, walnuts, flaxseeds, and oil
Avoid foods high in omega-6 fatty acids
   Margarine, sunflower, corn, and safflower oils
Avoid partially hydrogenated oils
Consume low-glycemic foods
Avoid refined grains and sugars; increase intake of whole grains, legumes,
   fruits, and vegetables
Increase intake of fruits and vegetables (goal four per day of each)
   Berries, apples, grapes, mangoes, etc.
   Dark green leafy, orange, red, and cruciferous vegetables
Decrease intake of red meat and high-fat dairy foods
Increase intake of white, black, or green teas
Increase intake of anti-inflammatory herbs
   Ginger, turmeric, capsaicin, boswellia

Food Allergies and Avoidance

Food allergy, as an exacerbating factor for asthma, is uncommon and occurs primarily in young children. Food avoidance should not be recommended before a double-blind food challenge has been made. When the outcome of such a challenge is positive, food allergen avoidance should be initiated, as it has been associated with a reduction in asthma exacerbations.

Sulfites (common food and drug preservatives found in foods such as processed potatoes, shrimp, dried fruits, beer, and wine) have often been implicated in causing severe asthma exacerbations and occasional deaths. They should be avoided by sensitive patients. Other dietary substances, such as the yellow dye tartrazine, benzoate, and monosodium glutamate, may have also been implicated, however, their role in asthma is unclear. Further clinical studies are needed to determine their relevance before making specific dietary restrictions.

Medication Usage

The incidence of osteoporosis in patients with asthma is similar to the population with COPD.[26] The chronic use of inhaled glucocorticoids for controlling inflammatory pathways is a primary cause. As in the COPD population, osteoporosis is underdiagnosed and under-treated in patients with asthma. Previously discussed strategies that reduce the risk for low bone density should be integrated into the overall plan for care for patients with asthma. Additionally, 1000 mg/day of calcium or 1000 mg/day in conjunction with cyclic etidronate has been shown to significantly increase lumbar spine BMD in patients chronically treated with glucocorticoids.[26]

COMPLEMENTARY AND ALTERNATIVE MEDICINE THERAPIES

Despite the lack of evidence supporting the efficacy of CAM modalities, the use of such therapies is popular in patients with asthma (see Table 17.5). Guidelines for use in clinical practice are also lacking due to the dearth of evidence from rigorous clinical trials.[111,123] In a

---

Textbox 17.1   Omega-3 Fatty Acids and Asthma

The Western diet has been implicated as a factor in the rising worldwide incidence of asthma due to the consumption of a diet high in the $(n - 6)$ PUFAs, *trans*-fatty acids, refined carbohydrates, and sugars. With the recommendation to decrease saturated fat intake to reduce coronary heart disease, the intake of omega-6 fatty acids, in the form of margarine and vegetable oils, increased in industrial countries. Furthermore, this has resulted in a lower omega-3 fatty acid intake. Given the proinflammatory nature of this diet, it would seem prudent that altering the intake of PUFAs in favor of increasing $(n - 3)$ fatty acids would be beneficial in reducing the prevalence and incidence of asthma. The benefits of $(n - 3)$ PUFA reportedly are derived due to the interference with early inflammatory signaling processes, reduction of AA in concentrations in neutrophils, decreased leukotriene generation, and reduced airway late response to allergen exposure.[105] Although there is increasing interest in using omega-3 fatty acid supplements (primarily as fish oils) as a potential therapeutic and pharmacologic intervention, the efficacy of using these supplements for the treatment of asthma is unclear. While some interventional studies have found no benefits, others have reported an improvement in asthmatic status.[118–121] Moreover, the Cochrane Database of Systematic Reviews also recently addressed the issue of efficacy regarding the use of fish oil supplements for children and adults, and was unable to determine if any benefits could be derived from supplementation.[108] The lack of clarity surrounding this issue is a result of the paucity of data in conjunction with the studies conducted to date having been poorly designed. Weaknesses in methodology include variability in fish oil dosage and grade, patient heterogeneity, and lack of outcome variables such as quality of life scores, and number of asthma exacerbations and hospital admissions, have been cited as study limitations.[105] While further studies are clearly needed to determine the efficacy of supplementation before global recommendations for use can be made, there is some evidence that suggests the omega-3 PUFA may have a protective impact on airway function in asthmatics. Since dietary guidelines published by many national organizations suggest eating fish at least two times per week, it seems prudent that individuals with asthma follow these recommendations.[126] Decreasing intake of omega-6 fatty acids, increasing consumption of fruits, vegetables, and whole grains, and avoiding consuming processed foods are also recommended in order to gain the benefits associated with the consumption of an anti-inflammatory diet. Foods high in omega-3 fatty acids include: cold-water oily fish, walnuts, pumpkin seeds, soy, some legumes, purslane, canola oil, and flaxseed seeds and oil. Studies, where fish oil supplementation has been linked with clinical benefits such as significant improvements in FEV_1, improved peak expiratory flow, reduced levels of TNF-α, and reduced medication use, have used low doses (1 g/day).[105]

---

review of the literature by Markham and Wilkinson,[123] very little evidence was found supporting the efficacy for various CAM modalities for improving outcome measures for asthma such as quality of life, pulmonary function, and immune function. Table 17.6 summarizes the results of the various studies that have evaluated the impact of CAM modalities on asthma. This clearly indicates that further research in this area is needed before CAM modalities can be recommended for widespread use for patients with asthma. Furthermore, the safety of these modalities also needs to be clarified. The use of herbal medicine reportedly was associated with an increased risk of hospitalization.[132] Side effects, such as pneumothorax and infection, have been associated with the use of acupuncture.[129]

TABLE 17.5
Popular CAM Modalities Used by Asthma Patients

Mind–body therapies
  Relaxation
  Buteyko breathing
  Yoga
  Music therapy
  Biofeedback
  Hypnosis
  Guided imaginary
Manual therapies
  Acupuncture
  Chiropractic
Herbal medicine or phytotherapy
  Traditional Chinese medicine
  Herbal remedies
  Propolis
Homeopathy
Others
  Speleotherapy
  Air ionizers

TUBERCULOSIS

Mycobacterium tuberculosis is the cause of the majority of TB in humans worldwide. The incidence of TB has increased since the 1980s, and the World Health Organization declared TB a global emergency in 1993. While present in developed countries, the spread of TB is most prevalent in sub-Saharan Africa, Asia, and the former Soviet Union. The increased incidence of TB in these countries is attributed to population growth, poverty, and drug resistance; other risk factors include diabetes, smoking, and poor nutritional intake. TB occurs more frequently in patients with HIV, and is a common cause of death in people with AIDS.[133]

The most common method of TB transmission is by inhalation of droplets from respiratory secretions. Active infection should be confirmed by the growth of *M. tuberculosis* from airway secretions, as chest x-rays can be normal in active TB. A positive purified protein derivative (PPD) skin test indicates exposure to the bacteria, but does not necessarily specify an active infection. Treatment of TB requires multidrug therapy, as monotherapy has been shown to be ineffective, and drug resistance is common. Proper treatment regimens and patient adherence are vital in improving response to therapy.[134] Liver toxicity is also a potential complication from these drugs and must be considered in the overall treatment of TB.[5]

MEDICAL NUTRITION THERAPY

Wasting is recognized as a common clinical feature in patients with TB. Malnutrition may be caused by a variety of factors, including poor intake resulting from reduced appetite, altered metabolism as a result of the inflammatory nature of the disease, and social factors common among patients with TB, such as poverty. Weight gain is typically seen with standard TB treatment, although some patients may remain underweight for months after completion of therapy, and much of the regained weight is often fat mass.[134] FFM, or lean mass, has been more closely associated with physical function and quality of life than fat mass or total body

TABLE 17.6
A Review of the Studies Assessing the Impact of CAM Modalities on Asthma

Modality	Sample Size	Outcome Measures Studied	Study Results
Mind–body therapies			
Biofeedback	$N = 16$	Immune function, medication use, lung function, and asthma severity	Significant reduction in white blood cells and neutrophils; significant increases in FEV_1 and FVC values; inhaler use decreased[127]
Relaxation	$N = 20$		
Buteyko breathing	$N = 36$	Asthma-related quality of life (QOL), peak expiratory flow, symptoms, and medication usage	Significant improvement in QOL, and significant reduction in bronchodilator usage[127,128]
Manual therapies			
Acupuncture (PRCT)[a]			
Single laser treatment	$N = 44$	Exercise-induced asthma; FEV_1	No protection against exercise-induced bronchoconstriction demonstrated[129]
Traditional acupuncture	$N = 23$	FEV_1, daily peak flow variability, symptom scores in patients with moderate persistent asthma	No significant differences or improvements were detected[130]
Traditional acupuncture	$N = 66$	Change in peak expiratory flow, changes in FEV_1, change in symptoms, medication usage, and QOL in patients with mild–moderate asthma	No significant differences in outcomes were noted[131]

[a]Prospective, randomized, controlled trials.

weight, so a gain in lean mass is desired. The relative lack of increased lean mass in this patient population may be a result of both reduced physical activity and altered protein metabolism.[134] However, a recent study has shown that nutritional counseling to increase intake, with the aid of commercially available nutrition supplements, resulted in a significant increase in lean body mass and improvement in physical function in patients in the early stages of treatment for TB.[135]

Isoniazid, a common drug used to treat both latent and active TB, increases the risk for peripheral neuropathy, especially in individuals with poor nutritional status. Vitamin B6 has been shown to prevent this complication, and may be supplemented in high-risk patients taking isoniazid, especially pregnant, malnourished, or alcoholic individuals.[136] Other micronutrient supplementation may be considered in cases of documented deficiency; commonly deficient nutrients in the TB population include iron, vitamin A, zinc, vitamin D, and niacin.[137–140] Studies have also suggested antioxidant levels are low in some patients with TB, however studies demonstrating benefit in the supplementation of nutrients such as vitamins E and C are lacking.[141]

Nutritional treatment of TB patients is further complicated in the presence of concomitant HIV infection; discussion of treatment for HIV or AIDS is discussed elsewhere in this text.

COMPLEMENTARY AND ALTERNATIVE MEDICINE THERAPIES

Little data are available regarding the prevalence of CAM modality use in patients with TB. As a high incidence of TB is found in developing nations, where traditional healers are the primary health care providers for a large part of the population, it can be surmised that the use of CAM may be high. Studies in Gambia, South Africa, Malawi, and India have suggested improvements in the number of TB patients treated successfully if traditional healers are educated on TB and then included in established TB programs.[142–145] Continuous education on the transmission and treatment of TB, for both the general population and health care providers, is essential in controlling TB internationally.

Some cultural medical beliefs prevalent in developing nations may hinder successful diagnosis and treatment of TB, especially in women, as they may face more barriers to receiving treatment, have different rates of compliance, and may fear the stigma associated with the disease more than men.[146] For example, delays in diagnosis and treatment have been reported in Nepalese women, as they are more likely to seek out traditional healers rather than government medical establishments.[147] In Vietnam, delays in treatment may occur due to beliefs in different types of TB, such as "physical" and "mental" TB, and the belief that men are more likely to contract TB than women.[148] This further underlines the necessity of continued education of both traditional healers and the general population.

As drug resistance is common, a great deal of current research on TB is focused on the development of new drugs. Hundreds of plant compounds have been identified as potentially toxic to *M. tuberculosis*, such as *Chamaedora tepejilote* hexane extract, extract of the stem bark of *Micromelum hirsutum*, and chemicals from the roots of *Engelhardia roxburghiana*, to name just a few.[149–151] While results of these studies are promising, more effort and research are necessary to develop new antitubercular drugs from these compounds.

SARCOIDOSIS

Sarcoidosis is a systemic disease of unknown etiology characterized by granulomatous inflammation of the lung in approximately 90% of patients.[2,142] However, multisystem involvement is characteristic and virtually any organ is vulnerable to this disease.[142] Incidence is highest in northern European whites and North American blacks; women are more affected than men among the black population. Onset is often in the third and fourth decade of life. The clinical presentation of patients with sarcoidosis usually include malaise, fever, and dyspnea, but 30–60% of patients are asymptomatic.[141] Among the patients who are asymptomatic, sarcoidosis is often discovered on chest x-ray. Pulmonary manifestations dominate the clinical course, although there is a wide variability among different patients regarding clinical course and prognosis. Spontaneous remissions occur in nearly two thirds of the patients while others experience chronic, persistent, progressive disease leading to severe loss of function of the affected organs.[142] Sarcoidosis is lethal in 1–4% of patients due to respiratory insufficiency or myocardial and central nervous system involvement.[142] Factors associated with a poorer prognosis include black race, onset after age of 40 years, hypercalcemia, splenomegaly, chronic uveitis, and osseous involvement.[142] Factors associated with an excellent prognosis include fever, polyarthritis, erythema nodosum, and bilateral hilar lymphadenopathy.[142]

Again, sarcoidosis is primarily a disease affecting the pulmonary system, which may have extrapulmonary manifestations involving the heart, brain, kidney, eye, or liver. Patients may be either symptomatic or asymptomatic with a vast range in prognosis dependent on several variables. Treatment is limited to steroids and immunosuppressive agents, but future studies are needed to assess the effectiveness of this medical treatment.

REFERENCES

1. Fauci, A.S. et al., *Harrison's Principles of Internal Medicine*, 14th ed., McGraw-Hill, New York, 1998.
2. Tierney, L.M. et al., *Current Medical Diagnosis and Treatment*, 39th ed., Lange Medical Books, McGraw-Hill, New York, 2000.
3. Thaler, D.E. et al., *Oxford of Clinical Medicine*, American ed., Oxford University Press, New York, 1999.
4. Mannino, D.M. et al., Chronic Obstructive Pulmonary disease surveillance — United States, 1971–2000, *MMWR Surveill. Summ.*, 51: 1–16, 2002.
5. Dambro, M.R., *Griffith's 5-minute Clinical Consult*, Lippincott, Williams & Wilkins, Philadelphia, 2001.
6. Wilson, J.D. et al., *Harrison's Principles of Internal Medicine*, 12th ed., McGraw-Hill, New York, 1991.
7. Ahya, S.N., Flood, K., and Paranjothi, S., *The Washington Manual of Medical Therapeutics*, 30th ed., Lippincott, Williams & Wilkins, Philadelphia, 2001.
8. Anthonisen, N.R. et al., Effects of smoking intervention and the use of inhaled anticholinergic bronchodilator on the rate of decline of FEVI. The Lung Health Study, *JAMA*, 272: 1497–1505, 1994.
9. Man, S.F.D. et al., Contemporary management of chronic obstructive pulmonary disease, *JAMA*, 290: 2313–2316, 2003.
10. Congleton, J., The pulmonary cachexia syndrome: aspects of energy balance, *Proc. Nutr. Soc.*, 58: 321–328, 1999.
11. Schols, A.M. et al., Prevalence and characteristics of nutritional depletion in patients with stable COPD eligible for pulmonary rehabilitation, *Am. Rev. Respir. Dis.*, 147: 1151–1156, 1993.
12. Wilson, D.O. et al., Body weight in chronic obstructive pulmonary disease: the National Institutes of Health Intermittent Positive Pressure Breathing Trial, *Am. Rev. Respir. Dis.*, 139: 1435–1438, 1989.
13. Landbo, C. et al., Prognostic value of nutritional status in chronic obstructive pulmonary disease, *Am. J. Respir. Crit. Care Med.*, 160: 1856–1861, 1999.
14. Foley, R. et al., The impact of nutritional depletion in chronic obstructive pulmonary disease, *J. Cardiopulm. Rehabil.*, 21: 188–195, 2001.
15. Sahebjami, H. and Sathianpitayakus, E., Influence of body weight on the severity of dyspnea in chronic obstructive pulmonary disease, *Am. J. Respir. Crit. Care Med.*, 161: 886–890, 2000.
16. Wouters, E., Nutrition and metabolism in COPD, *Chest*, 117, 274S–280S, 2000.
17. Engelen, M.P. et al., Nutritional depletion in relation to respiratory and peripheral skeletal muscle function in out patients with COPD, *Eur. Respir. J.*, 7: 1793–1797, 1994.
18. Berry, J.K. and Baum, C., Reversal of chronic obstructive pulmonary disease-associated weight loss. Are there pharmacological treatment options? *Druggist*, 64: 1041–1052, 2004.
19. Baarends, E.M. et al., Total free living energy expenditure in patients with severe chronic obstructive pulmonary disease, *Am. J. Respir. Crit. Care Med.*, 155: 549–554, 1997.
20. Tang, N.L. et al., Total daily energy expenditure in wasted chronic obstructive pulmonary disease patients, *Eur. J. Clin. Nutr.*, 56: 282–287, 2002.
21. Schols, A., Nutritional modulation as part of the integrated management of chronic obstructive pulmonary disease, *Proc. Nutr. Soc.*, 62: 783–791, 2003.
22. Schols, A.M. et al., Plasma leptin is related to proinflammatory status and dietary intake in patients with chronic obstructive pulmonary disease, *Am. J. Respir. Crit. Care Med.*, 160: 1220–1226, 1999.
23. Bolton, C.E. et al., Associated loss of fat-free mass and bone mineral density in chronic obstructive pulmonary disease, *Am. J. Respir. Crit. Care Med.*, 170: 1286–1293, 2004.
24. Schols, A.M.W.J. et al., Weight loss is a reversible factor in the prognosis of chronic obstructive pulmonary disease, *Am. J. Respir. Crit. Care Med.*, 157: 1791–1797, 1998.
25. Mallampalli, A., Nutritional management of the patient with chronic obstructive pulmonary disease, *Nutr. Clin. Pract.*, 19: 550–556, 2004.
26. Goldstein, M.F. et al., Chronic glucocorticoid therapy-induced osteoporosis in patients with obstructive lung disease, *Chest*, 116(6): 1733–1749, 1999, Review.

27. National Osteoporosis Foundation, Available at: www.nof.org (accessed: October 10, 2005).
28. Whittaker, J.S. et al., The effects of refeeding on peripheral and respiratory muscle function in malnourished chronic obstructive pulmonary disease patients, *Am. Rev. Respir. Dis.*, 142: 283–288, 1990.
29. Broek, R. et al., Optimizing oral nutritional drink supplementation in patients with chronic obstructive pulmonary disease, *Br. J. Nutr.*, 93(6): 965–971, 2005.
30. Fuenzalida, C.E. et al., The immune response to short-term nutritional intervention in advanced chronic obstructive pulmonary disease, *Am. Rev. Respir. Dis.*, 142(1): 49–56, 1990.
31. Efthimiou, J., The effect of supplementary oral nutrition in poorly nourished patients with chronic obstructive pulmonary disease, *Am. Rev. Respir. Dis.*, 137(5): 1075–1082, 1988.
32. Rogers, R.M., Donahoe, M., and Costantino, J., Physiologic effects of oral supplemental feeding in malnourished patients with chronic obstructive pulmonary disease. A randomized control study, *Am. Rev. Respir. Dis.*, 146: 1511–1517, 1992.
33. Ferreira, I.M. et al., Nutritional supplementation for stable chronic obstructive pulmonary disease, *Cochrane Database Syst. Rev.*, 2: CD000998, 2005.
34. Talpers, S.S. et al., Nutritionally associated increased carbon dioxide production: excess total calories vs. high proportion of carbohydrate calories, *Chest*, 102: 551–555, 1992.
35. Akrabawi, S.S. et al., Gastric emptying, pulmonary function, gas exchange, and respiratory quotient after feeding a moderate versus high fat enteral formula meal in chronic obstructive pulmonary disease patients, *Nutrition*, 12: 260–265, 1996.
36. Donahoe, M. et al., The effect of an aggressive nutritional support regimen on body composition in patients with severe COPD and weight loss, *Am. J. Respir. Crit. Care Med.*, 147: A313, 1994.
37. Borum, M.L. et al., The effect of nutritional supplementation on survival in seriously ill hospitalized adults: an evaluation of the SUPPORT data: study to understand prognoses and preferences for outcomes and risks of treatment, *J. Am. Geriatr. Soc.*, 48: S33–S38, 2000.
38. George, J. et al., Use of complementary and alternative medicines by patients with chronic obstructive pulmonary disease, *Med. J. Aust.*, 181: 248–251, 2004.
39. Maa, S.H. et al., Acupressure as an adjunct to a pulmonary rehabilitation program, *J. Cardiopulm. Rehabil.*, 17: 268–276, 1997.
40. Wu, H.S. et al., Effectiveness of acupressure in improving dyspnoea in chronic obstructive pulmonary disease, *J. Adv. Nurs.*, 45: 252–259, 2004.
41. Sliwinski, J. and Kulcj, M., Acupuncture induced immunoregulatory influence on the clinical state of patients suffering from chronic spastic bronchitis and undergoing long-term treatment with corticosteroids, *Acupunct. Electrother. Res.*, 14: 227–234, 1989.
42. Louie, S.W., The effects of guided imagery relaxation in people with COPD, *Occup. Ther. Int.*, 11: 145–159, 2004.
43. http://www.cff.org/UploadedFiles/publications/files/2003%20Patient%20Registry%20Report.pdf
44. Ren, C., Use of modulators of airways inflammation in patients with CF, *Clin. Rev. Allerg. Immunol.*, 23(1): 29–39, 2002.
45. Prescott, W.A. and Johnson, C.E., Antiinflammatory therapies for cystic fibrosis: past, present, and future, *Pharmacotherapy*, 25(4): 555–573, 2005.
46. Wood, L.G. et al., Circulating markers to assess nutritional therapy in cystic fibrosis, *Clin. Chim. Acta*, 353: 13–29, 2005.
47. Rust, P. et al., Long-term oral beta-carotene supplementation in patients with cystic fibrosis: effects on antioxidative status and pulmonary function, *Ann. Nutr. Metab.*, 44: 30–37, 2000.
48. Renner, S. et al., Effects of beta-carotene supplementation for six months on clinical and laboratory parameters in patients with cystic fibrosis, *Thorax*, 56: 48–52, 2001.
49. Freedman, S.D. et al., Fatty acids in cystic fibrosis, *Curr. Opin. Pulm. Med.*, 6: 530–532, 2000.
50. DeVizia, B. et al., Effect of an 8-month treatment with omega-3 fatty acids (eicosapentaenoic and docosahexaenoic) in patients with cystic fibrosis, *J. Parenter. Enteral Nutr.*, 27: 52–57, 2003.
51. Lawrence, R. and Sorrell, T., Eicosapentaenoic acid modulates neutrophils leukotriene B-4 receptor expressing in cystic fibrosis: evidence of a pathogenetic role for leukotriene B-4, *Lancet*, 342: 465–469, 1993.

52. Stern, R.C. et al., Use of nonmedical treatment by cystic fibrosis patients, *J. Adolesc. Health*, 13(7): 612–615, 1992.

53. Grasso, M.C. et al., Benefits of music therapy as an adjunct to chest physiotherapy in infants and toddlers with cystic fibrosis, *Pediatr. Pulmonol.*, 289(6): 371–381, 2000.

54. Holland, A.E. et al., Non-invasive ventilation assists chest physiotherapy in adults with acute exacerbations of cystic fibrosis, *Thorax*, 58(10): 880–884, 2003.

55. Faurox, B. et al., Chest physiotherapy in cystic fibrosis: improved tolerance with nasal pressure support ventilation, *Pediatrics*, 103: E32, 1999.

56. Enright, S. et al., Inspiratory muscle training improves lung function and exercise capacity in adults with cystic fibrosis, *Chest*, 126(2): 405–411, 2004.

57. De Jong, W. et al., Inspiratory muscle training in patients with cystic fibrosis, *Resp. Med.*, 95(1): 31–36, 2001.

58. Lin, Y.C. et al., Acupuncture pain management for patients with cystic fibrosis: a pilot study, *Am. J. Chin. Med.*, 33(1): 151–156, 2005.

59. Anbar, R.D., Self hypnosis for patients with cystic fibrosis, *Pediatr. Pulmonol.*, 30(6): 461–465, 2000.

60. Hernandez-Reif, M. et al., Children with cystic fibrosis benefit from massage therapy, *J. Pediatr. Psychol.*, 24(2): 175–181, 1999.

61. Hudson, V.M., New insights into the pathogenesis of cystic fibrosis: pivotal role of glutathione system dysfunction and implications for therapy, *Treat. Respir. Med.*, 3(6): 353–363, 2004.

62. http://www.cff.org/living_with_cf/nutrition_and_cf/

63. Skuladottir, H. et al., Does insufficient adjustment for smoking explain the preventive effects of fruit and vegetables on lung cancer? *Lung Cancer*, 45(1): 1–10, 2004.

64. Marchand, L.L. et al., Intake of flavonoids and lung cancer, *J. Natl. Cancer Inst.*, 92: 154–160, 2000.

65. The ATBC Cancer Prevention Study Group, The alpha-tocopherol, beta-carotene lung cancer prevention study: design, methods, participant characteristics, and compliance, *Ann. Epidemiol.*, 4(1): 1–10, 1994.

66. Wright, M.E. et al., Development of a comprehensive dietary antioxidant index and application to lung cancer risk in a cohort of male smokers, *Am. J. Epidemiol.*, 160: 68–76, 2004.

67. Fabricius, P. and Lange, P., Diet and lung cancer, *Monaldi Arch. Chest Dis.*, 59(3): 207–211, 2003.

68. Holick, C.N., Dietary carotenoids, serum beta-carotene, and retinol and risk of lung cancer in the alpha-tocopherol, beta-carotene cohort study, *Am. J. Epidemiol.*, 156(6): 536–547, 2002.

69. Lee, D.-H. and Jacobs, D.R., Jr., Interaction among heme iron, zinc, and supplemental vitamin C intake on the risk of lung cancer: Iowa Women's Health Study, *Nutr. Cancer*, 52: 130–137, 2005.

70. Donaldson, M.S., Nutrition and cancer: a review of the evidence for an anti-cancer diet, *Nutr. J.*, 3: 19, 2004.

71. Schabath, M.B. et al., Dietary phytoestrogens and lung cancer risk, *JAMA*, 294: 1493–1504, 2005.

72. DeWys, W.D., Prognostic effect of weight loss prior to chemotherapy in cancer patients. Eastern Cooperative Oncology Group, *Am. J. Med.*, 69(4): 491–497, 1980.

73. Grosvenor, M., Symptoms potentially influencing weight loss in a cancer population. Correlations with primary site, nutritional status, and chemotherapy administration, *Cancer*, 63(2): 330–334, 1989.

74. Harvie, M.N. et al., Energy balance in patients with advanced metastatic melanoma and metastatic breast cancer receiving chemotherapy — a longitudinal study, *Br. J. Cancer*, 92: 673–680, 2005.

75. Drisko, J.A. et al., The use of antioxidant therapies during chemotherapy, *Gynecol. Oncol.*, 88(3): 434–439, 2003. Review.

76. Spronck, J.B. and Kirkland, J.C., Niacin deficiency increases spontaneous and etoposide-induced chromosomal instability in rat bone marrow cells *in vivo*, *Mutat. Res.*, 508(1–2): 83–97, 2002.

77. Caffrey, P.B. and Frenkel, G.D., Selenium compounds prevent the induction of drug resistance by cisplatin in human ovarian tumor xenografts *in vivo*, *Cancer Chemother. Pharmacol.*, 46(1): 74–78, 2000.

78. Prasad, K.N. et al., Pros and cons of antioxidant use during radiation therapy, *Cancer Treat Rev.*, 28(2): 79–91, 2002. Review.

79. Agus, D.B. et al., Stromal cell oxidation: a mechanism by which tumors obtain vitamin C, *Cancer Res.*, 59(18): 4555–4558, 1999.
80. Langemann, H. et al., Quantitative determination of water- and lipid-soluble antioxidants in neoplastic and non-neoplastic human breast tissue, *Int. J. Cancer*, 43(6): 1169–1173, 1989.
81. http://mayoclinic.com/health/cancer-treatment/
82. Weiger, W.A. et al., Advising patients who seek complementary and alternative medical therapies for cancer, *Ann. Intern. Med.*, 137: 889–903, 2003.
83. Gottschlich, M.M., Ed., *The Science and Practice of Nutrition Support: A Case-Based Core Curriculum*, ASPEN, Kendall-Hunt, Dubuque, IA, 2001.
84. Gadek, J.E. et al., Effect of enteral feeding with eicosapentaenoic acid, gammalinoleic acid, and antioxidants with acute respiratory distress syndrome, *Crit. Care Med.*, 27: 1409–1420, 1999.
85. Ritz, M.A. et al., Impacts and patterns of disturbed gastrointestinal function in critically ill patients, *Am. J. Gastroenterol.*, 95: 3044–3052, 2000.
86. Reignier, J. et al., Early enteral nutrition in mechanically ventilated patients in the prone position, *Crit. Care Med.*, 32: 94–99, 2004.
87. Klein, Y. et al., Non-ventilatory-based strategies in the management of acute respiratory distress syndrome, *J. Trauma*, 57: 915–924, 2004.
88. Rance, M., Kinetic therapy positively influences oxygenation in patients with ALI/ARDS British Association of Critical Care Nurses, *Nurs. Crit. Care*, 10(1): 35–41, 2005.
89. Centers for Disease Control and Prevention. Severe Acute Respiratory Syndrome (SARS), Fact Sheet on Legal Authorities for Isolation/Quarantine, dated: April 23, 2003. http:www.cdc.gov/ncidod/sars/factsheetlegal.htm (accessed: October 21, 2003).
90. Lee, N. et al., A major outbreak of severe acute respiratory syndrome in Hong Kong, *N. Engl. J. Med.*, 348(20): 1986–1994, 2003.
91. Poutanen, S.M. et al., Identification of severe acute respiratory syndrome in Canada, *N. Engl. J. Med.*, 348(20): 1995–2005, 2003.
92. Tsang, K.W. et al., Severe acute respiratory syndrome (SARS) in Hong Kong, *Respirology*, 8: 259–265, 2003.
93. Nicholls, J.M. et al., Lung pathology of fatal severe acute respiratory syndrome, *Lancet*, 361: 1773–1778, 2003.
94. Tsang, K.W. et al., A cluster of cases of severe acute respiratory syndrome in Hong Kong, *N. Engl. J. Med.*, 348: 1977–1985, 2003.
95. Centers for Disease Control and Prevention. Severe Acute Respiratory Syndrome (SARS), Updated Interim U.S. Case Definition for Severe Acute Respiratory Syndrome (SARS), dated: July 18, 2003. http:www.cdc.gov/ncidod/sars/casedefinition.htm (accessed: October 21, 2003).
96. Anderson, K.N., Anderson, L.E., and Glanze, W.D., *Mosby's Dictionary*, 5th ed., C.V. Mosby, St. Louis, 1998.
97. Asthma and Allergy Foundation of America, Allergic Asthma, http://www.aafa.org/display.cfm?id=8&sub=16 (accessed: October 2003).
98. Samter, M. and Beers, R.F., Concerning the nature of intolerance to aspirin, *J. Allergy*, 40: 281–293, 1967.
99. Zeitz, H.J., Bronchial asthma, nasal polyps, and aspirin sensitivity: Samter syndrome, *Clin. Chest Med.*, 9: 567–576, 1988.
100. Roy, S.R. and Milgrom, H., Management of the acute exacerbation of asthma, *J. Asthma*, 40: 593–604, 2003.
101. O'Connor, R.D., Current approaches to asthma management: assessing clinical and economic evidence, *J. Manag. Care Pharm.*, 8(Suppl. 5): 8–17, 2002.
102. Soriano, J.B. et al., Predictors of poor asthma control in European adults, *J. Asthma*, 40: 803–813, 2003.
103. Mickleborough, T.D. and Gotshall, R.W., Dietary salt intake as a potential modifier to airway responsiveness in bronchial asthma, *J. Altern. Complement Med.*, 10: 633–642, 2004.
104. Devereux, G. and Seaton, A., Diet as a risk factor for atopy and asthma, *J. Allergy Clin. Immunol.*, 115: 1109–1117, 2005.

105. Mickleborough, T.D., Dietary omega-3 polyunsaturated fatty acid supplementation and airway hyperresponsiveness in asthma, *J. Asthma*, 42: 305–314, 2005.

106. Smit, H.A., Chronic obstructive pulmonary disease, asthma and protective effects of food intake: from hypothesis to evidence, *Respir. Res.*, 2: 261–264, 2001.

107. Black, P.N. and Sharpe, S., Dietary fat and asthma: is there a connection? *Eur. Respir. J.*, 10: 6–12, 1997.

108. Wood, L.G. et al., Carotenoid concentrations in asthmatics versus healthy controls, *Asia Pac. J. Clin. Nutr.*, 13: S74, 2004.

109. Gilliland, F.D. et al., Children's lung function and antioxidant vitamin, fruit, juice and vegetable intake, *Am. J. Epidemiol.*, 158: 576–584, 2003.

110. Hu, G. and Cassano, P., Antioxidants and pulmonary function: the third National Health and Nutrition Examination Survey (NHANES III), *Am. J. Epidemiol.*, 151: 975–981, 2000.

111. Györik, S.A. and Brutsche, M.T., Complementary and alternative medicine for bronchial asthma: is there new evidence? *Curr. Opin. Pulm. Med.*, 10: 37–43, 2004.

112. Kaur, B. et al., Vitamin C supplementation for asthma, *Cochrane Database Syst. Rev.*: CD00093, 2001.

113. Pearson, P.J.K. et al., Vitamin E supplements in asthma: a parallel group randomized placebo-controlled trial, *Thorax*, 59: 652–656, 2004.

114. Shaheen, S.O. et al., Dietary antioxidants and asthma in adults, *Am. J. Respir. Crit. Care Med.*, 164: 1823–1828, 2001.

115. Fogarty, A. et al., Oral magnesium and vitamin C supplements in asthma: a parallel group randomized placebo-controlled trial, *Clin. Exp. Allergy*, 33: 1355–1359, 2003.

116. Kelley, P.J. and Arney, T.D., Use of magnesium sulfate for pediatric patients with acute asthma exacerbations, *J. Infus. Nurs.*, 28: 329–336, 2005.

117. Broadfiled, E.C. et al., A case–control study of dietary and erythrocyte membrane fatty acids in asthma, *Clin. Exp. Allergy*, 34: 1232–1236, 2004.

118. Kirsch, C. et al., Effect of eicosapentaenoic acid in asthma, *Clin. Allergy*, 18: 177–187, 1988.

119. Picado, D. et al., Effects of a fish oil enriched diet on aspirin intolerant asthmatic patients: a pilot study, *Thorax*, 43: 93–97, 1988.

120. Dry, J. and Vincent, D., Effect of a fish oil diet on asthma: results of a 1-year double-blind study, *Int. Arch. Allergy Appl. Immunol.*, 95: 156–157, 1991.

121. Hodge, L. et al., Effect of dietary intake of omega-3 and omega-6 fatty acids on severity of asthma in children, *Eur. Respir. J.*, 11: 361–365, 1998.

122. Fogarty, A. and Britton, J., The role of diet in the aetiology of asthma, *Clin. Exp. Allergy*, 30: 615–627, 2000.

123. Markham, A.W. and Wilkinson, J.M., Complementary and alternative medicines (CAM) in the management of asthma: an examination of the evidence, *J. Asthma*, 41: 131–139, 2004.

124. McKeever, T.M. and Britton, J., Diet and asthma, *Am. J. Respir. Crit. Care Med.*, 170: 725–729, 2004.

125. 5 A Day The Color Way. Available at: http://5aday.com (accessed: October 10, 2005).

126. American Heart Association. Available at: www.americanheart.org

127. Kern-Buell, C.L. et al., Asthma severity, psychophysiological indicators of arousal, and immune function in asthma patients undergoing biofeedback-assisted relaxation, *Appl. Psychophysio. Biofeedback*, 25: 79–91, 2000.

128. Opat, A.J. et al., A clinical trial of the Buteyko breathing technique in asthma as taught by a video, *J. Asthma*, 37: 557–564, 2000.

129. Norheim, A.J., Adverse effects of acupuncture: a study of the literature for the years 1981–1994, *J. Altern. Complement Med.*, 2: 291–297, 1996.

130. Shapira, M.Y. et al., Short-term acupuncture therapy is of no benefit in patients with moderate persistent asthma, *Chest*, 121: 1396–1400, 2002.

131. Medici, T.C. et al., Acupuncture and bronchial asthma: a long-term randomized study of the effects of real versus sham acupuncture compared to controls in patients with bronchial asthma, *J. Altern. Complement Med.*, 8: 737–750, 2002.

132. Blanc, P.D. et al., Use of herbal products, coffee or black tea, and over-the-counter medications as self-treatments among adults with asthma, *J. Allergy Clin. Immunol.*, 100: 789–791, 1997.

133. Davies, P., The world-wide increase in tuberculosis: how demographic changes, HIV infection and increasing numbers in poverty are increasing tuberculosis, *Ann. Med.*, 35: 235–243, 2003.

134. Shwenk, A. et al., Nutrient partitioning during treatment of tuberculosis: gain in body fat mass but not in protein mass, *Am. J. Clin. Nutr.*, 79(6): 1006–1012, 2004.

135. Paton, N.I. et al., Randomized controlled trial of nutritional supplementation in patients with newly diagnosed tuberculosis and wasting, *Am. J. Clin. Nutr.*, 80(2): 460–465, 2004.

136. Sahbazian, B. and Weis, S., Treatment of active tuberculosis: challenges and prospects, *Clin. Chest Med.*, 26: 273–282, 2005.

137. Das, D.B. et al., Effect of iron supplementation on mild to moderate anaemia in pulmonary tuberculosis, *Br. J. Nutr.*, 90(3): 541–550, 2003.

138. Fugusi, F.M. et al., Vitamin A status of patients presenting with pulmonary tuberculosis and asymptomatic HIV-infected individuals, Dar es Salaam, Tanzania, *Int. J. Tuberc. Lung Dis.*, 7(8): 804–807, 2003.

139. Karyadi, E. et al., A double-blind, placebo-controlled study of vitamin A and zinc supplementation in persons with tuberculosis in Indonesia: effects on clinical response and nutritional status, *Am. J. Clin. Nutr.*, 75(4): 720–727, 2002.

140. Shils, M.E., Ed. et al., *Modern Nutrition in Health and Disease*, 9th ed., Lippincott, Williams & Wilkins, Philadelphia, 1999, p. 1634.

141. Madebo, T. et al., Circulating antioxidants and lipid peroxidation products in untreated tuberculosis patients in Ethiopia, *Am. J. Clin. Nutr.*, 78(1): 117–122, 2003.

142. Harper, M.E. et al., Traditional healers participate in tuberculosis control in The Gambia, *Int. J. Tuberc. Lung Dis.*, 8(10): 1266–1268, 2004.

143. Banerjee, A. et al., Acceptability of traditional healers as directly observed treatment providers in tuberculosis control in a tribal area of Andhra Pradesh, India, Int. *J. Tuberc. Lung Dis.*, 8(10): 1260–1265, 2004.

144. Colvin, M. et al., Contribution of traditional healers to a rural tuberculosis control programme in Hlabisa, South Africa, *Int. J. Tuberc. Lung Dis.*, 9(Suppl. 1): S86–S91, 2003.

145. Brouwer, J.A. et al., Traditional healers and pulmonary tuberculosis in Malawi, *Int. J. Tuberc. Lung Dis.*, 2(3): 231–234, 1998.

146. Hudelson, P., Gender differentials in tuberculosis: the role of socio-economic and cultural factors, *Tuberc. Lung Dis.*, 77(5): 391–400, 1996. Review.

147. Yamasaki-Nakagawa, M. et al., Gender difference in delays to diagnosis and health care seeking behaviour in a rural area of Nepal, *Int. J. Tuberc. Lung Dis.*, 5(1): 24–31, 2001. Erratum in: *Int. J. Tuberc. Lung Dis.*, 5(4): 390, 2001.

148. Long, N.H. et al., Different tuberculosis in men and women: beliefs from focus groups in Vietnam, *Soc. Sci. Med.*, 49(6): 815–822, 1999.

149. Jimenez, A. et al., Secondary metabolites from *Chamaedora tepejilote* (palmae) are active against *Mycobacterium tuberculosis*, *Phytother. Res.*, 19(4): 320–322, 2005.

150. Ma, C. et al., Anti-tuberculosis constituents from the stem bark of *Micromelum hirsutum*, *Planta Med.*, 71(3): 261–267, 2005.

151. Lin, W.Y. et al., Antitubercular constituents from the roots of *Engelhardia roxburghiana*, *Planta Med.*, 71(2): 171–175, 2005.

18 Ear Health

Duke Johnson

CONTENTS

INTRODUCTION

The ear with its associated vestibular system is a common source of health problems to which many conventional and alternative treatments are applied. In fact, otitis media (middle ear infection), which is already the most common diagnosis among preschool children, has increased during the last decade.[1] With rising healthcare costs and concern about antibiotic resistance, alternative treatments have become increasingly popular even though a great deal of research to support many of these practices is not currently available. In order to thoroughly comprehend the validity and effectiveness of current available approaches to prevent or ameliorate dysfunction, a brief review of normal pertinent anatomy and physiology will first be presented.

EAR ANATOMY

The ear is divided into three anatomical regions, namely, the external, middle, and inner ear (see Figure 18.1).

EXTERNAL EAR

The external ear consists of the auricle and external auditory canal. The auricle is designed to help capture and funnel sound waves into the external auditory canal. Its shape is maintained

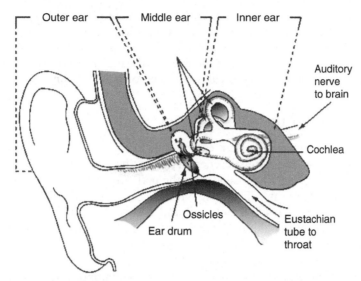

FIGURE 18.1 The outer, middle, and inner ear. Reference: http://weboflife.nasa.gov/learningResources/vestibularbrief.htm.

by elastic fibrocartilage. The cartilage is attached to the temporal bone and is covered by skin, which extends into the canal. There are eight different muscles that attach to the auricle. The lateral half of the external auditory canal is cartilaginous and has a thicker skin with subcutaneous tissue and ceruminous (wax producing) glands. The medial half of the external canal is bony with only epidermis lying on periosteum.

MIDDLE EAR

The middle ear (or tympanic cavity) consists of the eardrum (or tympanic membrane), three ossicles (malleus, incus, and stapes), and two muscles (tensor tympani and stapedius). The tympanic cavity is normally filled with air and communicates with the air cells or cavities within the mastoid bone. It also communicates with the nasopharynx (nose and throat) anteromedially by way of the auditory (Eustachian) tube. The tympanic cavity mucosa is continuous with the membrane that lines the air cells within the mastoid bone as well as the membrane within the Eustachian tube.

The tympanic membrane is 0.1-mm thick, is slightly oval with 9 mm × 11 mm dimensions, lies at an angle of 40° in the saggital plane, and is concave medially.

The manubrium of the malleus bone is attached to the tympanic membrane. The head of the malleus is attached to the body of the incus by small ligaments. The long body of the incus articulates with the stapes and the base of the stapes is directed toward the vestibular window of the inner ear.

INNER EAR

The inner ear is comprised of two major structures, namely, the cochlea (end organ for hearing) and the semicircular canals (end organ for balance), which are interconnected by the vestibule. The inner ear is compared to a series of tunnels or canals within the temporal bone referred to as bony labyrinth. Within the bony labyrinth is a membranous labyrinth, which conforms to the shape of the bony labyrinth and is filled with endolymph fluid.

Between the membranous labyrinth and bony labyrinth is another fluid called perilymph. The membranous labyrinth contains the nerve receptors. Nerve branches from the semicircular canals and associated structures form the vestibular division (balance) of the vestibulocochlear nerve. The cochlear nerve serving the cochlea (hearing) forms the rest of the vestibulocochlear (VIII cranial) nerve, which relays information to the brain.

PHYSIOLOGY OF THE EAR

As sound waves are funneled into the external auditory canal by the auricle and strike the tympanic membrane, the acoustic energy causes the tympanic membrane to vibrate. These mechanical vibrations are transferred to the perilymph of the inner ear via the ossicles stimulating the fluid to vibrate. The fluid vibration is detected by hair cell cilia of the membranous labyrinth or basilar membrane and these cells send out rapid-fire codes of electrical signals to the brain about the frequency, intensity, and duration of the sound. The fluid wave travels the length of the cochlea and is dissipated at the round window, which is back in the tympanic cavity.

The ossicles (malleus, incus, and stapes) are exceedingly important because they augment the acoustical energy that strikes the tympanic membrane. If sound waves were directed at the oval (water) window (where the base of the stapes rests), almost all of the sound would be reflected back to the middle ear (air) and only 1% of the energy would reach the cochlea.

The tympanic membrane is much larger than the oval window, therefore the ossicles concentrate the vibration force (thus increasing force applied per square area). Additionally, the ossicles act as levers, which increase the vibration force, resulting in an overall increase in sound energy by 20-fold. This mechanism is important to understand how infections or disease processes involving any part of the ear can diminish or alter the perception of hearing.

Signals from receptors within the semicircular canals, which are oriented along different planes transmit information interpreted by the brain related to orientation and balance.

The Eustachian tube functions as a pressure equalizing valve for the middle ear. When functioning properly, it opens for a fraction of a second periodically, equalizing pressure variances that may have occurred with altitude changes, etc. If the Eustachian tube does not function properly, fluid can collect within the middle ear, resulting in pain or diminished hearing.[2,3]

EAR DISORDERS

When the normal anatomy or physiology of the structures previously described is disrupted, this results in impairment of hearing or balance. The most common disorders will now be discussed.

HEARING LOSS OR DEAFNESS

There are four basic types of hearing loss:

1. *Conductive hearing loss*: In this type, sound waves are not able to get to and stimulate the inner ear. The problem lies in the outer or middle ear, such as impacted wax, perforation of the tympanic membrane, calcification of the bones of the middle ear, otitis externa (infection of the outer ear), and otitis media.
2. *Sensorneural hearing loss*: This occurs when the sensory cells of the cochlea of auditory nerve cells are dysfunctional. The sound wave is not capable of getting transformed

within the cochlea and transferred to the brain. Some common reasons for this type of hearing loss include normal aging, noise damage to cochlea, ototoxic medications and tumors, such as acoustic neuromas.

3. *Mixed hearing loss*: This loss is due to a combination of both conductive and sensorneural hearing loss.
4. *Central hearing loss*: The problem with this type is located in the brainstem or brain.

OTITIS EXTERNA (OUTER EAR INFECTION)

This is a bacterial and fungal infection in the outer ear. Otitis externa is caused by either a contamination of the canal with unclean water or an imbalance of the normal outer ear flora because of soap, hairspray, etc.

OTITIS MEDIA (MIDDLE EAR INFECTION)

Otitis media is an inflammation and infection of the middle ear. Usually, the Eustachian tube becomes inflamed or obstructed from allergies or throat infections. This disrupts the normal ventilation of the middle ear, leading to pressure changes and an accumulation of fluid inside the middle ear. Viruses and bacteria travel up the Eustachian tube, resulting in the middle ear infection. Viruses that enter through the nose or mouth through communication from other people (coughs, shared food, etc.) then travel up the Eustachian tube, resulting in a middle ear infection. Pressure builds within the region, leading to discomfort.

TINNITUS

Tinnitus is a condition where continuous noise sounds are perceived by an individual in one or both ears. The sounds are described as ringing, hissing, or roaring noises.

1. Outer ear causes are due to wax or foreign bodies lying against the eardrum.
2. Middle ear causes are due to fluid accumulation (chronic or acute), otosclerosis, infection, allergy, or arthritis.
3. Tinnitus from inner ear usually indicates a more permanent and serious disorder. This may be caused by repeated exposure to excessive sound levels, trauma to head or neck, medications (such as aspirin, quinine, streptomycin, neomycin, kanamycin, ethacrynic acid, and furosemide), aging, tumor, hypertension, anemia, diabetes, thyroid dysfunction, syphilis, and glucose metabolism abnormalities.

VERTIGO

This is the sensation where individuals feel as if they are spinning or their surroundings are moving. This is most commonly caused by inner ear viral infection but may also be caused by tumors, displacement of ear calcium crystals (otoliths) — commonly called benign positional vertigo, Meniere's disease, or vestibular nerve inflammation.

MENIERE'S DISEASE

This is a condition of the inner ear which causes attacks of true vertigo, tinnitus, and decreased hearing. It is believed to be due to an increase in inner ear fluid pressure. The attacks last from 1 to 24 h. As the condition progresses, the hearing gradually worsens over time.

CONVENTIONAL APPROACHES TO EAR DISORDERS

HEARING LOSS OR DEAFNESS

Conductive Hearing Loss

The conventional treatments are based upon the cause of hearing loss. If cerumen (wax) buildup has occurred, the treatment involves removing the wax with suction or irrigation and wax softening ear drops.

Perforations of the tympanic membranes very commonly heal spontaneously and are carefully observed to monitor healing and reduce possible infection. If healing does not occur spontaneously, then surgical correction may be necessary.

Calcification of the stapes, otosclerosis, with associated immobilization of the bone, usually occurs slowly over time. Conventionally, if hearing loss is minimal, no intervention is commonly done. For individuals with significant otosclerosis where age or significant health concerns prohibit surgery, hearing aids can be fitted to improve the condition. For significant otosclerosis in healthy patients, the stapes bone is removed (stapedectomy) and a small window is made to the inner ear. An artificial replacement made out of Teflon and platinum or other materials is then substituted for the nonfunctioning stapes bone.[4]

Otitis externa (infection of the outer ear) is treated with antimicrobial ear drops and occasionally oral antibiotics for severe conditions.

Otitis media (infection of the middle ear) is most commonly treated with antibiotics, topical analgesic drops, and decongestants. This will be discussed in greater detail below.

Sensorneural Hearing Loss

Conventionally, very little treatment can be done when the hearing loss is due to aging, noise damage, or ototoxic medications other than hearing aids. If tumors are the cause, surgery can be performed to remove the tumor.

Central Hearing Loss

Very little can be done except for surgery when appropriate.

OTITIS EXTERNA

The conventional treatments for this condition are antimicrobial drops and occasional oral antibiotics. If condition reoccurs because of swimming, etc. then ear plugs are recommended.

OTITIS MEDIA

The most common conventional treatments involve oral antibiotics, topical ear canal analgesics, and decongestants or antihistamines. There is some literature now that would indicate that otitis media should be perhaps treated with decongestants alone since the condition is believed to spontaneously resolve if enough time is provided. The risk here is that otitis media can lead to ruptured ear drums and recurrent and chronic otitis media may lead eventually to permanent hearing problems. Occasionally, despite above treatments, individuals with recurrent otitis media are treated with myringotony tubes placed in surgery in order to keep the congenitally small Eustachian tube open. Adenoidectomy may also help reduce chronic condition. Conventional prevention for otitis media would recommend avoiding second-hand smoke, breastfeeding for the first year of life if possible, and immunization with Pneumococcal and Haemophilus vaccine.[5]

Tinnitus

- *Outer ear*: Outer ear treatments would involve removing the foreign body or wax buildup as noted above.
- *Middle ear*: Fluid accumulation would be treated with decongestants, infection with antibiotics, allergies with antihistamines and otosclerosis as noted in the section "Conductive Hearing Loss" above.
- *Inner ear*: Conventionally, if medications are causative, then avoidance of these medicines would be the first step. Avoidance of caffeine may also be helpful.[6] Tumors that are causative would be removed if possible. Hypertension is controlled usually through weight loss, exercise, and medication. Anemia, if causative, would be corrected and glucose metabolism abnormalities would be corrected with smoking avoidance, weight loss, diet management, and possibly medications. Thyroid abnormalities would also be corrected if causative through medication or surgery.

Vertigo

If vertigo is due to viral labrynthitis (viral infection of the inner ear) conventional management would involve either nothing since condition is usually self-limiting or temporary antivertigo medications. Tumors would be removed if possible and benign positional vertigo is treated with positioning exercises. Vestibular nerve inflammation is sometimes treated with medication and Meniere's disease treatment is covered in the next section.

Meniere's Disease

There has been very little success treating Meniere's disease with surgery in order to prevent its progression. Most conventional treatment has involved diuretics and antivertigo medication. In severe cases, the inner ear may need to be destroyed and surgery or ototoxic medications have been used to perform this task.

ALTERNATIVE APPROACHES TO EAR DISORDERS

Alternative treatment use has increased over the last 20 years. Although there is not a great deal of research available concerning the use of many alternative approaches, there is an increasing amount of studies showing benefit of some treatments.

Hearing Loss

Conductive Hearing Loss

Hearing loss due to wax buildup is treated with oil drops to soften wax and irrigation. There are no alternative treatments for eardrum perforations or otosclerosis. Alternative approaches to otitis externa are usually from a prevention perspective using drying or antiseptic drops after swimming. There are extensive treatments in alternative medicine for otitis media and this will be discussed in the section on "Otitis Media."

Sensorneural Hearing Loss

Ginkgo has been reported to help with cochlear deafness[7] but there has not been significant research to support this claim. Its use for tinnitus and vertigo will be covered in the section on "Vertigo."

Central Hearing Loss

No treatments of note are recommended.

OTITIS EXTERNA

Most alternative treatments have focused on prevention of the condition. For repeat infections, drying or antiseptic eardrops of a few drops of vinegar diluted 50% has been recommended after swimming. Insufficient reliable information was found for alternative treatments of otitis externa.

OTITIS MEDIA

There are many alternative treatments for otitis media. Most have to do with their ability to reduce mucous membrane inflammation or boost immune system function in fighting upper respiratory infections. The following will discuss which botanicals have been used for the treatment of otitis media; safety and efficacy will also be discussed. Table 18.1 also describes the use of herbs and otitis media. These herbs are considered reasonably safe if used as directed.

Table 18.2 illustrates herbs that have been used for treatment of otitis media but are not recommended primarily because of safety concerns but also because of the lack of scientific literature to support their use. The herbs will be listed with corresponding risks.

German Chamomile (*Matricaria recutita*)

The azulene constituents found in German Chamomile inhibit the release of histamine. Unfortunately, it may cause contact dermatitis and anaphylaxis.[8,9] It can also increase anticoagulation[10] and is teratogenic and so should not be taken during pregnancy. It is possibly effective for topical skin inflammation.[10,11]

HOPS (*Humulus lupulus*)

HOPS (*Humulus lupulus*) is used topically as an antibacterial[10,12] but may cause a contact dermatitis. There is no reliable information about use with ear infections[13] and probably not worth using.

Mullein (*Verbascum densiflorum*)

Mucilage alleviates local irritation[8,11,14] and saponins have an expectorant effect[11,14–16] and may have activity against influenza.[17] It is probably safe orally[11,14,18] but topical use is without proven safety. It is possibly effective when treating respiratory tract mucous membrane inflammation, cough, and sore throat.[11,14] It is apparently a reliable alternative treatment.

Garlic (*Alllium sativum*)

Fresh garlic has been shown in laboratory to have some antibacterial and antiviral activity[10,11,19] but there is insufficient reliable information to support use for ear infections either topically or orally. It is possibly safe but without proven benefit. One article mentions that

TABLE 18.1
Reasonably Safe Herbs for Ear Health

1. Mullein (*Verbascum densiflorum*) — Mucilage alleviates local irritation[8,11,14] and saponins have an expectorant effect[11,14,15,16] and may have activity against influenza.[17] It is probably safe orally[11,14,18] but topical use is without proven safety. It is possibly effective when treating respiratory tract mucous membrane inflammation, cough, and sore throat.[11,14] It is apparently a reliable alternative treatment.

2. Garlic (*Allium sativum*) — Fresh garlic has been shown in laboratory to have some antibacterial and antiviral activity[10,11,19] but there is insufficient reliable information to support use for ear infections either topically or orally. It is possibly safe but without proven benefit. One article mentions that it may be helpful hypothetically for treating infections.[20] There is one study[21] that demonstrated that a natural ear drop containing garlic was as effective as conventional anesthetic drops in controlling pain associated with otitis media.

3. St. John's wort (*Hypericum perforatum*) — Its constituents hypericin and pseudohypericin have been shown to have antimicrobial action but there is insufficient reliable data about use for ear infections. It is likely safe at appropriate doses for short time[8,10,14,24] but not during pregnancy.[26] This may be a viable alternative treatment but not proven.[25]

4. Echinacea (*Echinacea pallida*, *Echinacea purpurea*) — It is probably effective when *Echinacea pallida* root extract is used orally as supportive therapy for influenza-like infections.[11] *Echinacea purpurea* above ground parts (herb) extract or 95% herb/5% root juice is possibly effective for shortening the duration of the common cold.[24,27,28] Some preparations might reduce the severity and duration of colds if taken when symptoms first develop.[27–30] It is likely safe when taken orally and appropriately[18,27,29,33] but daily use should be limited to eight consecutive weeks because of concern that long-term daily use may depress immunity.[10,11,18] Asthma worsening and allergic reaction have been noted. In light of effectiveness and safety, Echinacea may by helpful.[31]

5. Onion (*Allium cepa*) — Likely safe when used orally and appropriately.[11] A maximum of 35 mg of diphenylamine constituent is recommended per day if used over several months.[11] In folk medicine it has been used as cough and asthma treatment. There is unreliable sufficient research concerning its effects on cough but it has been shown to reduce significantly bronchial constriction and have antimicrobial effects.[16] This appears to be perhaps helpful.

6. Gumweed (*Grindelia robusta*) — Possibly safe when used orally and appropriately but may stimulate an allergic reaction or gastrointestinal problems.[11,18] It is possibly effective for the treatment of upper respiratory infections and has antimicrobial effects.[11]

7. Licorice (*Glycyrrhiza glabra*) — Possibly safe when used orally and appropriately for short term medicinal purposes but chronic use over 6 weeks or large amounts can cause hypertension, hypokalemia, rhabdomyolysis, and congestive heart failure.[8,10,11,22] It is possibly effective for upper respiratory tract mucous membrane inflammation. It is an expectorant[22] and cough suppressant.[22,24] It may be helpful and safe at appropriate doses short term.

8. Valerian (*Valeriana officinalis*) — Possibly safe when used orally and appropriately for medicinal purposes up to 14 days. Possibly effective when used to help with sleep short term.[11,38]

9. Eucalyptus (*Eucalyptus globulus*) — Possibly safe when used orally and appropriately[18] but is unsafe for children and possibly unsafe when oil is used near face because it can cause bronchospasm. It is possibly effective orally for respiratory tract mucous membrane inflammation but if used, should be used with caution.

10. Thyme flower and leaf (*Thymus vulgaris*) — Possibly safe orally at appropriate levels[11,18,39] but unsafe during pregnancy in large amounts. Effective when used topically for upper respiratory tract mucous membrane inflammation.[11]

11. Lavender (*Lavandula augustifolia*) — Possibly safe when used orally.[11,18] It is possibly effective to help with sleep.[11] May be considered to help with sleep during infections and illness.

TABLE 18.2
Herbs Not Recommended for Ear Health

1. German Chamomile (*Matricaria recutita*) — dermatitis, anaphylaxis,[8,9] increases anticoagulation[10]
2. HOPS (*Humulus lupulus*) — no reliable scientific support (NRSS)
3. Lobelia (*Lobelia inflata*) — unsafe[12,22]
4. Goldenseal (*Hydrastis canadensis*) — unsafe[8,10,16,18,23]
5. Apple Cider Vinegar — no significant scientific support although one study showed some effectiveness with granular myringitis[32]
6. American Elder, Elderberry, Elderflower (*Sambucus canadensis*) — cyanide risk[18]
7. Green Tea (*Camellia sinensis*) — caffeine controversial for children, infants, and pregnancy[16,34]
8. Fenugreek (*Trigonella foenum-graecum*) — unsafe in pregnancy,[10] NRSS, wheezing, allergic reactions
9. Pulsatilla (*Anemone pulsatilla*) — severe local irritant and unsafe for pregnancy[11] although one homeopathic remedy containing it was helpful[35]
10. Chickweed (*Stellaria media*) — NRSS, nervous system abnormalities[10,16]
11. Black Cohosh (*Cimicifuga racemosa*) — NRSS, unsafe for pregnancy[10,36,37]
12. Desert Tea, Brigham Tea, Morman Tea (*Silybum marianum*) — NRSS, kidney damage, liver damage[18]
13. Baikal Skullcap (*Scutellaria baicalensis*) — NRSS
14. Sage (*Salvia officinalis*) — tachicardia, kidney damage[10,11,14,18]
15. Thyme Oil (*Thymus vulgaris*) — unsafe, NRSS[10,18]
16. Aconite (*Aconitum napellus*) — fast-acting poison, cardiac toxicity, death[12,40,41]

it may be helpful hypothetically for treating infections.[20] There is one study[21] that demonstrated that a natural ear drop containing garlic was as effective as conventional anesthetic drops in controlling pain associated with otitis media.

Lobelia (*Lobelia inflata*)

Lobelia is likely unsafe when preparations of above ground parts are used orally.[12,22] No reliable topical safety is available. Effectiveness is not shown with reliable research and therefore not recommended.

Goldenseal (*Hydrastis canadensis*)

The alkaloids hydrastine and berberine found in Goldenseal are thought to be antimicrobial[8,10,22] but these effects have not been specifically proven for goldenseal. It is unsafe at high doses (500 mg of constituent or 8–10 g of dry root depending on the concentration of berberine), long-term use,[16,18] in children,[23] or during pregnancy[8,10] and so not recommended.

St. John's Wort (*Hypericum perforatum*)

The constituents of St. John's Wort, hypericin, and pseudohypericin, have been shown to have antimicrobial action but there is insufficient reliable data about use for ear infections. It is likely safe at appropriate doses for short time[8,10,14,24] but not during pregnancy.[26] This may be a viable alternative treatment but not proven.[25]

Echinacea (*Echinacea pallida, Echinacea purpurea*)

Echinacea is probably effective when *Echinacea pallida* root extract is used orally as supportive therapy for influenza-like infections.[11] *Echinacea purpurea* above ground parts (herb) extract or

95% herb/5% root juice is possibly effective for shortening the duration of the common cold.[24,27,28] Some preparations might reduce the severity and duration of colds if taken when symptoms first develop.[27–30] It is likely safe when taken orally and appropriately[18,27,29,33] but daily use should be limited to eight consecutive weeks because of concern that long-term daily use may depress immunity.[10,11,18] Asthma worsening and allergic reaction have been noted. In light of effectiveness and safety, Echinacea may be helpful.[31]

Apple Cider Vinegar

There is insufficient reliable data about effectiveness of apple cider vinegar although it does appears to be effective for the management of granular myringitis.[32]

American Elder, Elderberry, Elderflower (*Sambucus canadensis*)

American Elder and elderberry is probably safe when used for medicinal purposes.[12] Possibly unsafe when leaves, stems, and unripe fruit are used because of a cyanide poisoning risk.[18] Since its effectiveness has not been shown with reliable information and risks are significant, this is not recommended.

Onion (*Allium cepa*)

Onion is likely safe when used orally and appropriately.[11] A maximum of 35 mg of diphenylamine constituent is recommended per day if used over several months.[11] In folk medicine, it has been used for cough and asthma treatment. There is unreliable sufficient research concerning its effects on cough but it has been shown to significantly reduce bronchial constriction and have antimicrobial effects.[16] This appears to be perhaps helpful.

Gumweed (*Grindelia robusta*)

Gumweed is possibly safe when used orally and appropriately but may stimulate an allergic reaction or gastrointestinal problems.[11,18] It is possibly effective for the treatment of upper respiratory infections and has antimicrobial effects.[11]

Green Tea (*Camellia sinensis*)

Green tea is probably safe when used orally in moderate amounts[16,34] but possibly unsafe when over 5 cups used per day.[16] It is unsafe for children, infants, and during pregnancy because of the caffeine content. There is no reliable information about proven effectiveness for upper respiratory or ear infections and is therefore probably not a good alternative.

Fenugreek (*Trigonella foenum-grawcum*)

Fenugreek is possibly safe in medicinal amounts[10,11] but likely unsafe in pregnancy.[10] It is possibly effective when used topically for inflammation[11] but research on upper respiratory infection effectiveness is lacking. It may cause wheezing and allergic reactions.

Pulsatilla (*Anemome pulsatilla*)

Pulsatilla is likely unsafe when fresh ground parts are used orally or topically because it is a severe local irritant. Use during pregnancy is unsafe orally.[11] The available reliable data is insufficient about effectiveness and is therefore not recommended. One study looking at homeopathic treatment of otitis media involved a treatment containing pulsatilla. The homeopathic remedy was helpful.[35]

Chickweed (*Stellaria media*)

Chickweed has been used in folk medicine for asthma and lung disease. It is likely safe orally[16] but no reliable information is available about topical safety. Since there is no evidence of therapeutic value[9,10] and adverse reactions can include nervous system abnormalities,[10,16] it is probably not a good alternative.

Black Cohosh (*Cimicifuga racemosa*)

Black cohosh has been traditionally used for fever, sore throat, and cough.[8,10] It is likely safe when used orally and appropriately for up to 6 months[18] but is unsafe during pregnancy.[10,36,37] Since no reliable information is available about effectiveness, this is probably not recommended.

Desert Tea, Brigham Tea, Morman Tea (*Silybum marianum*)

There is insufficient reliable information about the safety of Desert, Brigham, or Morman tea for medicinal uses.[13] There is no reliable information about effectiveness and potential risks are great. Plants with at least 10% tannins can cause kidney damage and necrotic conditions of the liver[18]; so this is not recommended.

Licorice (*Glycyrrhiza glabra*)

Licorice is probably safe when used orally and appropriately short term for medicinal purposes but chronic use over 6 weeks or large amounts can cause hypertension, hypokalemia, rhabdomyolysis, and congestive heart failure.[8,10,11,22] It is possibly effective for upper respiratory tract mucous membrane inflammation. It is an expectorant[22] and cough suppressant.[22,24] It may be helpful and safe at appropriate doses in the short term.

Valerian (*Valeriana officinalis*)

Valerian is possibly safe when used orally and appropriately for medicinal purposes up to 14 days. Possibly effective when used to help with sleep short term.[11,38]

Baikal Skullcap (*Scutellaria baicalensis*)

There is insufficient reliable information for treating upper respiratory tract infections with Baikal Skullcap. Therefore, its use in not recommended.

Eucalyptis (*Eucalyptus globulus*)

Eucalyptis is possibly safe when used orally and appropriately[18] but is unsafe for children and possibly unsafe when oil is used near the face because it can cause bronchospasm. It is possibly effective orally for respiratory tract mucous membrane inflammation but if used, should be used with caution.

Sage (*Salvia officinalis*)

Sage is possibly effective for nasal inflammation[11] but possibly unsafe when used in amounts greater than that found in food or used for a long time.[10,14,18] Since some adverse effects are tachycardia and kidney damage,[10,11,14,18] it is not recommended.

Thyme Flower and Leaf (*Thymus vulgaris*)

The thyme flower and leaf is possibly safe orally at appropriate levels[11,18,39] but unsafe during pregnancy in large amounts. It is effective when used topically for upper respiratory tract mucous membrane inflammation.[11]

Thyme Oil (*Thymus vulgaris*)

Thyme oil is likely unsafe unless it is diluted. Unsafe in large amounts (maximum use levels are less than 0.003%) and should not be taken orally.[10,18] There is insufficient reliable information about effectiveness and should therefore probably not be used.

Lavender *(Lavandula augustifolia)*

Lavender is possibly safe when used orally.[11,18] It is possibly effective to help with sleep.[11] Lavender may be considered to help with sleep during infections and illness.

Aconite (*Aconitum napellus*)

Aconite is unsafe orally or topically. It is a strong, fast-acting poison that affects the heart and central nervous system.[12] It can cause palpitations, cardiac toxicity, and death[40,41] and so should not be used.

Otitis media develops when the Eustachian tube does not open normally usually from inflammation associated with allergy or infection. Many foods are suspected to cause allergic or inflammatory responses, which can result in chronic or recurrent infections. Avoidance or reduction of one or more of the following foods may be helpful, namely, dairy products, peanut products, oranges, wheat, corn, and eggs. Additionally, simple sugars may reduce immune functioning and should be reduced. Immune functioning will most likely be enhanced with an age-appropriate multivitamin. Second-hand smoke should be reduced around children. Infants who are breastfed for 1 year apparently have less infections as well.

Tinnitus

Outer ear — Causes would involve removing the foreign body or wax buildup as noted in the subsection "Conductive Hearing Loss" in the section "Conventional Approaches to Ear Disorders."

Middle ear — Infections, fluid buildup and allergic reactions would be approached as noted in the subsection "Otitis Media" in the section "Conventional Approaches to Ear Disorders."

Inner ear — Avoidance of substances is suspected to worsen the condition, such as caffeine. Alternative hypertension management if causative would be managed as noted in Chapter 10 and glucose metabolism abnormalities as discussed in Chapter 16. Ginkgo may be effective for the treatment of tinnitus.[16]

Vertigo

Ginkgo (leaf extract) has been shown to be possibly effective for vertigo.[11,43–45] Some herbs with antihistamine effects as noted in the subsection on "Conductive Hearing Loss" in the section "Conventional Approaches to Ear Disorders" may also be helpful.

Meniere's Disease

Inner ear fluids are affected by diet; therefore, dietary control is a very important part of the management of this disease. Patients should be counseled to avoid caffeine, alcohol, tobacco, and to eat foods low in salt and sugar. Careful adherence to the diet may reduce frequency and severity of attacks, which helps prevent attack-related hearing loss.

Integration of Conventional and Alternative Approaches

The best approach to potential or real ear disorders is an integration of the best of conventional and alternative approaches. It is in essence always better to prevent disease rather than to withhold treatment until disorders exist. Alternatives or complementary medicine's strong emphasis on preventive measures is prudent and should be incorporated when possible as part of any patient care. If integration leads to reduced antibiotic use and fewer surgeries, then antibiotic resistance and the costs of medicine will go down.

Challenges exist in that herbal or food-based therapies do have risks, adverse side effects, and may interact with medicines or other health conditions. These challenges can be overcome though with thorough knowledge of possible treatments. As research continues to add to our knowledge base, treatment options will expand and we will all benefit.

CASE STUDY

Mrs. A's 3-year-old son, Tommy, had a long history of recurrent ear infections treated with multiple strong antibiotics. His infections became almost continuous with visits to physician's offices approximately every 2 weeks. Mrs. A was very hesitant to see an ear, nose, and throat (ENT) specialist because she was informed that her son would most likely need myringotomy tubes. Despite her reluctance, Mrs. A finally brought Tommy to the specialist because her concerns of possible chronic hearing loss and antibiotic exposure exceeded her worries about a surgical procedure for him.

To her surprise, instead of immediately scheduling surgery for Tommy, the ENT specialist made one last attempt at a nonsurgical approach. Smoking was prohibited in her home and dietary modifications were made. Some of Tommy's dairy intake was replaced with rice milk. Peanut products, wheat, and eggs were significantly removed from his diet. Mrs. A attempted to introduce garlic into the family meals and simple sugars were almost eliminated. Tommy's infections decreased to only a few times per year over the next 2 years. At 6 years of age, he has apparently outgrown his problem because of increased Eustachian tube size and surgery is not anticipated for him in the future.

REFERENCES

1. Lanphear, B.P., et al., Increasing prevalence of recurrent otitis media among children in the United States, *Pediatrics*, 99(3), E1, 1997.
2. House Ear Clinic. www.houseearclinic.com/hdeust.htm
3. Otolaryngology. Queens University. http://meds.queensu.ca/medicine/otolaryngology/edu/ungrad/pa.htm
4. Levenson, M.J., Otosclerosis — a description. Ear Surgery Information Center Stapedectomy. www.earsurgery.org/otscl.html
5. InteliHealth. Harvard Medical Schools Consumer Health Information. http://www.intelihealth.com/IH/ihtIH/WSIHW000/408/408.html
6. www.kennedyseminars.com/handouts/tinnitus/html

7. Castleman, M., *Nature's Cures*, Emmaus, PA: Rodale Press, Inc., 1996.
8. *The Review of Natural Products by Facts and Comparisons*, St. Louis, MO: Wolters Kluwer Co., 1999.
9. Subiza, J., et al., Anaphylactic reaction after the ingestion of chamomile tea: a study of cross-reactivity with other composite pollens, *J. Allergy Clin. Immunol.*, 84, 353, 1989.
10. Newall, C.A., Anderson, L.A., and Philipson, J.D., *Herbal Medicine: A Guide for Healthcare Professionals,* London: The Pharmaceutical Press, 1996.
11. Blumenthal, M., et al. eds., *The Complete German Commission E Monographs: Therapeutic Guide to Herbal Medicines*, Translated by S. Klein., Boston, MA: American Botanical Council, 1998.
12. Leung, A.Y. and Foster, S., *Encyclopedia of Common Natural Ingredients Used in Food, Drugs and Cosmetics*, 2nd edn, New York, NY: Wiley, 1996.
13. Jellin, J.M., et al., *Pharmacist's Letter/Prescriber's Letter Natural Medicine's Comprehensive Database*, 3rd edn, Stockton, CA: Therapeutic Research Faculty, pp. 567–568, 2000.
14. Foster, S. and Tyler, V.E., *Tyler's Honest Herbal: A Sensible Guide to the Use of Herbals and Related Remedies*, 3rd edn, Binghamton, NY: Haworth Herbal Press, 1993.
15. Wichtl, M.W., In N.M. Bisset, ed. *Herbal Drugs and Pharmaceuticals*. Stuttgart: Med. Pharm. GmbH Scientific Publishers, 1994.
16. Gruenwald, J., et al., *PDR for Herbal Medicines*, 1st edn, Montvale, NJ: Medical Economics Company, Inc., 1998.
17. Zgorniak-Nowosielska, I., et al., Antiviral activity of *Flos verbasci* infusion against influenza and Herpes simplex viruses, *Arch. Immunol. Ther. Exp.* (Warsz), 39(1–2), 103, 1991.
18. McGuffin, M., et al. eds., *American Herbal Products Association's Botanical Safety Handbook*, Boca Raton, FL: CRC Press, 1997.
19. Weber, N.D., et al., *In vitro* virusidal effects of *Allium sativum* (garlic) extract and compounds, *Planta Med.*, 58, 417, 1992.
20. Klein, J.O., Management of acute otitis media in an era of increasing antibiotic resistance, *Int. J. Pediatr. Otorhinolaryngol.*, 49(Suppl. 1), S15, 1999.
21. Sarrell, E.M., et al., Efficacy of naturalpathic extracts in the management of ear pain associated with acute otitis media, *Arch. Pediatr. Adolesc. Med.*, 155(7), 796, 2001.
22. Tyler, V.E., *Herbs of Choice*, Binghamton, NY: Pharmaceutical Products Press, 1994.
23. Chan, E., Displacement of bilirubin from albumin by berberine, *Biol. Neonate*, 63(4), 201, 1993.
24. Schulz, V., Hansel, R., and Tyler, V.E., *Rational Phytotherapy: A Physician's Guide to Herbal Medicine*, Translated by Terry C. Telger, 3rd edn, Berlin: Springer, 1998.
25. Schempp, C., et al., Antibacterial activity of hyperforin from St. John's wort against multiresistant Staphylococcus aureus and gram-positive bacteria, *Lancet*, 353, 2129, 1999.
26. Lee, A., et al., Safety of St. John's wort during breastfeeding, *Clin. Pharmacol. Ther.*, 67(2), 130, 2000 (abstract PII-64).
27. Brinkeborn, R.M., Shah, D.V., and Degering, F.H., Echinaforce and other Echinacea fresh plant preparations in the treatment of the common cold. A randomized, placebo-controlled, double-blind clinical trial, *Phytomedicine*, 6, 1, 1996.
28. Barrett, B., Vohmann, M., and Calabrese, C., Echinacea for upper respiratory tract infection, *J. Fam. Pract.*, 48, 628, 1999.
29. Gunning, K., Echinacea in the treatment and prevention of upper respiratory tract infections, *West. J. Med.*, 171, 198, 1999.
30. Scolomicki, S., et al., The influence of active components of *Eleutherococcus senticosus* on cellular defense and physical fitness in man, *Phytother. Res.*, 14, 30, 2000.
31. Mark, J.D., et al., The use of dietay supplements in pediatrics: a study of Echinacea, *Clin. Pediatr.*, (Phila) 40(5), 265–269, 2001 May.
32. Jung, H.H., et al., Vinegar treatment in the management of granular myringitis. *J. Laryngol. Otol.*, 116(3), 176, 2002.
33. Chavez, M.I. and Chavez, P.I., Echinacea. *Hospital Pharmacy*, 1998, 33, 180, 1998.
34. Mitscher, L.A., et al., Chemoprotection: a review of the potential therapeutic antioxidant properties of green tea (*Camellia sinensis*) and certain of its constituents, *Med. Res. Rev.*, 17(4), 327, 1997.
35. Friese, K.H., et al., The homeopathic treatment of otitis media in children — comparisons with conventional therapy. *Int. J. Clin. Pharmacol.*, 35(7), 296, 1997.

36. Gennaro, A., *Remington: The Science and Practice of Pharmacy*, 19th edn, Baltimore: Lippincott Williams & Wilkins, 1996.
37. Brinker, F., *Herb Contraindications and Drug Interactions*, 2nd edn, Sandy, OR: Eclectic Medical Publications, 1998.
38. Donath, F., et al., Critical evaluation of the effect of valarian extract on sleep structure and sleep quality, *Pharmacopsychiatry*, 33, 47, 2000.
39. *Monographs of the Medicinal Uses of Plant Drugs*, Exeter, UK: European Scientific Cooperative on Phytotherapy, 1997.
40. Tai, Y.T., Adverse effects from traditional Chinese medicine, *Lancet*, 341, 892, 1993.
41. Tai, Y.T., et al., Cardiotoxicity after accidental herb-induced aconite poisoning, *Lancet*, 340, 1254, 1992.
42. Fatovich, D.M., Aconite: a lethal Chinese herb, *Ann. Emerg. Med.*, 21, 309, 1992.
43. Diamond, B.J., et al., *Ginkgo biloba* extract: mechanisms and clinical indications, *Arch. Phys. Med. Rehabil.*, 81, 668, 2000.
44. Cesarani, A., et al., *Ginkgo biloba* (EGb 761) in the treatment of equilibrium disorders, *Adv. Ther.*, 15, 291, 1998.
45. Haguenauer, J.P., et al., [Treatment of equilibrium disorders with Ginkgo biloba extract. A multicenter double-blind drug vs. placebo study.] *Presse. Med.*, 15, 1569, 1986.

19 Skin Health

Jennifer Doley and Joseph Genebriera

CONTENTS

NUTRITION AND THE SKIN

Nutrition plays an important role in the health of the skin. The symptoms of several nutritional deficiencies are expressed as changes in the skin. Diet alterations help to control the symptoms of such skin disorders as acne, and several types of dermatitis. Perhaps nutrition's most important relationship with the skin is seen in wound healing; adequate intake of many macro- and micronutrients are crucial to healing. Malnutrition increases the risk of some types of wounds, and severely inhibits the body's ability to heal damaged skin. This chapter describes the role of nutrition in skin health and in skin disorders, with particular emphasis on wound healing. Nontraditional methods to promote healing are explored as well.

ANATOMY AND PHYSIOLOGY

The skin is the body's largest organ. Its functions include protection from external injury, management of fluid and electrolyte balance, temperature control, absorption of UV radiation, production of vitamin D and epidermal lipids, and sensation. The skin also functions as part of the immune system. Skin thickness varies depending on anatomic location, gender, and age. Skin is thickest in the soles of the feet and palms of the hand, thinnest around the eyes, and is generally thicker in males than in females. The skin is comprised of three layers: the epidermis, dermis, and subcutis, each with specific functions (see Figure 19.1).

EPIDERMIS

The epidermis is the thin outer layer of the skin and is completely avascular; it is dependent on the dermal layer for nutrient delivery and waste removal through diffusion. The epidermis is composed of several sublayers. The stratum germinativum, or basal layer, is the deepest layer of the epidermis, and contains a single layer of basal cells. Basal cells continually divide, forming keratinocytes, pushing older keratinocytes up into the squamous cell layer. The outer layer of the skin, the stratum corneum, or horny layer, is comprised of fully mature keratinocytes, which are continuously shed as new keratinocytes are pushed up from the basal layer.

    The basal layer of the epidermis contains melanocytes, which produce the skin pigment melanin. Melanin absorbs radiant energy from the sun and protects against UV radiation. Chronic light exposure increases the production of melanin; body parts with little exposure to sunlight, such as the skin of the inner upper arm, are generally lighter than skin frequently exposed to sunlight, such as the skin of the outer upper arm. The number of melanocytes is the same in equivalent body sites in all skin colors, but the rate of pigment production and distribution varies. Darker skin has more active melanocytes, and distributes melanin to surrounding keratinocytes in smaller packages than is the case in pale-skinned individuals.

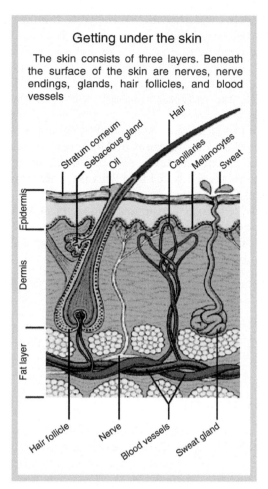

FIGURE 19.1 Illustrating the various layer components of the skin. (From "Getting under the skin," *The Merck Manual of Medical Information*, Second Home Edition, Mark H. Beers, Eds., p.1187. Copyright 2003 by Merck & Co., Whitehouse Station, N.J. With permission.)

The epidermal layer also contains Langerhans cells, which are produced in the bone marrow. Langerhans cells are a component of the skin immune system; they ingest foreign antigens and alert lymphocytes to activate the immune system.

DERMIS

The dermis is the middle layer of the skin, and contains blood vessels, lymph vessels, collagen bundles, fibroblasts, nerves, epidermal appendages, and pain and touch receptors. There are three main cell types in the dermis: fibroblasts, macrophages, and mast cells. The fibroblasts produce collagen, which holds the dermal layer together. Macrophages are immunological cells which act as scavengers. Mast cells function in type 1 immunological reactions and interactions with eosinophils.

Epidermal appendages include sweat glands, sebaceous glands, and hair follicles. Sweat glands, or eccrine glands, are found all over the body except on the lips, ear canal, and labia minora; they are most concentrated in the palms of the hands and soles of the feet.

They produce sweat, which cools the body via evaporation from the skin. Sebaceous glands, or holocrine glands, are also found all over the body except on the soles and dorsum of the feet. Sebaceous glands produce sebum, or oil, which helps to lubricate the skin and protects against excess moisture. Sebaceous glands often empty into hair follicles; this complex is called the pilosebaceous unit. Hair growth is cyclical, and the orientation of hair follicles in relation to the surface of the skin will determine how curly or straight the hair.

The vascular system of the dermis is complex, and functions as more than just a mode for oxygen and nutrient delivery and waste removal. Along with the sweat glands, the vascular network is a key factor in thermoregulation. Large amounts of heat can be exchanged via cutaneous blood flow, and this is controlled through vasoconstriction or vasodilation via the thermoregulatory center in the hypothalamus.

Nerves in the skin provide sensory perception, important in avoidance of noxious stimuli such as pressure, temperature extremes, and mechanical trauma. Several specialized nerve cells in the dermis detect different stimuli: Merkel and Meissner cells detect light touch, and Pacini corpuscles detect pressure.

SUBCUTIS

The subcutis is the deepest layer of skin, consisting of a network of collagen and fat cells. This network helps to conserve the body's heat and protects the body from injury by acting as a shock absorber.

NUTRITION AND SKIN HEALTH

Good nutrition, with an adequate intake of all macronutrients, micronutrients, and fluid, is essential to good skin health. Clinical deficiencies of some nutrients may manifest in the skin, described as follows.

VITAMIN A

Vitamin A deficiency produces primarily ocular symptoms, consisting of night blindness, conjunctival dryness, and Bitot's spots, an accumulation of keratinized epithelial conjunctiva cells. Vitamin A deficiency may also manifest in skin in the form of perifollicular hyperkeratosis, an accumulation of skin epithelium around hair follicles, seen particularly around the outer arms and thighs. Vitamin A deficiency is most common in children, as the liver contains little vitamin A stores at birth, and is more likely to occur in children in developing countries after being weaned from breast milk. Food sources rich in vitamin A include liver, milk, eggs, and yellow and leafy green vegetables.

RIBOFLAVIN

A deficiency in riboflavin produces a skin condition called oculo-orogenital syndrome. Skin areas with a high concentration of sebaceous glands, such as the nasolabial folds, eyelids, external ear, labia, and scrotum, are more highly affected. The skin becomes reddened, greasy, scaly, and painful. Plugs of sebum may accumulate in the hair follicles and produce a condition known as dyssebacia, or "shark skin." Angular stomatitis, horizontal fissures in the corners of the mouth, and cheilosis, vertical fissures around the mouth, also occur. Riboflavin deficiency generally occurs in combination with other nutrient deficiencies, usually caused by a severely restricted food intake. Malabsorption of the vitamin, as sometimes seen in celiac disease or other gastrointestinal (GI) disorders causing chronic diarrhea, can also lead to deficiency. Riboflavin is found in small amounts in most plant and animal foods; good sources include eggs, lean meats, milk, broccoli, and enriched breads and cereals.

NIACIN

Niacin deficiency, called pellagra, affects the skin as well. Dermatosis is usually the first symptom and affects areas of skin exposed to sunlight such as the hands, forearms, wrists, face, and neck. Erythema first occurs, followed by scaling, thickening, and pigmentation changes of the skin. Symptoms similar to riboflavin deficiency also occur, including stomatitis and magenta tongue. Neurological and GI effects, most notably dementia and diarrhea, are common as well. Pellagra, like riboflavin deficiency, is more likely to occur with other nutrient deficiencies. Vitamin B_6, riboflavin, and copper are all necessary for the metabolic conversion of the amino acid tryptophan to niacin; deficiencies of these nutrients will predispose an individual to pellagra. Isoniazid, a medication used to treat tuberculosis, causes depletion of vitamin B_6, and can therefore also lead to pellagra. Dietary sources of niacin include red meat, liver, legumes, milk, eggs, cereals, fish, and corn.

VITAMIN C

Adult scurvy is first exhibited by weakness and fatigue, progressing to joint, bone, and muscle aches, and then advancing to skin symptoms. Skin symptoms include acne, defects of body hair, and perifollicular hemorrhages or perifollicular hyperkeratosis, usually affecting the anterior thorax and abdominal wall, forearms, legs, and thighs. Ecchymoses, resulting from skin hemorrhages, may occur in the later stages of the disease. Deficiency of vitamin C is rare in developed countries, but may occur in individuals with diets devoid of fruits and vegetables. Particularly good sources of vitamin C are broccoli, Brussels sprouts, strawberries, citrus fruits, and spinach. Cooking significantly reduces the amount of vitamin C present in most foods.

ESSENTIAL FATTY ACIDS

Linoleic and alpha-linolenic acids cannot be synthesized by the body and are therefore considered essential fatty acids. Essential fatty acid deficiency is generally seen only in patients receiving long-term fat-free or very low-fat parenteral nutrition formulas, without any oral intake of fat. A deficiency can cause dry, flaky, or scaly skin, usually starting in the nasolabial folds and eyebrows and spreading across the face and neck. Additional symptoms may include growth retardation in children, increased susceptibility to infection, poor wound healing, anemia, and fatty liver.

NUTRITION AND SKIN DISORDERS

Certain diet components, while not the cause of some skin diseases, will certainly affect the symptoms of these disorders. Acne, when associated with polycystic ovarian syndrome (PCOS), may improve with diet management for weight loss and insulin resistance. Several forms of dermatitis are allergic in nature, and symptoms can be controlled in part with avoidance of certain dietary allergens. Even the effects of sunburn may be mitigated with dietary supplementation.

ACNE

Acne vulgaris is a common problem in adolescents and young adults, but can occur in individuals of any age. The disorder is caused by abnormal desquamation of follicular epithelium, resulting in obstruction of the pilosebaceous canal. This obstruction leads to the formation of microcomedones, or blocked pores, which can become inflamed due to overgrowth of the bacterium *Propionibacterium acnes*, and lead to open comedones, commonly known as "blackheads" or closed comedones, commonly called "whiteheads." An increase in sebum production is generally seen, however the degree of the disease is not related to the amount of sebum produced. Sebaceous glands are sensitive to androgens, thus explaining the increased incidence of acne in puberty.

Noninflammatory acne is most commonly managed through one or more topical treatments. One of the most commonly used ingredients in over-the-counter treatments, benzoyl peroxide, can be effective in treating mild cases of noninflammatory acne by destroying the *P. acnes* bacteria. It acts as an antiseptic and oxidizing agent, and reduces the number of comedones. Improvement may be seen after 2 to 3 weeks of benzoyl peroxide use.

Retinoids, derivatives of vitamin A, function by slowing the desquamation process, thereby decreasing the number of comedones and microcomedones. Retinoids are the most effective comedolytic agents in use. Topical retinoids, such as tretinoin, and topical retinoid analogs, such as adapalene and tazarotene, help to normalize the abnormal follicular keratinocyte desquamation — a key pathophysiologic factor in comedogenesis.

Other topical treatments are also available. Salicylic acid inhibits comedogenesis by promoting desquamation of follicular epithelium. It has been shown to be as effective as benzoyl peroxide in the treatment of comedonal acne. Topical azelaic acid cream helps both to normalize keratinization and to reduce the proliferation of *P. acnes*, and has proven to be effective against both noninflammatory and inflammatory lesions. Topical antibiotics, most commonly erythromycin and clindamycin, work directly by killing *P. acnes*. Through their bactericidal activity, they also have a mild indirect effect on comedogenesis.

Although topical therapy is generally adequate for comedonal acne, control of inflammatory acne may require systemic antibiotics. The antibiotics proven to be most effective include tetracycline, doxycycline, minocycline, and erythromycin. These drugs penetrate the follicle and sebaceous gland well and decrease colonization by *P. acnes*. They also have an anti-inflammatory effect independent of their antimicrobial properties.

Hormonal therapy, via oral contraceptives, has also proven to be effective in some female patients, and was approved by the Food and Drug Administration (FDA) in 1997 for the treatment of acne. Studies have shown that the use of some oral contraceptives can reduce acne lesions by more than 50% via a decrease in androgen production, which in turn reduces sebum secretion. Researchers report that results may not be seen for 3 to 4 months after starting therapy, with maximal results seen after 6 months.

Severe acne, if left untreated, may cause physical scarring and is unlikely to respond to topical therapy. Initially, patients may be treated with 6 months of oral antibiotics; if no improvement is seen, oral isotretinoin may be started. Isotretinoin, or Accutane, is an oral retinoid that decreases the size and secretion of the sebaceous glands, normalizes follicular keratinization, inhibits *P. acnes* growth, and exerts an anti-inflammatory effect. The potential side effects of isotretinoin are extensive, and physicians prescribing this medication should be advised about its potentially dangerous consequences. Patients should be evaluated frequently for adverse effects and to ensure compliance with therapy.

The most common side effects of isotretinoin are dry eyes, mouth, lips, nose, or skin. Other side effects include itching, nosebleeds, muscle aches, sun sensitivity, depression, and poor night vision. Skin and eye dryness can be prevented or treated with moisturizers, creams, and eye drops. Hypertriglyceridemia and hypercholesterolemia may occur in as many as 25% of patients treated with isotretinoin; triglyceride and cholesterol levels should be checked before and during treatment. Diet modification and reduced dosage of isotretinoin are usually effective in treating hyperlipidemia, but discontinuation of the drug may be considered in severe cases. Liver enzyme levels should be also monitored periodically. As isotretinoin is a derivative of vitamin A, patients are advised not to take supplemental vitamins containing vitamin A to avoid any additive toxic effects. All side effects of isotretinoin usually subside 1 to 3 weeks after cessation of the medication.

Isotretinoin can cause birth defects in the developing fetus, including defects of the central nervous system, skull, eyes, and cardiovascular system. It is important that women of childbearing age are not pregnant and do not get pregnant while taking this medication. Women must sign consent forms and take a pregnancy test before initiation of isotretinoin. Women must use two separate effective forms of birth control at the same time for 1 month before treatment begins, during the entire course of treatment, and for 1 full month after stopping the drug.[1–3]

Nutritional Management

Avoidance of chocolates, fats, sweets, and carbonated beverages was commonly recommended as part of the treatment for acne. However, these dietary restrictions are no longer part of standard medical treatment, as little evidence has been found to link the consumption of these foods and incidence of acne.[2,3] There has recently, however, been an indication that some forms of acne may be related to diet, as demonstrated in a study examining the incidence of acne in two nonwesternized societies. In over 1300 subjects, no cases of acne were found. The genetic background of these societies was similar to other groups who have a higher incidence of acne. Their lifestyles differed from traditional western lifestyles in their consumption of low-glycemic index foods and higher levels of physical activity. The lack of hyperinsulinemia has been postulated as the possible reason for the absence of acne in these populations. Hyperinsulinemia elicits endocrine responses that may affect the development of acne through mediators such as androgens, insulin-like growth factors (IGF), and retinoid signaling pathways.[4]

The link between hyperinsulinemia and acne is also demonstrated in individuals with PCOS. PCOS is characterized by obesity, androgen excess (producing hirsutism and acne), and menstrual irregularity. Insulin resistance and hyperinsulinemia is a common finding in women with PCOS. Treatment for hyperinsulinemia, as with type II diabetes, includes exercise, weight loss, and diet. Diet changes consist of shifting carbohydrate consumption from simple sugars and refined carbohydrates to complex carbohydrates found in whole grain products, legumes, fruits, and vegetables. If lifestyle changes are ineffective, metformin may enhance insulin sensitivity. Studies on metformin use in patients with PCOS demonstrated a reduction in androgens and a resultant reduction in acne, as well as a decline in weight.[5]

ATOPIC DERMATITIS

Dermatitis, or eczema, is an inflammation of the skin characterized by edema, redness, oozing, crusting, scaling, and pruritus. Atopic is a term applied to a group of hereditary diseases that are allergic in nature. An immunoglobulin-E (IgE)-mediated allergic reaction is responsible for the symptoms of AD. Symptoms result when an allergen binds to IgE antibodies, which causes the release of immune mediators and cytokines, triggering inflammatory responses in the skin.

AD usually affects individuals with a personal or family history of allergic disorders, such as hay fever and asthma, and is more common in infants and young children. The incidence of AD has increased significantly in the last 40 years, possibly indicating that unknown environmental factors play a part in its development, as well as the development of other atopic diseases. People who live in urban areas and in climates with low humidity seem to be at an increased risk for developing AD. Children with AD may experience an improvement of symptoms after age 3 to 4 years, although their skin may remain dry and easily irritated, and remissions or exacerbations can continue into adulthood. AD affects males and females equally and accounts for 10 to 20% of all referrals to dermatologists. Scientists estimate that 65% of patients develop symptoms in the first year of life, and 90% develop symptoms before the age of 5 years. Onset after the age of 30 years is less common and often occurs after exposure of skin to harsh conditions. Factors such as temperature and humidity changes, fragrances, bacterial skin infections, environmental irritants, stress, wool fabrics, and fabric softeners may worsen symptoms.

Research has been conducted on the prevention of AD in infants, with mixed results. Some research has suggested that the avoidance of common food allergens, such as eggs and peanuts, in pregnancy and during breastfeeding, may reduce sensitization to these allergens in infants, possibly reducing the development of food allergies and other atopic diseases.[6] Probiotics have been shown to promote intestinal immune function. Results of one study demonstrated supplementation of the probiotics *Bifidobacterium lactis* and *Lactobacillus GG* in infants with AD resulted in faster resolution of symptoms as compared to a control group.[7] Breastfeeding is perhaps the most important preventative measure to take, as it is known to enhance infants' immune function, although some studies have suggested that prolonged breastfeeding may encourage the prevalence of AD.[8]

Treatment of AD involves maintenance of a skin care routine, including daily application of lubricants within 3 min of bathing. Over-the-counter preparations may be used, but many cases warrant the prescription of a stronger corticosteroid cream or ointment. Side effects of long-term use of topical corticosteroids can include thinning of the skin, infections, growth suppression in children, and stretch marks on the skin.[8]

Phototherapy with the use of ultraviolet A or B light waves, or both together, can be an effective treatment for mild to moderate dermatitis in adults and children over 12 years of age. Photochemotherapy, a combination of ultraviolet light therapy and a drug called psoralen, can also be used in cases that are resistant to phototherapy alone. When phototherapy is utilized, the minimum amount of radiation is used to produce relief of symptoms, and the skin is monitored carefully. Possible long-term side effects of this treatment include premature skin aging and an increased risk of skin cancer. Another topical treatment, tacrolimus, an immunomodulator, has been found to be effective in treating moderate to severe AD without causing the atrophy that might occur with prolonged use of topical corticosteroids. Tacrolimus works equally well in children and adults, with more than two thirds of both groups having an improvement in symptoms of greater than 50%.[8]

Nutritional Management

Diet may play a part in the severity of symptoms in AD. Both $n-6$ and $n-3$ polyunsaturated fatty acids (PUFAs) have been studied. It has been suggested that individuals with AD have a defect in the enzyme that converts linoleic acid into gamma-linolenic acid. This inability to produce gamma-linolenic acid results in an altered ratio of plasma phosolipids in neutrophils and lymphocytes, and thereby alters the immunologic activity of these cells. Because of this hypothesis, evening primrose oil (EPO), which contains gamma-linolenic acid, has been a focus of AD research. Study results are mixed, but some evidence does suggest that supplementation of EPO improves gamma-linolenic acid concentrations in phosolipids in skin cells, thus increasing the production of the less inflammatory prostaglandin E1 (PGE1), which reduces the production of proinflammatory metabolites such as prostaglandin E2 (PGE2).[9]

Studies focusing on *n*–3 PUFAs, particularly eicosapentaenoic acid (EPA) and docosa-hexaenoic acid (DHA), have produced more definitive outcomes. One study, supplementing subjects with fish oil containing 180 mg of EPA/day and 120 mg of DHA/day for 8 weeks, showed improvement of symptoms and an increase in EPA and DHA ratio of cell lipids, particularly of neutrophils.[10] Another study supplemented subjects with 12 g of EPA/day for 6 weeks, resulting in a reduction of erythema and scaling in AD patients.[11] Two studies using lower doses of EPA, 1.8 g/day for 12 weeks, also demonstrated improvement in symptoms.[12,13] Two additional studies compared the effects of fish oil supplementation with corn oil supplementation. Interestingly, both the fish oil and corn oil supplemented groups experienced equally improved symptoms. Researchers suggested these results occurred because the increased *n*–3 PUFAs in both groups inhibited the proliferation of T-cells, thus reducing inflammatory responses.[14]

A study of the effects of a low-calorie, vegetarian diet on the symptoms of AD was conducted in Japan. Results showed a 50% decline in symptoms, possibly due to a significant reduction in the synthesis of PGE2. These results were achieved in 20 subjects consuming a vegetarian diet restricted to approximately 1085 cal/day over a 2-month period. While raising interesting points with regard to nutrition and AD, a diet of this nature is neither practical nor nutritionally adequate.[15]

In addition to more common food allergens, like egg, peanut, and milk proteins, other food chemicals have been found to be allergenic. These pseudoallergens include histamine, salicylates, benzoates, and other compounds found in fruits, vegetables, and spices. The allergenic mechanism of these compounds is not entirely understood, but does involve an increased production of proinflammatory mediators such as the cytokines interleukin (IL)-4, IL-10, and IL-13. As these mediators have been shown to play a part in AD, studies were conducted to determine the role of pseudoallergens in diet on symptoms of AD. Results suggested a potential sensitivity of some AD patients to pseudoallergens.[16]

DERMATITIS HERPETIFORMIS

Dermatitis herpetiformis (DH) is a relatively rare skin disease, also allergic in nature. Unlike AD, the symptoms of DH result from a non-IgE-mediated reaction. This reaction is triggered by ingestion of gluten. It has been shown that all patients with DH also suffer from gluten-sensitive enteropathy, a latent and usually asymptomatic form of celiac disease. The incidence of celiac disease is much more common than previously believed, many cases remain undiagnosed because patients do not exhibit the classic GI symptoms.

IgA antibodies are deposited in the dermal layer of the skin and a skin biopsy positive for IgA in unaffected skin denotes a positive diagnosis of DH. Patients with DH exhibit an increased incidence of other autoimmune disorders such as autoimmune thyroid disease and type I diabetes.

DH affects primarily Caucasians, males more than females. Usual age of onset is in young adulthood, although the disease can manifest itself at any age. Signs include vesicles, papules, and urticaria-like lesions seen primarily in the extensor surfaces of the body, such as the elbows, knees, forearms, and buttocks. Symptoms such as itching and burning are usually severe, and scratching can cause excoriation of skin and limit the number of intact blisters seen.

Nutritional Management

Treatment of DH includes adherence to a gluten-free diet and medication, most commonly dapsone, which relieves itching. Diet should be used in conjunction with medication, and medication doses may be reduced as symptoms improve. Adherence to the gluten-free diet must be strict, otherwise complete control of symptoms will not occur. Symptoms generally abate after the diet has been followed for 6 to 9 months.

Compliance with a gluten-free diet is difficult for most patients to maintain, as it eliminates all cereals of the species Triticeae, which include wheat, rye, and barley. The toxic agent of these cereals is the protein gliadin, which is high in the amino acids proline and glutamine. Oats have traditionally been eliminated from the gluten-free diet, however recent studies have shown that pure oats are not toxic to gliadin-sensitive patients, as they have a much lower concentration of the prolamines toxic to these individuals. Oats, however, may be contaminated with wheat products due to crop rotation or cereal milling procedures. Comprehensive diet education with a registered dietitian and involvement in celiac disease support groups may aid patients in diet compliance.[17,18]

SUNBURN

Sunburn results from overexposure to the sun's UVB rays. The amount of UV rays that reach the earth's surface varies greatly depending on the season and atmospheric conditions such as weather and degree of air pollution. Exposure to UV rays can be amplified by the reflection of light from sand, snow, water, and other surfaces. When the skin is exposed to UV rays, melanocytes increase production of melanin, temporarily enhancing protection against future sun exposure. The amount of melanin produced varies greatly among individuals; persons with darker skin tones are less sensitive to sun exposure due to an elevated quantity of melanin, however can still become sunburned with prolonged exposure. Symptoms, including mild erythema, pain, swelling, tenderness, and blisters, appear within 1 to 24 h of sun exposure and usually peak within 72 h. Consequences of prolonged and repeated exposure to sunlight include an increased risk of skin malignancies and premature aging.

A few simple precautions can prevent most cases of sunburn. Limited exposure (less than 30 min) to brighter midday sunlight is key. Sunlight is less intense before 10 a.m. and after 3 p.m. in most climates. If prolonged exposure to sunlight cannot be avoided, sunscreens containing P-aminobenzoic acid (PABA) and an sun protection factor (SPF) of at least 30 are recommended. Hats, clothing, and sunglasses are also invaluable in preventing exposure to damaging UVB rays.

Nutritional Management

While nature can help to prevent the damage caused by UV rays by raising melanin production, increasing epidermis thickness and providing antioxidants to superficial skin layers, some studies have suggested that supplementation of nutrients may aid these processes. Vitamins C and E, natural antioxidants, may have a photoprotective effect. Two studies have demonstrated that supplemented doses of 671 mg to 2 g of alpha-tocopherol/day and 2 to 3 g of ascorbic acid/day resulted in a reduction of skin changes with exposure to UV radiation.[19,20] These studies indicate that the combination of vitamins C and E is necessary for producing the desired effect, as they work synergistically.

The potential photoprotective effects of carotenoids have also been studied. Two studies, which supplemented subjects with doses of 60 and 90 mg/day of beta-carotene, for 28 and 23 days, respectively, did not show a beneficial effect of beta-carotene supplementation when subjects were irradiated.[21,22] However, another study supplementing subjects with 30 mg/day of beta-carotene for a longer time period, 10 weeks, showed a reduced incidence and severity of skin erythema after exposure to UV radiation.[23] One study investigated the carotenoid lycopene. Subjects ingested approximately 16 mg/day of lycopene in the form of tomato paste. Results showed a 40% reduction in erythema after UV exposure after 10 weeks of lycopene supplementation.[24] Additional studies have used natural carotenoid supplements, containing varying amounts of beta-carotene, alpha-carotene, cryptoxanthin, zeaxanthin, and lutein. Results of one study showed that higher doses of natural carotenoids (60 to 90 mg/day) exerted a photoprotective effect.[25] Another study suggested that concurrent natural caroten-oid (25 mg/day) and vitamin E (335 mg/day) supplementation produced a greater photopro-tective effect than did carotenoid supplementation alone.[26] Proposed mechanisms for the photoprotective properties of carotenoids include stimulation of melanogenesis, inhibition of serum lipid peroxidation, and increased reflection capacity of the skin.

The third nutrient studied for its photoprotective characteristics is $n-3$ PUFAs. Food sources of $n-3$ PUFAs are primarily fish oils, particularly those from higher fat fish such as mackerel, salmon, sardines, anchovy, and herring. Studies investigating both EPA and DHA have demonstrated photoprotective effects in varying doses, 1.8 to 4 g/day of EPA and 1.2 g/day of DHA. The effects were noted after 4, 10, and 12 weeks of supplementation respectively.[27–29] Scientists did note that despite a reduction of UV radiation-induced erythema, there was an increase in lipid peroxidation in the skin of irradiated subjects, perhaps because of the unstable nature of $n-3$ PUFAs.

It is unknown whether the amount of vitamins C and E, carotenoids, and $n-3$ PUFAs typically ingested by diet alone will protect skin from damage to UV radiation. Supplemen-tation above these typical amounts has been shown to have a small photoprotective effect, and therefore may be beneficial for light-skinned individuals at high risk for sun damage. Certainly, supplementation of these nutrients does not have nearly the same protective effect, and therefore should not replace the use of sunscreens and other UV radiation blockers.

WOUND HEALING

Skin damage appears in a number of forms, including scrapes and abrasions; shearing; venous, arterial and diabetic ulcerations; cellulitis; and dermatitis. Serious wounds, particu-larly deep pressure ulcers and burns, are the most challenging to treat, both medically and nutritionally. Malnutrition and a number of disease states, when poorly controlled, contrib-ute to the formation and impair the healing of wounds. Achieving and maintaining a good nutritional status is critical to maximize the healing of these types of wounds.

BURNS

Burns may occur from exposure to open flames, steam, electricity, hot liquids and surfaces, and radiation. The elderly may be at higher risk for burns due to decreased reaction time, poor vision, and decreased mobility. Young children may also be at higher risk for burns due to child abuse and unsupervised activities, leading to accidents. Electrical burns are more difficult to assess than other types of burns; the electrical current enters and exits the body at two different sites, causing damage to internal tissues. Assessment of burns involves an estimation of the percent of total body surface area (BSA) burned, and the degree of burn damage (see Table 19.1).

Healing of burns is generally divided into three periods: emergent (or inflammation) stage, acute (or proliferative) stage, and rehabilitative (or adaptive) stage. In the emergent phase, the first several days after injury, treatment involves fluid resuscitation, maintenance of pulmon-ary function, and management of burns. Fluid shifts occur after burn injuries, resulting in edema to the damaged tissues, or sometimes generalized edema. Fluid losses from wound

TABLE 19.1
Degree of Burn Damage

Burn Depth	Color/Vascularity	Appearance/Pain	Healing/Scarring
Stage I superficial	Pink or red	No blisters, delayed pain, tender	Healing in 3 to 5 days, no scars
Stage II superficial partial thickness	Pink or red, blanches with brisk capillary refill	Intact blisters, moist surface, weeping, very painful	Healing in 7 to 10 days, pigment discoloration
Stage II deep partial thickness	Mixed red, waxy white, blanches with slow capillary refill	Broken blisters, moist surface, sensitive to pressure, insensitive to light touch, marked edema	Healing in 2 to 3 weeks, hypertrophic scars
Stage III full thickness	White, black, red, tan, no blanching, thrombosed vessels, poor distal circulation	Eschar — dry, leathery, rigid. No sensation. Body hairs pull out easily	Skin grafts required for healing
Stage IV subdermal	Charred	Devitalized or mummified, subcutaneous tissue may be evident	Skin grafts or flaps required for healing

Source: From Richard, R., Assessment and diagnosis of burn wounds, *Adv. Wound Care*, 12, 468, 1999.

exudate can be significant, and fluid and electrolyte replacement is critical to maintain cell function and cardiac output. Pulmonary function can be impaired via damage to lung tissue from inhalation of smoke and carbon dioxide, edema of the throat and reduced cardiac output leading to hypoxia, and restricted breathing due to deep burns of the chest. Maintenance of pulmonary function often requires mechanical ventilation.

The acute phase of burn care occurs after the patient has been adequately fluid resuscitated and lasts until full thickness wounds have been skin grafted and partial thickness wounds are healed. Care during this period involves continued wound care, including mechanical and surgical debridement of wounds, and prevention of complications. Potential complications include continued pulmonary insufficiency, sepsis and localized infections, multiorgan failure, acid–base imbalances, and fluid and electrolyte imbalances.

The rehabilitation phase involves the patient's return to society and dealing with lasting complications from the burn injury, such as contractures, scar tissue, and psychological issues. The adaptation of healed wounds can continue for years. Collagen fibers are remodeled by macrophages, which maximizes the strength of the scar tissue. Patients with extensive healed burns may have difficulty with temperature regulation, as the skin's ability to sweat and shiver is affected by full thickness injuries. Normal pigmentation to scar tissue may not return, therefore protection from UV radiation is important.[31,32]

PRESSURE ULCERS

The incidence of pressure ulcers rises with increasing age, due to changes both in the skin as it ages and decreased mobility. Quantities of collagen and elastin continuously decline with age, resulting in thin, dry, and inelastic skin more prone to damage. Atrophy of all layers of the skin and reduced subcutaneous fat stores result in more pronounced bony prominences, and therefore an increased risk of pressure ulcers. Another major risk factor for pressure ulcers is immobility or inactivity. Bed- or chair-bound individuals, such as paraplegics or quadriplegics, are at risk, as well as those who are immobile due to physical illness or an impaired mental state. Incontinent persons are also at higher risk of pressure ulcers, as soiled skin is moist and exposed to more bacteria. Table 19.2 illustrates the four stages of pressure ulcers.

Prevention of pressure ulcers requires diligent nursing care and an interdisciplinary team effort. Patients who are bed-bound must be repositioned at least every 2 h. Patients who are chair-bound must be repositioned every hour at a minimum, ideally every 15 min. Special pressure reducing mattresses and cushions may be used. Other devices such as wedge cushions, pressure-relieving boots, and foam pillows should be used to relieve pressure on high-risk areas such as the heels, ankles, knees, and coccyx, or other areas with bony prominences.[33,34]

TABLE 19.2
Pressure Ulcer Stages

Stage I	Change in skin temperature, tissue consistency, and sensation as compared to surrounding skin. The ulcer appears as a defined area of redness, or in darker skin tones, may have a blue or purple color
Stage II	Partial thickness skin loss involving the epidermis and sometimes the dermis. The ulcer appears as an abrasion, blister, or shallow crater
Stage III	Full thickness skin loss involving loss or damage to the subcutaneous tissue. The ulcer appears as a deep crater
Stage IV	Full thickness skin loss involving loss or damage to muscle, bone, or supporting structures such as tendons and joints

Source: From Calianno, C., *Adv. Wound Care*, 13, 244, 2000.

> ### Textbox 19.1 Toxic Epidermal Necrolysis Syndrome and Stevens–Johnson Syndrome
>
> Toxic Epidermal Necrolysis Syndrome (TENS) and Stevens–Johnson Syndrome (SJS) are rare skin diseases, usually attributed to a hypersensitivity reaction to a drug or its metabolites. The drug reaction causes epidermal erythema, skin blisters, and peeling of the epidermis in large sheets, resulting in areas of denuded skin similar in appearance to second-degree burns. Body areas most commonly affected are the trunk, face, and proximal limbs. Reactions involving more than 30% loss of epidermis are classified as TENS, those involving less than 10% are classified as SJS, and those in between are classified as TENS–SJS overlap. The exact mechanism is unknown. The drugs most commonly associated with TENS and SJS are sulfonamides, barbiturates, nonsteroidal anti-inflammatory drugs (NSAIDs), phenytoin, allopurinol, and penicillin, although other drugs have been implicated. Mortality rate can be high in patients with TENS, and death is usually caused by fluid and electrolyte imbalances and sepsis.
>
> Treatment of TENS is similar to that of burn victims, including fluid replacement, temperature management, prevention and treatment of infection and other complications, and nutrition support. Steroids may be used with caution; some studies have suggested that steroids may reduce skin loss in the early stages of the disease, but also increase the risk of infection and sepsis. Immunoglobulin therapy has been used to reduce the severity of TENS symptoms, which anecdotally has resulted in positive results, however some studies have not proven a benefit of immunoglobulin therapy, and suggest a potentially detrimental effect. Ophthalmology consults are recommended as TENS may affect the eyes, and result in blindness if untreated. Nutritional needs are elevated and should be calculated similarly to those of burn patients. Nutrition support frequently includes tube feeding, as patients are often unable to meet their nutrition needs orally. Parenteral nutrition should be initiated only if the patient demonstrates intolerance to enteral feeds or if a GI complication, such as GI bleeding, precludes the use of the enteral route.[35,36]

PHYSIOLOGY OF WOUND HEALING

Normal wound healing occurs in three distinct phases: inflammation, proliferation, and maturation. The inflammation stage begins at the time of injury and continues for 3 to 10 days, depending on the severity of the wound, and may be prolonged if the wound is infected or necrotic. Inflammation begins with constriction of the blood vessels and initiation of blood coagulation to minimize blood loss. The local immune system is activated and leukocytes enter the wound and attack bacteria. Macrophages arrive after leukocytes and remove blood clots, bacteria, and other foreign bodies. Release of growth factors and other substances begins the process of re-epithelialization. The proliferative phase is characterized by the activity of fibroblasts, which synthesize collagen for the formation of new tissue. Two to three weeks postinjury, the maturation, or remodeling phase begins, which is characterized by maturation of collagen cross-linking, which increases the contraction and strength of the scar. Maturation can continue for months or years in severe injuries.

Several factors are necessary for normal wound healing. Adequate oxygenation of damaged tissues is vital; in a hypoxic environment, fibroblasts cannot replicate, and production of collagen is limited. Hypoxic wounds are also prone to bacterial invasion, which significantly increases the infection rate. Many diseases may cause wounds to become hypoxic. Cardiac disease, resulting in reduced cardiac output, diabetes, peripheral vascular disease (PVD), smoking, and chronic infections, will limit the body's ability to deliver adequately oxygenated blood to the wound.

Wound infection impairs healing, as bacteria release enzymes and other proteins that degrade fibrin and growth factors. Risk of infection increases in hypoxic wounds, wounds containing foreign bodies (i.e., sutures), and wounds with large amounts of necrotic tissue. Complete sterilization of a wound is unnecessary and unrealistic; a reduction in the number of bacteria in a wound to less than 10^5 organisms per gram of tissue will significantly increase the likelihood of successful healing. Attempts to completely sterilize a wound may also cause damage to healthy tissue. Reduction of wound bacteria can be accomplished by debridement of necrotic tissue and the use of topical antibiotic treatments.

Blood glucose management is critical to optimize wound healing. Hyperglycemia has a number of negative side effects, in both hospitalized ill patients and otherwise healthy individuals. Long-term poorly controlled blood glucose levels may lead to vascular disease, and therefore a predisposition to extremity ulcers and poor wound healing. Uncontrolled blood glucose levels can cause osmotic diuresis, making fluid management problematic. Hyperglycemia also has a negative impact on immune function; it has been associated with reduced granulocyte function, and decreased production of phagocytes and other immune cells. A higher incidence of infectious complications, including wound infections, has been noted in hospitalized hyperglycemic patients.[37]

A moist wound environment is also crucial to healing. Desiccation of a wound can cause an eschar to form, which inhibits epithelialization. Steroid use is detrimental to wound healing as well; steroids impair the inflammatory process, thus limiting the effects of macrophages and fibroblasts. Non-steroidal anti-inflammatory drugs may also delay wound healing, as they reduce collagen production. Use of tobacco products has a twofold effect on wound healing; tobacco impairs oxygen delivery to damaged tissues, and nicotine has a significant vasoconstricting effect.[38]

Nutritional Management

Malnutrition, including deficiencies in both macro- and micronutrients, considerably impairs wound healing, and is reviewed as follows.

Energy Requirements

Adequate calorie provision is critical for the facilitation of wound healing. Many studies have demonstrated that malnutrition and inadequate calorie intake result in delayed wound healing and an increased incidence of infection and other complications. Estimating calorie needs for patients with wounds is difficult without the use of indirect calorimetry, as needs vary depending on the severity of the wound, stage of healing, age, weight, comorbidities, and other factors. General recommended calorie needs for healing are 30 to 35 cal/kg, but estimations should be individualized to each patient and adjusted according to success of healing and changes in nutritional monitoring parameters.

In estimating calorie needs, it is important to recognize that overfeeding can be as detrimental to a patient as underfeeding. Overfeeding calories may result in excess CO_2 production, thus worsening respiratory status or making weaning from mechanical ventilation more difficult. Excessive calorie administration may also cause hyperglycemia, hepatic steatosis, refeeding syndrome, and hypertriglyceridemia.[39]

Estimating energy needs in burn patients is especially challenging. Burns induce a catabolic state, which significantly increases the body's energy needs. Calorie needs are dependent on the degree and extent of injury. It has been established that once burns exceed 50 to 60% of total BSA, energy needs do not increase significantly. An accurate body weight is frequently difficult to establish, as edema may be present. Ideally, energy expenditure should be

TABLE 19.3
Energy Calculations for Burn Patients

Curreri (revised 1989)	Males: 25 cal/kg × BMR[a] factor + (40 × BSAB)[b]
	Females: 22 cal/kg × BMR factor + (40 × BSAB)
	BMR factor = age 20–40 years = 1.0
	age 40–50 years = 0.95
	age 50–60 years = 0.90
	age 75–100 years = 0.80
Ireton-Jones (revised 1998)	Vent patient: 1784–11 (age) + 5 (kg) + 244 (males) + 239 (trauma) + 804(burns)
Zawacki (1970)	1440 cal/BSA[c]/day
Xie (1993)	(1000 cal/BSA/day) + (25 × BSAB)
Milner (1994)	{BMR × [0.274 + (0.0079 × BSAB) − (0.004 × DPB[d])]} + BMR

[a]Basal metabolic rate.
[b]% Body surface area burned.
[c]Total body surface area (in m^2).
[d]Days postburn.

measured with a metabolic cart. However, the cost of calorimeters is prohibitive for many institutions, so clinicians may need to rely on available formulas to calculate calorie needs. Many formulas have been developed to estimate energy needs in this patient population, however their accuracy is questionable, as they cannot account for daily fluctuations in the patient's clinical course, medications, temperature, and metabolic state. Calculated energy needs for the same patient vary depending on the formula used, and some formulas do not account for the extent of injury.[31]

The most commonly used formulas for calculating energy expenditure in burn patients are the Curreri and the Ireton-Jones formulas.[40] Research has indicated the Curreri formula may overestimate energy needs. Dickerson et al.[41] examined the use of 46 different formulas used to calculate energy expenditure in burn patients. The actual energy expenditure of 24 burn patients was measured via indirect calorimetry, and these numbers compared with the estimated energy expenditure derived from different formulas. The authors concluded that none of the methods tested were precise, but did advocate the use of the three most accurate formulas (Zawacki, Xie, and Milner), if indirect calorimetry was not available (see Table 19.3).[41]

Protein Requirements

In addition to calorie needs, protein needs also increase in patients with wounds. Recommended amounts vary from 1.25 to 2.0 g/kg, however, various factors such as the degree of injury and comorbidities must be taken into account when estimating protein needs. Like calorie needs, protein needs should also be adjusted based on wound healing response and nutritional monitoring parameters. Adequate calorie intake is critical to ensure that protein is used to build new tissue, and not utilized as an energy source.

Protein needs are highly elevated in burn patients, because of both increased needs for healing and protein losses from the wounds. The total amount of protein recommended varies from 1.5 to 3.0 g/kg, but 2.0 to 2.5 g/kg is generally utilized for most patients with significant burns. In thermal injury, catabolism will often result in a negative nitrogen balance despite the aggressive provision of protein and calories. Excessive protein administration has not been shown to be beneficial and may cause azotemia.[39]

In addition to total protein, specific amino acids have been studied in relation to wound healing. Research has shown that supplementation of these nutrients in certain patients with wounds may be beneficial.

Arginine

Arginine, an amino acid commonly found in both plant and animal proteins, is considered a semiessential amino acid. Arginine is involved in many metabolic processes, most notably the synthesis of ornithine and nitric oxide. Ornithine is necessary for the synthesis of proline, glutamate, and polyamines, which are converted to collagen. Nitric oxide, a vasodilator, helps to regulate infection and immune function. Arginine also influences the levels of IGF-I, a hormone that promotes wound healing. Arginine has been shown to improve blood flow to the liver and gut, and decrease the production of proinflammatory cytokines.[42,43]

Arginine needs increase in the presence of trauma, wounds, and growth. Studies of wound healing and arginine supplementation suggest that arginine improves wound healing via an increased production of hydroxyproline, collagen, and lymphocyte response. Suggested doses range from 14 to 25 g/day, and can be provided in both oral supplements and tube feeding formulas.[44,45] Standard enteral formulas contain small amounts of arginine; arginine-enriched formulas typically contain $\sim 2\%$ of total calories in the form of arginine. Some studies have found increased mortality in critically ill septic patients receiving supplemental arginine, possibly due to its effects on the immune system and excess production of nitric oxide. Arginine supplementation in these patients should be delayed until sepsis is resolved.[46]

Glutamine

Glutamine, like arginine, is also considered an essential amino acid in times of stress. Glutamine is the most abundant amino acid in the body, and is the primary fuel for rapidly dividing cells, such as enterocytes, lymphocytes, and fibroblasts. Oxidized glutamine provides substrates for the synthesis of DNA, RNA, and glutathione, an antioxidant. Glutamine supplementation in critical illness and injury has been shown to preserve gut integrity, decrease infection rate, and reduce nitrogen losses.

Most glutamine researchers have used supplemental doses of 0.35 to 0.5 g/kg/day. Parenteral sources of glutamine are expensive, unstable in solution, and not as effective as enterally supplemented glutamine. Glutamine is present in small amounts in most enteral nutrition formulas, with larger amounts available in specialty glutamine-rich formulas. Glutamine powder, usually in 10 g packets, is available as well.[47,48]

Ornithine

Supplementation of ornithine alpha-ketoglutarate (OKG), a precursor of glutamine and arginine, has been studied in burn patients. In addition to providing a fuel for the production of arginine, OKG may improve wound healing by reducing postburn catabolism by stimulating the release of growth hormone and insulin. Research has shown ornithine supplementation in burn patients to reduce wound healing time and nitrogen excretion, increase nutritional markers, and improve the quality of wound healing. Studied OKG doses range from 20 to 40 g/day.[49,50]

Fat Requirements

Some researchers have focused on the potential benefits of supplementing specific fatty acids in acutely ill patients. Patients with diets high in omega-6 fatty acids have a large concentration of arachadonic acid (AA) in their cell membranes. During injury or illness, AA is released from cell membranes and metabolized, producing proinflammatory eicosanoids. When the amount of omega-3 fatty acids such as EPA increases in the diet, EPA displaces AA in the cell membranes, thus reducing the production of proinflammatory eicosanoids during illness or injury. When EPA is metabolized the eicosanoids produced are less proinflammatory. This ability to modulate immune function may have an impact on wound healing, especially in burn patients, who are at high risk for infection and suffer from a highly catabolic state.[51]

Human studies have been conducted regarding the role of omega-3 fatty acids in wound healing. One study concluded that the provision of a modified immune-enhancing formula in burn patients resulted in a reduction in infection rate and length of hospital stay. The immune-enhancing formula differed from the control formulas in that it contained 5 g of omega-3 fatty acids per 1000 cal, as well as arginine and glutamine.[52] A second study concluded that the provision of an immune-enhancing formula did not make a difference in infection rate or length of hospital stay; however, both the study and control formulas contained significant amounts of omega-3 fatty acids (2.2 g and 1.75 g per 1000 cal, respectively).[53]

Another study conducted on rats suggested omega-3 fatty acid supplementation might impair the later stages of wound healing. Rats fed a 20% lipid diet comprised of omega-3 fatty acids demonstrated a reduction in wound tensile strength as compared to rats fed a 20% lipid diet comprised of corn oil. The authors hypothesized that this reduction in wound strength was due to changes in collagen cross-linking rather than total amount of collagen produced.[54]

Studies have suggested that burn patients have an altered fatty acid metabolism and an increased use of fatty acids for healing and immune function after burn injury. Although more research is needed, some initial data indicates a possible benefit for an increase in omega-3 fatty acid intake to help modulate immune function, thereby improving infection rates, a common and often life-threatening complication of burns and other wounds. This benefit must be weighed against the possible negative side effect of omega-3 fatty acid supplementation on later stages of healing.

Micronutrients

Vitamin C

The role of vitamin C in collagen formation is well known. Vitamin C, along with oxygen, iron, and alpha-ketoglutarate, is a necessary component for the hydroxylation of the amino acids proline and lysine during collagen formation. Vitamin C is also necessary for the production of other connective tissues, neurotransmitters, and carnitine; acts as an antioxidant; aids in the absorption of iron; and plays a role in immune function.

A minimum of 5 to 10 mg/day of vitamin C is necessary to prevent the symptoms of scurvy, however the recommended dietary allowance (RDA) for vitamin C is 75 mg/day for women, 90 mg/day for men, with an additional 35 mg/day for smokers. Studies have shown that vitamin C needs are also higher in pregnant or lactating women, and patients with increased oxidative stress, including individuals with burns and other wounds. Vitamin C needs are increased in thermally injured patients due to changes in metabolism, increased losses through the wounds, and changes in the absorption and excretion of vitamin C.

The benefit of supplemental vitamin C in the absence of deficiency is not proven. However, as patients with significant burns (more than 20% BSA) frequently present with some degree of vitamin C deficiency, it is generally recommended that this patient group be supplemented with 500 to 1000 mg/day of vitamin C. Supplementation may not be necessary for less severe wounds if the patient is receiving the RDA for vitamin C via oral intake, a standard multivitamin, or enteral or parenteral nutrition. Toxicity is unusual in healthy adults, as excess vitamin C is excreted in the urine; patients with renal dysfunction should avoid large doses. The recommended upper limit of vitamin C intake is 2000 mg/day; larger doses may cause GI side effects such as nausea and diarrhea. Supplemental use in wound healing should be re-evaluated for necessity at least every 30 days.[31,55,56]

Vitamin A

In addition to its role in vision, vitamin A also functions in cellular differentiation and immunity. Vitamin A has been shown to help counteract the catabolic effects of steroids. A deficiency of vitamin A results in a decline in immune responses, epithelialization, and collagen synthesis. Deficiency is rare in most countries, as vitamin A is fat-soluble and stored in the liver. The RDA for vitamin A is 1000 mcg/day, or 3333 international units (IU) per day. In cases of suspected deficiency, or for those receiving high-dose steroids, the recommended supplemental dose of vitamin A is 25,000 IU/day for 10 days. As the risk of toxicity is greater with fat-soluble vitamins, supplementation of vitamin A should be frequently re-evaluated, and supplementation should not be used in the presence of liver and renal failure unless fat malabsorption is also present.[55,56]

Vitamin E

Vitamin E functions primarily as an antioxidant; deficiency of vitamin E causes anemia and peripheral neuropathy due to free radical damage. Deficiency caused by inadequate dietary intake is extremely rare, as vitamin E is found in a variety of foods, especially oils and fats. Vitamin E deficiency can occur due to genetic defects in the vitamin E transfer protein, in patients with fat malabsorption, and in patients receiving long-term parenteral nutrition. The RDA for vitamin E is 15 mg/day. Studies have shown no benefit in the supplementation of vitamin E in wound healing; in some animal studies, vitamin E supplementation resulted in delayed wound healing via retardation of collagen synthesis and reduced wound tensile strength. Excessive vitamin E supplementation has also been shown to impede the absorption of vitamin A and inhibit the inflammatory process. Supplementation of vitamin E exceeding the RDA should not be used in wound healing unless a deficiency has been verified.[55] Supplemental vitamin E is sometimes used in patients receiving hyperbaric oxygen therapy (HBOT) to potentially decrease the risk of free radical damage, although definitive evidence for the efficacy of its use is lacking.[57] Topical vitamin E has been used to reduce the formation of scar tissue, but some studies suggest it may actually be detrimental to the cosmetic appearance of scars, and may cause contact dermatitis in some patients. Studies supporting its use are limited and largely anecdotal.[58]

Zinc

Zinc is the most abundant trace element in the body, and is a necessary component of many enzymes involved in DNA, RNA, protein and collagen synthesis, and cell proliferation. It is a vital nutrient in wound healing. Most dietary zinc comes in the form of animal proteins, although it is also found in legumes and cereals. Vegetarians are at higher risk for deficiency due to the lack of animal protein in their diets and an increased intake of phytates, which inhibit zinc absorption. Others at risk for zinc deficiency include pregnant and lactating women, infants, and children. Zinc deficiency is most commonly seen in malnutrition, malabsorption, and alcoholism, as well as those with increased needs due to infection or inflammation, growth, or healing, and those with increased losses from burns, wounds, and diarrhea. The RDA for zinc is 11 mg/day for men and 8 mg/day for women.

Early studies reported accelerated wound healing in patients supplemented with zinc, however these results have not been reproduced or confirmed. Zinc supplementation is not beneficial in patients with adequate zinc stores. Evaluation of zinc stores is difficult, however, as plasma zinc concentrations represent only 2% of nutritionally available total body zinc; concentrations may be altered due to stress, infection, and food intake.[59] The decision to supplement zinc should be based on either a clinical presentation of zinc deficiency or the presence of malnutrition and other risk factors for zinc deficiency. The generally recommended dose for supplementation is 220 mg/day of zinc sulfate orally or 10 mg/day intravenously (IV). Excessive intake of zinc, more than 150 mg/day, interferes with copper absorption. A copper deficiency, in turn, can inhibit wound healing by causing anemia and therefore decreasing oxygen delivery to damaged tissues. Consequently, zinc supplementation should be used with caution. Supplementation should be of limited duration, 10 to 30 days, and continued only when deficiency is still present or zinc losses remain high[55,59,60].

Textbox 19.2   Route of Nutrition Support — Parenteral versus Enteral

Nutrition support is sometimes necessary in patients with large wounds or burns. Burn patients, especially those with inhalation injuries, are frequently on mechanical ventilation and therefore cannot eat. Other patients may not be able to consume adequate oral nutrition to meet their increased needs for healing. If the GI tract is functional, enteral nutrition is always the first choice when nutrition support is needed. The benefits of enteral nutrition over parenteral nutrition are well documented. Enteral nutrition more closely mimics normal physiological feeding, reduces the risk of infectious complications, helps to maintain gut integrity, reduces the risk of bacterial translocation, and is less costly than parenteral nutrition. Parenteral nutrition is associated with higher infection rates, metabolic abnormalities such as hyperglycemia, electrolyte disturbances, and metabolic acidosis. Parenteral nutrition may be necessary if the GI tract is not functional, due to protracted ileus, malabsorption, or high-output GI fistulas. Whether parenteral or enteral nutrition is utilized, tight control of blood glucose, adequate supply of nutrients, avoidance of overfeeding and maintenance of fluid and electrolyte balance are essential to optimize wound healing.

Nutritional management in patients with wounds, especially burns and deep pressure ulcers, is crucial for healing. Not only are adequate intake of calories and protein essential, but specific macronutrient proponents such as arginine, glutamine, ornithine, and omega-3 fatty acids are also important in healing, both directly and indirectly by affecting immune function and other metabolic processes. Many micronutrients are also vital for healing wounds, especially in patients with pre-existing deficiencies and elevated losses, as seen in burn patients.

NONNUTRITIONAL MANAGEMENT

Many nonnutritional methods to promote wound healing, besides standard nursing and surgical care, have been studied. Some have become generally accepted as part of standard treatments, while other approaches continue to have limited use in conventional medicine due to a lack of supportive evidence of their efficacy. Some of these wound healing methods are described as follows.

Hormones and Steroids

Acute injury and illness results in increased stress hormone production, and decreased production of anabolic hormones, such as human growth hormone (HGH) and testosterone. The resultant catabolic state forces the body to break down lean tissue to supply fuel to meet increased demands for energy, leaving little protein available to create new tissue. Loss of lean body mass is associated with a number of negative effects on healing, including impaired immune function, increased infection, and delayed healing times. Studies have shown that the use of HGH in burn patients results in weight gain, reduced urinary nitrogen losses, and reduced protein catabolism. However, significant hyperglycemia is a common side effect, due to the anti-insulin action of HGH. HGH is also cost prohibitive, and is only approved by the FDA for use in short stature children. These issues limit its use as an anticatabolic agent.

Testosterone has also been tested as an anticatabolic agent, however its use is impractical due to its virilizing effects and short half-life. However, oxandrolone, a testosterone derivative with minimal virilizing effects, has been approved by the FDA for weight gain after involuntary weight loss and to offset protein catabolism associated with prolonged corticosteroid use. Studies of malnourished patients with wounds and lean body mass loss supplemented with oxandrolone showed a significant improvement in wound healing correlating with an increase in weight. The maximum dose to promote gain of lean tissue is 20 mg/day, however patient response to oxandrolone is variable, and lower doses may be adequate. The generally recommended duration of treatment is 2 to 4 weeks; longer courses of therapy may be necessary in patients with severe wounds or burns. Oxandrolone should not be used in patients with breast or prostate cancer, nephrosis, hypercalcemia, and in pregnant patients. It is important to maintain adequate nutritional intake with the use of any anabolic agent; anabolism will not occur if the body does not have the necessary substrates to create new tissue.[61–63]

Honey

Honey has been used as a topical wound treatment for centuries, as it has many properties that aid in wound healing. Honey provides a moist environment for healing and its osmotic effect causes fluid to be drawn up from underlying tissues, preventing dehydration of the wound. This moisture barrier prevents the dressings from adhering to the wound and therefore reduces removal of new tissue when dressings are changed. Research has also suggested that topical application of nutrients increases the rate of growth of granulation tissue. Honey's high osmolarity creates a poor environment for the growth of bacteria. Additionally, when honey is diluted with water, glucose oxidase produces hydrogen peroxide. Hydrogen peroxide is an effective antibacterial, but is no longer used as a standard treatment in wound care due to its inflammatory effects. However, the amount of hydrogen peroxide produced in diluted honey is about 1000 times less than a standard 3% hydrogen peroxide solution — not enough to produce inflammation, but enough to act as a mild antibacterial. Honey has also been shown to stimulate the production and function of lymphocytes and neutrophils. Reduction of pain and edema in wounds has been attributed to honey's anti-inflammatory properties. Reduced edema aids circulation and thus improves oxygenation of damaged tissues. Decreased inflammation reduces the production of free radicals, and the antioxidants present in honey help neutralize remaining free radicals. Free radical reduction helps to prevent further necrosis, and therefore may prevent partial thickness burns from converting to full thickness burns.

Culinary honey cannot be used for wound care treatment. Heat treatment of culinary honey, necessary to destroy *Clostridium botulinum* bacteria, will also destroy glucose oxidase, the enzyme responsible for producing hydrogen peroxide. Gamma-radiation is used to sterilize therapeutic honey. Other considerations must be taken into account when considering the use of honey in clinical practice. Honey will typically run off of a wound when applied directly; honey-impregnated dressings are more effective. If wounds produce a large amount of exudate, dressing changes should be frequent, as the beneficial properties of honey will be lost as the exudate dilutes the honey. Absorbent or occlusive secondary dressings are useful to prevent honey oozing out of the primary dressing.[64,65]

Aloe Vera and Other Plant Extracts

Aloe vera is a cactus whose extracts are found in many skin care products. Aloe vera gel consists of 96% water and a variety of polysaccharides, enzymes, minerals, vitamin sterols, and amino acids.[66] Evidence from animal studies suggests that the topical or oral use of aloe vera may be beneficial in the treatment of burns and wounds. These studies demonstrate aloe or its constituents' ability to stimulate the production of cytokines and nitric oxide, and improve collagen synthesis.[67] However, conflicting evidence suggests aloe gel may not be an effective wound care treatment. Studies conducted on humans with surgical wounds, chronic venous ulcers, and pressure ulcers showed either no difference or delayed wound healing in subjects treated with aloe as compared to control subjects. Several factors limit the practicality of aloe vera use in wound healing. Fresh aloe vera from a cut plant may maintain its biological activity for only a few hours. Factors such as growing, harvesting, the age of the plant, and extraction methods will also affect the potency of aloe. The FDA has approved topical aloe vera use for inflammation, however they do not regulate or investigate products claiming to contain aloe vera extracts, as it is a botanical product.[66]

In non-Western cultures, other plant products and extracts are used frequently for wound healing and other skin conditions. Papaya fruit, mashed and applied topically to wounds, has been shown in some studies to reduce necrotic tissue and increase granulation of healthy tissue. Most published reports are anecdotal and do not compare the use of papaya to that of commercial products or conventional wound care treatments.[68] Other plant extracts used for wound healing in non-Western cultures include *Buddleja globosa* leaves in Chile; Eupolin ointment, derived from the *Chromolaena odorata* plant, in Southeast Asia; and extracts from *Hypericum patulum* and *H. hookerianum* in India.[69] While there is scant or no data in the scientific literature to support the use of these treatments, they may be beneficial for those patients living in developing countries where the cost of conventional treatments is prohibitive and availability is limited or nonexistent.[67]

Oxygen Therapy

Adequate oxygenation of tissues is vital to successful wound healing, and ischemia contributes to the initial formation of some wounds. Two types of oxygen therapy are available for the treatment of wounds: topical oxygen therapy and total body HBOT. Topical oxygen is applied to extremity wounds via a limb-encasing device, and oxygen is delivered at pressures greater than atmospheric pressure. It has been demonstrated that oxygen will not penetrate far into a wound when applied topically, but some studies have shown positive outcomes with its use. Other research has suggested that topical oxygen therapy may destroy newly formed blood vessels in venous leg ulcers and reduce oxygen delivery in diabetic foot ulcers. Further research is needed to assess its effectiveness.

In HBOT, a patient is enclosed in a chamber pressurized at 2 to 3 atm., while breathing 100% oxygen for periods of 60 to 120 min a day for 10 to 60 treatments. Data suggests that patients whose wounds are not hypoxic will not benefit from HBOT; those with wound tissue oxygen concentrations of less than 20 mmHg will benefit the most. Patients with wound oxygen concentrations of 20 to 40 mmHg should demonstrate delayed healing despite sufficient wound care and good nutritional status before HBOT is considered. HBOT has been shown to be an effective tool to increase oxygen concentrations in ischemic wounds, even in patients with poor vascularization. Side effects of HBOT may include exacerbation of congestive heart failure, reversible myopia, claustrophobia, and hearing loss due to pressure changes, which is usually reversible. Long-term side effects of the use of HBOT have not been investigated; concerns include the possibility of increased oxidative stress in cells exposed to pure oxygen. Further studies are needed to determine ideal conditions of use, such as oxygen pressure, concentration, frequency, and duration of administration.[70–73]

Negative Pressure Therapy

Negative pressure therapy, or vacuum-assisted closure, is a common therapy used for healing a variety of wounds, including pressure ulcers, chronic ulcers, burns, and traumatic injuries. Negative pressure therapy may be used with wounds involving any type of tissue, including bone, tendon, muscle, fascia, and blood vessels; however, wounds must be free of necrotic tissue, well vascularized, and not actively bleeding. Medical grade foam, cut to the dimensions of the wound, is placed in the wound bed, and then sealed with an impermeable dressing. A noncollapsible evacuation tube is placed on the foam, and attached to a vacuum device. Pressure of 25 to 125 mmHg is applied, and wound exudate is collected in a sealed canister. Wound healing is promoted via improved blood flow, oxygenation and nutrient delivery, reduction of bacterial contamination, and reduction of trauma to damaged tissue from frequent dressing changes.

Complications from negative pressure therapy are minimal; maceration or pressure necrosis of skin due to poor positioning of the evacuation tube is possible, especially if the tube is placed over bony prominences. Excessive tissue granulation into the sponge may occur, and lead to bleeding when the sponge is changed; this may be avoided or limited by more frequent dressing changes or applying a lower suction pressure.[71,72]

Hydrotherapy

Hydrotherapy, or whirlpool, has been used extensively in the treatment of many kinds of wounds. Patients with extensive wounds, such as burns, may be immersed in full-body whirlpools, or extremities may be submerged in smaller tanks. Warm water injected with air is circulated at various rates; sessions typically last 20 to 30 min. Wounds are then sprayed with clean water to remove additional debris and remaining contaminated water. The agitation of the water and air around the wound helps to remove toxic debris, dilutes bacterial contamination, and the warmth of the water mildly aids blood circulation. Water helps to soften necrotic tissue, which facilitates mechanical debridement. Whirlpool therapy also allows for gentler and less painful removal of dressings. Pulsed lavage, another form of hydrotherapy, involves the delivery of an irrigation solution to a wound at pressures ranging from 10 to 15 psi. Lavage therapy has the same benefits as whirlpool therapy, and some studies have shown higher rates of granulation tissue production in patients receiving lavage therapy as compared to those receiving whirlpool therapy. Drawbacks associated with hydrotherapy include an increased risk of microbial cross-contamination from patient to patient due to inadequately sterilized hydrotherapy equipment.[72,73]

Laser Therapy

High-intensity laser therapy is used frequently in dermatology for the treatment of pigmented lesions, skin resurfacing, and hair removal. Low-intensity lasers, such as helium–neon (HeNe) and gallium arsenide (GaAs), have been used for wound healing. Some wounds are too large to make laser therapy practical, and optimum wavelength and beam width is difficult to achieve in a clinical setting. Therefore, an alternative to conventional lasers, light-emitting diodes, is becoming more common as a wound-healing tool. Diodes can produce multiple wavelengths and are arranged in an array, allowing for treatment of large wounds. Cell and animal studies have suggested that laser therapy may increase fibroblast, growth factor and mast cell production, and increase epithelial activity. Theoretically, exposure to the photon energy released by lasers enhances cellular migration or cellular proliferation. However, research has produced mixed results as to the efficacy of low-intensity laser therapy on wound healing.[74–77]

Ultrasound

Ultrasound, employed as a diagnostic tool for many years, is electrical energy converted to sound waves at frequencies above the range of human hearing (> 20,000 Hz). These sound waves are applied to tissues through a hydrated medium, such as a water bath, by a treatment applicator. Ultrasound is generally delivered to affected tissues for sessions of 1 to 10 min, 1 to 3 times per week for 4 to 12 weeks. High-frequency ultrasound transmits warmth to the tissue, and is used as a relaxant in musculoskeletal conditions. Low-frequency ultrasound has little thermal effects; it is utilized in wound care largely because of its mechanical effects. Mechanical debridement via ultrasound is thought to occur through the burst of micro-bubbles, produced in the liquid medium, on the wound. This mechanism is known as cavitation. Laboratory experiments have suggested that in the early stages of healing, ultrasound may stimulate collagen, fibroblast and macrophage synthesis, increase collagen tensile strength, reduce the inflammatory phase, and promote the proliferative phase of healing. Clinical studies, however, have provided limited evidence for the effectiveness of ultrasound in wound healing.[72–74,78]

Electrotherapy

Four different kinds of electrostimulation are available for wound care treatment: direct current, low-frequency pulsed current, high-voltage pulsed current, and pulsed electromagnetic fields. Methods for each treatment modality vary; in general, an electrode with a cathode and an anode are placed on the wound or on healthy tissue near the wound. A current of electricity is run through the electrode at varying voltages and frequencies. Potential benefits of electrotherapy include increased migration of neutrophils and macrophages, fibroblast stimulation, improved blood flow, and bacteriostasis. Research results show only indirect benefits of electrotherapy in wound healing, and optimum treatment protocols and timing are unclear.[72–74]

Maggots

Maggots, larvae of the green bottle fly, were used frequently for wound care in the United States in the 1930s and 1940s, and gained notice again in the 1990s. Up to 1000 sterile maggots are introduced into the wound and left for 1 to 3 days. The wound and maggots are covered with a cage-like dressing made of netting, allowing air to reach the larvae; larvae may suffocate if conventional dressings are applied. Care should be taken to limit maggot contact with peripheral wound tissue, as their digestive enzymes may cause cellulitis and erythema of healthy tissue. Some care must also be taken to avoid crushing the maggots; bed rest is sometimes recommended, depending on the location of the wound. Bed rest may also help to limit leg edema, which will reduce wound exudate and lessen the risk of the larvae drowning. Maggot therapy may fail due to larvae desiccation; this can occur when maggots cannot get underneath a dry eschar covering the wound. Softening of the edges of the eschar before placement of the maggots is recommended. Research has shown that most wounds can be effectively debrided with maggot therapy within 1 week.

Maggot therapy is most beneficial for wounds requiring debridement — wounds with necrotic tissue, and wounds with purulent drainage and slough. Maggots remove necrotic tissue, disinfect wounds, reduce wound odors, and promote the formulation of granulation tissue. Maggots excrete antibacterial substances and may digest bacteria themselves. Maggots also excrete ammonia, allantoin, calcium carbonate, and urea, causing an alkaline environment, which stimulates granulation and inhibits bacterial growth. Side effects are minimal; some patients complain of increased pain during treatment, which can be effectively treated with analgesics. Psychological and aesthetic issues in maggot therapy can largely be overcome with education of patients, their family, and medical staff.[79–82]

Psychological Factors

Growing interest in holistic medicine has led researchers to investigate the concept of mind or spirit in relation to measurable physiological changes in the body. Some studies have suggested that stress may have a detrimental effect on wound healing. Stressors can come from a variety of sources, including psychological stress, physical trauma, and pain. The stress or "fight or flight" response causes vasoconstriction, shunting blood to the heart and lungs, and away from the skin and peripheral tissues. Cortisol, released during the stress response, increases blood glucose levels, reduces lymphocyte production, and impairs collagen synthesis via a reduction in fibroblast proliferation. Research has also shown that psychological stress reduces formation of proinflammatory cytokines at the wound site. These physiological changes may account for study results demonstrating delayed healing in stressed patients. Use of strategies to reduce stress and pain, such as relaxation, meditation, guided imagery, healing touch, massage, prayer, and hypnosis, have not been studied extensively and their efficacy is largely theoretical. Further research in this area is needed.[83–85]

CASE STUDY 1

An 87-year-old female is admitted from a nursing home to the hospital with urosepsis and dehydration. She has a large stage IV sacral decubitis. Her previous medical history includes type 2 diabetes for 12 years, chronic obstructive pulmonary disease (COPD), and PVD. Records from the nursing home indicate she has limited mobility due to debility, chronic shortness of breath and arthritis, and her nutritional intake is poor. She is started on a diabetic diet. Medications include glyburide and prednisone.

• Height	5'2"
• Weight	86 lb
	• Usual weight 123 lb, gradual weight loss over 2 years
• Laboratory results	• Na 145 mmol/l
	• K 4.5 mmol/l
	• Cl 112 mmol/l
	• BUN 45 mg/dl
	• Creatinine 1.4 mg/dl
	• CO_2 26 mmol/l
	• Albumin 2.3 g/dl
	• Finger stick blood glucoses 187–274 mg/dl

What Factors May Have Led to This Patient's Development of a Pressure Ulcer, and Will Impede Her Ability to Heal?

The patient is significantly underweight, creating bony prominences; she lacks fat stores to cushion her skin as pressure is applied when sitting or lying down. Her limited mobility impedes her ability to reposition herself and therefore increases the amount of time pressure is applied to high-risk areas of her body. Low weight, albumin, and poor intake reveal malnutrition, and indicate possible micronutrient deficiencies, which limits her body's ability to heal. The patient has diabetes and PVD; vascular damage impairs delivery of adequately oxygenated blood to damaged tissues. She is also on prednisone, a steroid medication causing thinning of the skin. Poorly controlled blood glucose and steroid therapy will result in impaired immune function, thereby increasing her risk of infections and further delaying wound healing.

What Are the Patient's Nutritional Needs?

Nutritional needs

- 1172–1370 cal/day (30–35 cal/kg)
- 59–78 g protein per day (1.5–2.0 g/kg)
- Arginine 14–25 g/day
- Vitamin C 1000 mg/day
- Zinc sulfate 220 mg/day (in presence of deficiency)
- 100% RDA of other vitamins and minerals

The patient's calorie needs appear quite low due to her extremely low body weight. Her true energy needs may be higher depending on her metabolic rate; nutritional parameters such as prealbumin should be monitored frequently (once or twice weekly) to ensure the patient is meeting her needs. Estimated energy requirements may be titrated upward if the patient is not meeting her healing and nutrition goals at the current calorie level.

What Interventions Should Be Utilized to Improve This Patient's Nutritional Status?

Nutritional goals

- Maintain adequate nutritional intake to maximize healing
- Maintain prealbumin levels within normal ranges (~ 20–40 mg/dl)
- Prevent further weight loss
- Optimize blood glucose management
- After wounds are healed, weight gain of 1–2 pounds per week until target weight reached

These goals may be reached with a number of nutritional interventions. Improved intake may occur by implementing simple measures, such as an alteration in diet consistency, extra assistance with meals, a high-calorie/high-protein diet and snacks, and addition of commercial nutritional supplements. An ideal oral supplement would contain extra protein, arginine, vitamin C, and other micronutrients. An appetite stimulant may be considered if intake is limited due to poor appetite. Enteral nutrition support should be utilized if these measures are unsuccessful in improving the patient's oral intake. Tube feeding can be infused overnight and held during the day to continue to encourage oral intake. Due to the patient's degree of malnutrition, she should be monitored closely for signs of refeeding syndrome. Blood glucose control may be achieved with medications and modification of the amount and type of carbohydrate eaten; management will be difficult if steroid therapy continues.

Prealbumin levels and weights should be monitored once or twice weekly to evaluate changes in nutritional status. A multivitamin and additional vitamin C should be considered if the patient is not receiving adequate amounts from enteral or oral nutrition. Zinc supplementation is only beneficial if a deficiency is present or suspected. Vitamin A supplementation may also be considered as the patient is taking steroid medications. All micronutrient supplementation should be reevaluated every 2 weeks to avoid toxicities.

WHAT OTHER NONNUTRITIONAL INTERVENTIONS ARE KEY TO HEALING THE PATIENT'S WOUND?

Proper nursing care is essential — the patient must be turned or repositioned frequently to relieve pressure to high-risk areas. Proper mattress and wheelchair cushions are also essential in relieving pressure. If the wound is clean — free of necrotic tissue — a wound vac may be applied to help improve blood flow to the area and facilitate healing. Blood glucose levels need to be maintained within normal range via diet and medication.

If wound healing is delayed despite the intake of adequate nutrition, an anabolic agent may be beneficial in this patient to promote the synthesis of lean body tissue and therefore wound healing. A low dose of 5 mg/day may be trialed; the dose may be increased up to 20 mg/day, and the duration of treatment is usually 2 to 4 weeks, although additional intermittent treatments may be used if needed.

CASE STUDY 2

A 38-year-old man is admitted to the intensive care unit (ICU) with 40% TBSA second- and third-degree burns to his trunk, back, and arms after a house fire. He has significant inhalation injuries and is intubated. The patient has no prior medical history. The patient's height is 6'2", usual and admit weight is 202 lbs.

WHAT ARE THE PATIENT'S CALORIE AND PROTEIN NEEDS?

Ideally, the patient's estimated calorie expenditure should be measured via indirect calorimetry. If this method is unavailable, a number of formulas may be utilized:

Curreri: Males: 25 cal/kg $\times$ BMR factor $+ (40 \times$ BSAB)
$25(91.8) \times 1.0 + (40 \times 40) = \mathbf{3895}$

Ireton-Jones: $1784 - 11\,(\text{age}) + 5\,(\text{kg}) + 224\,(\text{males}) + 239\,(\text{trauma}) + 804\,(\text{burns})$
$1784 - 11(38) + 5(91.8) + 244 + 804 = \mathbf{2873}$

Zawacki: 1440 cal/BSA/day
$1440 \times 2.16 = \mathbf{3110}$

Xie: $(1000 \text{ cal/BSA/day}) + (25 \times \text{BSAB})$
$(1000 \times 2.16) + (25 \times 40) = \mathbf{3160}$

Milner: BMR may be calculated by the Fleisch equation:
$\text{BMR} = \{37 - [(\text{age} - 20)/10]\} \times \text{BSA} \times 24$
$\text{BMR} = 1825$

$\{\text{BMR} \times [0.274 \times (0.0079 \times \text{BSAB}) - (0.004 \times \text{DPB})]\} + \text{BMR}$
$\{1825 \times [0.274 \times (0.0079 \times 40) - (0.004 \times 1)]\} + 1825 = \mathbf{2895}$

Results of the comparison of the five estimates show, as literature suggests, that the Curreri formula may overestimate energy requirements. Calculating a number of different estimates of calorie needs is cumbersome; most practitioners find it more practical to use one formula. A second formula may be used to verify results of the first. Clinical judgment must be exercised, taking into account factors such as the patient's temperature, medical complications, and metabolic state. We will use an average estimate of 3000 cal for this patient.

Protein needs are $\sim$ 2.0–2.5 g/kg or 184–230 g/day.

WHAT IS THE APPROPRIATE ROUTE OF NUTRITION SUPPORT FOR THIS PATIENT?

The patient is unable to eat due to mechanical ventilation. If the patient is hemodynamically stable, i.e., able to maintain adequate blood pressure, enteral nutrition should be initiated, ideally within 12 to 24 h of injury. Tolerance of enteral nutrition in burn patients can be difficult to achieve, especially immediately postinjury when blood pressure may be low. Some research has suggested enterally feeding hypotensive patients may cause gut necrosis.[86,87] Tolerance of tube feedings in hypotensive patients is certainly problematic, as blood supply to the gut is limited. If blood pressure is maintained with or without pressor agents, however, enteral nutrition should be started immediately to help maintain gut and immune function. Some experts suggest the use of an isotonic low-fiber formula, fed into the small bowel, and advanced slowly. The patient should be monitored closely for signs of tube feeding intolerance, such as increased nasogastric output, and abdominal distention or pain.[86]

There are several factors in the care of burn patients that can make it difficult to meet nutrition needs. Burn patients undergo frequent surgeries; enteral feeds are often discontinued the night before surgeries are performed, thus limiting the amount of nutrition received. Some studies have indicated that continued enteral feeding immediately before and during surgery might be safe if certain precautions are taken to reduce the risk of aspiration. If tube feeding is to be given during surgery, the tube should be placed postpylorically, and gastric decompression via nasal or oral tube should be administered.[88] Further research is needed to ensure the safety of this practice, and most institutions still hold enteral feedings for a significant period of time before and after surgery. Tube feedings may also be held for nursing interventions such as medication administration and dressing changes.

Several enteral formulas marketed specifically for wound healing are available; these contain higher amounts of total protein, vitamin A, vitamin C, zinc, and arginine compared to standard formulas. If a 1 cal/ml formula is used for our patient, and the feeding runs 24 h/day, the goal rate will be 125 ml/h. The tube feeding can be initiated at 30 to 50 ml/h and advanced as tolerated by 20 ml every 4 to 6 h to goal rate. A higher goal rate should be considered to account for times the feeding will be held; some clinicians may calculate the feeding to run at 20 h/day. This would make the goal rate for our patient 150 ml/h. Some patients may not tolerate a volume this high. More calorically dense formulas are available, however they may not be tailored for patients with wounds; supplemental protein, arginine, vitamins, and minerals may be needed. To help with tolerance issues related to volume, postpyloric feedings and prokinetic medications may be useful. Some patients may better tolerate a semielemental formula with peptides and medium-chain triglycerides, as these forms of protein and fat are more easily absorbed. If the calorie and protein needs cannot be met by tube feeding alone, parenteral nutrition should be utilized to supplement enteral nutrition.

HOW CAN ADEQUACY OF NUTRITION SUPPORT BE MEASURED?

Body weight should be measured regularly, but will not be an indicator of nutrition status immediately postburn due to changes in fluid status. Long-term, weight measurements are more indicative of nutrition status, however some weight loss is expected with extensive burns. Severe catabolism and inactivity will reduce lean body mass even if adequate nutrition is provided.

Visceral protein levels are indicators of degree of illness, and more useful to clinicians as a tool to determine a patient's risk of developing malnutrition.[89] However, trends in visceral protein levels are still of some use in determining if the nutrition regimen is sufficient. Prealbumin levels are generally recognized as the most sensitive to changes in nutritional intake, however, like any hepatic protein, production of prealbumin will be reduced in catabolic and inflammatory states. C-reactive protein may be measured to gauge the level of inflammation; if C-reactive protein is elevated, prealbumin will be depressed. If inflammatory indicators are declining and prealbumin is not improving, calorie intake may be inadequate. Prealbumin levels are generally measured once or twice weekly.

Assessing the patient's overall progress, especially the rate and degree of healing, may give a better picture of the response to nutrition support. If wounds are not healing as expected, despite good wound care and lack of complications, malnutrition may be the cause. Monitoring for signs of overfeeding, such as hyperglycemia and hypercapnia, is also important. Nutrition needs will decrease as the burns heal; regular reassessment of energy, protein, and micronutrient needs is important to avoid overfeeding.

THREE WEEKS POSTBURN, THE PATIENT HAS BEEN EXTUBATED AND STARTED ON ORAL NUTRITION. WHAT STRATEGIES SHOULD BE UTILIZED TO MEET NUTRITION NEEDS?

Due to the patient's prolonged intubation, a swallow evaluation by the speech language pathologist is beneficial to determine the appropriate consistency of the patient's diet and provide the patient with strategies to improve swallowing and prevent aspiration. If the patient's swallow function is adequate, the diet may be rapidly progressed, as tolerated, to a high calorie, high-protein diet. Calorie-dense oral supplements should be used to meet the patient's nutrient needs. Ideally, the patient's tube feeding should continue until he is able to demonstrate adequate nutritional intake by mouth. The tube feeding may be held for several hours around mealtime to allow the stomach to empty and improve appetite. When the patient is able to take 25 to 50% of estimated calorie needs by diet, the tube feeding can be changed to a nocturnal schedule, running only at night for 10 to 12 h, to provide approximately 50% of nutrient needs. Nocturnal feedings may be discontinued when the patient is able to meet more than 75% of needs by mouth. Nutritional parameters should be monitored until complete recovery is achieved.

GLOSSARY

Azotemia: Presence of nitrogenous bodies, especially urea in the blood.

Conjunctiva: Mucous membrane that lines the eyelids.

Contractures: A condition of fixed high resistance to the passive stretch of a muscle, sometimes as a result of fibrosis of tissues surrounding a joint.

Cytokines: Proteins produced by white blood cells that helps to regulate immunological aspects of cell function during inflammation and other immune responses.

Denuded: Removal of a protecting layer of tissue.

Dermatosis: Any condition of the skin in which inflammation is not a feature.

Desquamation: Shedding of the epidermis.

Ecchymoses: Large irregularly formed hemorrhagic areas on the skin.

Eicosanoids: The products of metabolism of arachadonic acid.

Erythema: Diffuse area of redness on the skin.

Eschar: Slough (necrotic tissue) on the skin especially resulting from a burn.

Exudate: Pus-like or serous fluid seeping out of vessel walls into adjoining tissue.
Granulation: Formation of new blood-rich tissue on the healing surface of a wound.
Immunomodulation: The use of nutrients to alter the body's immune responses.
Papules: Red elevated area on the skin, often preceding vesicle or pustule formation.
Pruritus: Severe itching.
Purulent: Forming or containing pus.
Stomatitis: Inflammation of the mouth.
Urticaria: A vascular reaction of the skin characterized by wheals and severe itching.
Vesicles: A blister-like elevation of the skin containing serous fluid.
Virilizing: Development of physical masculine characteristics.

REFERENCES

1. Liao, D.C., Management of acne, *J. Fam. Pract.*, 52, 43 2003.
2. Bershad, S.V., The modern age of acne therapy: a review of current treatment options, *The Mount Sinai J. Med.*, 68, 279, 2001.
3. Webster, G.F., Acne vulgaris, *BMJ*, 325, 475, 2002.
4. Cordain, L. et al., Acne vulgaris: a disease of western civilization, *Arch. Dermatol.*, 138, 1584, 2002.
5. Kazerooni, T. and Dehghan-Kooshkghazi, M., Effects of metformin on hyperandrogenism in women with polycystic ovarian syndrome, *Gynecol. Endocrinol.*, 17, 51, 2003.
6. Moneret-Vautrin, D.A., Optimal management of atopic dermatitis in infancy, *Allerg. Immunol.*, 34, 325, 2002.
7. Isolauri, T. et al., Probiotics in the management of atopic eczema, *Clin. Exp. Allergy*, 30, 1604, 2000.
8. Thestrup-Pedersen, K., Treatment principles of atopic dermatitis, *J. Eur. Acad. Dermatol. Venereol.*, 16, 1, 2002.
9. Boelsma, E., Hendriks, H., and Roza, L., Nutritional skin care: health effects of micronutrients and fatty acids, *Am. J. Clin. Nutr.*, 73, 853, 2001.
10. Ziboh, V.A. et al., Effects of dietary supplementation of fish oil on neutrophils and epidermal fatty acids, *Arch. Dermatol.*, 122, 1277, 1986.
11. Maurice, P.D. et al., Effects of dietary supplementation with eicosapentaenoic acid in patients with psoriasis, *Adv. Prostaglandin Thromboxane Leukot. Res.*, 17B, 647, 1987.
12. Bjornboe, A. et al., Effect of dietary supplementation with eicosapentaenoic acid in the treatment of atopic dermatitis, *Br. J. Dermatol.*, 117, 463, 1987.
13. Bittiner, S.B. et al., A double-blind, randomized, placebo-controlled trial of fish oil in psoriasis, *Lancet*, 1, 378, 1998.
14. Soyland, E. et al., Effect of dietary supplementation with very long-chain n–3 fatty acids in patients with psoriasis, *N. Engl. J. Med.*, 328, 1812, 1993.
15. Tanaka, T. et al., Vegetarian diet ameliorates symptoms of atopic dermatitis through reduction of the number of peripheral eosinophils and of PGE2 synthesis by monocytes, *J. Physiol. Anthropol. Appl. Hum. Sci.*, 20, 353, 2001.
16. Worm, M. et al., Clinical relevance of food additives in adult patients with atopic dermatitis, *Clin. Exp. Allergy*, 30, 407, 2000.
17. Fry, L., Dermatitis herpetiformis: problems, progress and prospects, *Eur. J. Dermatol.*, 12, 523, 2002.
18. Shils, M. et al., *Modern Nutrition in Health and Disease*, 9th ed., Lippincott, Williams & Wilkins, Philadelphia, 1999, pp. 1504–1507, 1163–1167.
19. Fuchs, J. and Kern, H., Modulation of UV-light-induced skin inflammation by D-alpha-tocopherol and L-ascorbic acid: a clinical study using solar simulated radiation, *Free Radic. Biol. Med.*, 25, 1006, 1998.
20. Eberlein-Konig, B., Placzek, M., and Przybilla, B., Protective effect against sunburn of combined systemic ascorbic acid (vitamin C) and D-alpha-tocopherol (vitamin E), *J. Am. Acad. Dermatol.*, 38, 45, 1998.

21. Wolf, C., Steiner, A., and Honigsmann, H., Do oral carotenoids protect human skin against ultraviolet erythema, psorales phototoxicity, and ultraviolet-induced DNA-damage? *J. Invest. Dermatol.*, 90, 55, 1988.

22. Garmyn, M. et al., Effect of beta-carotene supplementation on the human sunburn reaction, *Exp. Dermatol.*, 4, 101, 1995.

23. Gollnick, H.P.M. et al., Systemic beta carotene plus topical UV-sunscreen are in optimal protection against harmful effects of natural UV-sunlight: results of the Berlin-Eilath study, *Eur. J. Dermatol.*, 6, 200, 1996.

24. Stahl, W. et al., Dietary tomato paste protects against ultraviolet light-induced erythema in humans, *J. Nutr.*, 131, 1449, 2001.

25. Lee, J. et al., Carotenoid supplementation reduces erythema in human skin after simulated solar radiation exposure, *Proc. Soc. Exp. Biol. Med.*, 223, 170, 2000.

26. Stahl, W. et al., Carotenoids and carotenoids plus vitamin E protect against ultraviolet light-induced erythema in humans, *Am. J. Clin. Nutr.*, 71, 795, 2000.

27. Orengo, I.F., Black, H.S., and Wolf, J.E., Influence of fish oil supplementation on the minimal erythema dose in humans, *Arch. Dermatol. Res.*, 284, 219, 1992.

28. Rhodes, L.E. et al., Dietary fish oil supplementation in humans reduces UVB-erythemal sensitivity but increases epidermal lipid peroxidation, *J. Invest. Dermatol.*, 103, 151, 1994.

29. Rhodes, L.E. et al., Effect of eicosapentaenoic acid, an omega-3 polyunsaturated fatty acid, on UVR-related cancer risk in humans. An assessment of early genotoxic markers, *Carcinogenesis*, 24, 919, 2003.

30. Richard, R., Assessment and diagnosis of burn wounds, *Adv. Wound Care*, 12, 468, 1999.

31. Gottschlich, M., Ed., *The Science and Practice of Nutrition Support: A Case-Based Core Curriculum*, Kendall/Hunt Publishing, Dubuque, 2001, pp. 395–401.

32. Wilson, R.E., Care of the burn patient, *Ostomy Wound Manage.*, 42, 16, 1996.

33. Calianno, C., Assessing and preventing pressure ulcers, *Adv. Wound Care*, 13, 244, 2000.

34. Mathus-Vliegen, E.M.H., Nutritional status, nutrition and pressure ulcers, *Nutr. Clin. Pract.*, 16, 286, 2001.

35. Craven, N.M., Management of toxic epidermal necrolysis, *Hosp. Med.*, 61, 778, 2000.

36. Coss-Bu, J.A. et al., Nutrition requirements in patients with toxic epidermal necrolysis, *Nutr. Clin. Pract.*, 12, 81, 1997.

37. Van Den Berghe, G. et al., Intensive insulin therapy in the critically ill patients, *N. Engl. J. Med.*, 345, 1359, 2001.

38. Stadelmann, W.K. et al., Impediments to wound healing, *Am. J. Surg.*, 176, 39S, 1998.

39. Klein, C.J., Stanek, G.S., and Wiles, C.E., Overfeeding macronutrients to critically ill adults: metabolic complications, *JADA*, 98, 795, 1998.

40. Ireton-Jones, C. and Jones, J.D., Improved equations for predicating energy expenditure in patients: the Ireton-Jones equations, *Nutr. Clin. Pract.*, 17, 29, 2002.

41. Dickerson, R.N. et al., Accuracy of predictive methods to estimate resting energy expenditure of thermally-injured patients, *JPEN*, 26, 17, 2002.

42. Collins, N., Arginine and wound healing, *Adv. Wound Care*, 14, 16, 2001.

43. Flynn, N.E. et al., The metabolic basis of arginine nutrition and pharmacotherapy, *Biomed. Pharmacother.*, 56, 427, 2002.

44. Ochoa, J.B. et al., A rational use of immune enhancing diets: when should we use dietary arginine supplementation? *Nutr. Clin. Pract.*, 19, 216, 2004.

45. Williams, J.Z., Naji, A., and Barbul, A., Effect of specialized amino acid mixture on human collagen deposition, *Ann. Surg.*, 236, 369, 2002.

46. Basu, H.N. and Liepa, G.U., Arginine: a clinical perspective, *Nutr. Clin. Pract.*, 17, 218, 2002.

47. Zhou, Y. et al., The effect of supplemental enteral glutamine on plasma levels, gut function, and outcome in severe burn patients: a randomized, double-blind, controlled clinical trial, *JPEN*, 27, 241, 2003.

48. Savy, G., Everything you ever wanted to know about glutamine, *Today's Dietitian*, 1, 52, 1999.

49. Donati, L. et al., Nutritional and clinical efficacy of ornithine alpha-ketogluterate in severe burn patients, *Clin. Nutr.*, 18, 307, 1999.

50. Coudray-Lucas, C. et al., Ornithine alpha-ketoglutarate improves wound healing in severe burn patients: a prospective randomized double-blind trial versus isonitrogenous controls, *Crit. Care Med.*, 28, 1772, 2000.

51. Pratt, V.C. et al., Fatty acid content of plasma lipids and erythrocyte phospholipids are altered following burn injury, *Lipids*, 36, 675, 2001.

52. Gottschlich, M. et al., Differential effects of three enteral dietary regimens on selected outcome variables in burn patients, *JPEN*, 14, 225, 1990.

53. Saffle, J.R. et al., Randomized trial of immune-enhancing nutrition in burn patients, *J. Trauma*, 42, 793, 1997.

54. Albina, J.E. et al., Detrimental effects of an omega-3 fatty acid-enriched diet on wound healing, *JPEN*, 17, 519, 1993.

55. Ross, V., Micronutrient recommendations for wound healing, *Support Line*, 24, 3, 2002.

56. Thomas, D.R., Specific nutritional factors in wound healing, *Adv. Wound Care*, 10, 40, 1997.

57. Etlik, O. et al., The effect of antioxidant vitamins E and C on lipoperoxidation of erythrocyte membranes during hyperbaric oxygenation, *J. Basic Clin. Physiol. Pharmacol.*, 8, 269, 1997.

58. Baumann, L.S. and Spencer, J., The effects of topical vitamin E on the cosmetic appearance of scars, *Dermatol. Surg.*, 25, 311, 1999.

59. Shils, M. et al., *Modern Nutrition in Health and Disease*, 9th ed., Lippincott, Williams & Wilkins, Philadelphia, 1999, p. 233.

60. Andrews, M. and Gallagher-Allred, C., The role of zinc in wound healing, *Adv. Wound Care*, 12, 137, 1999.

61. Himes, D., Protein-calorie malnutrition and involuntary weight loss: the role of aggressive nutritional intervention in wound healing, *Ostomy Wound Manage.*, 45, 46, 1999.

62. Chang, D.W., DeSanti, L., and Demling, R.H., Anticatabolic and anabolic strategies in critical illness: a review of current treatment modalities, *Shock*, 10, 155, 1998.

63. Williams, G.J.P. and Herndon, D.N., Modulating the hypermetabolic response to burn injuries, *J. Wound Care*, 11, 87, 2002.

64. Molan, P.C., Potential of honey in the treatment of wounds and burns, *Am. J. Clin. Dermatol.*, 2, 13, 2001.

65. Lusby, P.E., Coombes, A., and Wilkinson, J.M., Honey: a potent agent for wound healing? *J. Wound Ostomy Continence Nurs.*, 29, 295, 2002.

66. Gallagher, J. and Gray, M., Is aloe vera effective for healing chronic wounds? *J. Wound Ostomy Continence Nurs.*, 30, 68, 2003.

67. Mantle, D., Gok, M.A., and Lennard, T.W.J., Adverse and beneficial effects of plant extracts on skin and skin disorders, *Adverse Drug React. Toxicol. Rev.*, 20, 89, 2001.

68. Pieper, B. and Caliri, M.H.L., Nontraditional wound care: a review of the evidence for the use of sugar, papaya/papain, and fatty acids, *J. Wound Ostomy Continence Nurs.*, 30, 175, 2003.

69. Mensah, A.Y. et al., Effects of *Buddleja globosa* leaf and its constituents relevant to wound healing, *J. Ethnopharmacol.*, 77, 219, 2001.

70. Gordillo, G.M. and Sen, C.K., Revisiting the essential role of oxygen in wound healing, *Am. J. Surg.*, 186, 259, 2003.

71. Hopf, H.W. et al., Adjuncts to preparing wounds for closure: hyperbaric oxygen, growth factors, skin substitutes, negative pressure wound therapy (vacuum assisted closure), *Foot Ankle Clin. North Am.*, 6, 661, 2001.

72. Hess, C.L., Howard, M.A., and Attinger, C.E., A review of mechanical adjuncts in wound healing: hydrotherapy, ultrasound, negative pressure therapy, hyperbaric oxygen, and electrostimulation, *Ann. Plast. Surg.*, 51, 210, 2003.

73. Frantz, R.A., Adjuvant therapy for ulcer care, *Clin. Geriatr. Med.*, 13, 553, 1997.

74. Cullum, N. et al., Systematic reviews of wound care management: beds, compression, laser therapy, therapeutic ultrasound, electrotherapy, and electromagnetic therapy, *Health Technol. Assess.*, 5, 1, 2001.

75. Whelan, H.T. et al., Effect of NASA light-emitting diode irradiation on wound healing, *J. Clin. Laser Med. Surg.*, 19, 305, 2001.

76. Lucas, C. et al., Wound healing in cell-studies and animal model experiments by low level laser therapy: were clinical studies justified? A systematic review, *Lasers Med. Sci.*, 17, 110, 2002.
77. Schindl, A. et al., Low-intensity laser therapy: a review, *J. Invest. Med.*, 48, 312, 2002.
78. Johnson, S., Low-frequency ultrasound to manage chronic venous leg ulcers, *Br. J. Nursing*, 12, S14, 2003.
79. Wolff, H. and Hansson, C., Larval therapy — an effective method of ulcer debridement, *Clin. Exp. Dermatol.*, 28, 134, 2003.
80. Horobin, A.J., Maggots and wound healing: an investigation of the effects of secretions from *Lucilia sericata* larvae upon interactions between human dermal fibroblasts and extracellular matrix components, *Br. J. Dermatol.*, 148, 923, 2003.
81. Mumcuoglu, K., Clinical applications for maggots in wound care, *Am. J. Clin. Dermatol.*, 2, 219, 2001.
82. Dossey, L., Maggots and leeches: when science and aesthetics collide, *Alternative Ther.*, 8, 12, 2002.
83. Whitney, J.D. and Heitkemper, M.M., Modifying perfusion, nutrition, and stress to promote wound healing in patients with acute wounds, *Heart and Lung*, 28, 123, 1999.
84. Kiecolt-Glaser, J.K. and Glaser, R., Psychological stress and wound healing, *Adv. Mind-Body Med.*, 17, 15, 2001.
85. Wientjes, K., Mind-body techniques in wound healing, *Ostomy Wound Manage.*, 48, 62, 2002.
86. McClave, S.A. and Chang, W., Feeding the hypotensive patient: does enteral feeding precipitate or protect against ischemic bowel? *Nutr. Clin. Pract.*, 18, 279, 2003.
87. Zaloga, G.P., Roberts, P.A., and Marik, P., Feeding the hemodynamically unstable patient: a critical evaluation of the evidence, *Nutr. Clin. Pract.*, 18, 285, 2003.
88. Jenkins, M.E. et al., Enteral feeding during operative procedures in thermal injuries, *J. Burn Care Rehabil.*, 15, 1999, 1994.
89. Mueller, C., True or false: serum hepatic proteins concentrations measure nutritional status, *Support Line*, 26, 8, 2004.

Appendix A. Bioavailability

John Stroster and Jennifer Muir Bowers

CONTENTS

BIOAVAILABILITY DEFINED

The definition of bioavailability of a nutrient has developed from the related concept of the bioavailability of a drug. The U.S. Food and Drug Administration (FDA) states that "the term 'bioavailability' means the rate and extent to which the active ingredient or therapeutic ingredient is absorbed from a drug and becomes available at the site of drug action" (Federal Food, Drug and Cosmetic Act, Section 505, j, 8A). Although the drug model is analogous for some nutrients, it may not always be suitable when considering the different absorption and conversion patterns that many nutrients display. For this reason, an expanded assortment of terms has evolved to better describe the bioavailability of nutrients in the body.

- *Bioavailability* is the proportion of an ingested nutrient available for utilization in normal physiologic functions and for storage.[1]
- *Bioconversion* is the proportion of a bioavailable nutrient converted to its active form.[2]
- *Bioefficacy* is the proportion of an ingested nutrient that is absorbed and converted to the active form.[2]
- *Functional bioefficacy* is the proportion of an ingested nutrient performing a particular metabolic function.[3]

FACTORS IMPACTING BIOAVAILABILITY

Factors that may synergistically impact the bioavailability of a nutrient can be categorized as either present within the individual host (intrinsic) or unique to the nutrient and matrix consumed (extrinsic).[1–8]

HOST-RELATED FACTORS

- Hormonal changes induced by events such as pregnancy or menopause
- Efficiency of the gastrointestinal tract
- Coexisting pathologies (e.g., atrophic gastritis)
- Current nutrient status is often inversely associated with bioavailability
- Age-related changes to normal physiology, including declining renal function
- Genetic factors

EXTRINSIC FACTORS

- Food, drug, or nutrient interactions upon consumption
- Rate-limiting processes related to nutrient transport and metabolism
- Formulation and dosage of nutrient

CHOOSING A MICRONUTRIENT SUPPLEMENT

The percentage of American adults who report using some type of vitamin and mineral supplement has been increasing.[9] With abundant food fortification and decreased incidence of nutritional deficiencies, this growing trend in supplement use is by consumers in search for more optimal health and morbidity reduction. Unable to control for the various host-related factors, the manufacturers of micronutrient supplements have often focused on differences in bioavailability to promote their particular product formulation. Unfortunately, bioavailability has become more of a marketing strategy than a reliable benchmark when comparing supplements. Consider the following:

- Successful absorption across the gastrointestinal tract does not guarantee conversion to an active form (when applicable), nor whether the nutrient will perform a desired metabolic function.[3]
- There are some instances when decreased bioavailability is favored, as seen with calcium reducing the risk of colorectal lesions.[8,10] In this case, bioavailability and functional bioefficacy are disengaged.
- Many of the conclusions on this topic have been a result of extrapolations from *in vitro* solubility data or animal studies, and should not be generalized to humans.
- The cost of a nutritional supplement must be measured against the adequacy of the supplement. A supplement may cost twice as much as its competitor, but be otherwise adequate for the individual.
- Several methodologies used to measure bioavailability exhibit limited sensitivity and reproducibility.[8]
- If nutritional supplements fell under the same federal status as pharmaceuticals, it is possible that many of the different formulations for a particular nutrient would be deemed bioequivalent.

Table A.1 and Table A.2 outline a number of human intervention studies involving the bioavailability of some commonly used micronutrients.

BETA-CAROTENE

Beta-carotene can be supplemented as either all-*trans*-β-carotene or 9-*cis*-β-carotene. There are few studies that compare the bioavailability of the two forms, but evidence suggests that the 9-*cis*-β-carotene is bioconverted to all-*trans*-β-carotene before or during absorption, making a direct comparison impractical.[22]

TABLE A.1
Effect of Methodology on the Bioavailability of Calcium Citrate and Calcium Carbonate (Human Intervention Studies)

Author (year)	Design	Conclusions
Heller et al.[11] (2002)	*Subjects:* 25 postmenopausal women (10 on estrogen, 15 not treated) (age range: 44–80 years; median: 61.8 years) (23 Caucasian, 2 Hispanic) *Design:* Randomized, three-phase crossover *Treatments:* 1. Two tablets Citracal® 250 mg + D 2. One tablet Os-Cal® 500 mg + D 3. Two tablets of a placebo *Measurement:* Blood drawn hourly between 0800 and 1400 through heparin lock: • ΔAUC in serum calcium • 25OHD status • 1,25-(OH)$_2$ D status	The authors hypothesized that estrogen treatment or vitamin D status would impact the bioavailability of two commonly used calcium supplements differently, as reflected by ΔAUC of the serum calcium after subtraction of the placebo phase. In subjects treated with estrogen, there was essentially no difference in bioavailability between calcium carbonate and calcium citrate. In subjects who did not receive estrogen treatment, the bioavailability was significantly higher for calcium citrate.
Heaney et al.[12] (1999)	*Experiment 1:* High-load urinary increment	For both salts, calcium bioavailability tended to be higher in subgroups with higher serum vitamin D metabolites. While measuring the serum concentration of a nutrient is an analog of classical pharmacokinetic studies, this technique demonstrates limited sensitivity when the test substance is found normally in the body and cannot be differentiated from the amount absorbed.[8] Future studies should further explore the relationship hormone status has on calcium bioavailability and functional bioefficacy, using a more sensitive technique. The methodology employed to determine the bioavailability of calcium supplements may explain some of the inconsistencies found in the literature. The authors had previously noted many studies that reported differences between the absorption of calcium citrate and carbonate used the urinary increment method, while other studies that used tracer methodology often found no difference. This group of researchers utilized both methodologies in the same subjects and two different loading doses to compare the two calcium salts.

Continued

TABLE A.1 (Continued)
Effect of Methodology on the Bioavailability of Calcium Citrate and Calcium Carbonate (Human Intervention Studies)

Author (year)	Design	Conclusions
	Subjects: 20 healthy men and women (10 postmenopausal women) (all women treated with estrogen) *Design:* Randomized, two-phase crossover *Treatments:* 1. Control day with a standardized meal 2. Calcium citrate 1000 mg labeled with ^{45}Ca 3. Calcium carbonate 1000 mg labeled with ^{45}Ca Urine was collected for a 5 h period; blood drawn at the fifth hour Paired-tests were separated by 1 week and dosing was administered with the standardized meal *Measurement:* Blood and urine were collected: • Stable and radioactive calcium • Urinary creatinine *Experiment 2:* Low-load serum concentration *Subjects:* 17 premenopausal women *Treatments:* Identical to high-load, only no urine component or control day and a 4-week interval between phases.	The 1000 mg load was chosen because it was identical to previous studies; the 300 mg load was considered atypical of a serving of dairy foods. The authors concluded that, "when taken with food, calcium from the carbonate salt is fully as absorbable as from citrate, and that the urinary increment is not sufficiently sensitive to be useful in comparing sources in free-living subjects." Unlike the urinary increment or serum concentration methods, biotracer techniques are much more sensitive since the labeled molecule is present in the body only in miniscule quantities. In this study, over 99% of the added tracer was recovered in the prepared carbonate salt and approximately 90% for the citrate preparation. Given the bioequivalence of the two salts, the cost benefit analysis favors the less expensive carbonate product.[13,14]

TABLE A.2
Effect of Source Factors on the Bioavailability and Bioefficacy of Vitamin E and Folic Acid (Human Intervention Studies)

Author (year)	Design	Conclusions
Beta-carotene You et al.[22] (1996)	*Subjects:* 2 men and 1 woman	The authors wished to obtain qualitative information on the bioavailability and bioefficacy of two forms of beta-carotene, all-*trans*-β-carotene and 9-*cis*-β-carotene.
	Treatments: Single dose of 992–994 μg 9-*cis*-β-carotene and 6–8 μg of all-*trans*-β-carotene, both labeled with [^{13}C] 8 months later, dosing procedure was repeated, but with unlabeled 9-*cis*-β-carotene	Substantial amounts of the [^{13}C] all-*trans*-β-carotene and [^{13}C] retinol appeared in the plasma after ingestion of an oral dose containing >99% [^{13}C] 9-*cis*-β-carotene, whereas only small amounts of the [^{13}C] 9-*cis*-β-carotene appear to be secreted in the blood stream.
	Measurement: Plasma saponified, purified using HPLC, and analyzed using GC-IRMS	The authors conclude that *cis*-β-carotene in part is isomerized to all-*trans*-β-carotene before or during digestion.
Vitamin E Huang and Appel[15] (2003)	*Subjects:* 184 adult nonsmokers	The authors studied the effects of supplementing diets with RRR-α-tocopherol acetate on serum concentrations of γ- and δ-tocopherol in 184 nonsmoking men and women.
	Design: Human intervention study (2 × 2 factorial) Randomized, double-blind, placebo-controlled Placebo (*n* = 93) and α-tocopherol (*n* = 91)	After 2 months of supplementation, concentration of α-tocopherol increased compared to placebo, but both γ- and δ-tocopherol concentrations were significantly reduced. Adjustment for baseline variables did not alter this pattern.
	Treatments: 1. Placebo (dicalcium phosphate + soybean oil) 2. Vitamin C alone (500 mg/tablet) 3. Vitamin E alone (400 IU RRR-α-tocopherol acetate) 4. Vitamin C + vitamin E	The characteristics of the participants between the two groups were similar and compliance was achieved, with 93% of the study participants taking over 90% of the study pills.
		There is research to support the beneficial effects of the other tocopherols like γ-tocopherol and related tocotrienols. These properties include more effective chemoprevention and antioxidant capabilities than α-tocopherol.

Continued

TABLE A.2 (Continued)
Effect of Source Factors on the Bioavailability and Bioefficacy of Vitamin E and Folic Acid (Human Intervention Studies)

	Measurement: Blood drawn 2 months after randomization. Compliance measured by pill counts and changes in serum concentrations: • (alpha) α-tocopherol • (gamma) γ-tocopherol • (delta) δ-tocopherol	The bioefficacy of vitamin E supplements may be less, due to the reduced concentrations of circulating γ- and δ-tocopherol caused by high doses of α-tocopherol.
Folate Melse-Boonstra et al.[16] (2004)	*Subjects:* 180 men and women aged 50–75 years *Design:* Human intervention study (parallel) Randomized, double-blind, placebo-controlled *Treatments:* 1. Placebo ($n = 60$) 2. Monoglutamyl folic acid ($n = 59$) 3. Polyglutamyl folic acid ($n = 61$) *Measurement:* Compliance measured by pill counts and a diary: • Serum folate • Erythrocyte folate • Plasma homocysteine	Natural folates from food sources are in the form of conjugated polyglutamyl chains, and their bioavailability is lower than the monoglutamyl form found in supplements and fortified food products. There are few studies that have investigated the effect of different species of folate on plasma total homocysteine. The researchers wished to quantify the bioavailability and bioefficacy of low doses of polyglutamyl folic acid relative to that of monoglutamyl folic acid. The study demonstrated that the bioavailability of polyglutamyl folic acid was 66% of that of the monoglutamyl form, based on serum and erythrocyte concentrations of the vitamin after 12 weeks. The purity of the capsules used was lower than expected (71% monoglutamyl and 58% polyglutamyl), but this was taken into account when calculations were made. No difference was seen between the two forms with respect to plasma homocysteine concentrations, showing equivalent functional bioefficacy. There are studies that have concluded no additional homocysteine-lowering effects beyond 500 μg folic acid, despite high levels of bioavailability and bioconversion.[3] Future studies should continue to utilize more sensitive techniques to explore the impact different species of folate have on the functional bioefficacy of the vitamin.

Vitamin C

Ascorbic acid and its oxidized form (dehydroascorbic acid) possess roughly equivalent bioavailability and maximal rates of intestinal uptake.[23] In food products, the relative bioavailability of the oxidized form would be increased, because glucose inhibits ascorbate but not dehydroascorbic acid.[24] When given orally, the absorption of ascorbic acid is inversely related to dosage, ranging from 80% (at 100 mg) to 63% (at 500 mg) to <50% (at 1250 mg with most of the absorbed dose excreted in the urine).[25,26] Calcium ascorbate is used mainly as a buffered vitamin C supplement to overcome gut irritation. While there are studies using rodents that indicate good bioavailability of the calcium in this supplement, rats endogenously synthesize vitamin C and to date no studies have compared the bioavailability of the three forms of vitamin C in humans.[27]

When administered intravenously, the limiting absorption mechanism is bypassed and very high levels in plasma can be attained. *In vitro* research has shown that ascorbic acid is cytotoxic to many malignant cell lines, and these concentrations are achievable through intravenous, though not oral dosing.[28] A few clinical studies used high-dose intravenous vitamin C treatment to treat terminal cancer patients. The researchers reported clinical benefits and improved survival, though these trials were neither randomized nor placebo-controlled.[29]

Vitamin B$_{12}$

While the forms of vitamin B$_{12}$ derived from the diet are the methyl, deoxyadenosyl, and hydroxy forms, cyanocobalamin is the form frequently used in therapeutic preparations.[20] For people with normal gastrointestinal function, the oral bioavailability between the cyano and methyl forms are equivalent, but significantly more cobalamin accumulates in liver tissue upon intake of methylcobalamin.[21,30] Due to the high incidence of malabsorption of dietary vitamin B$_{12}$ by elderly people, the recommendation for all adults over 50 is that they derive their vitamin B$_{12}$ requirement primarily from crystalline vitamin B$_{12}$, found in fortified foods or supplements. Such sources do not depend on the acid necessary to release the vitamin bound to proteins for the combination with intrinsic factor.[31]

Chromium

There is some evidence that organic sources of chromium, such as picolinate and brewer's yeast have greater bioavailability than inorganic complexes, such as chromium chloride.[17] It should be noted that the comparative analysis above was conducted in a rat model, and presently there is no reliable biomarker of dietary chromium or chromium status in humans.[18] Absorption of chromium is inversely related to intake, but may be enhanced by vitamin C.[19]

REFERENCES

1. Jackson, M.J., The assessment of bioavailability of micronutrients: introduction, *Eur. J. Clin. Nutr.*, 51(suppl), S1, 1997.
2. van Lieshout, M., West, C.E., and van Breemen, R.B., Isotopic tracer techniques for studying the bioavailability and bioefficacy of dietary carotenoids, particularly β-carotene, in humans: a review, *Am. J. Clin. Nutr.*, 77, 12, 2003.
3. Brouwer, I.A. et al., Bioavailability and bioefficacy of folate and folic acid in man, *Nutr. Res. Rev.*, 14, 267, 2001.
4. Russell, R.M., Factors in aging that effect the bioavailability of nutrients, *J. Nutr.*, 131, 1359S, 2001.
5. Krebs, N.F., Bioavailability of dietary supplements and impact on physiologic state: infants, children, and adolescents, *J. Nutr.*, 131, 1351S, 2001.

6. Guéguen, L. and Pointillart, A., The bioavailability of dietary calcium, *J. Am. Coll. Nutr.*, 19, 119S, 2000.

7. Shigematsu, N. et al., Effect of difructose anhydride III on calcium absorption in humans, *Biosci. Biotechnol. Biochem.*, 68, 1011, 2004.

8. Heaney, R.P., Factors influencing the measurement of bioavailability, taking calcium as a model, *J. Nutr.*, 131, 1344S, 2001.

9. Millen, A.E., Dodd, K.W., and Subar, A.F., Use of vitamin, mineral, nonvitamin, and nonmineral supplements in the United States: the 1987, 1992, and 2000 national health interview survey results, *J. Am. Diet Assoc.*, 104, 942, 2004.

10. Wallace, K. et al., Effect of calcium supplementation on the risk of large bowel polyps, *J. Natl. Cancer Inst.*, 96, 921, 2004.

11. Heller, H.J., Poindexter, J.R., and Adams-Huet, B., Effect of estrogen treatment and vitamin D status on differing bioavailabilities of calcium carbonate and calcium citrate, *J. Clin. Pharmacol.*, 42, 1251, 2002.

12. Heaney, R.P., Dowell, M.S., and Barger-Lux, M.J., Absorption of calcium as the carbonate and citrate salts, with some observations on method, *Osteoporos. Int.*, 9, 19, 1999.

13. Heaney, R.P. et al., Absorbability and cost effectiveness in calcium supplementation, *J. Am. Coll. Nutr.*, 20, 239, 2001.

14. Keller, J.L., Lanou, A.J., and Barnard, N.D., The consumer cost of calcium from food and supplements, *J. Am. Diet Assoc.*, 102, 1669, 2002.

15. Huang, H. and Appel, L.J., Supplementation of diets with α-tocopherol reduces serum concentrations of γ- and δ-tocopherol in humans, *J. Nutr.*, 133, 3137, 2003.

16. Melse-Boonstra, A. et al., Bioavailability of heptaglutamyl to monoglutamyl folic acid in healthy adults, *Am. J. Clin. Nutr.*, 79, 424, 2004.

17. Olin, K.L. et al., Comparative retention/absorption of [51]chromium (^{51}Cr) from ^{51}Cr chloride, ^{51}Cr nicotinate, and ^{51}Cr picolinate in a rat model, *J. Trace Elem. Electrolytes Health Dis.*, 11, 182, 1994.

18. Hambidge, M., Biomarkers of trace mineral intake and status, *J. Nutr.*, 133, 948S, 2003.

19. Seaborn, C.D. and Stoecker, B.J., Effects of antacid or ascorbic acid on tissue accumulation and urinary excretion of [51]chromium, *Nutr. Res.*, 10, 1401, 1990.

20. Scott, J.M., Bioavailability of vitamin B12, *Eur. J. Clin. Nutr.*, 51, S49, 1997.

21. Okuda, K. et al., Intestinal absorption and concurrent chemical changes of methylcobalamin, *J. Lab Clin. Med.*, 81, 557, 1973.

22. You, C.S. et al., Evidence of *cis–trans* isomerization of 9-*cis*-β-carotene during absorption in humans, *Am. J. Clin. Nutr.*, 64, 177, 1996.

23. Wilson, J.X., Bioavailability of oxidized vitamin C (dehydroascorbic acid) (Letter), *J. Am. Diet Assoc.*, 102, 1222, 2002.

24. Malo, C. and Wilson, J.X., Glucose modulates vitamin C transport in adult human small intestinal brush border membrane vesicles, *J. Nutr.*, 130, 63, 2000.

25. Padayatty, S.J. and Levine, M., New insights into the physiology and pharmacology of vitamin C. *CMAJ.*, 164, 3553, 2001.

26. Levine, M. et al., Vitamin C pharmokinetics in healthy volunteers: evidence for a recommended dietary allowance, *Proc. Natl. Acad. Sci.*, 93, 3704, 1996.

27. Cai, J. et al., Calcium bioavailability and kinetics of calcium ascorbate and calcium acetate in rats, *Exp. Biol. Med.*, 229, 40, 2004.

28. Koh, W.S. et al., Differential effects and transport kinetics of ascorbate derivatives in leukemia cell lines, *Anticancer Res.*, 18, 2487, 1998.

29. Cameron, E. and Pauling, L., Supplemental ascorbate in the supportive treatment of cancer: prolongation of survival times in terminal human cancer, *Proc. Natl. Acad. Sci.*, 73, 3685, 1976.

30. Anonymous, Methylcobalamin, *Altern. Med. Rev.*, 3, 461, 1998.

31. Yates, A.A., National nutrition and public health policies: issues related to bioavailability of nutrients when developing dietary reference intakes, *J. Nutr.*, 31, 1331S, 2001.

Appendix B. Integrative Nutrition in Surgical Patients

Douglas W. Wilmore

CONTENTS

INTRODUCTION

Nutritional care, whether provided by using traditional approaches or by incorporating complementary methods, is of fundamental importance to the surgical patient. A normal nutritional state, which insures an adequate macro- and micronutrient status, is essential for normal wound healing. Following an operation, the patient becomes more susceptible to infections, and undernutrition is a risk factor for this common and serious morbidity. Interest in this area has recently been directed toward utilizing specific nutrients to modify the immune response and enhance resistance to infection as one strategy to improve surgical outcomes. Finally, a major operation is a well-known physiological stress, and nutritional state correlates closely with performance status and other physiological responses, which are called into play to aid immediate recovery and shorten convalescence.

Thus, nutritional assessment, correction of nutritional deficits and possibly even nutrient prophylaxis is central to this aspect of care of the patient undergoing a planned elective of semielective procedure. Nutritional support in the patient requiring an emergency operation and intensive postoperative care is important in the long term to attenuate the catabolic response and minimize the erosion of lean body mass.

WHO IS AT RISK? — WHAT IS KNOWN

Despite the large number of patients undergoing elective surgical procedures and the increasing number of these operations performed in an elderly high-risk population, very few major intervention trials have been performed to document the effects of integrated nutritional therapy in this patient group. The available data reflecting patients at risk follows.

MALNOURISHED PATIENT

Percent weight loss has served as an indicator of undernutrition. An absolute level of risk has been associated with a weight loss of 15% or greater, but selected patients with a 10–15% weight loss may also be at risk and benefit from preoperative supplementation. The most often cited contemporary study to describe this relationship is the Veteran's Administration Cooperative trial of preoperative feeding of patients with gastrointestinal disease and associated weight loss.[1] While the overall trial results failed to demonstrate beneficial effects of 7 to 10 days of preoperative intravenous feeding, a subgroup of malnourished patients with a significant weight loss were identified as those who benefited from this intervention. Noninfectious complications were reduced in this subgroup receiving preoperative nutritional support, and infectious complications were not increased. Since both macro- and micronutrients were provided to these patients, it is not known if the improvement was related to increased availability of energy, partial resolution of protein malnutrition, correction of vitamin and other micronutrient deficiencies, or all of the above factors working in combination.

Identification of high-risk patients was well described in an exceedingly thorough study by Windsor and Hill.[2] Before major surgery, 102 patients were evaluated. Physical examination included determination of weight loss, assessment of mood, measurement of skeletal and respiratory muscle function, and evaluation of wound healing. Patients were placed into three groups: those who were normal ($n = 43$), those with weight loss >10% but with no physiological impairment ($n = 17$) and those with the same degree of weight loss with evidence of physiological impairment ($n = 42$). Following operation, the latter group had more postoperative complications, more septic complications, more postoperative pneumonia, and a longer hospital stay than the other two groups. The authors conclude that weight loss is an indicator of surgical risk providing that it is associated with clinically obvious impairment of organ function. Note that over two thirds of the group with weight loss had documented functional impairments.

ELDERLY

Nutritional surveys in middle class groups of individuals 65 years of age and older show that these free-living individuals as a group consume inadequate quantities of vitamins and micronutrients.[3] They are also a group of individuals who more frequently undergo elective operative procedures and as such represent a group at nutritional risk.

PATIENTS WITH BOWEL DISEASE

Several years ago European investigators studied the nutritional status of patients diagnosed with Crohn's disease who were stable and in remission.[4] These individuals had a surprisingly high incidence of vitamin and mineral deficiencies, to the extent that wound healing, resistance to infection, and the inflammatory responses would be compromised. Further studies demonstrated that specific supplements could correct these nutritional deficiencies.[5] Preoperative supplementation should be considered in these and other patients with malabsorption associated with bowel disease.

OTHER HIGH-RISK PATIENT GROUPS

Smokers have low vitamin C levels; those who consume alcohol in excess and have marginal food intake demonstrate signs of vitamin B deficiencies. If specific supplements above the usual requirements are not provided, patients receiving parenteral nutrition with short bowel syndrome have vitamin, mineral, and essential fatty acid deficiencies. Other nutrient deficiencies have been documented in patients with diabetes, renal failure, and other major chronic diseases and patients with these disorders should be evaluated and supplemented before operation if necessary.

WHAT INTERVENTIONS HELP?

PERIOPERATIVE FEEDINGS

Preoperative feedings for 7 to 10 days in the malnourished patient (defined as an individual with a >15% weight loss or >10% weight loss with signs of organ dysfunction) reduce postoperative complications. Cost–benefit studies using this approach are lacking. The effect of postoperative feedings has been evaluated in a large meta-analysis and this approach has not been found to be effective, and in fact may be harmful.[6]

Standard intravenous feedings have not been found to reduce mortality in the intensive care setting, although it is suggested that morbidity is decreased in malnourished patients.[7] A firm scientific basis for the use of tube feedings in intensive care unit (ICU) patients has also not been established.[8]

POSTOPERATIVE PROTEIN SUPPLEMENTS

Intervention by providing protein-enriched supplements for 10 to 16 weeks after discharge following abdominal surgery has increased body weight and lean body mass while the effect on recovery, handgrip strength, and quality of life could only be demonstrated in depleted patients.[9,10] These findings suggest that prolonged nutritional therapy has no major benefit except in depleted individuals.[10]

DIETS SUPPLEMENTED IN OMEGA-3 FATS, ARGININE, AND RNA

A large number of studies using a tube feeding diet fortified with these substances have recently appeared in the literature. Many claim that this diet has immunomodulatory effects. A recent meta-analysis shows a reduction in infection rate in patients undergoing elective operation who received these diets,[11] although there is no consistent agreement as to the timing of diet administration (should it be given pre- or postoperatively). More troubling, however, is data that suggests the diet is associated with increased mortality in critically ill patients.[11] Therefore, caution in prescribing these diets is warranted.

Few studies are available to evaluate the individual active components of these diets. In one study, diets were enriched with omega-3 fatty acids and vitamin E, and provided to patients with end-stage pancreatic cancer.[12] Survival was prolonged in this randomized blinded study when compared to a nonsupplemented control group. Other studies have evaluated the effects of vitamin E and other nutrients in the interaction with a variety of cancer therapies. Most involve small groups of patients and do not support clinical utility of the nutrient studied.

GLUTAMINE

This amino acid, which is thought to be nonessential in healthy individuals, has unique pharmacological properties that exert beneficial effects to the gastrointestinal tract, the immunological system, and other key tissues. Perioperative glutamine administration has been shown to reduce both postoperative infections and length of stay.[13] These effects are also observed in both critically ill patients and premature infants. Glutamine also exerts anabolic effects in both postoperative patients and individuals with AIDS wasting. A recent meta-analysis concluded that glutamine supplementation reduced mortality in intensive care patients, a characteristic which has not been associated with other single nutrients in modern times.[14] These many desirable effects combined with an exceedingly low complication rate and low cost make this an extremely important nutrient for administration to surgical patients in the perioperative period.

Most of the data in hospitalized patients involves the administration of glutamine intravenously as a dipeptide or as the L-amino acid. One study supplied a glutamine-supplemented enteral diet providing approximately 40 g glutamine/day, and infectious complication was greatly reduced in the treatment group.[15] Since other studies reporting benefits of oral glutamine use doses in adults between 30 and 40 g/day (given in divided doses), this is at present the suggested amount for supplementation. The supplement should be started 5 to 7 days before operation and continued in the postoperative until adequate diet and activity levels are achieved (this may be a month or more).

OTHER SUBSTANCES

A recent report evaluates the effect of a mixture of arginine, β-hydroxy-β-methylbutyrate, and glutamine on wound healing in healthy controls. Indices of healing were improved in the volunteers taking this mixture, but this product has yet to undergo clinical evaluation.[16]

OTHER APPROACHES

Patient education and knowledge of the postoperative care plan greatly reduces the stress of the procedure and has been found to limit pain, the need for analgesia, and reduce the length of stay.[17] Other techniques such as relaxation training, hypnosis, guided imagery, and other methods to reduce anxiety and aid coping have been studied in limited trials and found to be helpful.[18] These approaches are rarely taught by the primary surgeon, and hence the complementary and alternative medicine (CAM) providers who see the patient may have an opportunity to introduce and teach such techniques.

RECOMMENDATIONS ON THE USE OF HERBALS IN SURGICAL PATIENTS

Because of the widespread use of these agents, anesthesiologists have recently reviewed their activities and possible interactions with anesthetic agents and treatment provided in the postoperative period.[19] Of the eight herbal medicines studied, it was recommended that all be discontinued before surgery (Table B.1). No compelling evidence was cited that would indicate that these agents would benefit surgical patients and many examples were referenced that showed an association between the agent and a specific complication. Until more data is available, discontinuing herbals before operation represents the present standard of care.

TABLE B.1
Perioperative Concerns for Eight Commonly Used Herbal Agents

Herb	Perioperative Concern	Discontinuation before Operation
Echinacea	Allergic reaction, immunosuppression	No data
Ephedra	Myocardial ischemia, stroke, hypertension	24 h
Garlic	Increases risk of bleeding	7 days
Ginkgo	Increases risk of bleeding	36 h
Ginseng	Hypoglycemia, bleeding	7 days
Kava	Sedation, potential addiction potential	24 h
St. John's wort	Alters drug metabolism	5 days
Valerian	Sedative effect, increases anesthetic requirements	No data

Source: From Ang-Lee, M.K., Moss, J., and Yuan, C-S, *JAMA*, 286, 208, 2001.

It has been suggested that other substances may increase the risk of perioperative bleeding, and these nutrients include vitamin E and possibly fish oil. Little data is available to confirm this notion, but interaction of these nutrients with other agents (aspirin, herbals, and anticoagulants) may prolong bleeding time over what is expected. A careful history is necessary to assess this risk. If a variety of supplements are taken, then the safe approach would be to discontinue the fat-soluble agents a week before the operation and document the other drugs that the patient is taking.

CONCLUSIONS

The following points should be emphasized:

1. Preoperative nutritional supplementation for 7 to 10 days reduces postoperative complications in malnourished patients.
2. Short-term postoperative support in the hospitalized patient has not been shown to be valuable.
3. Long-term postoperative supplementation in depleted patients is helpful for convalescent rehabilitation.
4. Groups at high risk for vitamin and mineral deficiency should be supplemented for approximately 3 weeks before operation (a time necessary to replete fat-soluble vitamin stores). Trials have not been performed in this area, but few would advocate withholding these low-cost low-risk supplements to depleted individuals.
5. Glutamine should be supplemented in patients undergoing operation. Most investigators have studied glutamine administered by the intravenous route and this data is quite strong. A few studies suggest that this effect can be sustained with the use of oral glutamine (dose, 30–40 g/day administered throughout the perioperative period).
6. Patient education and other coping techniques are helpful to reduce the stress of operations and length of stay. These approaches should be utilized in elective surgical patients whenever possible.
7. Herbals should be discontinued before surgery in patients undergoing an elective operation. Vitamin E and omega-3 fats may interact with other substances which alter coagulation and if taken together or with other substances should probably be discontinued a week before operation.

8. Because of the time pressures on physicians and surgeons, these assessments and treatments should be performed by a dietitian, nurse, or physician's assistant in the preoperative period to optimize nutritional state before an elective operation.

REFERENCES

1. Veterans Affairs Total Parenteral Nutrition Study Group. Perioperative total parenteral nutrition in surgical patients, *N. Engl. J. Med.*, 325, 525, 1991.
2. Windsor, J.A. and Hill, G.L. Weight loss with physiologic impairment. A basic indicator of surgical risk, *Ann. Surg.*, 207, 290, 1988.
3. Payette, H. and Gray-Donald, K. Dietary intake and biochemical indices of nutritional status in an elderly population, with estimates of the precision of the 7-day food record, *Am. J. Clin. Nutr.*, 54, 478, 1991.
4. Geerling, B.J. et. al. Comprehensive nutritional status in patients with long-standing Crohn's disease currently in remission, *Am. J. Clin. Nutr.*, 67, 919, 1998.
5. Geerling, B.J. et al. Nutritional supplementation with $n-3$ fatty acids and antioxidants in patients with Crohn's disease in remission: effects on antioxidant status and fatty acid profile, *Inflamm. Bowel Dis.*, 6, 77, 2000.
6. Klein, S. et al. Nutritional support in clinical practice: review of published data and recommendations for future research directions, *Am. J. Clin. Nutr.*, 66, 683, 1997.
7. Heyland, D.K. et al. TPN in the critically ill patient: a meta-analysis, *JAMA*, 208, 2013, 1998.
8. Carlson, G. Nutritional support of the surgical patient: is it worth while? Adult patients, *Proc. Nutr. Soc.*, 59, 477, 2000.
9. Jensen, M.B. and Hessov, I. Randomization to nutritional intervention at home did not improve postoperative function, fatigue or well-being, *Br. J. Surg.*, 84, 113, 1997.
10. Beattie, A.H. et al. A randomized controlled trial evaluating the use of enteral nutritional supplements postoperatively in malnourished surgical patients, *Gut*, 46, 813, 2000.
11. Heyland, D.K. et al. Should immunonutrition become routine in critically ill patients? A systematic review of the evidence, *JAMA*, 286, 944, 2001.
12. Gogos, C.A. et al. Dietary omega-3 polyunsaturated fatty acids plus vitamin E restore immunodeficiency and prolong survival for severely ill patients with generalized malignancy: a randomized controlled trial, *Cancer*, 82, 395, 1998.
13. Wilmore, D.W. The effect of glutamine supplementation in patients following elective surgery and accidental injury, *J. Nutr.*, 131, 2543S, 2001.
14. Novak, F. et al. Glutamine supplementation in critically ill adults: a meta-analysis, *Clin. Nutr.*, 20, 54, 2001.
15. Houdijk, A.P. et al. Randomised trial of glutamine-enriched enteral nutrition on infectious morbidity in patients with multiple trauma, *Lancet*, 352, 772, 1998.
16. Williams, J.Z., Abumarad, N., and Barbul, A. Effect of a specialized amino acid mixture on human collagen deposition, *Ann. Surg.*, 236, 369, 2002.
17. Egbert, L.D. et al. Reduction of postoperative pain by encouragement and instruction of patients, *N. Engl. J. Med.*, 207, 824, 1964.
18. Petry, J.J. The role of the mind and emotions of patient and surgeon in the outcome of surgery, *Plast. Reconstr. Surg.*, 105, 636, 2000.
19. Ang-Lee, M.K., Moss, J., and Yuan, C-S. Herbal medicines and perioperative care, *JAMA*, 286, 208, 2001.

Appendix C. Herb–Drug Interactions

Philip J. Gregory

CONTENTS

Dietary supplements including herbs, vitamins, amino acids, and other natural products can interact with drugs and other supplements. Like drug–drug interactions, drug–supplement interactions can increase or decrease pharmacologic and toxic effects. Interactions can vary in clinical significance depending on patient-specific factors such as comorbid diseases, renal and hepatic function, and genetic variability. Nonetheless, knowledge of interaction mechanisms can help in anticipating the time course of an interaction and devising ways to avoid it.[1]

Drug–supplement interactions can be divided into two categories: pharmacodynamic and pharmacokinetic. Pharmacodynamic interactions involve the effect of the drug–supplement combination on the body. Pharmacokinetic interactions involve the effect of the body on the drug–supplement combination. Interactions that involve both pharmacodynamic and pharmacokinetic mechanisms can also occur.[1,2]

Pharmacodynamic interactions result from the similarity of the pharmacologic effects of a drug and supplement. For example, if a drug used to treat diabetes is taken with a supplement that also lowers blood sugar, the effect on blood sugar will be greater than taking either the drug or supplement alone. The additive or synergistic effect of the drug–supplement combination could be beneficial with appropriate management or could result in symptomatic hypoglycemia. Conversely, combinations of supplements and drugs can be antagonistic. For example, the effect of antihypertensive drugs can be attenuated by supplements that increase blood pressure.[1–3]

Pharmacokinetic interactions cause changes in the absorption, distribution, metabolism, or excretion of drugs or supplements. Pharmacokinetic interactions can increase or decrease the clinical effect and can increase risk of adverse reactions. The onset of pharmacokinetic interactions can be almost immediate or can be delayed for a week or more, depending on the mechanism of the interaction.[1,2]

Absorption of drugs and supplements from the gastrointestinal tract can change with concurrent administration of other drugs and supplements. Absorption interactions can occur as the result of binding or chelating a drug or supplement, such as the chelation of fluoroquinolone antibiotics by iron supplements. Other mechanisms of absorption interactions include changes in gastric pH, gastrointestinal motility, and drug transport systems, such as p-glycoprotein. These mechanisms can affect the extent of absorption, which can cause subtherapeutic serum levels, as well as the rate of absorption, which is usually clinically unimportant.[1–3]

TABLE C.1

Pharmacodynamic Interactions Causing Increased Pharmacologic Effect or Toxicity

Supplement	Drug	Comment
Dong quai	Coumadin (warfarin) and other drugs affecting clotting (aspirin; Plavix [clopidogrel]; nonsteroidal anti-inflammatory drugs [NSAIDs] such as Advil, Motrin [ibuprofen], others; Anaprox, Naprosyn [naproxen], others; Fragmin [dalteparin]; Lovenox [enoxaparin]; heparin; others)	Inhibits platelet aggregation; increases the effect of warfarin.[3,4]
Ephedra (Ma Huang, others)	Caffeine (guarana, cola nut, maté, coffee, tea)	Additive stimulant effect; increased risk of adverse effects.[6,7]
Kava	Hepatotoxic drugs ("statin" drugs; Cordarone [amiodarone]; Imuran [azathioprine]; Tegretol [carbamazepine]; isoniazid; niacin; alcohol; and many others)	Kava may adversely affect the liver. Other potentially hepatotoxic drugs may increase the risk of liver damage.[8,9]
Kava	Central nervous system (CNS) depressants (alcohol, barbiturates, benzodiazepines, narcotics, and others)	Concomitant use of kava and CNS depressants can increase the risk of drowsiness and motor reflex depression.[10–12]
Licorice	Digoxin	Higher doses of licorice can cause potassium loss and increase the risk for digoxin toxicity.[2]
S-adenosyl-L-methionine (SAMe)	Antidepressants (Serzone [nefazodone]; Paxil [paroxetine]; Zoloft [sertraline]; Nardil [phenelzine]; others)	Both SAMe and antidepressants increase the levels of the neurotransmitter serotonin, increasing the risk of serotonin side effects and serotonin syndrome.[13,14]
Saw palmetto	Coumadin (warfarin) and other drugs affecting clotting (aspirin; Plavix [clopidogrel]; NSAIDs such as Advil, Motrin [ibuprofen], others; Anaprox, Naprosyn [naproxen], others; Fragmin [dalteparin]; Lovenox [enoxaparin]; heparin; others)	Saw palmetto seems to slow clotting time and might increase the risk of bleeding when used with other anticoagulant or antiplatelet drugs.[15]
St. John's wort (SJW)	Antidepressants (Serzone [nefazodone]; Paxil [paroxetine]; Zoloft [sertraline]; others)	Both SJW and antidepressants increase the levels of the neurotransmitter serotonin, increasing the risk of serotonin side effects and serotonin syndrome.[16–18]
SJW	Narcotics	SJW can increase narcotic-induced sleep time and might also increase analgesic effects.[19,20]
Valerian	Sedative and hypnotic drugs	Valerian in combination with other drugs that cause drowsiness may have an additive sedative effect.[21–23]

Source: Adapted from Jellin JM, Gregory P, Batz F, et al., Eds. Natural Medicines Comprehensive Database (www.naturaldatabase.com). With permission.

TABLE C.2
Pharmacodynamic Interactions Causing Decreased Pharmacologic Effect

Supplement	Drug	Comment
Coenzyme Q10	Coumadin (warfarin)	May reduce the anticoagulant effect of warfarin; structurally similar to vitamin K.[5,24,25]
Glucosamine	Insulin, antidiabetic drugs (Amaryl [glimepiride]; DiaBeta, Glynase, Micronase [glyburide]; Actos [pioglitazone]; Avandia [rosiglitazone]; and others)	Glucosamine might cause insulin resistance and reduce the effectiveness of diabetes drugs.[28–32]
Soy	Nolvadex (tamoxifen)	Theoretically, the estrogenic effects of soy might interfere with the antiestrogen effects of tamoxifen.[33]

Source: Adapted from Jellin JM, Gregory P, Batz F, et al., Eds. Natural Medicines Comprehensive Database (www.naturaldatabase.com). With permission.

Distribution interactions can also affect drug and supplement pharmacokinetics. A drug or supplement might increase the free (active) concentration of another drug or supplement by competition or displacement from tissue-binding sites, such as plasma proteins. Distribution interactions are more theoretical than clinically relevant. Theoretically, the increased blood levels of a displaced drug or supplement could increase pharmacologic effect, but adverse effects are unlikely because of simultaneous increases in metabolism and elimination.[1,2]

Metabolism interactions of drugs and supplements can increase or decrease pharmacologic effects and increase the risk for adverse reactions. Many of these interactions involve the cytochrome P-450 (CYP) enzymes in the liver and small intestine. The CYP isoenzymes that most commonly affect drug and supplement metabolism are CYP 3A4, CYP 2D6, CYP 1A2, CYP 2C9, and CYP 2C19. If the drug or supplement inhibits CYP enzymatic activity, metabolism and elimination of that agent is slowed, which can increase the pharmacological

TABLE C.3
Pharmacokinetic Interactions Causing Increased Pharmacologic Effect or Toxicity

Supplement	Drug	Comment
Ephedra (Ma Huang, others)	Urinary alkalinizers (citrate products)	Decreased ephedra excretion; increased half-life.[38]
Ginkgo	Coumadin (warfarin)	Increased anticoagulant effects and bleeding risk. Ginkgo might alter the distribution of warfarin.[5,39]
Grapefruit	Calcium channel blockers	Grapefruit juice variably increases serum levels of calcium channel blockers, possibly decreasing intestinal metabolism by CYP 3A4 and increasing absorption.[40,41]
Ipriflavone	Theo-Dur, Slo-Phyllin, others [theophylline]	Ipriflavone can increase serum theophylline levels, possibly by decreasing theophylline metabolism by CYP 1A2.[42,43]

Source: Adapted from Jellin JM, Gregory P, Batz F, et al., Eds. Natural Medicines Comprehensive Database (www.naturaldatabase.com). With permission.

TABLE C.4
Pharmacokinetic Interactions Causing Decreased Pharmacologic Effect

Supplement	Drug	Comment
Calcium	Fluoroquinolones (Cipro [ciprofloxacin]; Levaquin [levofloxacin]; others)	Calcium decreases absorption.[44,45]
Calcium	Tetracyclines	Calcium decreases absorption.[44,45]
Calcium	Synthroid, Levoxyl, others [levothyroxine]	Calcium decreases absorption.[44,46]
Coenzyme Q10	HMG COA reductase inhibitors — "Statins" (Mevacor [lovastatin]; Zocor [simvastatin]; others)	May reduce levels of coenzyme Q10; decreased synthesis of coenzyme Q10 precursor.[26,27]
Garlic	Protease inhibitors (PI) (Fortovase, Invirase [saquinavir]; Viracept [nelfinavir]; Norvir [ritonavir]; others)	May reduce the antiviral effect of PI. Garlic induces CYP 3A4 and increases metabolism of PI.[47]
Garlic	Nonnucleoside reverse transcriptase inhibitors (NNRTI) (Viramune [nevirapine]; Rescriptor [delavirdine]; Sustiva [efavirenz]; others)	May reduce the antiviral effect of NNRTI. Garlic induces CYP 3A4 and may increase metabolism of NNRTI.[47]
Garlic	Neoral, Sandimmune [cyclosporin]	May reduce the immunosuppressive effect of cyclosporin. Garlic induces CYP 3A4 and may increase metabolism of cyclosporin.[47]
Garlic	Oral contraceptives (OCs)	May reduce the effect of OCs. Garlic induces CYP 3A4 and may increase metabolism of steroid drugs such as OCs.[47]
Ginger	Acid-inhibiting drugs (antacids; H_2 antagonists, Tagamet [cimetidine], Zantac [ranitidine], others; proton pump inhibitors, Prevacid [lansoprazole], Prilosec [omeprazole], others)	Theoretically, due to claims that ginger rhizome increases stomach acid, it might interfere with drugs that reduce gastric acidity.[48]
Soy	Antibiotics	Antibiotics may interfere with conversion of soy to its active forms.[49]
St. John's wort (SJW)	Lanoxin [digoxin]	SJW reduces digoxin serum levels. SJW seems to affect the multidrug transporter, p-glycoprotein, which mediates the absorption and elimination of digoxin and other drugs.[34–37]
SJW	PI (Fortovase, Invirase [saquinavir]; Viracept [nelfinavir]; Norvir [ritonavir]; others)	May reduce the antiviral effect of PI. SJW induces CYP 3A4 and increases metabolism of PI.[35,50,51]
SJW	NNRTI (Viramune [nevirapine]; Rescriptor [delavirdine]; Sustiva [efavirenz]; others)	May reduce the antiviral effect of NNRTI. SJW induces CYP 3A4 and may increase metabolism of NNRTI.[50–53]
SJW	Neoral, Sandimmune (cyclosporin)	May reduce the immunosuppressive effect of cyclosporin. SJW induces CYP 3A4 and may increase metabolism of cyclosporin.[35,54–58]
SJW	Prograf (tacrolimus)	May reduce the immunosuppressive effect of tacrolimus. SJW induces several CYP isoenzymes and may increase metabolism of tacrolimus.[59]

TABLE C.4 (Continued)
Pharmacokinetic Interactions Causing Decreased Pharmacologic Effect

Supplement	Drug	Comment
SJW	OCs	May reduce the effect of OCs. SJW induces CYP 3A4 and may increase metabolism of steroid drugs such as OCs.[60,61]
SJW	Theo-Dur, Slo-Phyllin, others (theophylline)	SJW may increase the metabolism of theophylline and lower serum theophylline levels.[35,62]
SJW	Coumadin (warfarin)	SJW reduces the anticoagulant effect of warfarin, possibly by increasing metabolism by CYP 2C9 enzyme.[60]

Source: Adapted from Jellin JM, Gregory P, Batz F, et al., Eds. Natural Medicines Comprehensive Database (www.naturaldatabase.com). With permission.

effect or potential for toxicity. Typically, inhibition interactions occur within hours to a few days. Drugs and supplements can also induce (increase) the expression of CYP isoenzymes, resulting in faster metabolism and elimination, which can decrease therapeutic effect. The clinical effects of induction interactions occur more slowly than inhibition interactions, usually occurring within 7 to 10 days. Drugs and supplements can affect or be affected by multiple CYP isoenzymes.[1,2]

Elimination interactions can also increase or decrease pharmacologic effects and increase the risk for adverse reactions, although this occurs less frequently than metabolism interactions. Drugs or supplements that adversely affect renal function can decrease elimination and prolong the pharmacologic effects. Some drugs and supplements can change the pH of the urine or affect active secretion into the renal tubules, which may increase or decrease excretion. Increased excretion can reduce pharmacologic effects, and decreased excretion can increase pharmacologic effects or adverse effects.[1,2]

REFERENCES

1. Scott GN, Elmer GW. Update on natural product–drug interactions. *Am. J. Health Syst. Pharm.*, 2002;59:339–47.
2. Hansten PD, Horn JR. *Hansten's and Horn's Drug Interactions Analysis and Management*, St. Louis, Missouri: Facts and Comparisons, 1999.
3. Jellin JM, Gregory P, Batz F, et al., Eds. Natural Medicines Comprehensive Database. www.naturaldatabase.com (accessed 6 December 2002).
4. Page RL II, Lawrence JD. Potentiation of warfarin by dong quai. *Pharmacotherapy*, 1999;19(7):870–6.
5. Heck AM, DeWitt BA, Lukes AL. Potential interactions between alternative therapies and warfarin. *Am. J. Health Syst. Pharm.*, 2000;57:1221–7.
6. Schulz V, Hansel R, Tyler VE. *Rational Phytotherapy: A Physician's Guide to Herbal Medicine*, Terry C. Telger, transl. 3rd ed, Berlin, Germany: Springer, 1998.
7. Haller CA, Benowitz NL. Adverse cardiovascular and central nervous system events associated with dietary supplements containing ephedra alkaloids. *N. Engl. J. Med.*, 2000;343(25):1833–8.
8. Escher M, et al. Drug points: hepatitis associated with kava, a herbal remedy for anxiety. *BMJ*, 2001;322:139.
9. Russmann S, Lauterberg BH, Hebling A. Kava hepatotoxicity [letter]. *Ann. Intern. Med.*, 2001;135:68–9.
10. Jussofie A, Schmiz A, Hiemke C. Kavapyrone enriched extract from *Piper methysticum* as modulator of the GABA binding site in different regions of rat brain. *Psychopharmacology*, 1994;116:469–74.

11. Schelosky L, Raffaup C, Jendroska K, Poewe W. Kava and dopamine antagonism. *J. Neurol. Neurosurg. Psychiatry*, 1995;58:639–40.

12. Boonen G, Pramanik A, Rigler R, Haberlein H. Evidence for specific interactions between kava in and human cortical neurons monitored by fluorescence correlation spectroscopy. *Planta. Med.*, 2000;66:7–10.

13. Iruela LM, et al. Toxic interaction of *S*-adenosylmethionine and clomipramine. *Am. J. Psychiatry*, 1993;150:522.

14. Berlanga C, et al. Efficacy of *S*-adenosyl-L-methionine in speeding the onset of action of imipramine. *Psychiatry Res.*, 1992;44(3):257–62.

15. Cheema P, El-Mefty O, Jazieh AR. Intraoperative haemorrhage associated with the use of extract of Saw palmetto herb: a case report and review of literature. *J. Intern. Med.*, 2001;250:167–9.

16. Miller LG. Herbal Medicinals. Selected clinical considerations focusing on known or potential drug–herb interactions. *Arch. Intern. Med.*, 1998;158:2200–11.

17. Gordon JB. SSRIs and St. John's wort: possible toxicity? *Am. Fam. Physician*, 1998;57(5):950–3.

18. Beckman SE, Sommi RW, Switzer J. Consumer use of St. John's wort: a survey of effectiveness, safety, and tolerability. *Pharmacotherapy*, 2000;20:568–74.

19. Upton R, Ed. St. John's wort, *Hypericum perforatum*: quality control, analytical and therapeutic monograph. *Am. Herbal Pharmacopoeia*, 1997;1–32.

20. Hussain MD, Teixeira MG. Saint John's wort and analgesia: effect of Saint John's wort on morphine induced analgesia. AAPS Ann Mtg & Expo Indianapolis, IN:2000;Oct 29–Nov 2: presentation 3453. URL: view.abstractonline.com/aaps/abstractViewer.asp (accessed 30 October 2000).

21. Klepser TB, Klepser ME. Unsafe and potentially safe herbal therapies. *Am. J. Health Syst. Pharm.*, 1999;56:125–38.

22. Plushner SL. Valerian: *Valeriana officinalis*. *Am. J. Health Syst. Pharm.*, 2000;57:328,333–5.

23. Houghton PJ. The scientific basis for the reputed activity of Valerian. *J. Pharm. Pharmacol.*, 1999;51(5):505–12.

24. Spigset O. Reduced effect of warfarin caused by ubidecarenone. *Lancet*, 1994;334:1372–3.

25. Landbo C, Almdal TP. [Interaction between warfarin and coenzyme Q10]. [Article in Danish]. *Ugeskr Laeger*, 1998;160(22):3226–7.

26. Mortensen SA, Leth A, Agner E, et al. Dose-related decrease of serum coenzyme Q10 during treatment with HMG-CoA reductase inhibitors. *Mol. Aspects Med.*, 1997;18(Suppl):S137–44.

27. De Pinieux G, Chariot P, Ammi-Said M, et al. Lipid-lowering drugs and mitochondrial function: effects of HMG-CoA Reductase inhibitors on serum ubiquinone and blood lactate/pyruvate ratio. *Br. J. Clin. Pharmacol.*, 1996;42(3):333–7.

28. Balkan B, Dunning BE. Glucosamine inhibits glucokinase *in vitro* and produces a glucose-specific impairment of *in vivo* insulin secretion in rats. *Diabetes*, 1994;43(10):1173–9.

29. Giaccari A, Morviducci L, Zorretta D, et al. *In vivo* effects of glucosamine on insulin secretion and insulin sensitivity in the rat: possible relevance to the maladaptive responses to chronic hyperglycaemia. *Diabetologia*, 1995;38(5):518–24.

30. Shankar RR, Zhu JS, Baron AD. Glucosamine infusion in rats mimics the beta-cell dysfunction of non-insulin-dependent diabetes mellitus. *Metabolism*, 1998;47(5):573–7.

31. Monauni T, Zenti MG, Cretti A, et al. Effects of glucosamine infusion on insulin secretion and insulin action in humans. *Diabetes*, 2000;49:926–35.

32. Pouwels MJ, Jacobs JR, Span PN, et al. Short-term glucosamine infusion does not affect insulin sensitivity in humans. *J. Clin. Endocrinol. Metab.*, 2001;86:2099–103.

33. de Lemos ML. Effects of soy phytoestrogens genistein and daidzein on breast cancer growth. *Ann. Pharmacother.*, 2001;35:1118–21.

34. Johne A, Brockmoller J, Bauer S, et al. Pharmacokinetic interaction of digoxin with an herbal extract from St. John's wort (*Hypericum perforatum*). *Clin. Pharmacol. Ther.*, 1999;66(4):338–45.

35. Schulz V. Incidence and clinical relevance of the interactions and side effects of Hypericum preparations. *Phytomedicine*, 2001;8:152–60.

36. Cheng TO. St. John's wort interaction with digoxin [letter]. *Arch. Intern. Med.*, 2000;160:2548.

37. Hennessy M, Kelleher D, Spiers JP, et al. St. John's wort increases expression of p-glycoprotein: implications for drug interactions. *Br. J. Clin. Pharmacol.*, 2002;53:75–82.

38. Haller CA, Jacob P III, Benowitz NL. Pharmacology of ephedra alkaloids and caffeine after single-dose dietary supplement use. *Clin. Pharmacol. Ther.*, 2002;71:421–32.

39. Matthews, MK. Association of *Ginkgo biloba* with intracerebral hemorrhage. *Neurology*, 1998;50:1934.

40. Ho PC, Ghose K, Saville D, et al. Effect of grapefruit juice on pharmacokinetics and pharmacodynamics of verapamil enantiomers in healthy volunteers. *Eur. J. Clin. Pharmacol.*, 2000;56:693–8.

41. Uno T, Ohkubo T, Sugawara K, et al. Effects of grapefruit juice on the stereoselective disposition of nicardipine in humans: evidence for dominant presystemic elimination at the gut site. *Eur. J. Clin. Pharmacol.*, 2000;56:643–9.

42. Monostory K, Vereczkey L, Levai F, et al. Ipriflavone as an inhibitor of human cytochrome P450 enzymes. *Br. J. Pharmacol.*, 1998;123(4):605–10.

43. Takahashi J, Kawakatsu K, Wakayama T, Sawaoka H. Elevation of serum theophylline levels by ipriflavone in a patient with chronic obstructive pulmonary disease. *Eur. J. Clin. Pharmacol.*, 1992;43(2):207–8.

44. Martindale W. *Martindale The Extra Pharmacopoeia*, London: Pharmaceutical Press, 1999.

45. *Micromedex Healthcare Series*, Englewood, CO: MICROMEDEX Inc.

46. Schneyer CR. Calcium carbonate and reduction of levothyroxine efficacy. *JAMA*, 1998;279(10): 750.

47. Piscitelli SC, Burstein AH, Welden N, et al. The effect of garlic supplements on the pharmacokinetics of saquinavir. *Clin. Infect. Dis.*, 2002;34:234–8.

48. Brinker F. *Herb Contraindications and Drug Interactions*, 2nd ed, Sandy, OR: Eclectic Medical Publications, 1998.

49. Morito K, Hirose T, Kinjo J, et al. Interaction of phytoestrogens with estrogen receptors alpha and beta. *Biol. Pharm. Bull.*, 2001;24:351–6.

50. Piscitelli SC, Burstein AH, Chaitt D, et al. Indinavir concentrations and St. John's wort. *Lancet*, 2000;355(9203):547–8.

51. Risk of drug interactions with St. John's wort and indinavir and other drugs. www.fda.gov/cder/drug/advisory/stjwort.html (accessed 11 February 2000).

52. Durr D, Stieger B, Kullak-Ublick GA, et al. St. John's wort induces intestinal p-glycoprotein/MDR1 and intestinal and hepatic CYP3A4. *Clin. Pharmacol. Ther.*, 2000;68:598–604.

53. de Maat M, Hoetelmans R, Mathot R, et al. Drug interaction between St. John's wort and nevirapine. *AIDS*, 2001;15:420–1.

54. Abul-Ezz SR, Barone GW, Gurley BJ, et al. Effect of herbal supplements on cyclosporine blood levels and associated acute rejection. American Society of Nephrology Annual Meeting, 2000;Oct 11–16: abstract A3754. www.abstracts-on-line.com/abstracts/ASN/search/results.asp?Num = 0% 2E3418788 (accessed 17 October 2000).

55. Ruschitzka F, Meier PJ, Turina M, et al. Acute heart transplant rejection due to Saint John's wort. *Lancet*, 2000;355(9203):548–9.

56. Gurley BJ, Barone GW. Herb–drug interaction involving St. John's wort and cyclosporine. AAPS Ann Mtg & Expo Indianapolis, IN:2000;Oct 29–Nov 2: presentation 3443. URL: view.abstractonline.com/aaps/abstractViewer.asp (Accessed 30 October 2000).

57. Breidenbach T, Hoffmann MW, Becker T, et al. Drug interaction of St. John's wort with cyclosporin. *Lancet*, 2000;355(9218):1912.

58. Barone GW, Gurley BJ, Ketel BL, et al. Drug interaction between St. John's wort and cyclosporin. *Ann. Pharmacother.*, 2000;34:1013–6.

59. Mai I, Bauer S, Krueger H, et al. Wechselwirkungen von Johaniskraut mit tacrolismus bei nierentransplantierten patienten. Symposium Phytopharmaka VII. Forschung und Klinische Anwendung, Berlin, October, 2001.

60. Yue QY, Bergquist C, Gerden B. Safety of St. John's wort (*Hypericum perforatum*). *Lancet*, 2000;355(9203):576–7.

61. Gorski JC, Hamman MA, Wang Z, et al. The effect of St. John's wort on the efficacy of oral contraceptives (abstract MPI-80). *Clin. Pharmacol. Ther.*, 2001;71:P25.

62. Nebel A, Schneider BJ, Baker RA, et al. Potential metabolic interaction between St. John's wort and theophylline. *Ann. Pharmacother.*, 1999;33:502.

Appendix D. Complementary and Alternative Medicine Practices Relative to Dentistry — Issues and Challenges

Riva Touger-Decker

CONTENTS

It is common knowledge among dietetics professionals that nutrition only cures malnutrition despite claims that exist in the consumer press about nutrients that strengthen teeth and prevent oral infectious diseases. An intact oral cavity is critical for eating, drinking, swallowing foods and fluids among other functions. Any compromise in the integrity of the oral cavity and its structures can impact oral functions including biting, chewing, swallowing and tasting foods, and beverages. A balanced diet with representation from all food groups and nutrients in amounts consistent with the dietary reference intakes provides adequate nutrition for oral health.

As far back as the time of the early Romans (25 BC to AD 50), healers were prescribing herbal remedies such as mustard seed for toothaches.[1] In the 18th century, Pierre Fauchard prescribed oil of cloves and cinnamon for infections of the pulp of the tooth.[1] More recently in the 20th century, the potential for lysine, an essential amino acid, used topically and systemically to treat and prevent herpes labialis was studied.[2] Additional research is needed particularly because there may be benefits and there are little known risks to supplemental lysine. In contrast, the role of vitamin C in curing or preventing periodontal disease has not been proven.[3] Excess amounts of this supplement in tablet form could contribute to gastrointestinal problems; in a chewable form, vitamin C supplements may contribute to caries risk.

The impact of other dietary supplements, notably antioxidants and foods such as green tea and black tea, on the oral cavity has also been documented.[4–6] The evidence in support of antioxidant use for oral disease/infection/surgery is scant. Select components of green and black teas have been shown to have anticariogenic properties.[4] The catechins in tea have antistreptococcal activity against *Streptococcus mutans* and *Streptococcus sobrinus*. Although the evidence on the degree of activity is varied, it does suggest that these catechins may have inhibitory and bactericidal action. Large clinical trials and strategies for addressing the myriad of confounding factors in humans are needed prior to making any practical recommendations regarding tea[5,6] and dental caries. Green tea polyphenols may have chemopreventive effects against oral leukoplakia and oral and gastrointestinal cancers.[7,8] Clinical applications warrant further investigation prior to any statements regarding the chemopreventive effects in humans, however.

Select supplements have been suggested as playing a role in managing periodontal disease, an oral infectious disease. Dietary supplements have no scientifically evidenced role in the management or treatment of periodontal disease. While there may be some relationships between periodontal disease and osteoporosis, vitamin D and calcium supplementation alone would not be a sound treatment for the disease, only the associated osteoporosis.[9,10] A frank vitamin C or folate deficiency would be the only situation in which either of these nutrients should be prescribed for soft tissue disorders.

As with every other aspect of health care, the use of complementary and alternative medicine by patients seeking dental care has increased. Due to the myriad of potential known and unknown complications associated with dietary supplements, dietetics and dental professionals should, at a minimum, find out which supplements patients use as well as reasons for use, have resources available to find out more about supplements and guide patients as needed regarding safety, risk, and benefit issues associated with supplements. The need for dietetics and dental professionals to be familiar with dietary supplements is underscored by three primary issues: (1) the potential for some supplements to affect the integrity of the oral cavity, (2) for others to interact with prescription medications, and (3) for potential systemic side effects, particularly with ergogenic supplements.

Although several vitamin, mineral, and other dietary supplements have been promoted for "optimal oral health and well-being," they are unnecessary and potentially harmful to prescribe before determining the presence of nutrition risk and potential nutrient deficits. Dietary supplements may interact with other orally administered medications and have a direct impact on the oral cavity.

The pharmacokinetic and pharmacodynamic interactions of medications and dietary supplements can impact the patient's health condition while in the dental chair, such as with the stimulatory effects of ephedrine-containing products, the impact of glucosamine or chondroitin on blood glucose in individuals taking oral hypoglycemic agents or the anticoagulant impact of vitamin E, garlic, and ginseng as well as other supplements and blood-thinning medications. Echinacea may interfere with the actions of immuno-suppressing medications secondary to its immune-enhancing effects.[11,12] The principal alkaloids of ephedra (ma huang) are ephedrine and pseudoephedrine[12]; when epinephrine and ephedrine-containing supplements are taken simultaneously, the resultant stimulatory effects including increased blood pressure and heart rate and central nervous system stimulation may be additive (Philip Gregory, PharmD, personal communication, April 2002). The impact of the combination is difficult to estimate as it would depend on how much of each agent is taken and the actual ephedrine content of the ephedra supplement consumed. According to the Natural Medicines Comprehensive Database,[12] ephedrine has a short half-life (2.5 to 3.6 h); the recommendation then to withhold consumption of ephedrine-containing supplements for 24 h prior to a dental procedure in which a local anesthetic with epinephrine would be administered would, therefore, be prudent (Philip Gregory, PharmD, personal communication, April 2002). While the impact of other stimulatory supplements, such as guarana and maté, with epinephrine-containing anesthetics used by dentists has not been published, it is certainly prudent to recommend that the dental professional exercise caution by asking patients about use of such products and making the recommendation that such use be suspended on days when dental treatment would include an oral anesthetic containing epinephrine.

Several dietary supplements have anticoagulant effects in individuals taking prescription anticoagulants. While this author was unable to find any published cases of patients taking both supplements with anticoagulant effects and prescription anticoagulants, it is likewise prudent in this situation as well to follow the recommendations of the literature[12] to avoid supplements with such impacts, such as black cohosh, garlic, vitamin E, red clover, sweet clover, passion flower, ginseng, *Ginkgo biloba*, and other supplements with this known impact.

The direct impact of select supplements on the oral mucosa has received limited study. However, supplements such as feverfew, *G. biloba*, echinacea, and St. John's wort can impact oral soft tissue and salivary function.[12] Feverfew can cause ulcers in the oral cavity when taken in tablet or fresh leaf form.[12]

ISSUES FOR THE PRACTITIONER

What does this all mean for the health care provider? Ask, ask, and ask again. It is imperative to ask the "what," "why," "when," "what else" to patients; *what* do they take, including dosage patterns and duration of use, *why* do they take the products instead of or in addition to conventional therapies, *when* do they take them (with or without meals, time relative to dental appointments), and *what else* do they take (inevitably there is something else). These questions should be asked of all new patients and others routinely. When one asks about prescription and over the counter drug use, ask about supplement use.

What do you do when you find out the products? Every health professional should have resources, either on the Internet (see box) or in hard copy form. There is the Natural Medicines Comprehensive Database available online, in print, and in PDA format.[12] A quick literature search will reveal review papers on herbal medicines for health and disease.[8,13] Recommendations regarding use of supplements should be limited to those for which there is valid, reliable, scientifically sound information available. Patients interested in learning more about supplements should be referred to appropriately credentialed professionals such as integrative medicine physicians and registered dietitians. The additional few minutes required to obtain this information from patients may help to prevent problems and is consistent with comprehensive health care.

The Natural Medicines Comprehensive Database[12] can be used to evaluate potential symptoms and side effects of these products. To address the potential consequences of these and other interactions, health care practitioners including dentists must have a knowledge foundation in dietary supplements. It is incumbent upon dental professionals to hold open discussions with patients, asking about use of herbs, vitamins, and other dietary supplements. Dentists should become familiar with resources on these products so as to guide patients appropriately about any potential side effects and risks due to disease, medication, or oral manifestations as a result of their use.

REFERENCES

1. Wilwerding T. *History of Dentistry* (online book). http://cudental.creighton.edu/HTM/history2001 PDF. Accessed August 10, 2004.
2. Griffith RS, Walsh DE, Myrmet KH, et al. Success of L-lysine therapy in frequently recurrent herpes simplex infection. Treatment and prophylaxis. *Dermatologica*, 1987;175:183–190.
3. Nishida M, Grossi S, Dunford R, et al. Dietary vitamin C and the risk for periodontal disease. *J. Periodontal.*, 2000;71:1215–1223.
4. Hamilton-Miller JMT. Anti-cariogenic properties of tea. *J. Med. Microbiol.*, 2001;50:299–302.
5. Zhang J, Kashket S. Inhibition of salivary amylase by black and green teas and their effects on the intraoral hydrolysis of starch. *Caries. Res.*, 1998;32:233–238.

6. Hsu S, Singh B, Lewis J, et al. Chemoprevention of oral cancer by green tea. *Gen. Dent.*, 2002;March/April:140–144.
7. Cohan R, Jacobson P. Herbal supplements: considerations in dental practice. *CDA J.*, 2000;28:600–610.
8. Wood A. Herbal remedies. *N. Engl. J. Med.*, 2002;347:2046–2056.
9. Wactawski-Wende J. Periodontal diseases and osteoporosis: association and mechanisms. *Ann. Periodontol.*, 2001;6:197–208.
10. Krall EA, Wehler C, Garcia RI, Harris SS, Dawson-Hughes B. Calcium and vitamin D supplements reduce tooth loss in the elderly. *Am. J. Med.*, 2001;111:452–456.
11. American Botanical Council. The Complete German Commission E Monographs: Therapeutic Guide to Herbal Medicines. Newton, MA: Integrative Medicine Communications, 1998.
12. Jellin JM, Gregory P, Batz F, Hitchens K, et al. Pharmacist's Letter/Prescriber's Letter Natural Medicines Comprehensive Database, 4th ed. Stockton, CA: Therapeutic Research Faculty; 2002; http://www.naturaldatabase.com (updated daily).
13. Yeh G, Kaptchuk T, Eisenberg D, Phillips R. Systematic review of herbs and dietary supplements for glycemic control in diabetes. *Diabetes Care*, 2003;26:1277–1294.

Appendix E. Phytochemicals and Disease Prevention

Mary Marian and Cynthia A. Thomson

TABLE E.1

Most Common Classes of Phytochemicals: Food Sources and Potential Clinical Benefits Associated with Consumption

- Carotenoids (over 600)
  - α-Carotene
  - Lycopene
  - Cryptoxanthin
  - β-Carotene
  - Lutein/zeaxanthin
- Flavonoids
  - Quercetin
  - Phytoestrogens
  - Isoflavoids
  - Lignans
- Indoles
- Isothiocyanates
  - Sulforaphane
- Monoterpenes
  - α-Limonene
- Organosulfide
  - Allylic sulfide
- Plant phenols
  - Phenols
  - Polyphenols

Phytochemical	Food Source(s)	Clinical Significance
Allylic sulfides	Garlic, onion, shallots chives, leeks	Anticancer activity, may ↓ risk for colon and stomach cancers; ↓ lipid peroxidation; ↓ cholesterol levels total and LDL
α-Linoleic acid	Flaxseed, soy, walnuts	Reduces inflammation, lowers blood cholesterol, may protect against breast cancer, enhanced immunity
Anthocyanins	Blackberries, blueberries, berries, strawberries	Antioxidants; inhibits HMG-CoA reductase
Ascorbic acid	Green and yellow vegetables, fruits	Antioxidant
β-Carotene	Green yellow fruits and vegetables	Reduces risk of cataracts, coronary artery disease, lung and breast cancers, enhanced immunity (elderly)
Capsaicin	Chili peppers	Antioxidant; reduces risk for colon, gastric, and rectal cancer
Catechin (flavonoid), theaflavins, thearubigins	Green and black tea, berries	Reduce risk of gastric cancer; antioxidant; increased immune function; ↓ cholesterol production

Continued

TABLE E.1 (Continued)

Most Common Classes of Phytochemicals: Food Sources and Potential Clinical Benefits Associated with Consumption

Phytochemical	Food Source(s)	Clinical Significance
Coumarin	Parsley, carrots, citrus	Reduces risk of cancers
Curcumin (plant phenol)	Turmeric, curry, cumin	Lowers cholesterol; reduces risk of skin cancer
Cynarin	Artichoke	↓ cholesterol levels
Ellagic acid (polyphenol)	Wine, grapes, currants, nuts (pecans), berries (strawberries, blackberries, raspberries), seeds	Reduces cancer risk; reduces LDL cholesterol while ↑ HDL cholesterol
Flavonoids and polyphenolic acids. Other phenolic compounds: caffeic–ferulic acids; sesame vanillin	Parsley, carrots, citrus fruits, broccoli, cabbage, cucumbers, squash, yams, tomatoes, eggplant, peppers, soy products, berries, potatoes, broad beans, pea pods, colored onions, radishes, horseradish, tea, onions, apples, red wine, grape juice	Extend activity of vitamin C; act as antioxidants; inhibit platelet aggregation anticarcinogenic activity and inhibit atherosclerosis
Genistein (phytoestrogen or isoflavone)	Soybean	Reduces risk of hormone-dependent cancers; reduces cholesterol levels; reduces thrombi formation, osteoporosis, menopausal symptoms
Indoles	Cabbage, broccoli, brussel sprouts, spinach, watercress, cauliflower, turnip, kohlrabi, kale, rutabaga, horseradish, mustard greens	Reduce risk of hormone-related cancers, may "inactivate" estrogen
Isoflavones and saponins	Soybeans and soybean products	↓ risks of certain cancers, potential ↓ risks for CAD and osteoporosis
Isothiocyanates. Sulforaphane (release during chewing of cruciferous vegetables)	Cabbage, cauliflower, broccoli and broccoli sprouts, brussels sprouts, mustard greens, horseradish, radish	Reduce risk of tobacco-induced tumors; stimulate GST activity
Lignans (phytoestrogen)	High fiber foods, especially seeds; flax	Reduce cancer risk (colon), reduce blood glucose and cholesterol; bind to estrogen receptor sites and may decrease the risk of estrogen-stimulated breast cancer
Lignin	Soybean products, flaxseed	
Lycopene (carotenoid)	Tomato sauce, catsup, red grapefruit, guava, dried apricots, watermelon	Antioxidant; reduces risk of prostate cancer, may reduce cardiovascular disease
d-Limonene	Citrus, citrus oils	Antioxidant; reduces cancer risk; reduces cholesterol production; reduces premenstrual symptoms
Monoterpenes	Parsley, carrots, celery, broccoli, cabbage, cauliflower, cucumbers, squash, yams, tomatoes, eggplant, peppers, mint, basil, caraway seed oil	Anticancer activity
Organosulfur compounds. Allylic acid	Garlic, onion, watercress, cruciferous vegetables, leeks	↓ lipid peroxidation; reduce risk of gastric cancer, antithrombotic; reduce cholesterol
Plant sterols	Broccoli, cabbage, cucumbers, squash, yams, tomatoes, eggplant, peppers, soy products, whole grains	↓ total and LDL cholesterol levels

TABLE E.1 (Continued)
Most Common Classes of Phytochemicals

Phytochemical	Food Source(s)	Clinical Significance
Polyacetylene	Parsley, carrots, celery	↓ risk for tobacco-induced tumors; alters prostaglandin formation
Phenolic acid	Cruciferous vegetables, eggplant, peppers, tomatoes, celery, parsley, soy, licorice root, flaxseed, citrus, whole grains, berries	Inhibits cancer through inhibition of nitrosamine formation; reduces risk for lung and skin cancers
Retinol	Green and yellow vegetables, fruits	Potentially ↓ risk for certain cancers
Selenium	Seafood, garlic	Antioxidant
Tocopherol (vitamin E)	Nuts, wheat germ, oils	Antioxidant

LDL, low-density lipoprotein; HDL, high-density lipoprotein; CAD, coronary artery disease; GST, glutathione-S-transferase.
↓decreased; ↑increased.

TABLE E.2
Foods and Cancer Activity

Highest levels of anticancer activity
  Garlic
  Soybeans
  Licorice
  Ginger
  Cabbage
  Umbelliferous vegetables
    Carrots
    Celery
    Cilantro
    Parsley
    Parsnips
Modest levels of anticancer activity
  Onions
  Flax
  Citrus
  Turmeric
  Tomatoes
  Peppers
  Brown rice
  Whole wheat
  Cruciferous vegetables
    Broccoli
    Brussels sprouts
    Cauliflower

Low levels of anticancer activity
  Oats and barley
  Mints
  Rosemary
  Thyme
  Organo
  Sage
  Basil
  Cantaloupe
  Berries

Appendix F. Clinical Growth Charts for the Assessment of Growth and Body Weight

2 to 20 Years: Girls
Stature-for-Age and Weight-for-Age Percentiles

NAME _____

RECORD # _____

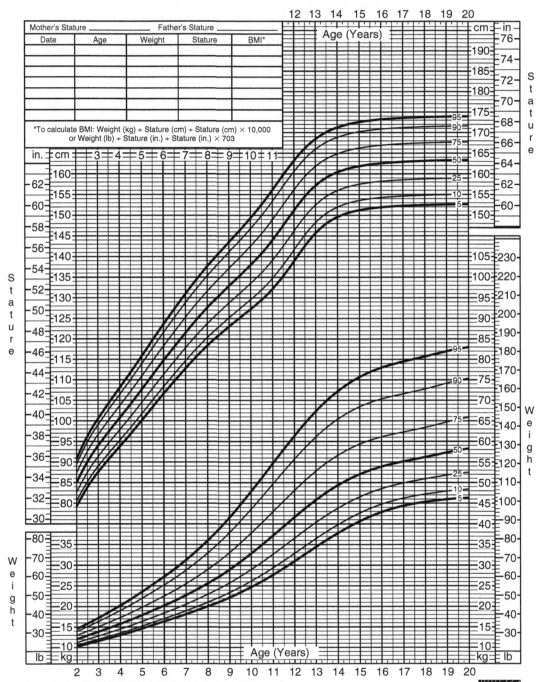

Source: Developed by the National Center for Health Statistics in collaboration with
the National Center for Chronic Disease Prevention and Health Promotion (2000).
http://www.cdc.gov/growthcharts

CDC

SAFER • HEALTHIER • PEOPLE™

2 to 20 Years: Boys
Stature-for-Age and Weight-for-Age Percentiles

NAME _____

RECORD # _____

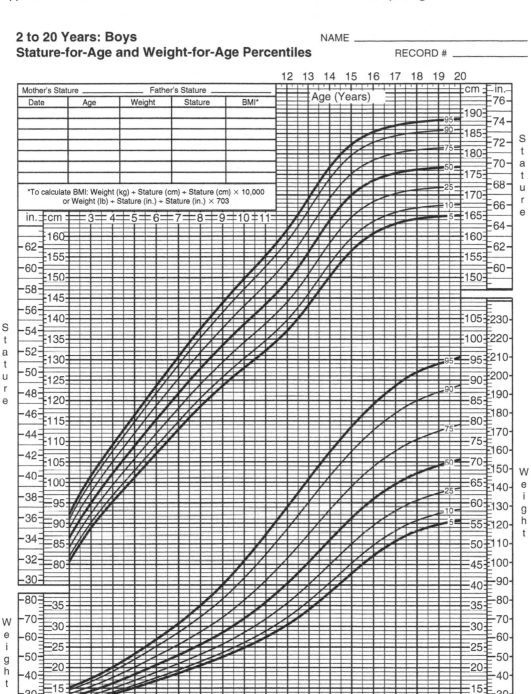

SAFER • HEALTHIER • PEOPLE™

Appendix G. MyPyramid: Steps to a Healthier You

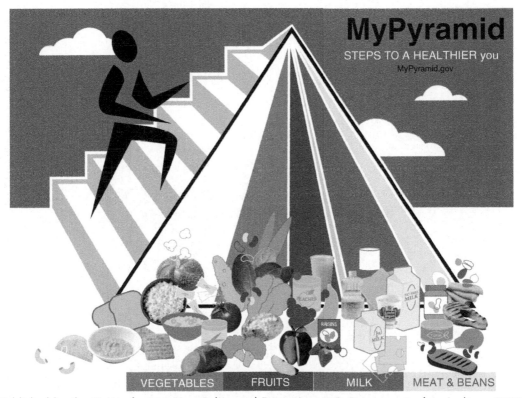

Published by the Center for Nutrition Policy and Promotion, U.S. Department of Agriculture, 2005. MyPyramid is an interactive food guidance system provides information for making healthier food choices. www.mypyramid.gov.

GRAINS
Make half your grains whole

Eat at least 3 oz of whole-grain cereals, breads, crackers, rice, or pasta every day

1 oz is about 1 slice of bread, about 1 cup of breakfast cereal, or 1/2 cup of cooked rice, cereal, or pasta

VEGETABLES
Vary your veggies

Eat more dark-green veggies like broccoli, spinach, and other dark leafy greens

Eat more orange vegetables like carrots and sweetpotatoes

Eat more dry beans and peas like pinto beans, kidney beans, and lentils

FRUITS
Focus on fruits

Eat a variety of fruit

Choose fresh, frozen, canned, or dried fruit

Go easy on fruit juices

MILK
Get your calcium-rich foods

Go low-fat or fat-free when you choose milk, yogurt, and other milk products

If you do not or cannot consume milk, choose lactose-free products or other calcium sources such as fortified foods and beverages

MEAT & BEANS
Go lean with protein

Choose low-fat or lean meats and poultry

Bake it, broil it, or grill it

Vary your protein routine — choose more fish, beans, peas, nuts, and seeds

For a 2,000-calorie diet, you need the amounts below from each food group. To find the amounts that are right for you, go to MyPyramid.gov.

| Eat 6 oz everyday | Eat 2½ cups everyday | Eat 2 cups everyday | Get 3 cups everyday; for kids aged 2 to 8, it's 2 | Eat 5½ oz. everyday |

Find your balance between food and physical activity

- Be sure to stay within your daily calorie needs.
- Be physically active for at least 30 min most days of the week.
- About 60 min a day of physical activity may be needed to prevent weight gain.
- For sustaining weight loss, at least 60 to 90 min a day of physical activity may be required.
- Children and teenagers should be physically active for 60 min everyday, or most days.

Know the limits on fats, sugars, and salt (sodium)

- Make most of your fat sources from fish, nuts, and vegetable oils.
- Limit solid fats like butter, stick margarine, shortening, and lard, as well as foods that contain these.
- Check the Nutrition Facts label to keep saturated fats, *trans* fats, and sodium low.
- Choose food and beverages low in added sugars. Added sugars contribute calories with few, if any, nutrients.

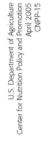

U.S. Department of Agriculture
Center for Nutrition Policy and Promotion
April 2005
CNPP-15

USDA is an equal opportunity provider and employer.

MyPyramid.gov
STEPS TO A HEALTHIER YOU

MyPyramid provides basic messages about healthy eating and physical activity that apply to everyone. These messages mirror the messages described by the 2005 Dietary Guidelines.

Appendix H. Summary and Comparison of Popular Diets

TABLE H.1
Summary and Comparison of Popular Diets

	South Beach Diet[1]	Dr. Atkins' New Diet Revolution[2]	The Zone: A Dietary Road Map[3]	Sugar Busters[4]
Authors	A Agatston, M.D.	RC Atkins, M.D.	B Sears, Ph.D.	HL Steward, MC Bethea, M.D., SS Andrews, M.D., LA Balart, M.D.
Premise	Is different from the Atkins diet with emphasis on the "right" carbs instead of no carbs and emphasizing good fats versus just any fat. After Phase 1 (2 weeks), your cravings for sugars and starches will disappear as will insulin resistance.	Obesity is a result of high insulin levels due to carbohydrate consumption. CHO restriction and ketosis are the keys to weight loss and total wellness.	"Enter and maintain the *Zone*" — the metabolic state in which the body works at peak efficiency — by consuming the right combinations of foods to reduce insulin levels and produce desirable eicosanoid balance.	"Sugar is toxic!" It causes increased insulin secretion leading to excessive fat storage. A "low-glycemic" diet is the key to control insulin and to promote weight loss.
Health claims	*The South Beach Diet* has consistently resulted in 8–13 lb weight loss in the first 2 weeks. Teaches you to avoid the bad carbs and eat the right fats. You lose weight, particularly the "belly" weight.	The Atkins diet will produce rapid weight loss by "sneaking calories out of the body unused" and will treat or prevent several health problems including heart disease, high blood pressure, diabetes, and chronic fatigue.	Numerous health problems are attributable to an eicosanoid imbalance. The Zone diet will produce "good eicosanoids" leading to weight loss and will reduce, prevent, or even cure conditions such as chronic fatigue, heart disease, cancer, HIV/AIDS, depression, and alcoholism.	The Sugar Busters diet will produce weight loss and treat or prevent conditions such as heart disease, dyslipidemia, and diabetes.
Diet patterns	*Phase 1*: Low CHOs: restricts intake of carbs high on the glycemic index; no dairy. *Phase 2*: Reintroducing carbs – good carbs (fruit, whole grains) are reintroduced with gradual weight loss continuing. Continue on Phase 2 until reaching goal weight. Still recommends restriction of high glycemic carbs. *Phase 3*: Maintenance: A diet for life. Recommends restriction of foods high on the glycemic index.	*Induction phase*: <20 g CHO/day *Ongoing weight loss*: 0–60 g CHO *Pre-maintenance*: Increase CHO until losing <1 pound/week *Maintenance*: Continuation of diet without weight loss (25–90 g CHO/day).	3 meals + 2 snacks per day. PRO:CHO:Fat = 1:1:1 ratio PRO "block" = 7 g CHO "block" = 9 g Fat "block" = 1.5 g Keep calories to ≤500 at each meal and ≤100 for snacks. "The best time to eat is when you are not hungry."	Consume 3 balanced meals a day. Portion size is important; foods should fit nicely on plate, no 2nd or 3rd helpings. Finish eating by 8:00 p.m.

TABLE H.1 (Continued)
Summary and Comparison of Popular Diets

The Carbohydrate Addict's Diet[5]	Dieting for Dummies[6]	Volumetrics[7]	Eat More, Weigh Less[8]
RF Heller, Ph.D. and RF Heller, Ph.D.	J Kirby, R.D. — for the American Dietetics Association	B Rolls, Ph.D. and RA Barnett	D Ornish, M.D.
Obesity is the result of "carbohydrate addiction" caused by too much insulin. Reducing the frequency of CHO consumption each day will reduce the intensity and frequency of carbohydrate "cravings" and promote weight loss.	Overweight and obesity is a result of excess calories and inadequate exercise. Reducing total calories, restricting consumption of sugar and sugary foods, saturated and total fat, and regular exercise will promote a healthy body weight.	Weight of food consumed is more constant than total energy intake or fat intake and with appropriate food choices more food can be consumed while keeping calories low to achieve optimal body weight.	"Eating fat makes you fat and gives you heart disease." Employing *intensive lifestyle changes*[8] (exercise and stress management) with a very low fat diet will promote weight loss.
The Carbohydrate Addict's diet will reduce cravings and produce weight loss. The authors state that the diet is "compatible with the diet recommendations of the American Heart Association."	Weight loss can reduce the risk of numerous health conditions including heart disease, diabetes, and hypertension.	Following the Volumetrics diet plan will promote and sustain weight loss while providing a nutritionally balanced diet.	The diet plan with *intensive lifestyle changes* will produce weight loss and reverse heart disease.
2 *Complementary Meals* + 1 *Reward Meal* each day. *Complementary meals* should be low in CHO and fat. All foods, including CHO, are allowed in the *Reward Meal*, but must be eaten within 1 h! Snacks in-between meals are not allowed.	Establish a personal food plan that takes into account current eating habits, lifestyle, ethnicity and culture, and energy needs. The diet is based on the Dietary Guidelines for Healthy Americans and should contain adequate amounts of food and nutrients from a variety of food groups from the Food Guide Pyramid.	The diet does not require structured eating pattern. Meals should not be skipped and snacks are allowed. Emphasizes food choice over timing or specific food combinations.	Eat whenever you are hungry and eat until you are satisfied. Appropriate in-between meal snacks are encouraged.

Continued

TABLE H.1 (Continued)
Summary and Comparison of Popular Diets

	South Beach Diet[1]	Dr. Atkins' New Diet Revolution[2]	The Zone: A Dietary Road Map[3]	Sugar Busters[4]
Foods to include	Lean proteins, healthy fats, and low-glycemic carbs.	Pure proteins and fats (meat, fish, eggs, cheese, butter and oil) and low-CHO vegetables.	Pure proteins and fats (primarily monounsaturated fat) and low-glycemic fruits and vegetables. Alcohol in moderation.	Lean meats, olive and canola oil, low-glycemic fruits, vegetables, and grains. Alcohol in moderation.
Foods to avoid	CHO—Phase I: all starchy foods, all dairy, all alcohol, full-fat cheeses, dark meat poultry products, fatty beef cuts, all fruits or juices, and starchy vegetables. Some legumes okay (no pinto beans).	CHO — pasta, breads, refined sugar products (soda, cookies, cake, etc.), milk, yogurt, most fruits and vegetables and alcohol.	High-glycemic CHO including breads, pasta, and certain fruits and vegetables. Saturated fat.	White bread, rice, pasta, potatoes, carrots, and all refined sugar products (soda, cookies, cake, etc.).
Weight loss?	*Yes*. Large weight loss initially due to loss of fluids, probable ketosis resulting in decreased caloric intake.	*Yes*. Initial weight loss is due to fluid loss, ketosis-induced appetite suppression, and caloric restriction.	*Yes*. Weight loss is due primarily to caloric restriction.	*Probable*. Weight loss is due to caloric restriction that is dependent on portion control.
Nutritionally adequate?	*Borderline*. Phase 1 is low in fiber and potentially calcium. Consumption of a variety of vegetables. and acceptable legumes could provide other needed vitamins and minerals. May be high in saturated fat.	*No*.[a] Diet low in fiber, fruits and vegetables. Low in many vitamins, minerals, and phytochemicals. May be high in saturated fat and cholesterol.	*Borderline*. May be low in fiber and some vitamins, minerals, and phytochemicals.	*Borderline*. May be low in fiber and some vitamins, minerals, and phytochemicals.
Health claims scientifically proven?	*No*. Dr. Agatston only presented the results of one study he conducted. Studies validating this approach to weight loss are nonexistent.	*Limited evidence*.[b] Studies confirm that "Atkins-type" diets result in significant weight loss.[9–11] Two published studies found that ketogenic weight loss diets increased TC[9] and LDL-C.[10] However, a more recent study found that an "Atkins-type" diet produced weight loss without any serious adverse effects (see *Potential health hazards*) and reduced TC, LDL-C, and TG and increased HDL-C.[11]	*No*. Studies cited in the book have not been validated or published in any peer-reviewed scientific journals.	*No*.

TABLE H.1 (Continued)
Summary and Comparison of Popular Diets

The Carbohydrate Addict's Diet[5]	Dieting for Dummies[6]	Volumetrics[7]	Eat More, Weigh Less[8]
Lean meats, poultry, seafood, butter, margarine, eggs, dairy products, selected fruits and vegetables. Alcohol in moderation.	Fiber-rich, complex CHO (whole grains, fruits, vegetables), and lean meats and dairy. Alcohol in moderation. Moderate intake of foods containing high amounts of sugar, fat, saturated fat and cholesterol, and salt. None.	Water and foods with high-water content (whole fruits and vegetables, broth-based soups). Fiber-rich grain and cereals. Lean meats, fish and poultry, and beans. Alcohol in moderation.	Complex CHO and vegetarian foods. Limit alcohol consumption. Vegetarian omega-3 fatty acid sources (whole grains, beans, seaweed, soybean foods, and purslane).
(*Complementary Meals*) Starchy and refined foods such as bread, pasta, potatoes, potato chips, desserts, selected fruits and vegetables.		High-fat foods and sugary drinks. Energy dense foods and snacks.	All fats and oils. High-fat meats and dairy sugar and refined sugar products (soda, cookies, cake, etc.). Salt and high sodium foods. Caffeine.
Probable. Weight loss is due to caloric restriction. However, if portions are not controlled for the *Complementary and Reward Meals* weight loss may not occur. *Borderline.* Recipes are high in saturated fat. Based on sample meal plans the diet may be low in fiber and some vitamins, minerals, and phytochemicals.	*Yes.* If followed correctly, weight loss is due to caloric restriction (and exercise). Weight loss may be more gradual than other popular diets. *Yes.* If followed correctly this diet meets current dietary recommendations.	*Yes.* If followed correctly, weight loss is due primarily to caloric restriction. Weight loss may be more gradual than other popular diets. *Yes.* If followed correctly this diet meets current dietary recommendations.	*Probable.* If followed correctly, weight loss is due to caloric restriction (and exercise). Weight loss may be more gradual than other popular diets. *Borderline.* May be low in B-vitamins and zinc. If fat intake falls below 10% of total calories the diet may not provide adequate amounts of essential fatty acids.
No.	*Yes.* Weight loss can be achieved as long as total calories are controlled. The recommended diet pattern facilitates weight loss and ensures a nutritionally balanced diet.[18,19]	*Limited evidence.* Short-term studies support the Volumetrics concept that greater amounts of low-energy dense foods can be consumed while still keeping calories low.[20,21] However, evidence to support the long-term effectiveness of this weight management approach is not available.	*Yes.* When combined (long-term) with the *intensive lifestyle changes* (exercise and stress management) the diet promotes weight loss and reduces coronary artery stenosis.[22,23]

Continued

TABLE H.1 (Continued)
Summary and Comparison of popular Diets

	South Beach Diet[1]	Dr. Atkins' New Diet Revolution[2]	The Zone: A Dietary Road Map[3]	Sugar Busters[4]
Potential health hazards[c]	Potentially high intake of *trans*-fatty acids and saturated fat. Low fiber and micronutrient intake if diet is not varied.	↑ TC, LDL-C[9,10] ↑ BP,[12]Orthostatic Hypotension,[13]gout/ kidney stones,[14,15] osteoporosis,[16] renal insufficiency.[17]	Unknown.	Unknown.
Is the diet practical?	*May be.* If the diet is liberated as recommended and individuals consume a varied diet, could be successful for long-term weight loss through healthy eating.	*No.* Requires severe food restrictions. Dining out is difficult. If weight gain occurs recommends returning to *Induction Phase* of diet until the weight is lost.	*No.* Requires a complicated and rigid diet plan. PRO:Fat:CHO ratios must be calculated for every meal and snack. Based on sample meal plans, the diet may not be palatable to everyone.	*No.* Restricts many foods and requires that certain foods be consumed together.

TABLE H.1 (Continued)
Summary and Comparison of popular Diets

The Carbohydrate Addict's Diet[5]	Dieting for Dummies[6]	Volumetrics[7]	Eat More, Weigh Less[8]
Unknown.	None.[d]	None.[d]	Plasma TG and VLDL-C levels may increase due to the high-CHO content of the diet.
No. The diet plan is not flexible. Sample menus for *Complementary Meals* are very low in calories and may lead to overeating at the *Reward Meal.*	*Yes.* The diet is flexible allowing for personal food preferences and does not restrict certain foods or food groups.	*Yes.* The diet is flexible allowing for personal food preferences and does not restrict certain foods or food groups.	*No.* The vegetarian diet may not be palatable to everyone. Individuals with high-energy needs may feel that it is too much food.

CHO, Carbohydrate; PRO, Protein; TC, Total cholesterol; LDL-C, Low-density lipoprotein cholesterol; VLDL-C, Very low-density lipoprotein cholesterol; TG, Triglycerides.

[a] Author recommends use of dietary supplements.

[b] No control groups were included for comparison in the studies by Rickman et al.,[9] or LaRosa et al.[10]

[c] Long-term research concerning the safety of most popular diets is not available.

[d] In susceptible individuals, high-CHO intake may increase VLDL-C levels.

REFERENCES

1. Agatston A. *The South Beach Diet*. New York, Random House; 2003.
2. Atkins RC. *Dr. Atkins' New Diet Revolution*. New York, National Book Network; 1999.
3. Sears B, Lawren B. *Enter The Zone: A Dietary Road Map*. New York, Regan Books; 1995.
4. Steward HL, Bethea MC, Andrews SS, et al. *Sugar Busters! Cut Sugar to Trim Fat*. New York, Ballantine Books; 1998.
5. Heller RF, Heller RF. *The Carbohydrate Addict's Diet: The lifelong solution to yo–yo dieting*. New York, Penguin Books; 1992.
6. Kirby J. *Dieting for Dummies*. Foster City, CA, IDG Books Worldwide; 1998.
7. Rolls B, Barnett RA. *Volumetrics: Feel Full on Fewer Calories*. New York, Harper Collins Publishers; 2000.
8. Ornish D. *Eat More Weigh Less: Dr Dean Ornish's Life Choice Program for Losing Weight Safely While Eating Abundantly*. New York, HarperCollins; 1997.
9. Rickman F, Mitchell N, Dingman J, et al. Changes in serum cholesterol during the Stillman Diet. *JAMA*, 1974;228:54–58.
10. LaRosa JC, Fry AG, Muesing R, et al. Effects of high-protein, low-carbohydrate dieting on plasma lipoproteins and body weight. *J. Am. Diet. Assoc.*, 1980;77:264–270.
11. Westman EC, Yancy WS, Edman JS, et al. Effect of 6-month adherence to a very low carbohydrate diet program. *Am. J. Med.*, 2002;113(1):30–36.
12. St Jeor ST, Howard BV, Prewitt E, et al. Dietary protein and weight loss: a statement for healthcare professionals from the Nutrition Committee of the Council on Nutrition, Physical Activity, and Metabolism of the American Heart Association. *Circulation*, 2001;104:1869–1874.
13. DeHaven J, Sherwin R, Hendler R, et al. Nitrogen and sodium balance and sympathetic-nervous-system activity in obese subjects treated with a low-calorie protein or mixed diet. *N. Engl. J. Med.*, 1980;302:477–482.
14. Franzese T. Medical nutrition therapy for rheumatic disorders. In: Mahan LK, Escott-Stump S, eds. *Krause's Food, Nutrition, & Diet Therapy*, 10th ed. Philadephia, PA, WB Saunders; 2000, pp. 970–986.
15. Reddy ST, Wang CY, Sakhaee K, et al. Effect of low-carbohydrate high-protein diets on acid–base balance, stone-forming propensity, and calcium metabolism. *Am. J. Kidney. Dis.*, 2002;40(2): 265–274.
16. Barzel US, Massey LK. Excess dietary protein can adversely affect bone. *J. Nutr.*, 1998;128: 1051–1053.
17. Brenner BM, Meyer TW, Hostetter TH, et al. Dietary protein intake and the progressive nature of kidney disease: the role of hemodynamically mediated glomerular injury in the pathogenesis of progressive glomerular sclerosis in aging, renal ablation, and intrinsic renal disease. *N. Engl. J. Med.*, 1982;307:652–659.
18. *Clinical Guidelines on the Identification, Evaluation, and Treatment of Overweight and Obesity in Adults. The Evidence Report*. National Institutes of Health, National Heart, Lung, and Blood Institute, 1998.
19. Klem ML, Wing RR, McGuire MT, Seagle HM, Hill JO. A descriptive study of individuals successful at long-term maintenance of substantial weight loss. *Am. J. Clin. Nutr.*, 1997;66:239–246.
20. Stubbs RJ, Johnstone AM, O'Reilly J, et al. The effect of covertly manipulating the energy density of mixed diets on *ad libitum* food intake in "pseudo free-living" humans. *Int. J. Obes.*, 1998;22: 980–987.
21. Rolls BJ, Bell EA. Dietary approaches to the treatment of obesity. *Med. Clin. North Am.*, 2000;84:401–418.
22. Ornish D, Brown SE, Scherwitz LW, et al. Can lifestyle changes reverse coronary heart disease? The lifestyle heart trial. *Lancet*, 1990;336:129–133.
23. Ornish D, Scherwitz LW, Billings JH, et al. Intensive lifestyle changes for reversal of coronary heart disease. *JAMA*, 1998;280:2001–2007.

Index